Acute Pain Management Essentials

AN INTERDISCIPLINARY APPROACH

Acute Pain Management Essentials

AN INTERDISCIPLINARY APPROACH

Alan David Kaye, MD, PhD, DABA, DABPM, DABIPP, FASA

Vice Chancellor of Academic Affairs,
Chief Academic Officer, and Provost
Pain Program Fellowship Director
Professor
Departments of Anesthesiology and Pharmacology,
Toxicology, and Neurosciences
Louisiana State University Health Sciences Center
Shreveport, Louisiana

Richard D. Urman, MD, MBA, FASA

Associate Professor of Anesthesia
Department of Anesthesiology, Perioperative and Pain Medicine
Brigham and Women's Hospital
Boston, Massachusetts

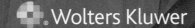

Wolters Kluwer

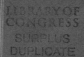

Philadelphia • Baltimore • New York • London
Buenos Aires • Hong Kong • Sydney • Tokyo

Acquisitions Editor: Keith Donnellan
Development Editor: Ariel S. Winter
Editorial Coordinator: Christopher Rodgers
Marketing Manager: Kirsten Watrud
Production Project Manager: David Saltzberg
Design Coordinator: Stephen Druding
Manufacturing Coordinator: Beth Welsh
Prepress Vendor: Straive

9 8 7 6 5 4 3 2 1

Printed in Mexico

Cataloging-in-Publication Data available on request from the Publisher

ISBN: 978-1-9751-6483-6

shop.lww.com

QUADM0622

To my wife Dr. Kim Kaye for being the best spouse a man could ask for in his life.

To my mother Florence Feldman who while enduring a lifetime of pain and suffering with seven back surgeries, taught me tremendous things about pain, to accomplish tasks with the highest of quality, and to reach my dreams and goals.

To my brother Dr. Adam M. Kaye, Pharm D, for his loving support and help over the past 50 plus years.

To all my teachers and colleagues at the University of Arizona in Tucson, Ochsner Clinic in New Orleans, Massachusetts General Hospital/Harvard School of Medicine in Boston, Tulane School of Medicine in New Orleans, Texas Tech Health Sciences Center in Lubbock, LSU School of Medicine in New Orleans, and LSU School of Medicine in Shreveport.

Alan David Kaye, MD, PhD, DABA, DABPM, DABIPP, FASA
Vice Chancellor of Academic Affairs, Chief Academic Officer, and Provost
Pain Program Fellowship Director
Professor, Department of Anesthesiology and Pharmacology, Toxicology, and Neurosciences
Louisiana State University School of Medicine
Shreveport, Louisiana

To my patients who inspired me to write this book to help other practitioners improve their care.

To my mentors for their encouragement and support.

To my students and trainees so that they can use this guide to better understand the needs of these patients.

To my family: my wife Dr. Zina Matlyuk, MD, and my daughters Abigail and Isabelle who make it all possible and worth it, every day.

Richard D. Urman, MD, MBA
Associate Professor of Anesthesia
Department of Anesthesiology, Perioperative and Pain Medicine
Harvard Medical School/Brigham and Women's Hospital
Boston, Massachusetts

Contributors

ASSOCIATE EDITOR

Elyse M. Cornett, PhD
Assistant Professor and Director of Research
Department of Anesthesiology
Department of Pharmacology, Toxicology & Neuroscience
LSU Health Shreveport
Shreveport, Louisiana

CONTRIBUTORS

Priya Agrawal, DO
Anesthesiologist, Pain Management Physician
Department of Anesthesiology, and Perioperative and Pain Medicine
Alameda Health System
Oakland, California

Oscar A. Alam Mendez, MD
Assistant Professor
Department of Anesthesiology
The University of Mississippi Medical Center
Jackson, Mississippi

Belal Alammar, MD
Resident
Department of Anesthesiology
Tulane University School of Medicine
New Orleans, Louisiana

Mahmoud Alkholany, MD
Consultant in Pain Medicine and Anaesthesia
Liverpool University Hospitals
Liverpool, United Kingdom

Varsha D. Allampalli, MD
Assistant Professor
Department of Anesthesiology
Louisiana State University Health Sciences
Shreveport, Louisiana

Matthew B. Allen, MD
Instructor
Department of Anaesthesia
Harvard Medical School
Boston, Massachusetts

Amy S. Aloysi, MD, MPH
Associate Professor
Department of Psychiatry
Icahn School of Medicine at Mount Sinai
New York, New York

Mark R. Alvarez, BS
Medical Student (4th year)
School of Medicine
Louisiana State University Health Sciences Center at Shreveport
Shreveport, Louisiana

Kapil Anand, MD, MBA
Associate Clinical Professor
Department of Anesthesiology, Perioperative & Pain Medicine
Stanford University School of Medicine
Stanford, California

Samuel P. Ang, MD
Resident Physician
Department of Anesthesiology, Perioperative Care, and Pain Medicine
NYU Langone Health
New York, New York

Boris C. Anyama, MD
Resident Physician
Department of Anesthesiology & Perioperative Medicine
University of Pittsburgh Medical Center
Pittsburgh, Pennsylvania

Melinda Aquino, MD
Assistant Professor
Department of Anesthesiology
Albert Einstein College of Medicine
Montefiore Medical Center
Bronx, New York

Brett L. Arron, MD
East Coast Surgery Center
Daytona Beach, Florida

Katherine C. Babin, BS, MD
Medical Student
LSU Health Shreveport
Shreveport, Louisiana

William C. Bidwell, MD
Resident Physician
Department of Emergency Medicine & Family Medicine
Louisiana State University Health Sciences–Shreveport
Shreveport, Louisiana

Megan A. Boudreaux, BS
Medical Student
Medical School
Louisiana State University School of Medicine–Shreveport
Shreveport, Louisiana

Taylor Marie Boudreaux, BS
Medical Student
School of Medicine
Louisiana State University
New Orleans, Louisiana

Carley E. Boyce, BS
Medical Student
Louisiana State University, HSC New Orleans
New Orleans, Louisiana

Joel Castellanos, MD, FAAPMR
Assistant Professor of Pain Medicine and Medical Director of Inpatient Rehabilitation
Department of Anesthesiology
University of California, San Diego
San Diego, California

John N. Cefalu, MD, MS
Anesthesiologist
Case Western University/University Hospitals and Clinics
School of Medicine
Case Western Reserve University
Cleveland, Ohio

Kheng Sze Chan, MD, PhD
Resident
Department of Anesthesiology, Perioperative, and Pain Medicine
Brigham and Women's Hospital
Harvard Medical School
Boston, Massachusetts

Melissa Chao, MD, MPH
Anesthesiology
Columbia University Irving Medical Center
New York, New York

Erica V. Chemtob, BS
Medical Student
School of Medicine and Health Sciences
The George Washington University
Washington, District of Columbia

Lindsey Cieslinski, DO
Resident Physician
Department of Anesthesiology
Tulane University School of Medicine
New Orleans, Louisiana

Alexandra Cloutet, BS
Medical Student
Department of Anesthesiology
Louisiana State University Health Sciences
Shreveport, Louisiana

Oren Cohen, MD
PGY3 Resident
Department of Anesthesiology
Louisiana State University
New Orleans, Louisiana

Elyse M. Cornett, PhD
Assistant Professor and Director of Research
Department of Anesthesiology
Department of Pharmacology, Toxicology & Neuroscience
LSU Health Shreveport
Shreveport, Louisiana

Madelyn K. Craig, MD
Resident Physician
Department of Anesthesia
Louisiana State University Health Science Center
New Orleans, Louisiana

Kelly S. Davidson, MD
Staff Anesthesiologist
Department of Anesthesia
United States Air Force
Eglin Air Force Base, Florida

Kelsey De Silva, MD
Resident Physician
Department of Anesthesiology
University of North Carolina Hospitals
Chapel Hill, North Carolina

Anis Dizdarevic, MD
Assistant Clinical Professor
Department of Anesthesiology and Pain Medicine
Columbia University Irving Medical Center
New York, New York

Randi E. Domingue, BS
School of Medicine
Louisiana State University Health Sciences Center Shreveport
Shreveport, Louisiana

Kevin A. Elaahi, MD
Resident
Department of Anesthesiology
Montefiore Medical Center/Albert Einstein COM
Bronx, New York

Ahmad Elsharydah, MD, MBA
Professor of Anesthesiology and Pain Management
Department of Anesthesiology and Pain Management
University of Texas Southwestern Medical Center at Dallas
Dallas, Texas

Lauren K. Eng, MD
Resident Physician
Department of Ophthalmology
Tulane University
New Orleans, Louisiana

Matthew R. Eng, MD
Associate Professor
Department of Anesthesiology
Louisiana State University Health Science Center
New Orleans, Louisiana

Kiana Fahimipour, MD
Resident Physician
Department of Anesthesiology
LSU Health Sciences Center New Orleans
New Orleans, Louisiana

Maged D. Fam, MBChB, MSc
Resident Physician
Department of Anesthesiology
Virginia Commonwealth University
Richmond, Virginia

Fadi Farah, MD
Assistant Professor
Department of Anesthesiology
Albert Einstein School of Medicine
Montefiore Medical Center
Bronx, New York

John J. Finneran IV, MD
Associate Professor of Anesthesiology and Associate Program Director, Anesthesiology Residency
Department of Anesthesiology
University of California, San Diego
San Diego, California

Antolin S. Flores, MD
Associate Professor
Anesthesiology
Wexner Medical Center at the Olio State University
Columbus, Ohio

Anna Formanek, MD
Pediatric Anesthesia Fellow
Boston Children's Hospital
Boston, Massachusetts

Caroline Galliano, BS
Medical Student
Louisiana State University School of Medicine
New Orleans, Louisiana

Juan Gabriel Garcia, MD
Anesthesiology Resident
Department of Anesthesiology and Pain Management
University of Texas Southwestern Medical Center
Dallas, Texas

Sonja A. Gennuso, MD
Assistant Professor
Department of Anesthesiology
LSU Health Shreveport
Shreveport, Louisiana

Clifford Gevirtz, MD, MPH
Adjunct Associate Professor
Department of Anesthesiology
Louisiana State University
New Orleans, Louisiana

Sameer K. Goel, MD
Resident
Department of Anesthesia
Virginia Commonwealth University
Richmond, Virginia

Savitri Gopaul, FNP-BC
Nurse Practitioner
VCU Health System
Richmond, Virginia

Leonid Gorelik, MD
Associate Professor
Anesthesiology
Ohio State University Wexner Medical Center
Columbus, Ohio

Karina Gritsenko, MD
Program Director, Regional Anesthesia and Acute Pain Medicine Fellowship
Director of Medical Student Regional Anesthesia and Inpatient Pain Medicine Rotation
Associate Professor
Departments of Anesthesiology, Family, & Social Medicine, and Physical Medicine & Rehabilitation
Montefiore Medical Center
Albert Einstein College of Medicine
Bronx, New York

Stephanie Guzman, MD
Assistant Professor of Clinical Anesthesiology
Department of Anesthesiology
Louisiana State University Health Sciences Center
New Orleans, Louisiana

Hannah W. Haddad, BS
Medical Student
Kansas City University
Kansas City, Missouri

Tyson Hamilton, DO
College of Osteopathic Medicine
Rocky Vista University
Ivins, Utah

Chance M. Hebert
Medical Student
Louisiana State University Health–Shreveport
Shreveport, Louisiana

Aimee Homra, MD
Clinical Assistant Professor
Department of Anesthesiology
Louisiana State University
New Orleans, Louisiana

Sarahbeth R. Howes, BS
Medical Student, Class of 2022
Louisiana State University Medical Center–Shreveport
Shreveport, Louisiana

G. Jason Huang, MD
Division of Family Medicine
HCA Houston Healthcare West
Houston, Texas

Jake Huntzinger, DO
Resident Physician
Department of Anesthesiology and Perioperative Medicine
Medical University of South Carolina
Charleston, South Carolina

Farees Hyatali, MD
Montefiore Medical Center
Jamaica, Queens, New York

Jonathan S. Jahr, MD, PhD
Professor Emeritus of Anesthesiology and Perioperative Medicine
David Geffen School of Medicine at UCLA
Ronald Reagan UCLA Medical Center
Los Angeles, California

Dominika James, MD
Associate Professor of Anesthesiology & Pain Medicine
Anesthesiology
University of North Carolina, Chapel Hill
Chapel Hill, North Carolina

Vijayakumar Javalkar, MD
Assistant Professor
Department of Neurology
LSU Health Shreveport
Shreveport, Louisiana

Mark R. Jones, MD
Interventional Pain Medicine of the South
Knoxville, Tennessee

Maryam Jowza, MD
Associate Professor
Department of Anesthesiology
University of North Carolina
Chapel Hill, North Carolina

Vijay Kata, MS
Medical Student
Department of Anesthesiology
LSUHSC New Orleans
New Orleans, Louisiana

Simrat Kaur, DO
Department of Anesthesiology
Virginia Commonwealth University Medical Center
Richmond, Virginia

Alan David Kaye, MD, PhD, DABA, DABPM, DABIPP, FASA
Vice-Chancellor of Academic Affairs, Chief Academic Officer, and Provost
Tenured Professor of Anesthesiology and Pharmacology, Toxicology, and Neurosciences
Pain Fellowship Program Director
LSU School of Medicine
Shreveport, Louisiana

Neil Kelkar, BS
College of Medicine – Phoenix
University of Arizona
Phoenix, Arizona

Jamie Kitzman, MD
Assistant Professor
Department of Anesthesiology and Pediatrics
Emory University
Atlanta, Georgia

Gopal Kodumudi, MD, MS
Anesthesiology Resident
Department of Anesthesiology
Louisiana State University
New Orleans, Louisiana

Carmen Labrie-Brown, MD
Associate Professor of Anesthesiology
LSU
New Orleans, Louisiana

Olabisi Lane, MD, PharmD
Assistant Professor
Department of Anesthesiology
Emory University School of Medicine
Atlanta, Georgia

Victoria L. Lassiegne, BS
Medical Student
Department of Anesthesiology
LSUHSC New Orleans
New Orleans, Louisiana

Ken Lee, MD
Fellow
Department of Anesthesiology
Brigham and Women's Hospital
Boston, Massachusetts

Henry Liu, MD
Professor of Anesthesiology and Perioperative Medicine
Department of Anesthesiology and Perioperative Medicine
Pennsylvania State University College of Medicine
Milton S. Hershey Medical Center
Hershey, Pennsylvania

Stewart J. Lockett, BS, MD
Medical Student
School of Medicine
Louisiana State University
Shreveport, Louisiana

Franciscka Macieiski, MD
LSU Shreveport Medical Center
Shreveport, Louisiana

Kunal Mandavawala, MD
Resident
Department of Anesthesiology, Perioperative, and Pain Medicine
Brigham and Women's Hospital
Clinical Fellow
Harvard Medical School
Boston, Massachusetts

Caitlin E. Martin, MD, MPH, FACOG
Director of OBGYN Addiction Services
Virginia Commonwealth University
Richmond, Virginia

Maria Michaelis, MD, FASA
Associate Professor
University of Nebraska Medical Center
Omaha, Nebraska

Benjamin Cole Miller, MS
Medical Student
Department of Anesthesiology
LSUHS Shreveport
Shreveport, Louisiana

Sumitra Miriyala, MPH, PhD, MBA, FAHA
Associate Professor
Department of Cellular Biology and Anatomy
Louisiana State University Health Sciences
Shreveport, Louisiana

Luke Mosel, DO
Resident Anesthesiologist
Department of Anesthesia
Ochsner LSU Shreveport
Shreveport, Louisiana

Brian M. Nelson, MD
Family Medicine Resident
Fort Belvoir Community Hospital
Fort Belvoir, Virginia

Linh T. Nguyen, BS
Medical Student
LSU Health Shreveport
Shreveport, Louisiana

Yvonne Nguyen, MD
Resident Physician
Department of Anesthesiology
Virginia Commonwealth University Health System
Richmond, Virginia

Chikezie N. Okeagu, MD
Resident Physician
Department of Anesthesiology
Louisiana State University Health Sciences Center
New Orleans, Louisiana

Aimee Pak, MD
Assistant Professor
Department of Anesthesiology
University of Oklahoma Health Sciences Center
Oklahoma City, Oklahoma

Wesley R. Pate, MD
Resident Physician
Department of Urology
Boston Medical Center
Boston, Massachusetts

Dharti Patel, PharmD
Pain Management Clinical Pharmacist
Department of Pharmacy
Virginia Commonwealth University Health System
Richmond, Virginia

Stephen P. Patin, MPH
Medical Student (MS4)
School of Medicine
LSU Health Shreveport
Shreveport, Louisiana

Alex D. Pham, MD
Anesthesiologist
Department of Anesthesiology
Louisiana State University School of Medicine
New Orleans, Louisiana

Taylor L. Powell, MS
Medical Student, Class of 2024
School of Medicine
Louisiana State University Health Shreveport
Shreveport, Louisiana

Praveen Dharmapalan Prasanna, MBBS, FCARCSI
Associate Professor
Department of Anesthesiology
Virginia Commonwealth University
Richmond, Virginia

Anand M. Prem, MD
Associate Professor of Anesthesiology
Medical Director, University Pain Clinic
Department of Anesthesiology
University of Mississippi Medical Center
Jackson, Mississippi

Devin S. Reed, MD
Resident
Department of Anesthesiology
University of Mississippi
Jackson, Mississippi

Christopher Reid, MD
Assistant Professor of Surgery and Director of Medical Student Plastic Surgery Education
Division of Plastic Surgery
Department of Surgery
University of California, San Diego
San Diego, California

Beth Ren, BS
MS4
Department of Anesthesiology
Tulane University
New Orleans, Louisiana

Nicole Rose Rueb, BS
Department of Medicine
School of Medicine
Louisiana State University Health Science Center
New Orleans, Louisiana

Stuart M. Sacks, MD
Resident Physician
Department of Anesthesiology, Perioperative, and Pain Medicine
Brigham and Women's Hospital
Boston, Massachusetts

Orlando John Salinas, MD, DABA
Associate Professor–Clinical Anesthesiology
Department of Anesthesiology
Louisiana State University
New Orleans, Louisiana

Karla Samaniego, MD
Intern
Department of Surgery
Texas Tech University Health Sciences Center School of Medicine
Lubbock, Texas

Scott A. Scharfenstein, MD
Physician
Anesthesiology
LSU Health New Orleans
New Orleans, Louisiana

Erica Seligson, MD
Resident Physician
Department of Anesthesiology, Perioperative, and Pain Medicine
Brigham and Women's Hospital
Boston, Massachusetts

Naum Shaparin, MD, MBA
Professor and Vice Chair, Business Affairs
Director, Multidisciplinary Pain Program
Department of Anesthesiology
Montefiore Medical Center/Albert Einstein College of Medicine
Bronx, New York

Meredith K. Shaw, MD
Resident Physician
Department of Anesthesiology
Louisiana State University Health Sciences Center
New Orleans, Louisiana

Islam Mohammad Shehata, MD
Assistant Lecturer
Department of Anesthesia
Faculty of Medicine
Ain Shams University
Cairo, Egypt

Sahar Shekoohi, PhD
Post Doctoral Fellow
Department of Anesthesiology
Louisiana State University Health Sciences Center
Shreveport, Louisiana

Marian Sherman, MD
Assistant Professor
Department of Anesthesiology and Critical Care Medicine
George Washington University School of Medicine and Health Sciences
Washington, District of Columbia

Harish Siddaiah, MD, FASA
Associate Professor
Department of Anesthesiology and Critical Care
Ochsner LSU Health
Shreveport, Louisiana

Andrea E. Stoltz, BS
Medical Student
Louisiana State University School of Medicine, New Orleans
New Orleans, Louisiana

Winston Suh, BS
Medical Student
LSU Health Shreveport
Shreveport, Louisiana

Shilen P. Thakrar, MD
Assistant Professor
Department of Anesthesiology
VCU Health System
Richmond, Virginia

Tina S. Thakrar, MD, MBA
Child and Adolescent and Adult Psychiatrist
Clinical Psychiatry Lead
Nystrom & Associates, Ltd.
New Brighton, Minnesota

George Thomas, BS
Medical Student
Department of Neurosurgery
George Washington University
Washington, District of Columbia

Lisa To, MD
Assistant Professor
Department of Anesthesia and Pain Management
University of Texas Southwestern
Dallas, Texas

Bryant W. Tran, MD
Associate Professor
Department of Anesthesiology
Virginia Commonwealth University
Richmond, Virginia

Natalie P. Tukan, MD
Resident Physician
Department of Anesthesiology
Brigham and Women's Hospital
Boston, Massachusetts

Richard D. Urman, MD, MBA
Associate Professor of Anesthesia
Director, Center for Perioperative Research
Harvard Medical School/Brigham and Women's Hospital
Boston, Massachusetts

Stephanie G. Vanterpool, MD, MBA, FASA
Assistant Professor
Department of Anesthesiology
University of Tennessee Graduate School of Medicine
Knoxville, Tennessee

Dev Vyas, MD
Anesthesia Resident
Department of Anesthesiology
Tulane University School of Medicine
New Orleans, Louisiana

William A. Wall, BS
MD Candidate
LSU School of Medicine
New Orleans, Louisiana

Eileen A. Wang, MD
Clinical Fellow
Department of Anesthesiology and Pain Medicine
UC Davis Health
Sacramento, California

Marissa Webber, MD
Clinical Instructor of Anesthesiology
Department of Anesthesiology
Weill Cornell Medical College/New York Presbyterian Hospital
New York, New York

Cassandra M. Armstead-Williams, MD
Assistant Professor
Department of Anesthesiology
Louisiana State University, Health Science Center
New Orleans, Louisiana

Blake Winston, DO
Resident Physician
Department of Anesthesiology
Tulane University
New Orleans, Louisiana

Ashley Wong, DO
Fellow Physician
Department of Anesthesiology
Montefiore Medical Center/Albert Einstein College of Medicine
Bronx, New York

Anna Woodbury, MD, MSCR, CAc
Associate Professor
Department of Anesthesiology and Pain Medicine
Emory University
Atlanta, Georgia

Jennifer S. Xiong, MD
Resident Physician
Department of Anesthesiology, Perioperative, and Pain Medicine
Harvard Medical School
Boston, Massachusetts

Lindsey K. Xiong, MS
Medical Student, Class of 2023
Tulane University School of Medicine
New Orleans, Louisiana

Nellab Yakuby, MD
Clinical Faculty and RAAPM Fellow
Department of Anesthesiology
University of California, Irvine
Orange, California

Justin Y. Yan, MD
Resident Physician
Department of Anesthesiology
LSU Health New Orleans
New Orleans, Louisiana

Foreword for Essentials of Acute Pain Book

It is estimated that over 230 million surgical procedures are performed worldwide annually. In the surgical patient, acute pain is directly involved in patient satisfaction, recovery, morbidity, and even mortality. For many years, acute pain lagged in effective treatments and side effects of opioids, a major treatment strategy, were well known to potentially result in respiratory depression, delayed recovery and discharge, and unwanted effects such as nausea and vomiting and opioid addiction.

It was not long ago that our life spans were much shorter and surgical treatments that are now commonplace were not available. Historically, tens of thousands of people died from the plague, caused by an organism easily treated with sulfonamide antibiotics. It is an amazing fact that dysentery was the single greatest cause of death of Confederate and Union soldiers during the American Civil War. Some of our greatest figures in history had shortened lives related to what we would now consider treatable states. George Washington died from acute bacterial epiglottis and poet Lord Byron died at an early age from an epileptic seizure. Harry Houdini died from acute appendicitis and Arthur Ashe died from a blood transfusion which caused him to be infected with the human immune deficiency virus. In the past year alone, it is estimated that 16,500 people in the United States died from nonsteroidal anti-inflammatory drug-mediated silent gastrointestinal bleeding, showing that at present, we still have a long way to go.

Principally during the last 50 years, we have dramatically increased our understanding of disease, surgical treatments, and pain states. In this regard, the technology to provide effective pain management also has grown significantly. Drug development has resulted in an increasing patient's life span, reducing pain, and enhancing quality of life. Drug-mediated miracles and procedures are commonplace and routine in our medical practices.

In the last decade, we have seen complete cataloging of the entire human genome and an increase in drug targets to well over one thousand sites. We find ourselves constantly at a new beginning with drugs, including in our fields of anesthesia and pain medicine. Structural activity relationships and complex three-dimensional analyses of therapeutic targets have produced further advances. Less than 50 years ago, the first opiate receptor was identified. In recent years, we have made substantial increases in understanding of endogenous opiates and subgroup opioid receptors throughout the body. Liposomal bupivacaine allows for pain relief for approximately 4 days. With all of these understandings, our future will ultimately see better targeting agents for acute and chronic pain states. It is an exciting time filled with hope in modern medicine and in our field. Anesthesia has never been safer thanks, in part, to drug development.

In recent years, we have seen considerable changes in acute pain management that have resulted in reduced opioid consumption and shorter hospital stays through a variety of strategies including enhanced recovery after surgery techniques and ultrasound-guided nerve blocks. The evolution of these techniques is simply remarkable with support coming from stakeholders including surgeons, administrators, nursing, and of course, anesthesia personnel.

Ongoing research has allowed for even newer drugs and technologies in the management of acute pain. Given that many patients historically were given large opioid prescriptions, and a subset of these people would end up hooked on analgesics, this is all noteworthy and important for society. The government has stepped in and all 50 states have passed legislature to limit analgesics in the first 1-2 weeks after surgical procedures. As a result, this has further heightened the need for effective acute pain management in all surgical disciplines.

In this state-of-the-art acute pain management book, we have created an easy-to-read book divided into many chapter topics not just for the practicing clinicians in different disciplines but also for medical students, interns, residents, and fellows. History affords us lessons and clues to be better prepared for our present and future. We must remain critical about expectations regarding quality and standardization of our drugs to maintain appropriate bioavailability and therapeutic outcomes. It is a golden age for drugs and technology directly affecting acute pain management. We should continue to improve the quality of life on this planet, one patient at a time.

Alan David Kaye, MD, PhD, DABA, DABPM, DABIPP, FASA
Vice Chancellor of Academic Affairs, Chief Academic Officer, and Provost
Pain Program Fellowship Director
Professor, Department of Anesthesiology and Pharmacology, Toxicology, and Neurosciences
Louisiana State University School of Medicine
Shreveport, Louisiana

Richard D. Urman, MD, MBA
Associate Professor of Anesthesia
Director, Center for Perioperative Research
Harvard Medical School/Brigham and Women's Hospital
Boston, Massachusetts

Preface

The first edition of *Acute Pain Management Essentials: An Interdisciplinary Approach* is intended to provide a timely update in the field of acute pain management and continue the mission of providing a concise, up-to-date, evidence-based, and richly illustrated book for students, trainees, and practicing clinicians. The book comprehensively covers a robust list of topics focused to improve understanding in the field of acute pain management with emphasis on recent developments in clinical practices, technology, and procedures. We strived for simple, accessible format that avoids encyclopedic language and lengthy discussions focused on anesthesia and pain management strategies.

As the practice of acute pain management becomes increasingly recognized as a major subspecialty of anesthesia, there is a growing interest from current practitioners to evolve their neuraxial, regional, and anesthesia techniques and understanding to optimize clinical skills and practice. This book contains all the essential topics that are required for the practitioner to quickly assess the patient and risk stratify them, decide on the type of analgesic plan that is most appropriate for the patient, its feasibility and safety, and provide expert consultation to other team members. We placed particular emphasis on clear, detailed images, latest techniques and illustrations, and an easy-to-read format with clinically relevant, practical aspects of acute pain management. The chapter contributors are national and international experts in the field, and the book's compact size makes it easy to carry around in the clinical setting.

We as clinicians must consistently strive to improve ourselves to deliver the best care for our many patients each day. We hope you enjoy our book!

Alan David Kaye, MD, PhD
Shreveport, Louisiana

Richard D. Urman, MD, MBA, FASA
Boston, Massachusetts

Acknowledgments

To Dr. Elyse Cornett, PhD, for her many contributions to help create this book.

Contents

UNIT II Organ Systems 105

UNIT III Special Populations 227

SECTION I

Basic Principles

1

Anatomy & Physiology of Acute Pain: Pain Pathways and Neurotransmitters

Alex D. Pham, Orlando John Salinas, Matthew R. Eng, Samuel P. Ang, Mark Jones, Elyse M. Cornett, and Alan David Kaye

Introduction

Pain is the human body's subjective experience in response to actual or potential tissue damage.[1] This unpleasant response has a protective role in alerting the body to potential danger and providing a means for self-preservation.[2] Pain can be classified as acute or chronic. While definitions may vary, acute pain usually lasts <3-6 months and is limited in duration. Acute pain typically has a sudden onset caused by noxious stimuli and follows some form of injury to the body. This type of pain resolves as soon as the initial injury heals. Acute pain can result from surgery, illness, or specific injuries to the body.

Noxious stimuli from the environment can lead to the activation of various nociceptors. Activation of these nociceptors then causes the transmission of a signal to the spinal cord's dorsal horn by neurons. At this location, the signal may be modulated before being sent to the central nervous system and further modified by various neurotransmitters. The result is the perception of pain by the brain.[3]

Knowledge of the basic anatomy, physiology, and neurotransmitters involved in the perception of acute pain allows for the proper diagnosis, treatment of, and resolution of acute pain. Additionally, understanding these mechanisms is valuable in guiding the development of new treatment interventions by targeting various parts of the pain pathway.[3]

Basic Concepts: Perception of Pain

Pain is the result of an activated pathway that is signaled by noxious stimuli and nociceptors. Nociceptors are receptors that occur throughout the body to sense noxious stimuli. The nociceptors then activate and transmit action potentials by nerves that connect to the spinal cord. The processing of potentially dangerous stimuli to the body by the nociceptors and nerve pathways is performed by the central nervous system and peripheral nervous system. This is referred to as the concept of nociception and can communicate noxious mechanical, thermal, or chemical stimulation stimuli.

The perception and interpretation of pain is described as a four-part process: transduction, transmission, modulation, perception.[4] The transduction of pain is the stimulation of the nociceptor to the activation of the sensory nerve ending. The transmission of pain refers to the pain signal transmitted along the nerve and spinal cord pathway from the nociceptor toward the brain. The modulation process describes the alteration of the pain signal as it ascends the spinal cord and through the brain. A contextualization of the noxious stimuli and circumstances may alter the pain signal through this modulation process. Finally, the perception of pain is the reception of the brain's pain signal and results in an understanding of the message and a concurrent physical or emotional response.

Pain signals travel as action potential impulses along a nociceptive pathway that courses the peripheral nerve, spinal cord, and brain.[5] A voltage-gated sodium channel mediates the conduction of these pain signals along an afferent axon. Each of the primary afferent neurons terminates in the dorsal horn of the spinal cord. At this location, they activate second-order pain-transmitting cells in the dorsal horn of the gray matter. The signal then decussates or crosses over to the other side of the spinal cord, traveling up the spinothalamic tract toward the thalamus and brain. The spinothalamic tract is the main pathway that pain signals travel along the spinal cord.

Primary Nociceptor Afferents

Nociceptors throughout the body give rise to two different types of pain fibers: unmyelinated C fibers and A delta (Aδ) fibers.[4] Unmyelinated C fibers are smaller in diameter, 0.4-1.2 mm, and conduct at a slow velocity, 0.5-2.0 m/s.[6] Slower than the Aδ fibers, C fibers transmit aching, imprecise localization, burning pain.[7] Responsible for about 70% of pain transmission, the C fibers are much more numerous than Aδ fibers. Aδ fibers are thicker myelinated fibers with a fast conduction velocity.[8] The Aδ fibers transmit the exact localization of sharp, stinging pain.[4]

The nociceptors activate action potentials based on a variety of substances that are released from damaged tissue. In response to mechanical, thermal, or chemical stimuli, the following substances are released: globulin and protein kinases, arachidonic acid, histamine, nerve growth factor, substance P, calcitonin gene-related peptide, potassium, serotonin, acetylcholine, acidic solution, ATP, and lactic acid.[4] Globulin and protein kinases may be released to cause severe pain in damaged tissue. Arachidonic acid is also released in response to damaged tissue. Through a biochemical pathway, metabolism to prostaglandins results in a G protein–mediated protein kinase A cascade. Aspirin works to block the arachidonic acid from forming prostaglandins. Histamine release from tissue damage also activates nociceptors to activate pain action potentials. Tissue damage and inflammation may also lead to the release of substance P and calcitonin gene-related peptide. In addition to the activation of nociceptors, they also cause vasodilation and, subsequently, tissue edema. Tissue damage also results in potassium release and a decrease in tissue pH. Serotonin, acetylcholine, and ATP are also released during tissue damage and cause nociceptors to become excited. Finally, muscle spasms and lactic acid can cause nociceptor activation during hyperactive muscle use or restricted blood flow to a muscle.

After nociceptors respond to noxious stimuli, an action potential transmits a pain signal to the central nervous system. Within the central nervous system's gray matter, there is a system of ten layers called the Rexed laminae.[5] The nociceptive axons enter the spinal cord through the dorsal roots and project toward the dorsal horn. The signals then branch, forming the Lissauer tract, which branches toward ascending and descending spinal cord tracts before entering the dorsal horn. Within the dorsal horn, the pain neurons are organized into different Rexed laminae. Rexed laminae I is called the marginal zone and relays pain and temperature sensation. Rexed laminae II are called the substantia gelatinosa and relays pain, temperature, and light touch sensation. Rexed laminae III/IV are the nucleus proprius and relays mechanical and temperature sensation to the brain. The first-order neurons of the spinothalamic tract synapse in these areas.

Pain Transmission at the level of the Spinal Cord, Brainstem, and Cerebral Cortex

The spinothalamic pathways include the anterolateral spinothalamic, spinoreticular, and spinomesencephalic tracts. Fast (Aδ) and slow (C) nerve fibers constitute two main pathways within the spinothalamic tract. The fast- and slow-conducting pathways are also known as the neospinothalamic and paleospinothalamic tracts[9] (see Fig. 1.1).

Primary (first-order neuron) nociceptive afferents carry information regarding pain and temperature from the periphery to the spinal cord. These primary afferents are fast-conducting myelinated Aδ fibers or slow-conducting unmyelinated C fibers. Fast (~20 m/s) Aδ fibers transmit information about sharp, pricking, or well-localized pain. Slow (~0.5-2 m/s) C fibers transmit information about crude touch, temperature, chemical, or poorly localized pain. Both fast and slow primary nociceptive afferents synapse in the dorsal horn of the spinal cord. The dorsal horn is divided into six cytologically distinct areas known as Rexed lamina.[10] Lamina I contains the secondary (second-order) neurons of the marginal zone nucleus. Lamina II contains the secondary neurons of the substantia gelatinosa. Lamina III & IV contain tertiary (third-order) neurons of the nucleus proprius.

Fast Aδ nociceptive afferents synapse in or near lamina I (marginal zone); secondary afferent axons arising from the marginal zone neurons cross the anterior white commissure and ascend in the contralateral lateral (mostly) and anterior spinothalamic tract and synapse on

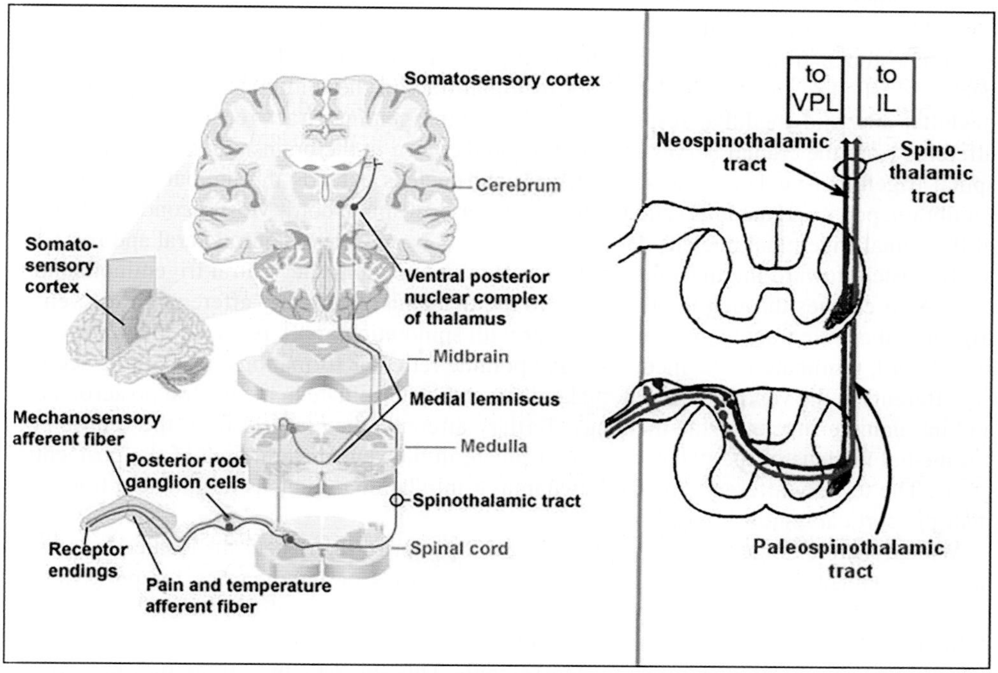

FIGURE 1.1 Spinothalamic tract, including peripheral nociceptors ascending through the spinal cord and brainstem to the somatosensory cortex. Dorsal column/medial lemniscus (proprioception/mechanosensory) is also shown in *yellow*. VPL, ventral posterolateral nucleus; IL, intralaminar nucleus; neospinothalamic, fast/Aδ fibers; paleospinothalamic, slow/C fibers. (Byrne JH, Dafny N, eds. *Neuroanatomy Online: An Electronic Laboratory for the Neurosciences*. Department of Neurobiology and Anatomy, McGovern Medical School at The University of Texas Health Science Center at Houston [UTHealth]. http://nba.uth.tmc.edu/neuroanatomy. © 2014 to present, all rights reserved.)

tertiary neurons located in the ventral posterolateral nucleus of the thalamus. The tertiary axons projecting from the ventral posterolateral nucleus then travel to the primary somatosensory cortex in the postcentral gyrus of the parietal lobe.

Slow primary C nociceptive afferents synapse in dorsal horn lamina II (substantia gelatinosa). Second-order axons then project from the substantia gelatinosa neurons a short distance to synapse in or near the ipsilateral nucleus proprius of lamina III & IV. Tertiary afferent axons then project from the nucleus proprius and cross the anterior white commissure to enter the contralateral anterior (mainly) and lateral spinothalamic tracts. Tertiary afferents from the nucleus proprius that comprise the spinoreticular tract exit to terminate in the medullary and pontine reticular formation. The reticular formation is thought to be responsible for levels of attention and consciousness and may play a role in modulating the response to pain.[11] Many of the tertiary afferents from the nucleus proprius that comprise the spinomesencephalic tract leave the spinothalamic tract to terminate in the midbrain periaqueductal gray (PAG) zone in the rostral pons and lower midbrain. The spinomesencephalic tract is thought to play an important role in the inhibition of pain. When PAG cells are activated, they are thought to act as a pain suppression system that releases endogenous opioids and other neurotransmitters to inhibit pain transmission at the spinal cord level (substantia gelatinosa).[12] The remaining tertiary afferents of the spinomesencephalic tract continue to the thalamus, where they synapse in either the centromedial nuclei or the nucleus parafascicularis within the intralaminar nuclei of the thalamus. The 4° (fourth-order neuron) afferent axons of the intralaminar nuclei then project diffusely throughout the cerebral cortex, hence their association with poorly localized sensory pain.

The spinal trigeminal pathway of the brain is an analog to the spinothalamic tract of the cord. The spinal trigeminal pathway conveys sensory information about pain, temperature, and crude touch from the head and neck. Primary nociceptive afferents carried by cranial nerves V, VII, IX, and X join the spinotrigeminal tract in the mid pons, caudal pons, upper medulla, and mid medulla, respectively. The spinotrigeminal tract receives these primary afferents from the cranial nerves during its caudal course in the brainstem, terminating in the spinal trigeminal nucleus. The spinal trigeminal nucleus extends throughout the brainstem (midbrain, pons, and medulla) and into the high cervical spinal cord. Most secondary afferents of the spinal trigeminal nucleus decussate immediately and travel contralateral and rostral in the brainstem toward the thalamus in the nerve tract known as the ventral trigeminothalamic tract. As it courses through the brainstem to the thalamus, secondary afferents of the ventral trigeminothalamic tract branch and, together with spinoreticular afferents ascending from the spinal cord, terminate in the medullary and pontine reticular formations. Remaining secondary afferents in the ventral trigeminothalamic tract then terminate in the ventral posteromedial and intralaminar nuclei of the thalamus. Tertiary afferents then project from the ventral posteromedial nucleus of the thalamus and terminate in the ventrolateral area of the postcentral gyrus. The tertiary afferents from the thalamus's intralaminar nucleus terminate diffusely in multiple cortical regions[13] (see Fig. 1.2).

Wide dynamic range neurons are found in and comprise many neurons located in the spinal cord's dorsal horn. They may be projection neurons or interneurons for polysynaptic responses. They receive input from a broad range of sensory modalities (Aδ, C, nonnoxious A-fiber) and continuously process environmental (ie, nociceptors/proprioception) and internal (ie, interneurons/descending brainstem) signals. This somesthetic activity may help to discriminate between varying degrees of nociceptive input. Wide dynamic range neurons possess large receptive fields with both low and high threshold areas. They demonstrate plasticity that allows them to modify their receptive field size. Nociceptive-specific fibers, in contrast, have a smaller receptive field that does not demonstrate plasticity, and they receive inputs only from Aδ and C fibers.[14]

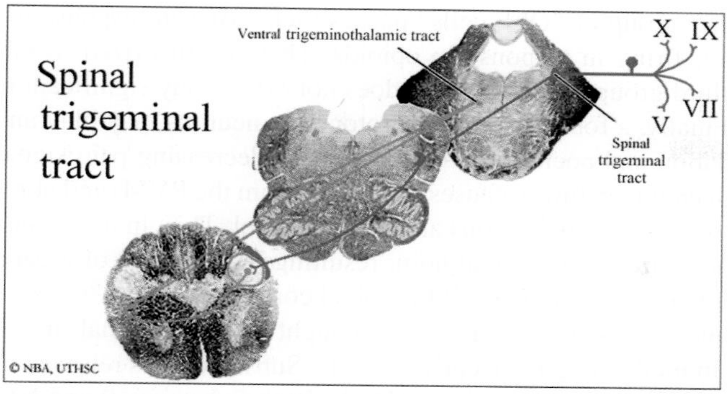

FIGURE 1.2 The spinal trigeminal tract of the brainstem. Primary nociceptors synapse in the trigeminal nucleus of the caudal medulla, and secondary afferents project rostral through medulla and pons. (Byrne JH, Dafny N, eds. *Neuroanatomy Online: An Electronic Laboratory for the Neurosciences*. Department of Neurobiology and Anatomy, McGovern Medical School at The University of Texas Health Science Center at Houston [UTHealth]. http://nba.uth.tmc.edu/neuroanatomy. © 2014 to present, all rights reserved.)

Pain perception is not limited to one specific area of the brain. It involves multiple neural structures including nociceptors, spinothalamic tracts, somatosensory cortex, thalamic projections (sensory relay), prefrontal cortex (planning of complex behavior and decision making), cingulate cortex (provides an emotional description of pain and helps to coordinate response), and insula cortex (links emotion to action). It can be viewed as a fluid system that may explain why pain experiences are individualized. Chronic pain from nociceptive or nonnociceptive factors can cause prolonged pain matrix activation.[15] Second-order neurons are not nociceptive specific, while third-order neurons associated with orbitofrontal and limbic systems modify the pain experience based upon various factors, including beliefs, emotions, and expectations.[16] This multifactorial and unique individual interpretation of nociceptive stimuli is termed the pain matrix.

Pain Modulation: Increase or Decrease Pain Signals?

Both ascending and descending pathways can modulate nociceptive signals. Opiate receptors exist at the spinal cord's dorsal horn and binding to these receptors causes hyperpolarization of these neurons. This results in inhibition of firing and preventing the release of substance P, thus blocking ascending nociceptive signal transmission.[17]

Together, the PAG and rostral ventromedial medulla (RVM) form a regulatory loop controlling the descending pain modulation pathway. This regulatory loop may facilitate or inhibit pain, depending on which cells in the system are activated. The PAG is an area of gray matter in the midbrain surrounding the cerebral aqueduct. It receives input from various limbic system regions and plays a significant role in controlling descending pain modulation. The PAG projects to the serotonergic neurons of the RVM and locus coeruleus (LC), a part of the brain involved in physiological responses to stress. The RVM includes the nucleus raphe magnus (a member of the rostral group of raphe nuclei, the primary location for serotonin production within the brain), and other adjacent nuclei. The RVM receives input from the hypothalamus, amygdala, insula, and PAG. RVM cells project to the spinal cord's dorsal horn, the preganglionic sympathetic neurons, and the central canal.[18] By utilizing these connections, the RVM works in conjunction with the PAG to act as the primary control center modulating descending pathways of nociceptive transmission.[19]

The RVM contains four types of cells. One group of cells known as "ON-cells" increases firing rates when associated with a nociceptive signal, facilitating pain perception. On the other hand, another group of "OFF-cells" pauses their firing in response to noxious stimuli and increases their firing in response to opioids. They are theorized to inhibit nociceptive transmission. A third group of neutral cells does not exhibit any significant response to nociceptive stimuli. Finally, a fourth group of serotonergic neurons may play an essential role in emotional modulation and nociceptive modulation by decreasing pain signals. Activation of the inhibitory descending pathway causes serotonin (from the RVM) and norepinephrine (produced from the LC) release from axons at the spinal level. This, in turn, causes the release of enkephalins at the spinal cord's dorsal horn, resulting in inhibition of ascending nociceptive signal transmission at the dorsal horn of the spinal cord.[20]

Substance P and neurokinin-1 (NK-1) are thought to be additional important neurotransmitters involved in modulating nociceptive signals. Substance P is released at the dorsal horn of the spinal cord in response to noxious stimuli. Both Substance P and NK-1 receptors are found in high levels within the RVM and thought to be involved in descending modulation of nociceptive signals.[21]

It is theorized that for a healthy functioning body, there is a significant amount of descending inhibitory modulation, preventing pain perception at baseline. However, there may be either an increase in facilitatory modulation or a decrease in descending inhibitory modulation of nociceptive signals in specific individuals, resulting in an imbalance of nociceptive signal transmission. Recent studies suggest that decreased descending inhibitory modulation is found in individuals with chronic pain. Furthermore, a loss of descending inhibition may result in dysfunctional pain.[22]

Inhibitory and Excitatory Neurotransmitters/ Neuropeptides of Pain

The somatosensory system can be incredibly complex, involving several pain pathways and neurotransmitters. In this chapter, we will discuss the most important neurotransmitters involved in the process of acute pain. The primary excitatory neurotransmitters that we will discuss are glutamate and aspartate. In conjunction, we will discuss the main inhibitory neurons, including GABA and glycine. We will discuss different types of neuropeptides that can be inhibitory and excitatory. Given evolving research with pain pathways and potential novel targets in the peripheral and central nervous system, we hope to gain improved insight into the acute pain pathway's neurotransmitters.

Excitatory Neurotransmitter of Pain

The main excitatory neurons involved with pain transmission include glutamate and aspartate. These neurotransmitters can be found throughout the somatosensory pathway beginning from the afferent neurons to second-order neurons and the thalamus.[23] Other excitatory neurotransmitters that will be discussed include ATP.

There are several pain synapses that utilize multiple types of glutamate receptors, including four total classes: NMDA, AMPA, kainate, and metabotropic receptors.[24] The AMPA, kainate, and NMDA receptors are ionotropic receptors.[24] The metabotropic receptors are G protein–coupled receptors, which means they exert their effects through second messenger systems.[25] Activation of these receptors leads to neuromodulatory actions. The metabotropic receptors are present at different levels of the pain pathways regulating nociceptive signaling transmission.[26] The kainate and AMPA receptors are ionotropic receptors meaning that when activated, they increase membrane permeability for sodium and potassium.[24] Both receptor types are responsible for mediating a large portion of rapid afferent pain signaling for any stimulus.[23] Glutamate facilitates pain signaling transmission through Aδ and C fibers.[27]

NMDA receptors are also widely distributed throughout the somatosensory pathway and expressed on several types of sensory neurons.[28] NMDA receptors are both ionotropic and voltage-gated, which increase membrane permeability for calcium.[24] They are activated through extensive or prolonged stimulation through the somatosensory pathways, eventually removing magnesium from the channel, thus blocking its inhibition.[23] NMDA receptors are involved in central sensitization, including leading to increased sensitization at dorsal horn neurons. This leads to a rise in prolonged depolarization, lower threshold activation, and larger receptive field size.

Prior studies have shown that presynaptic NMDA receptor activity can strengthen excitatory signaling to dorsal horn neurons in the spine at primary afferent terminals. Additionally, postsynaptically, NMDA receptors can potentiate excitability while decreasing inhibition at synapses via increasing K^+–Cl^- cotransporter-2 proteolysis.[29] The NMDA and glutamate sensitization relationship can be influenced by other factors, including the release of bradykinin, causing increased glutamate release by neurons and astrocytes. This can further exacerbate a severe pain sensitivity state known as central sensitization pain.[23]

Glutamate transporters are found on glial membranes and can contribute to worsening glutamate release.[23,30] For instance, glutamate transporters, glutamate transporter –1 (GLT-1), and glutamate-aspartate transporter (GLAST) are suppressed in the chemotherapy-induced neuropathy leading to increased spinal glutamate. This eventually leads to increased levels in the extracellular space meeting cellular synapses.[23]

Metabotropic glutamate receptors are G protein–coupled receptors that are activated by glutamate.[24] They are involved in long-term changes and are not ion channels but instead activate a biochemical chain altering proteins, including ion channels. These events can eventually lead to alterations in synapse excitability. These receptors can be found in pre- and postsynaptic neurons, including the cerebellum, cerebral cortex, and hippocampus.[31] Notably, all metabotropic glutamate receptors (except mGlu6 receptor) are within the nociceptive pathways to modulate pain transmission. They are also involved in the induction and maintenance of central sensitization.[32]

Metabotropic glutamate receptors are categorized into three primary groups (I, II, III). Group I's primary function is to increase NMDA receptor activity. Group I involves Gq/11 leading to the release of inositol trisphosphate (IP3) and diacyl glycerol (DAG), eventually leading to calcium release and activating of protein kinase C (PKC), respectively. Group II and II metabotropic receptors lead to a decrease in NMDA receptor activity. They are involved through Gi/Go leading to a reduction of AMP and PKA activity.[23]

It is widely accepted that activation of Group I metabotropic receptors at nociceptor afferents in the periphery and spinal cord promotes pain. However, prior studies have implicated that Group I receptors in the supraspinal region can lead to an increase or decrease in nociception. For instance, Class I agonists decrease nociception in the amygdala. The antagonist in this area had similar effects. In the thalamus, Class I agonist potentiated nociceptive response of the thalamus. In the PAG, positive allosteric modulators decreased the nociceptive response.[32]

Aspartate is an excitatory neurotransmitter involved with pain.[23] Prior studies support its role in modulating nociceptive-specific neurons and altering the threshold in inflammation and neuropathic pain in mice.[33] D-Aspartate is defined as an agonist of the NMDA receptor. Boccella et al. had conducted a study with mice lacking an aspartate-metabolizing enzyme, D-aspartate oxidase, leading to elevated D-aspartate concentrations in these mice.[33] They found that mice lacking the enzyme had an increased evoked activity of neurons involved in nociception located at the dorsal horn of the spinal cord in the lumbar area.[33] Furthermore, they were found to have a notable decrease in the threshold for mechanical and thermal domains. Mice lacking this enzyme appeared to have worsened nocifensive behavior to the formalin test in this study.[33]

ATP has also been implicated in the role of pain transmission, particularly through the P2X receptors.[34] The P2X receptors are distributed among the central and peripheral pain fibers. Specifically, they are located on primary afferent fibers that synapse in neurons of the dorsal horn (lamina V and lamina II). This leads to an increase in glutamate release.[23] Prior studies involving P2 receptor-selective antagonist support the concept of ATP initiating and maintaining chronic pain.[35] Tsuda et al. 2003 had shown that P2X4 receptor stimulation of microglial cells is required for tactile allodynia. The increase in P2X4 receptors was also observed in microglial cells in neuropathic pain states.[34] When ATP binds to the P2 receptors on microglial cells, the cells undergo a morphological change. This change leads to an upregulation of cytokine receptors and P2 receptors. Subsequently, these activated glial cells release inflammatory molecules (NGF, NO, and cytokines), leading to prolonged pain. Prior studies have shown that knockout mice that do not have P2X4 and P2X7 have a reduced response to thermal and mechanical sensation. P2X2 and P2X3 have been implicated in nerve fibers involved in cancers of the head and neck.[23]

Inhibitory Neurotransmitters

The two main inhibitory neurotransmitters for the somatosensory system are GABA and glycine. Anatomically, at the level of the spine, glycine is the most active.[27] In comparison, GABA is dominant above these levels.[23]

GABA can be found in the spinal cord in lamina I, II, and III. The three classes of GABA receptors are $GABA_A$, $GABA_B$, and $GABA_C$. The $GABA_A$ receptor is a ligand-gated ion channel that is attached to a chloride channel that can be affected by alcohol, benzodiazepines, and barbiturates.[23,36] This receptor can be affected by $GABA_A$ agonist such as muscimol and an antagonist such as gabazine.[23] Of note, $GABA_A$ receptors are associated with C-fiber nociceptors and large myelinated fibers leading to allodynia postintradermal injection of capsaicin.[23] In prior animal studies, in *naïve* animals, $GABA_A$ receptor agonists and antagonists led to antinociception and pronociception states, respectively.[37] Furthermore, $GABA_A$ receptors can be found presynaptically at afferent terminals and postsynaptically on dorsal horn neurons. Inhibiting these receptors can produce pain involving allodynia.[38]

$GABA_B$ receptors are G-protein–coupled receptors that are associated with opening potassium influx channels, calcium channel inhibition, and activation of adenylyl cyclase. $GABA_B$ receptors can be found in a variety of locations, including peripherally and centrally. Examples include the spinal cord, thalamus, and brainstem. GABA can alter nociceptive signaling at the level of the dorsal horn through $GABA_A$ and $GABA_B$ receptors. $GABA_B$ receptors located in the spinal cord modulate the activity of neurons in the dorsal horn and peptidergic primary afferent terminals. Presynaptically, when $GABA_B$ receptors are activated, they can block glutamate and substance P receptors. Of note, in a study involving mice lacking $GABA_B$ receptors, they displayed decreased sensitivity to mechanical nociceptive and hot stimulation and solidified the presence of $GABA_B$-mediated pain. Additionally, $GABA_B$ receptor activation in the spinal cord and ventrolateral thalamus is associated with baclofen's antinociceptive effects. Lastly, it was found that inhibition by GABA was reduced at the level of the spinal cord in neuropathic pain states, eventually leading to elevated excitation and contributing to central sensitization. It was demonstrated that baclofen leads to antinociception in neuropathic animals. Interestingly, it was found that intraspinal transplantation of precursors of interneurons that release GABA positively affected neuropathic allodynia.[39]

Neuropeptides

Neuropeptides also contribute to the somatosensory pathway and pain. These compounds can be either excitatory or inhibitory and are markedly diverse. Compared to neurotransmitters' actions, neuropeptides do not act as quickly and have a slower onset of action and longer duration of effect. Key neuropeptides involved in pain are substance P, neurokinin A, enkephalins, and somatostatin.[23]

Substance P (SP) and neurokinin A are classified as the two main excitatory neuropeptides. They exert their effects through the neurokinin 1 and 2 receptors known as NK1R and NK2R, respectively. Both peptides can be found in the neurons at the levels of the spinal cord and supraspinal levels, including the thalamus, with notable concentrations at primary afferent neurons.[23] Substance P and neurokinin A belong to the tachykinin family. Although both bind to neurokinin receptors (NKR), substance P preferably binds to neurokinin 1 receptors (NK1), and neurokinin A binds preferably to NK2—both of which belong to the GPCR family.[40] With noxious stimuli, these neuropeptides are released after the continued stimulation of C-nociceptors. The mechanism of action is through the spreading of these neuropeptides in the dorsal horn leading to possible interaction with several synapses.[23] Although both neuropeptides are heavily involved in nociceptive pain signaling, much research in substance P has revealed its major involvement in pain signaling.

Substance P can be found at the dorsal horn of the spinal cord, the amygdala, and substantia nigra. Substance P is created by neurons of the dorsal root ganglion, stored in vesicles, and rapidly transferred down the axon toward spinal and peripheral nerves. During inflammatory states and injury to peripheral nerves, it was shown that phenotypes of neurons change. Primary afferent fibers that are responsible for releasing substance P upregulate NK1 receptors in the dorsal horn. NKR interacts with phospholipase C leading to second messenger pathways, ultimately generating depolarization of membranes and contributing to AMPA and NMDA receptor activity. SP has also been found to affect the expression of inflammatory molecules, cytokines, and transcription factors such as nuclear factors kappa-light chain enhancer of activated B cells (NF-KB), a factor that leads to activation of proinflammatory compounds and development of hyperalgesia. In rat models of pain, NK1 receptor expression was upregulated in neurons of the spinal cord. Furthermore, in inflammatory states, capsaicin stimulation lead to NKR endocytosis of spinal cord neurons leading to prolonged release of substance P.[40]

The main inhibitory neuropeptides are somatostatin and enkephalins. These inhibitory neuropeptides can be found in various locations, including descending tracts from various nuclei of the brainstem projecting to the dorsal horn and at the spinal levels, including dorsal horn neurons.[23] Somatostatin inhibits neurogenic inflammation. Pharmacologic analogs of somatostatin elicited acute anti-inflammatory effects speculated through inhibiting the release of inflammatory mediators at peptidergic sensory nerve terminals and from mast cells.[41] Somatostatin inhibitory neurons reduced cortical V pyramidal neuron activity, one of the markers of neuropathic pain in this study. It was found that pharmacologic activation of somatostatin-expressing cells reduced pyramidal neuron hyperactivity and allodynia.[42]

Enkephalins belong to the endogenous opioid peptide families. Neurons producing enkephalins can be found in a wide distribution of the body. They can be found in the spinal cord in lamina I, II, and V and the PAG. They can also be found concentrated in areas of the hypothalamus and globus pallidus. They are involved in many physiologic processes and affect the gastrointestinal, respiratory, cardiovascular, and somatosensory system.[43]

Enkephalins exert their effect through mu, delta, and kappa receptors. Mu receptors are mainly found in the central nervous system, delta receptors are distributed in the spinal cord, and kappa receptors are found in the spinal cord. Enkephalins have a higher affinity for the delta-opioid receptor, with mu- and kappa-opioid receptors following affinity. The receptors are G protein–coupled receptors with downstream effects leading to the reduction of potassium and calcium influx. Activation of mu receptors in the midbrain leads to inhibitory descending pathway activation of the nucleus reticular paragigantocellularis and PAG.[44]

There are several neurotransmitters and neuropeptides that are involved in pain. Essential excitatory peptides include glutamate, aspartate, with the addition of ATP as a contributing factor. Primary inhibitory neurotransmitters include GBA and glycine. Neuropeptides are also involved, including substance P, neurokinin A, enkephalins, and somatostatin. Neurotransmitters and neuropeptides involved in acute pain can be complex, and continued research is tantamount if we are to understand the acute pain and nociceptive pathways fully.

Conclusion

From an evolutionary standpoint, pain is a protective mechanism developed to prevent tissue damage and communicating threats to the human body. This unpleasant, subjective experience can alter behavior to prevent further damage and promote healing. Pain is often classified into either acute or chronic pain. Acute pain is a normal, immediate response to noxious stimuli and most commonly results from some form of injury to the body.[2] This type of pain characteristically arises suddenly after a particular insult and is self-limited in duration (<3-6 months).

Noxious stimuli from the environment can activate complex pathways in the human body that ultimately lead to the perception of pain in the central nervous system. The anatomy and physiology involved in the perception of pain are quite complex. Numerous pathways and neurotransmitters have been described, which relay and modify pain signals in various parts of the body. These modified signals are eventually transmitted to the brain and perceived as a painful experience.[3]

It is important to have a fundamental understanding of the anatomy, physiology, and neurotransmitters involved in acute pain. This understanding allows the proper diagnosis of injury location and severity. Furthermore, it helps guide treatment plans and allows us to monitor for the resolution of injuries and tissue damage. Finally, a thorough understanding of these mechanisms will aid in the future development and improvement of treatment interventions available for acute pain.[45]

REFERENCES

1. Williams ACDC, Craig KD. Updating the definition of pain. *Pain*. 2016;157:2420-2423. https://pubmed.ncbi.nlm.nih.gov/27200490/
2. Nesse RM, Schulkin J. An evolutionary medicine perspective on pain and its disorders. *Philos Trans R Soc B Biol Sci*. 2019;374(1785):20190288. https://royalsocietypublishing.org/doi/10.1098/rstb.2019.0288
3. Meyr AJ, Steinberg JS. The physiology of the acute pain pathway. *Clin Podiatr Med Surg*. 2008;25:305-326. https://pubmed.ncbi.nlm.nih.gov/18486847/
4. Lee GI, Neumeister MW. Pain: pathways and physiology. *Clin Plast Surg*. 2020;47(2):173-180.
5. Steeds CE. The anatomy and physiology of pain. *Surgery*. 2016;34(2):55-59.
6. Hudspith MJ. Anatomy, physiology and pharmacology of pain. *Anaesthesia & Intensive Care Medicine*. 2016;17:425-430.
7. Steeds CE. The anatomy and physiology of pain. *Surgery (Oxford)*. 2009:507-511.
8. Bourne S, Machado AG, Nagel SJ. Basic anatomy and physiology of pain pathways. *Neurosurg Clin N Am*. 2014;25(4):629-638.
9. Byrne JH, Dafny N, eds. *Neuroanatomy Online: An Open Access Electronic Laboratory for the Neurosciences* [Internet]. Department of Neurobiology and Anatomy—The University of Texas Medical School at Houston. Accessed November 10, 2020. https://nba.uth.tmc.edu/neuroanatomy/
10. Rexed B. The cytoarchitectonic organization of the spinal cord in the cat. *J Comp Neurol*. 1952;96(3):415-495. https://pubmed.ncbi.nlm.nih.gov/14946260/
11. Martins I, Tavares I. Reticular formation and pain: the past and the future. *Front Neuroanat*. 2017;11:51. www.frontiersin.org
12. Hemington KS, Coulombe MA. The periaqueductal gray and descending pain modulation: why should we study them and what role do they play in chronic pain? *J Neurophysiol*. 2015;114(4):2080-2083. https://pubmed.ncbi.nlm.nih.gov/25673745/
13. Brodal P. *The Central Nervous System* [Internet]. Oxford University Press; 2010:196-200. Accessed November 10, 2020. http://oxfordmedicine.com/view/10.1093/med/9780190228958.001.0001/med-9780190228958
14. AI B. *The Senses: A Comprehensive Reference*. Vol. 5. Elsevier; 2008:331-338. Accessed November 10, 2020. https://www.elsevier.com/books/the-senses-a-comprehensive-reference/basbaum/978-0-12-370880-9

15. Moseley GL. A pain neuromatrix approach to patients with chronic pain. *Man Ther*. 2003;8(3):130-140.
16. Garcia-Larrea L, Peyron R. Pain matrices and neuropathic pain matrices: a review. *Pain*. 2013;154(suppl 1):S29-S43. https://pubmed.ncbi.nlm.nih.gov/24021862/
17. Kline IV RH, Wiley RG. Spinal μ-opioid receptor-expressing dorsal horn neurons: role in nociception and morphine antinociception. *J Neurosci*. 2008;28(4):904-913. https://www.jneurosci.org/content/28/4/904
18. Mason P. Rostral ventromedial medulla. In: *Encyclopedia of Pain* [Internet]. Springer; 2013:3419-3421. Accessed November 10, 2020. https://link.springer.com/referenceworkentry/10.1007/978-3-642-28753-4_3849
19. Heinricher MM. Pain modulation and the transition from acute to chronic pain. *Adv Exp Med Biol*. 2016;904:105-115.
20. Budai D, Khasabov SG, Mantyh PW, Simone DA. NK-1 receptors modulate the excitability of on cells in the rostral ventromedial medulla. *J Neurophysiol*. 2007;97(2):1388-1395. https://pubmed.ncbi.nlm.nih.gov/17182914/
21. Brink TS, Pacharinsak C, Khasabov SG, Beitz AJ, Simone DA. Differential modulation of neurons in the rostral ventromedial medulla by neurokinin-1 receptors. *J Neurophysiol*. 2012;107(4):1210-1221. https://pubmed.ncbi.nlm.nih.gov/22031765/
22. Ossipov MH, Morimura K, Porreca F. Descending pain modulation and chronification of pain. *Curr Opin Support Palliat Care*. 2014;8:143-151. ncbi.nlm.nih.gov/pmc/articles/PMC4301419/?report=abstract
23. Nouri KH, Osuagwu U, Boyette-Davis J, Ringkamp M, Raja SN, Dougherty PM. Neurochemistry of somatosensory and pain processing. In: Benzon HT, Raja SN, Liu SS, Fishman SM, Cohen SP, eds. *Essentials of Pain Medicine*. 4th ed. Elsevier; 2018:11-20.e2.
24. Purves D, Augustine GJ, Fitzpatrick D, et al. *Neuroscience*. 2nd ed. Sinauer Associates; 2001.
25. Niswender CM, Conn PJ. Metabotropic glutamate receptors: physiology, pharmacology, and disease. *Annu Rev Pharmacol Toxicol*. 2010;50:295-322.
26. Goudet C, Magnaghi V, Landry M, Nagy F, Gereau RW IV, Pin JP. Metabotropic receptors for glutamate and GABA in pain. *Brain Res Rev*. 2009;60(1):43-56.
27. Goud DJ. *Neuroanatomy*. 5th ed. Lippincott Williams and Wilkins;2014.
28. Raja SN, Sivanesan E, Guan Y. Central Sensitization, *N*-methyl-D-aspartate receptors, and human experimental pain models: bridging the gap between target discovery and drug development. *Anesthesiology*. 2019;131(2):233-235.
29. Laumet GO, Chen S-R, Pan H-L. *NMDA Receptors and Signaling in Chronic Neuropathic Pain*. Humana Press Inc; 2017:103-110.
30. Shigeri Y, Seal RP, Shimamoto K. Molecular pharmacology of glutamate transporters, EAATs and VGLUTs. *Brain Res Rev*. 2004;45(3):250-265.
31. López-Bendito G, Shigemoto R, Fairén A, Luján R. Differential distribution of group I metabotropic glutamate receptors during rat cortical development. *Cereb Cortex*. 2002;12(6):625-638.
32. Pereira V, Goudet C. Emerging trends in pain modulation by metabotropic glutamate receptors. *Front Mol Neurosci*. 2019;11:464.
33. Boccella S, Vacca V, Errico F, et al. D-Aspartate modulates nociceptive-specific neuron activity and pain threshold in inflammatory and neuropathic pain condition in mice. *Biomed Res Int*. 2015;2015:905906.
34. Toulme E, Tsuda M, Khakh BS, et al. On the role of ATP-Gated P2X receptors in acute, inflammatory and neuropathic pain. In: Kruger L, Light AR, eds. *Translational Pain Research: From Mouse to Man*. CRC Press/Taylor & Francis; 2010. Chapter 10. https://www.ncbi.nlm.nih.gov/books/NBK57271/
35. Gerevich Z, Illes P. P2Y receptors and pain transmission. *Purinergic Signal*. 2004;1(1):3-10.
36. Sigel E, Steinmann ME. Structure, function, and modulation of GABAA receptors. *J Biol Chem*. 2012;287:40224-40231.
37. Potes CS, Neto FL, Castro-Lopes JM. Inhibition of pain behavior by GABA(B) receptors in the thalamic ventrobasal complex: effect on normal rats subjected to the formalin test of nociception. *Brain Res*. 2006;1115(1):37-47. doi:10.1016/j.brainres.2006.07.089
38. Price TJ, Prescott SA. Inhibitory regulation of the pain gate and how its failure causes pathological pain. *Pain*. 2015;156(5):789-792.
39. Malcangio M. GABAB receptors and pain. *Neuropharmacology*. 2018;136:102-105.
40. Zieglgänsberger W. Substance P and pain chronicity. *Cell Tissue Res*. 2019;375(1):227-241.
41. Helyes Z, Pintér E, Németh J, et al. Anti-inflammatory effect of synthetic somatostatin analogues in the rat. *Br J Pharmacol*. 2001;134(7):1571-1579.
42. Cichon J, Blanck TJJ, Gan W-B, Yang G. Activation of cortical somatostatin interneurons prevents the development of neuropathic pain. *Physiol Behav*. 2018;176(1):139-148.
43. Shenoy SS, Lui F. Biochemistry, endogenous opioids. In: *StatPearls* [Internet]. StatPearls Publishing; 2021.
44. Cullen JM, Cascella M. Physiology, enkephalin. In: *StatPearls* [Internet]. StatPearls Publishing; 2021.
45. Bell A. The neurobiology of acute pain. *Vet J*. 2018;237:55-62. https://pubmed.ncbi.nlm.nih.gov/30089546/

2

Neurobiology of Acute Pain

Alex D. Pham, Madelyn K. Craig, Devin S. Reed, William C. Bidwell, William A. Wall, Kiana Fahimipour, Brian M. Nelson, Alan David Kaye, and Richard D. Urman

Introduction

Pain, although subjective, can objectively follow the nociceptive pathway beginning from the initial stimulus leading to what we perceive as pain. This phenomenon can be described as nociception, which is defined as "the encoding and processing of noxious stimuli in the nervous system."[1] Although pain offers our system protection from threats, it can also be unwanted. Stimuli can be chemical, thermal, mechanical, neurogenic, and inflammatory leading to activation of the somatosensory and nociceptive pathways and eventually to the central nervous system (CNS).[1] Pain is an incredibly complex phenomenon, which is why it is tantamount that we explain the neurobiology of acute pain and its intricacies. We will explore the physiologic process from initial stimuli in the periphery from transduction to transmission through the spinal cord to supraspinal levels. We will explain the biology of inflammatory states and acute pain. Furthermore, we will also explain descending pain modulation and the detrimental phenomena of central sensitization involving neuroplasticity with associated hyperalgesia and allodynia.[1,2] It is our hope that through this chapter, we can offer our readers a comprehensive understanding of nociceptive pathways to improve treatment for acute pain.[1,3]

Neurobiology of Pain at the Periphery to the Spinal Cord

Nociception is defined as the peripheral process of encoding and processing noxious stimuli. These stimuli activate a nociceptor or peripherally located neuron leading to the eventual realization of pain. The nociceptors are characterized based on the type of stimuli they respond to, with a classification based on whether they respond generally to thermal, mechanical, or chemical stimuli, but can also be classified as polymodal, silent, and mechano-thermal.[4] The type of receptor is based upon its location, including the skin, joints, and viscera. Nociception is further broken down and characterized by the nerve fiber type with its properties based on the speed of transmission of the axon and diameter of the fiber.[5]

The presence or absence of myelin, which acts as an insulator, is responsible for faster transmission. The degree of myelination can vary. Myelinated fibers act as an insulator that sends a signal that is interrupted at the nodes of Ranvier but has a faster speed of transmission. Unmyelinated fibers provide slower continuous conduction. A-fibers are myelinated, and C-fibers are unmyelinated.[5] C-fibers are small diameter unmyelinated axons bundled in fascicles, which are surrounded by Schwann cells and support slower conduction velocities, whereas A-fibers are myelinated axons and support faster conduction velocities and mediate fast onset pain.[5] A-fibers are further characterized based on motor and sensory properties, breaking down into alpha, beta, delta, and omega, which corresponds to their properties and relating to velocity based on myelination and axon thickness. Alternately, sensory properties are characterized toward which receptors the fibers are related to, characterized as type 1a, type 1b, type II, type III, and type IV.

The process by which a noxious stimulus turns into a painful signal is a multistep process. Peripheral nerve endings are unencapsulated, pseudounipolar, and arise from the dorsal root ganglion (DRG) or trigeminal ganglion with innervation peripherally at the skin and centrally on a second-order neuron.[5] The process of signal transduction takes place when this noxious stimuli involving free nerve endings (C and A delta fibers) lead to the opening of ion gated channels, which in turn convert it to an electrochemical signal by making changes in membrane potential, then opening additional channels, and the eventual depolarization of the afferent nerve These primary afferents carry this stimulus from the periphery to the CNS where they terminate predominantly in laminae I, II, and V of the dorsal horn on relay neurons and local interneurons.[4,5] The main nociceptive pain transducing channels include acid-sensing ion channels (ASICs), transient receptor potential (TRP), cation channels, and voltage-gated sodium channels. ASICs are nonvoltage sensitive, protein-induced sodium channels that detect changes in pH and have been associated with epilepsy, depression, migraines, and neuropathic pain.[6] TRP channels are a group of channels with different roles and responses to modulators. Examples include TRPV1, which responds by allowing the passage of calcium ions and is potentiated by heat, acidity, and capsaicin, and TRPA1, which is sensitive to thermal, mechanical, and chemical stimuli.[7] Voltage-gated sodium (Nav) channels play a principal role in the generation of an action potential by being heavily involved in the transformation from transduction to transmission.[7] Other common voltage-gated channels include calcium and potassium.[5] The previously mentioned ASIC and TRP depolarize Nav channels leading to the formation of an action potential. Membrane depolarization leads to extracellular sodium ion influx, which in turn causes an increase in membrane potential leading to a threshold whereby an action potential is generated.[7]

Nociceptors are responsive to many different mediators, both inflammatory and noninflammatory, which corresponds to both the receptor type and the location within the body. Common inflammatory mediators include 5-HT, kinins, histamine, nerve growth factors, adenosine triphosphate, PG, glutamate, leukotrienes, nitric oxide, NE, and protons, while noninflammatory mediators include calcitonin gene–related peptide, GABA, opioid peptides, glycine, and cannabinoids.[6]

Biology of Peripheral Pain Signals—Transmission of the Signal

For noxious stimuli to be perceived, it must first be transduced at the nerve endings in the periphery then transmitted along the nerve axon to the dorsal horn of the spinal cord. Numerous ion channels and G-protein–linked receptors have been identified and thought to play a role in the transduction and transmission of noxious stimuli. One group of ion channels called transient receptor potential ion channels (TRP channels) transduce noxious stimuli by allowing entry of cations leading to depolarization and generation of an action potential that is then transmitted down the axon to the spinal cord. Different types of stimuli (eg, temperature, chemical, and mechanical/intense pressure) activate different subtypes of TRP channels. TRP vanilloid 1 (TRPV1) channel and TRP melastatin 8 (TRPM8) channel respond to heat and cold stimuli, respectively. Several TRP channels are polymodal responding to temperature and chemical stimuli. The following TRP channels also respond to potentially noxious chemical stimuli: TRPV1, the receptor for capsaicin, and TRPM8, the receptor for menthol. Isoflurane's pungent odor is transduced by TRP ankyrin 1 (TRPA1) channel, the receptor for mustards and garlic.[1] Two-pore potassium (K2P-KCNK) channels, voltage-gated potassium channels, and voltage-gated sodium channels are other thermotransducers that modulate the response to temperature stimuli. TREK-1 and TRAAK, both part of the KCNK potassium channel family, are found in some C fibers and are proposed to modulate receptor excitability.[8] Several classes of sodium channels are expressed on sensory neurons; however, Nav 1.7, 1.8, and 1.9 are predominantly found on nociceptors. Mutations within these receptors have been found in painful disorders and insensitivities to pain. Mechanosensory transducers have not been positively identified, although a number of channels have been proposed. Degenerin/epithelial sodium (DEG/ENac) channels; TRPV1, TRPV4, and TRPA1 channels; KCNK channels; and acid-sensitive ion channels (ASICs) are candidate proteins thought to play a role in mechanical hypersensitivity.[8] Opioid, cannabinoid, $GABA_b$, and alpha-2 receptors are a few of the G-protein–linked receptors involved in antinociception that work by reducing calcium entry via modulation of calcium channels.[1] Voltage-gated sodium and potassium channels are also involved in signal modulation. Upregulation of the action potential occurs via sodium channels, while downregulation occurs via potassium channels.[9] A set of action potentials encodes the intensity of the noxious stimulus.[5] Voltage-gated calcium channels are also involved in transmission of noxious stimuli. A modulatory subunit of the calcium channel is found highly expressed in C fibers especially after nerve injury. This is the target of gabapentin.[1] N- and T-type calcium channels found on C fibers are upregulated after nerve injury in disorders such as diabetic neuropathy.[8] Once the action potential has reached the dorsal horn, the signal is again transduced to be transmitted to the brain.

Biology of Inflammatory Process and How It Affects Pain Sensorium

During inflammation, cells of the immune system and circulatory system migrate to the sites of injury releasing inflammatory mediators. These mediators include cytokines; chemokines; acute phase proteins; peptides, such as bradykinin; eicosanoids, such as prostaglandins; and vasoactive amines, such as serotonin (Table 2.1). Activated macrophages involved in the upregulation of inflammation secrete proinflammatory cytokines IL-1beta, IL-6, and tumor

TABLE 2.1 INFLAMMATORY MEDIATORS INVOLVED IN PAIN

1. Cytokines:
   - IL-1beta
   - IL-6
   - TNF-alpha
2. Chemokines
3. Acute phase proteins
4. Peptides:
   - Bradykinin
5. Eicosanoids
   - Prostaglandins
   - PGE_2
   - PGI_2
6. Vasoactive amines
   - Serotonin

From Zhang JM, An J. Cytokines, inflammation, and pain. *Int Anesthesiol Clin*. 2007;45:27-37. https://doi.org/10.1097/AIA.0b013e318034194e; Choi SI, Hwang SW. Depolarizing effectors of bradykinin signaling in nociceptor excitation in pain perception. *Biomol Ther*. 2018;26:255-267. https://doi.org/10.4062/biomolther.2017.127.

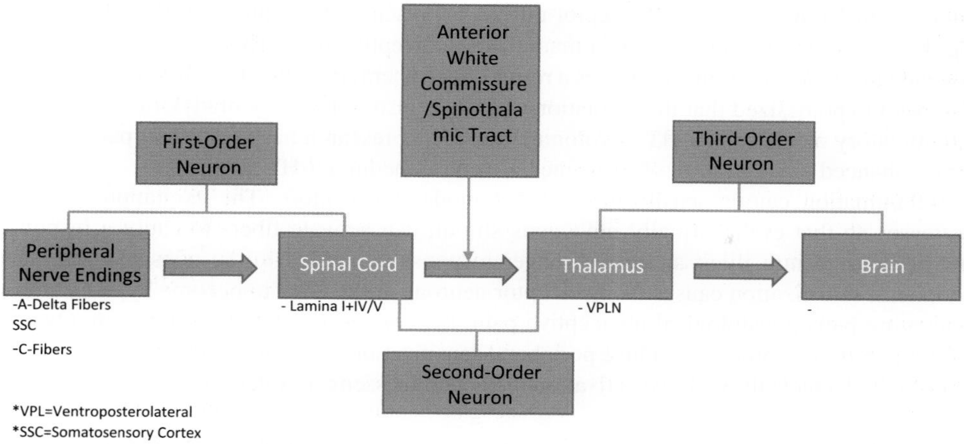

FIGURE 2.1 Inflammatory process from macrophages to pathologic pain. (From Zhang JM, An J. Cytokines, inflammation, and pain. *Int Anesthesiol Clin.* 2007;45:27-37. https://doi.org/10.1097/AIA.0b013e318034194e; Choi SI, Hwang SW. Depolarizing effectors of bradykinin signaling in nociceptor excitation in pain perception. *Biomol Ther.* 2018;26:255-267. https://doi.org/10.4062/biomolther.2017.127.)

necrosis factor (TNF)-alpha (Fig. 2.1). These three cytokines are known to be involved in process of pathologic pain by activating nociceptive sensory receptors. IL-1beta, for example, is expressed in nociceptive DRG neurons and is found to increase PGE_2 and substance P in glial and neuronal cells.[10] Bradykinin, one of the major mediators of pain during inflammation, alters the electrical functions of nociceptor sensory neurons by enhancing their excitability, therefore greatly contributing to pain generation and exacerbation. Bradykinin also electrically sensitizes the pain-mediating nociceptor neurons. It has been hypothesized that bradykinin may augment the depolarization of specific effector ion channels expressed in nociceptor neurons through intracellular signaling via G-protein–coupled receptors. The opening of ion channels TRPV1, TRPA1, and ANO1 is involved in the role as a depolarizing effector in the direct induction of neuronal firing by bradykinin.[11]

Prostaglandins, another important inflammatory mediator of pain, are formed when arachidonic acid is released from the plasma membrane by phospholipase A_2 and further metabolized through the cyclooxygenase pathway (COX-1/COX-2) to release prostaglandins. Prostaglandin E_2 (PGE_2) and PGI_2 have the greatest impact among prostanoids in processing of pain signals. PGE_2, an abundant prostaglandin, displays versatile biological activities such as involvement in blood pressure regulation, fertility, and immune responses. In inflammatory processes, PGE_2 plays a great role in all processes that leads to the classic signs of inflammation: pain, redness, and swelling.[12] The four identified subtypes of PGE_2 receptors are EP_1, EP_2, EP_3, and EP_4. These receptors work through the G-protein–coupled signaling. EP_1 causes activation of phospholipase C, producing IP_3 and diacylglycerol, followed by calcium mobilization and activation of protein kinase C. Whereas agonist stimulation of EP_2 and EP_4 receptors, which are coupled to G_s protein, activates adenylyl cyclase generating AMP (cAMP) and then protein kinase A. PGE_2 action on central sites (brain and spinal cord) and peripheral sensory neuron results in pain. Interestingly, there is increased expression of EP_1 receptors during brachial plexus nerve injury, avulsion of injured DRG, and painful neuromas. Activating EP_1 pathway can cause mobilization of cytosolic calcium in this spinal dorsal horn, which is involved in the late phase of carrageenan-induced inflammatory pain. Pharmacologic interventions targeting upstream and downstream PGE_2 signals are used as therapeutic strategies for alleviating pain.[12] PGI_2 is another inflammatory mediator, which causes edema and pain. Its actions work through IP receptors-cAMP signaling pathway, which can mediate pain during acute inflammation. The IP receptor mRNA is present in the neurons of the DRG including those that express substance P, a marker for nociceptive pain. This receptor may also be involved in spinal pain transmission as a result of peripheral inflammation. Interestingly, it has also been hypothesized that the formation of PGI_2 is also induced by bradykinin.[12,13] Another inflammatory mediator is 5-HT (serotonin), and recent research has shown that pain sensitivity is enhanced via activation of rostromedial ventral medulla 5-HT neurons.[13]

Inflammation causes sensitization of polymodal nociceptors. The excitation threshold decreases so that even normally innocuous stimuli can activate fibers to cause a response, and noxious stimuli illicit an even stronger response compared to the nonsensitized state. Peripheral sensitization causes the nociceptor neurons in the CNS to become hyperexcitable, generating pathophysiological nociceptive pain: hyperalgesia and nociceptive pain. Overall, inflammatory mediators can induce peripheral sensitization by changing the response properties of ion channels through the activation of second messenger system.[14]

Neurobiology at Level of Spinal Cord Transmission

Pain signal transmission is part of the survival response. Nociceptive transmission is an afferent cycle, initiating in the peripheral primary neuron based upon noxious stimuli. Peripheral stimuli must cause threshold depolarization to generate an axon potential. These primary afferent neurons, whose cell bodies reside in neighboring dorsal root ganglia, enter the spinal cord as dorsal roots—traveling rostrally or caudally several levels in the tracts of Lissauer—before synapsing with secondary neurons at the dorsal horn.

Primary afferent neurons have a distinctive termination pattern within the spinal cord dorsal horn. The dorsal horn is classically divided into lamina, which correspond with specific afferent synaptic sites. Nonnoxious stimuli—such as stretch—travel by A-beta fibers and synapse with interneurons at lamina III.[6] Noxious stimuli from thermal or mechanical nociceptors travel by A-delta fibers or unmyelinated C fibers. A-delta fibers terminate in lamina I and lamina IV/V. C fibers terminate at laminae II, or substantia gelatinosa, where they stimulate the neurotransmitter substance P.[6] These fibers influence pain signals and response by modulating ascending and descending neurons that cross in the dorsal horn of the spinal cord. Both types of nociceptor neurons remain silent in homeostasis during absence of pain stimuli.

The majority of primary afferent neurons synapse to interneurons in these dorsal horn laminae, allowing extensive modulation of input signals to occur. Interneuron synapses are a point where several neurotransmitters are released and can stimulate a range of reactions, defined by the pharmacological effects from the signal. Excitatory exchange may cause release of substance P, which binds postsynaptic NK1 receptors, or release of glutamate, which may bind to a variety of receptors.[6,15] Ultimately, these excitations trigger massive influx of calcium and depolarization of the interneuron.[15] Inhibitory neurotransmitters—such as glycine, GABA, endocannabinoids, and enkephalins—provide tonic inhibition at the dorsal horn. Glycine and GABA can attenuate the excitatory pathways. Inhibitory enkephalins bind mu-receptors on primary afferents at the dorsal horn allowing direct attenuation of input signals.[15] Additional exogenous opioids are often the mainstay of analgesic therapy. The summation of this dynamic complex communication within the dorsal horn determines the output signal along ascending pathways to the brain.

Ascending pathways from lamina I and IV/V of the dorsal horn decussate in the anterior white commissure and ascend cranially in the spinothalamic tract to the contralateral ventral posterolateral nucleus of the thalamus and on to the somatosensory cortex. The spinothalamic tract consists of two parts: the lateral spinothalamic tract—which focuses on pain and temperature sensation—and the anterior spinothalamic tract—which carries pressure sensation information.[15] Other afferent signals that synapse in the superficial dorsal horn are propagated through the parabrachial tract toward the hippocampal regions of the brain. These tracts are responsible for memory and emotional components associated with nociception.[15]

Descending tracts—such as the corticospinal and rubrospinal tracts—decussate at the caudal aspect of the medulla, travelling caudally in the posterior column to the dorsal horn before exiting as the spinal nerve. The rubrospinal tracts integrate information with the initial withdrawal reflex at lamina VI. This initial spinal reflex enables rapid motor withdrawal to noxious stimuli even prior to conscious recognition of the damage to protect further damage. The rubrospinal tract indirectly carries regulatory signals from the cerebrum and cerebellum to inhibit extensor muscles and promote flexor activity, ultimately leading to a retraction from the noxious stimuli.[15]

Concept of Central Sensitization

The modern medical understanding of central sensitization started in 1983 where experiments demonstrated increased excitability of motor neurons beyond the anticipated response.[16] Understanding central sensitization often requires unintuitive insight that a repeated exposure to a stimulus has the potential to actually increase the response and further amplify a baseline. This is now fundamentally defined by the International Association for the Study of Pain as "increased responsiveness of nociceptive neurons in the CNS to their normal or subthreshold afferent input."[16]

Central sensitization likely occurs as part of the larger protective mechanism of pain to generate a reflex withdrawal in order ultimately allows the body time to heal.[16,17] Yet when applied to chronic pain, the CNS has the potential to create the experience of heightened sensitivity through hyperalgesia and allodynia and thus the pain response is no longer protective.[16] These increased sensitivities are a part of neural plasticity that promote an increase in synaptic efficacy and membrane excitability. The effects can then recruit many nociceptive pathways to include the overactivation of ascending A-beta fibers leading to an increased pain response.[16]

This dysfunctional phenomenon can largely be attributed to the dorsal horn by looking at molecular changes within primary afferent neurons. The cumulative changes increase membrane excitability, facilitate synaptic strength, and decrease inhibitory influences in dorsal horn neurons.[16,17] These changes are a result of two distinct phases. First, glutamate, the transmitter of primary afferent neurons, is phosphorylation dependent and binds to multiple receptors on postsynaptic neurons. The most applicable to sensitization is glutamates activation of the *N*-methyl-D-aspartate receptor. Glutamate removes the voltage block of Mg^{2+} on the NMDAR and allows an influx of Ca^{2+} to then depolarize and activate numerous intracellular pathways. This is because the released Ca^{2+} further phosphorylates NMDA receptors increasing both the activity and density of receptors leading to postsynaptic hyperexcitability. The second phase that promotes a longer lasting change in hypersensitivity is the transcription of new proteins and is described in pathological injury. As an example, sustained inflammation can generate the production of excess cyclooxygenase-2 also in dorsal horn neurons with subsequent production of prostaglandin E2 resulting in inflammatory hyperalgesia. This is not an isolated example as inflammation can induce a phenotypic switch in primary sensory neurons when exposed to excess nerve growth factor. At the level of transcription, there is a shift in the α-amino-3-hydroxy-5-methyl-4-isoxazolepropionic acid (AMPA) receptor from the Ca^{2+} impermeable GluR2 to the Ca^{2+} permeable GluR1. The now activated AMPAR with increased Ca^{2+} availability can then activate previously silent signaling pathways to an active state and potentiate lasting central sensitization.[16,17]

The Concept of Pain Modulation

As pain signals are propagated throughout the body, they may become altered before pain is ultimately interpreted and perceived in the brain. This is the basis for why certain noxious stimuli produce varying responses in different individuals and why nociception does not always correlate with the experience of pain. There are many ways by which pain signals can be modulated, but in this section, we will focus on some of the main theories such as the gate control theory and modulatory mechanisms of endogenous and exogenous opioids, autonomic function, and amino acids.

In 1965, a revolutionary theory was put forward by Ronald Melzack and Charles Patrick Wall that sought to provide a model of pain encompassing many of the opposing theories of their day.[18] The model was deemed "The Gate Control Theory" and included many aspects from popular pain models such as the Specificity and Pattern theories. Melzack and Wall believed that pain and touch fibers synapsed in two different regions within the dorsal horn of the spinal cord, the substantia gelatinosa and a group of cells they referred to as "transmission" cells. Stimulation at the level of the skin will produce a signal that is elicited through primary afferents and transmitted to either the substantia gelatinosa or cells within the dorsal horn of the spinal cord. It is suggested that the substantia gelatinosa acts as a gate modulating the transmission of signals from primary afferent neurons to the transmission cells. This gate is acted on by many cortical and subcortical structures in addition to both large and small fibers that carry antinociceptive and pronociceptive signals, respectively. If nociceptive signals from small fibers outweigh and overcome the inhibition brought on by large fibers, the sensation of pain can be experienced.[19]

One of the earliest and most studied mechanisms of pain modulation is the effect of endogenous and exogenous opioids. Endogenous and exogenous opioids exert an analgesic effect through interactions with various opioid receptors: μ-, δ-, and κ-opioid receptors, nociception or orphan FQ receptors, and opioid receptor–like orphan receptors.[19] Once bound to these receptors, opioids inhibit calcium and potassium channels ultimately preventing the release of pain neurotransmitters. There are several endogenous opioids in the brain such as endorphins, enkephalins, and dynorphins that produce antinociceptive effects when acting on their respective opioid receptors. The release of these endogenous brain molecules is part of the reason behind why individuals who have just undergone traumatic experiences such as motor vehicle collisions do not experience pain initially.[19] Conversely, exogenous opioids have become extremely useful in the treatment of inflammatory pain. By the peripheral activation of opioid receptors on A-delta and C fibers in the dorsal root ganglia, these drugs cause a powerful analgesic response; however, when acting centrally, they lead to significant side effects and addictive properties that are concerning.

The autonomic nervous system is linked to the modulation of pain through the dopaminergic, serotonergic, and noradrenergic pathways. Although dopamine is thought to play a vital role in pain modulation, the specificities of its action are still unclear and actively being researched. It is believed that dopamine acts on D2-like and potassium receptors in the amygdala leading to a decrease in the release of glutamate. Decreasing glutamate secretion in turn leads to the closing of intracellular calcium channels and decreased nociception.[19] As for the serotonergic and noradrenergic pathways, they serve as key players in the descending pathways of pain modulation; to truly understand how cortical and subcortical areas influence pain modulation through these pathways, the roles of the periaqueductal gray (PAG) region of the midbrain and the rostroventromedial (RVM) medulla must be explained. Recognized as one of the first brain regions implicated in pain modulation, the PAG region of the midbrain can to exert an endogenous antinociceptive effect. After many early studies involving the use of opioids and electrical stimulation of this region in animals, this PAG has established itself as the source of opioid-mediated pain inhibition. It receives inputs from cortical sites as well as the dorsal horns of the spinal cord via parabrachial nuclei and has reciprocal interactions with the RVM medulla.

The RVM is equally important to descending pain modulation. Apart from its interaction with the PAG, the RVM medulla also receives inputs from the thalamus, noradrenergic locus coeruleus, and parabrachial region and transmits signals to the dorsal horns and trigeminal nucleus caudalis. This region's impact on descending pain modulation is multifaceted with systems that both inhibit and facilitate pain. An imbalance between these systems has been shown in animal studies to be the underlying cause of pathologic pain.[20] While the RVM contains serotonergic, GABAergic, and glycinergic pathways that all project to the spinal cord, it is speculated that the release of serotonin is responsible for the pronociceptive and antinociceptive effects. The effect of spinal 5-hydroxytryptamine is entirely reliant upon the receptor subtype for which the molecule binds with 5-HT_{1A}, 5-HT_{1B}, 5-HT_{1D}, and 5-HT_7 receptors inhibiting pain and 5-HT_{2A} and 5-HT_3 facilitating pain.[20]

Noradrenergic projections act in descending pain modulation and originate from regions such as the locus coeruleus and the Kölliker-Fuse pontine noradrenergic nuclei. Upon stimulation of these regions, norepinephrine is released into the cerebrospinal fluid of the spine, which modulates an antinociceptive effect via presynaptic and postsynaptic $\alpha 2$ adrenergic receptors. Studies show that the analgesic response found from $\alpha 2$ agonist activity in the spine is synergistic with opioid administration and that activation of $\alpha 1$ receptors may even promote pain.[20] All in all, the various descending pathways that both facilitate and inhibit pain are constantly working in unison to create a baseline state of nociception that can be easily influenced by illness, injury, and inflammation.

The last modulatory mechanism that will be discussed is that of inhibitory amino acids mainly GABA and CCK. GABA, an inhibitory amino acid found in the CNS, is believed to inhibit nociception through descending modulatory processes. Loss of GABA and therefore its nociceptive inhibition leads to development of certain types of pain such as inflammatory and neuropathic.[19] In contrast, CCK, which is an inhibitory amino acid that is often released after the intake of food, may facilitate pain through its interactions in the RVM and certain molecules such as cannabinoids and opioids.

Conclusion

The neurobiology of acute pain can involve complex cellular and molecular mechanisms.[1] Beginning from the initial stimulus from the periphery, pain involves several phases including transduction, transmission, modulation, and perception leading to noxious stimuli.[1-3] Peripheral receptors respond to different stimuli transmitting different types of information (temperature, mechanical, nociception) to different lamina of the dorsal horn.[1,2] There are a variety of ascending and descending tracts involved in pain transmission and modulation that we must continue to explore. Furthermore, there are supraspinal regions involved including primary and secondary somatosensory cortices.[2] The neurobiology of acute pain is complex and continues to evolve. It is our aim to offer a comprehensive understanding of the nociceptive pathways leading to acute pain.

REFERENCES

1. Bell A. The neurobiology of acute pain. *Vet J.* 2018;237:55-62. https://doi.org/10.1016/j.tvjl.2018.05.004
2. Ringkamp M, Dougherty PM, Raja SN. Anatomy and physiology of the pain signaling process. In: *Essentials of Pain Medicine*. 4th ed. Elsevier; 2018:3-10.e1. http://dx.doi.org/10.1016/B978-0-323-40196-8.00001-2
3. Giordano J. The neurobiology of pain. *Pain Manag A Pract Guid Clin Sixth Ed.* 2001;353:1089-1100.
4. *Pain Principles (Section 2, Chapter 6) Neuroscience Online: An Electronic Textbook for the Neurosciences*. Department of Neurobiology and Anatomy—The University of Texas Medical School at Houston. n.d. Accessed October 21, 2020. https://nba.uth.tmc.edu/neuroscience/m/s2/chapter06.html

5. Dubin AE, Patapoutian A. Nociceptors: the sensors of the pain pathway. *J Clin Investig*. 2010;120:3760-3772. https://doi.org/10.1172/JCI42843
6. Yam MF, Loh YC, Tan CS, Adam SK, Manan NA, Basir R. General pathways of pain sensation and the major neurotransmitters involved in pain regulation. *Int J Mol Sci*. 2018;19. https://doi.org/10.3390/ijms19082164
7. McEntire DM, Kirkpatrick DR, Dueck NP, et al. Pain transduction: a pharmacologic perspective. *Expert Rev Clin Pharmacol*. 2016;9:1069-1080. https://doi.org/10.1080/17512433.2016.1183481
8. Basabaum AI, Bautista DM, Scherrer G, Julius D. Cellular and molecular mechanisms of pain. *Cell*. 2009;2:267-284. https://doi.org/10.1016/j.cell.2009.09.028.Cellular
9. Fenton BW, Shih E, Zolton J. The neurobiology of pain perception in normal and persistent pain. *Pain Manag*. 2015;5:297-317. https://doi.org/10.2217/pmt.15.27
10. Zhang JM, An J. Cytokines, inflammation, and pain. *Int Anesthesiol Clin*. 2007;45:27-37. https://doi.org/10.1097/AIA.0b013e318034194e
11. Choi SI, Hwang SW. Depolarizing effectors of bradykinin signaling in nociceptor excitation in pain perception. *Biomol Ther*. 2018;26:255-267. https://doi.org/10.4062/biomolther.2017.127
12. Ricciotti E, Fitzgerald GA. Prostaglandins and inflammation. *Arterioscler Thromb Vasc Biol*. 2011;31:986-1000. https://doi.org/10.1161/ATVBAHA.110.207449
13. Bannister K, Dickenson AH. What do monoamines do in pain modulation? *Curr Opin Support Palliat Care*. 2016;10:143-148. https://doi.org/10.1097/SPC.0000000000000207
14. Schaible HG, Ebersberger A, Natura G. Update on peripheral mechanisms of pain: beyond prostaglandins and cytokines. *Arthritis Res Ther*. 2011;13:210. https://doi.org/10.1186/ar3305
15. Urch DC. Normal pain transmission. *Rev Pain*. 2007;1:2. https://doi.org/10.1177/204946370700100102
16. Latremoliere A, Woolf CJ. Central sensitization: a generator of pain hypersensitivity by central neural plasticity. *J Pain*. 2009;10:895-926. https://doi.org/10.1016/j.jpain.2009.06.012
17. Woolf CJ. Central sensitization: implications for the diagnosis and treatment of pain. *Pain*. 2011;152:S2. https://doi.org/10.1016/j.pain.2010.09.030
18. Moayedi M, Davis KD. Theories of pain: from specificity to gate control. *J Neurophysiol*. 2013;109(1):5-12. https://doi.org/10.1152/jn.00457.2012
19. Kirkpatrick DR, Mcentire DM, Hambsch ZJ, et al. Therapeutic basis of clinical pain modulation. *Clin Transl Sci*. 2015;8(6):848-856. https://doi.org/10.1111/cts.12282
20. Isenberg-Grzeda E, Ellis J. Editorial supportive care and psychological issues around cancer. *Curr Opin Support Palliat Care*. 2015;9(1):38-39. https://doi.org/10.1097/SPC.0000000000000055

3

Evaluation and Measurement of Pain

Alan David Kaye, Alex D. Pham, Chikezie N. Okeagu, and Elyse M. Cornett

Introduction

Assessing pain can be a difficult task. Because of the subjective nature of pain and the challenges of selecting and applying various types of pain evaluation instruments, assessing pain may result in unreliable or biased results.[1] Indeed, pain assessment and reporting can be a fluid process and can be influenced by the patient, observer, conduction of the test, socioeconomic status, the ethnic background of the patient, comfort level of the patient, and other variables.[2] Given these difficulties, a study of existing pain assessment methods is essential. In the following chapter, we evaluate current pain assessment modalities for adults, the pediatric population, and special populations, including cognitively impaired/nonverbal patients.

Common Adult Population Assessment Tools

Visual Analog Scale

The Visual Analog Scale (VAS) is a linear scale that measures the magnitude of pain severity (Fig. 3.1). It is designed for patients >8 years old. It encompasses a horizontal line scaled as a spectrum from mild pain beginning from the left to increasing severity to the right end of the horizontal line.[2] The line is commonly 10 cm in length, with each side of the line ending in extremes—either no pain or intense pain. Of note, the line may be present as a horizontal or vertical line.[1] In terms of utilization, the patient marks his or her pain on the line of the spectrum of the scale.[3]

The results of a majority of studies imply that there is little difference among pain scales; however, VAS has been demonstrated to be superior compared to the Numerical Rating Scale (NRS) or Verbal Rating Scale (VRS).[1] VAS has shown to be associated with different behaviors of pain and ratio-level scoring.[1] Furthermore, VAS has been demonstrated to be sensitive to treatment modalities.[1] It has also been noted that through VAS, pain severity assessed at two separate time points displays an accurate difference in magnitude of pain.[3]

There are other versions of the VAS. One such version is known as the mechanical VAS, which utilizes a marker that is slidable and is "superimposed" on the horizontal line. This horizontal VAS is described as being drawn on a ruler and can be scored based on the back, which has numbers for the scale.[1] Prior studies have revealed that the mechanical VAS has promising test-retest reliability.[3]

The VAS does have its own disadvantages. First it is difficult to apply the VAS to individuals who are experiencing perceptual-motor difficulties.[1] This is present in patients

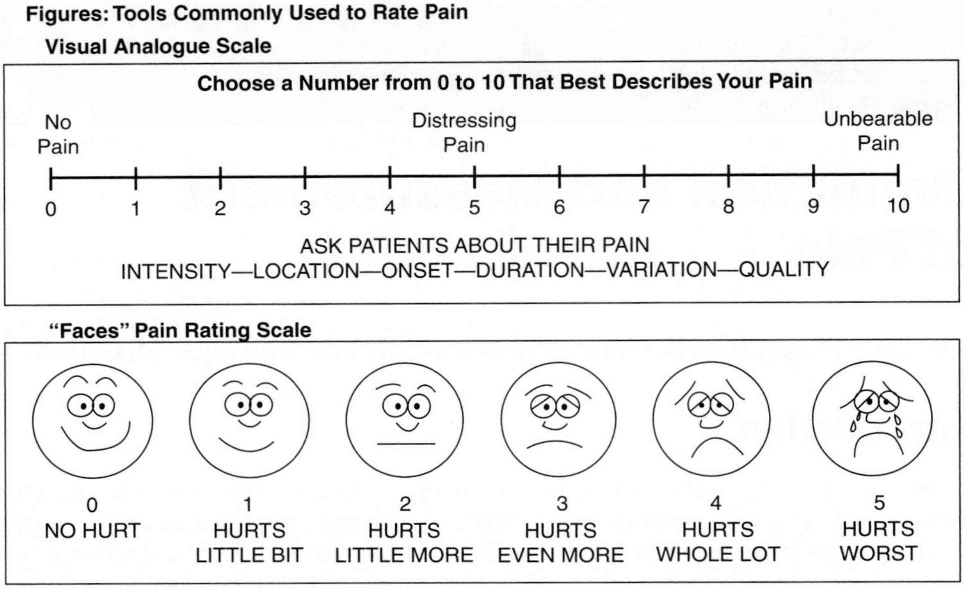

FIGURE 3.1 VAS image. (Gould D, et al. Visual Analogue Scale (VAS). *J Clin Nurs.* 2001;10:697-706.)

experiencing chronic pain. Second, individuals commonly utilize a ruler as measuring pain intensity must account for centimeters or millimeters to assess their pain magnitude.[1] This can be time-consuming with the chance of introducing bias into the scale. Additionally, patients suffering from a cognitive disability may increase rates of incompletion.[1]

The Visual Analog Scale has been used to measure pain in adults. The Visual Analog Scale has above-average noncompletion events with elderly patients.[1] Prior studies attribute failure rates among older populations toward three major categories: extent of motor abilities, level of impairment of cognitive ability, and level of education.[4] The VAS does indeed require the conceptual thought of pain and the ability to move a pencil marking toward the area representing their appropriate level of pain.[4] In the elderly population, it is recommended that VRS be utilized instead of VAS as prior studies have shown it has fewer failure responses.[1]

Numerical Rating Scale

The NRS allows the measurement of pain by having the user circle numbers (Fig. 3.2). These numbers can vary and range from 0 to 10, 0 to 20, or 0 to 100. The extremes of each scale

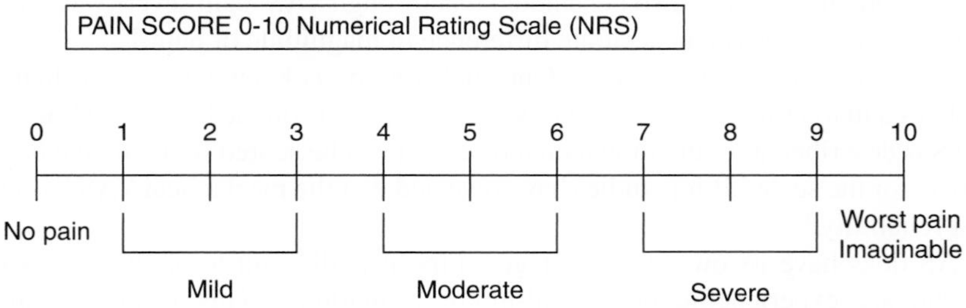

FIGURE 3.2 NRS image. (Melzack R. The McGill Pain Questionnaire: major properties and scoring methods. *Pain*. 1975;1(3):277-299. doi:10.1016/0304-3959(75)90044-5)

include 0 meaning a state of no pain and with the highest number correlating with a high pain intensity state.[3] The NRS is akin to the VRS in that it has positive data supporting its validity. Past studies have shown that NRS corresponds well with measuring treatments for pain. This scale can be given as a written scale or orally. Positive benefits to this scale are that it is well understood, is not difficult to use, and can be scored with ease.[1] Patients who suffer from multiple pain symptoms appear to prefer NRS.[2]

The disadvantages of this test are that it lacks ratio qualities compared to VAS or Graphic Rating Scale (GRS).[3] An example of this is cited by Lazaridou et al. in that equal intervals on the NRS may possibly not reflect the intensity of the pain.[1] This means that the interval distance between 9 and 7 may not be equivalent to the interval distance of 3 and 1.[1] Another disadvantage is "anchoring," entailing that patients may sometimes "anchor" their pain at the higher limit of the scale, which can change the way they rate their pain intensities.[1]

Verbal Rating Scales

The VRS measures pain through a spectrum of adjectives (Fig. 3.3). These adjectives are listed from the least intensity of pain to the most severe intensity of pain.[3] Those taking the test are requested to choose the appropriate adjective that accurately represents their pain.[1] Each adjective is associated with a scoring system.[1] Furthermore, the VRS is not just limited

Anxiety Category	Patient Evaluation	Anesthesiologist Evaluation
Mild	**VRS** **Mean:** 2.46 **Median:** 2 **Range:** 0–7 **SD:** ±1.71	**VRS** **Mean:** 2.43 **Median:** 2 **Range:** 0–6 **SD:** ±1.49
	VFAS **Most common face:** 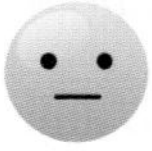	**VFAS** **Most common face:** 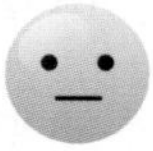
Moderate	**VRS:** **Mean:** 5.61 **Median:** 5 **Range:** 2–8 **SD:** ±1.52	**VRS** **Mean:** 5.82 **Median:** 6 **Range:** 3–9 **SD:** ±1.30
	VFAS **Most common face:** 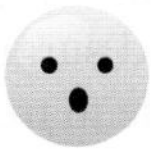	**VFAS** **Most common face:** 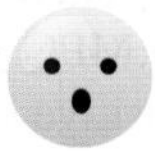
Severe	**VRS** **Mean:** 8.82 **Median:** 9 **Range:** 6–10 **SD:** ±1.33	**VRS** **Mean:** 9 **Median:** 9 **Range:** 7–10 **SD:** ±0.93
	VFAS **Most common face:** 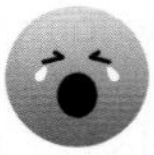	**VFAS** **Most common face:** 

SD = Standard deviation

FIGURE 3.3 Example of VRS.

by adjectives. Other forms of VRS encompass the use of phrases and a behavioral rating scale where the patient can describe their pain intensity by sentences.[1,3]

The Verbal Rating Scale has many advantages. First, it is simple to use and is easy to administer and score. Second, the validity of VRS to measure pain is supported.[1] Third, compliance rates are positive and are reportedly due to the fact that it is not difficult to comprehend.[1] This can be applied to the elderly population. The results of the VRS correlate well with different types of pain measuring tools.[1] Verbal Rating Scale is analogs to VAS in this sense.[3]

The Verbal Rating Scale does have some disadvantages. The VRS may not have an appropriate number of responses to choose from as patients may run into difficulty in choosing the most accurate response to represent their pain.[3] Additionally, accuracy of the test can be compromised as intervals between each word on the scale may not be weighted differently from the perspective of the patient. This can lead to difficulties in accurately rating pain intensity and changes in pain.[3] Another limitation of the VRS is that in order for this test to work, the patient must know and understand the words given by this pain assessment.[1]

McGill Pain Questionnaire

The McGill Pain Questionnaire (MPQ) measures pain through several aspects and is considered comprehensive. It tests patients' pain based on three aspects: cognitive-evaluative, affective, and sensory. This questionnaire comprises a list of 78 words that can be divided into 20 sections.[1] Each section consists of descriptors that are arranged from least intense to most intense. The sections are numbered based on the three aspects mentioned previously. For example, sections 1-10 are for sensory. Sections 11 through 15 represent the affective component.[1] Sections 16 is the evaluative arm of the questionnaire.[1] Sections 17 through 20 are the miscellaneous aspects of pain. Patients are asked to choose the words that best correlate with their pain severity.[1] Once chosen, the selected words are translated to a pain index. The words chosen by the patients are summed and assigned a ranking.[1] The MPQ also includes measuring the present pain severity based on an intensity scale of 1 to 5.[2]

A shorter version of the MPQ is also utilized in clinical practice. This involves 15 words or descriptors that belong to the sensory and affective category. The sensory category is composed of 11 descriptors, and the affective category consists of 4 descriptors. They are rated on a magnitude scale from 0 to 3—0 being "none" to 3 being the most "severe" experience of pain.[1,2]

The short MPQ has reportedly been comparable to the original MPQ.[2] The short MPQ may be easier to use compared to the original MPQ as it is shorter to administer.[2] This version of the MPQ is beneficial for obstetrics and surgical patients.[2] The short MPQ has shown to be sensitive enough to show differences due to treatments.[2] Lastly, this version may be easier for geriatric patients.[1]

Brief Pain Inventory

The Brief Pain Inventory (BPI) was created to evaluate patients with cancer. However, as time progressed, this assessment tool began to be utilized for generic/chronic pain patients. It is available in a long and short version. The long version includes 17 items, and the short version encompasses 9 items[5] (Fig. 3.4).

The long form required a longer period of 1 week to gauge pain interference and severity. This version inquired use of medications and to evaluate for descriptors that may accurately report their pain.[6] Questions from the long version included techniques to mitigate pain and

Date: _____ /_____ /_____ Time: ____________

Name: ________________ ________________ ____________

Last First Middle initial

1) Throughout our lives, most of us have had pain from time to time (such as minor headaches, sprains, and toothaches) have you had pain other than these everyday kinds of pain today?

1. Yes 2. No

2) On the diagram, shade in the areas where you feet pain, Put an X on the area that hurts the most.

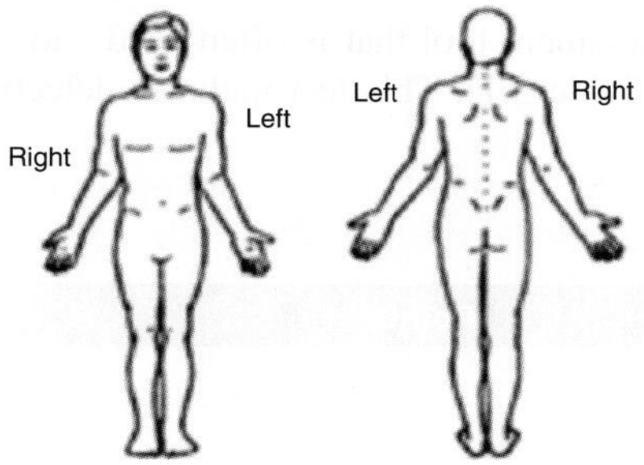

3) Please rate your by circling the one number that best describes your pain at its **worst** in the past 24 hours.

0	1	2	3	4	5	6	7	8	9	10
No pain										Pain as bad as you can imagine

4) Please rate your pain by circling the one number that best describes your pain at its least in the past 24 hours.

0	1	2	3	4	5	6	7	8	9	10
No pain										Pain as bad as you can imagine

5) Please rate your pain by circling the one number that best describes your pain on **average**.

0	1	2	3	4	5	6	7	8	9	10
No pain										Pain as bad as you can imagine

6) Please rate your pain by circling the one number that tells how much pain you have **right now**.

0	1	2	3	4	5	6	7	8	9	10
No pain										Pain as bad as you can imagine

7) What treatments or medications are you receiving for your pain?

____

____

8) In the past 24 hours, how much **relief** have pain treatments or medications provided? Please circle the one percentage that most shows how much relief you have received.

0%	10	20	30	40	50	60	70	80	90	100%
No relief										Complete relief

9) Circle the one number that describes how, during the past 24 hours, pain has **interfered** with your:

A. General activity

0	1	2	3	4	5	6	7	8	9	10
Does not interfere										Completely interferes

B. Mood

0	1	2	3	4	5	6	7	8	9	10
Does not interfere										Completely interferes

C. Walking ability

0	1	2	3	4	5	6	7	8	9	10
Does not interfere										Completely interferes

D. Normal work (includes both work outside the home and housework)

0	1	2	3	4	5	6	7	8	9	10
Does not interfere										Completely interferes

E. Relations with other people

0	1	2	3	4	5	6	7	8	9	10
Does not interfere										Completely interferes

F. Sleep

0	1	2	3	4	5	6	7	8	9	10
Does not interfere										Completely interferes

G. Enjoyment of life

0	1	2	3	4	5	6	7	8	9	10
Does not interfere										Completely interferes

FIGURE 3.4 Example of BPI scale. The Brief Pain Inventory is a medical questionnaire used to measure pain, developed by the Pain Research Group of the WHO Collaborating Centre for Symptom Evaluation in Cancer Care.

associated length and percentage of pain relief.[6] Because this version was found to take too long, especially if used repeatedly, the shorter version was produced.[6]

The shorter version is more common and will be described as follows.[5] This version of the BPI assesses pain through two major categories. The first category is by pain score severity, and the second category is the pain interference score.[5] The pain severity score draws from the four options describing pain severity. This includes current pain, average pain, least pain, and worst pain. Each of these options is then rated with a score of 0, meaning without pain, or to a high score of 10, which means the most severe pain.[5] The total possible score can be from either 0 to the max score of 40.[5] The pain interference portion of the inventory is designed through seven categories. These categories include work, general activity, mood activity, ability to walk, relationships, enjoyment of life, and sleep.[6] These categories are assigned a value of 0, meaning no interference, or 10, meaning interferes completely. The total score can be from 0 to 70 on this inventory.[5]

Pediatric Population

Neonatal Infant Pain Scale

The Neonatal Infant Pain Scale (NIPS) is a pain assessment tool that is often used and has been shown to be dependable with high validity[1,2] (Table 3.1). This test includes detecting

TABLE 3.1 EXAMPLE OF NIPS

Parameter	Finding	Points
Facial expression		
	Relaxed	0
	Grimace	1
Cry		
	No cry	0
	Whimper	1
	Vigorous crying	2
Breathing patterns		
	Relaxed	0
	Change in breathing	1
Arms		
	Restrained	0
	Relaxed	0
	Flexed	1
	Extended	1
Legs		
	Restrained	0
	Relaxed	0
	Flexed	1
	Extended	1
State of arousal		
	Sleeping	0
	Awake	0
	Fussy	1

NIPS: Total points for the 6 parameters, where minimum score is 0 and maximum score is 7.

Motta Gde C, Schardosim JM, Cunha ML. Neonatal Infant Pain Scale: cross-cultural adaptation and validation in Brazil. *J Pain Symptom Manage*. 2015;50(3):394-401. https://doi.org/10.1016/j.jpainsymman.2015.03.019

and measuring behaviors of pain. This includes arousal state, arm movement, breathing, leg movement, facial expression, and crying.[1] Each category consists of its own subcategories. For example, the facial expression category includes relaxed with a score of 0 and grimace with a score of 1.[2] The category for "cry" consists of "no cry" with a score of 0 to "vigorous" with a score of 2.[2] The NIPS can range from 0 to 7. A summation score of >3 is an indicator for the presence of pain.[2]

Oucher Scale

The Oucher scale is a self-reporting tool that is indicated for children aged 3-12 years[7] (Fig. 3.5). This tool includes a pain scale from 0 to 10 and a scale of pictures consisting of children's faces expressing different painful states.[7] Older children (8-12 years) can use this scale as they can utilize the numerated rating scale. Zero means "no hurt," and 10 is the most severe, meaning "the biggest hurt you could ever have." The photographic scale is utilized for younger children.[7] The bottom picture shows a picture of a child's face with no painful expression, while the picture at the very top of the scale shows a child's expression in severe pain.[7]

The Oucher scale includes several diverse versions to include other ethnic backgrounds for the photographic portion. These versions include faces of Caucasians, African Americans, and Hispanic ethnicity.[7] It was shown that the Oucher pain scale showed high validity, especially with the Hispanic and African American versions.[7] There have been positive reports of the African American version with children who have sickle cell anemia. Test results had a positive consistency with other pain assessment tools, including Visual Analogue Scales and the

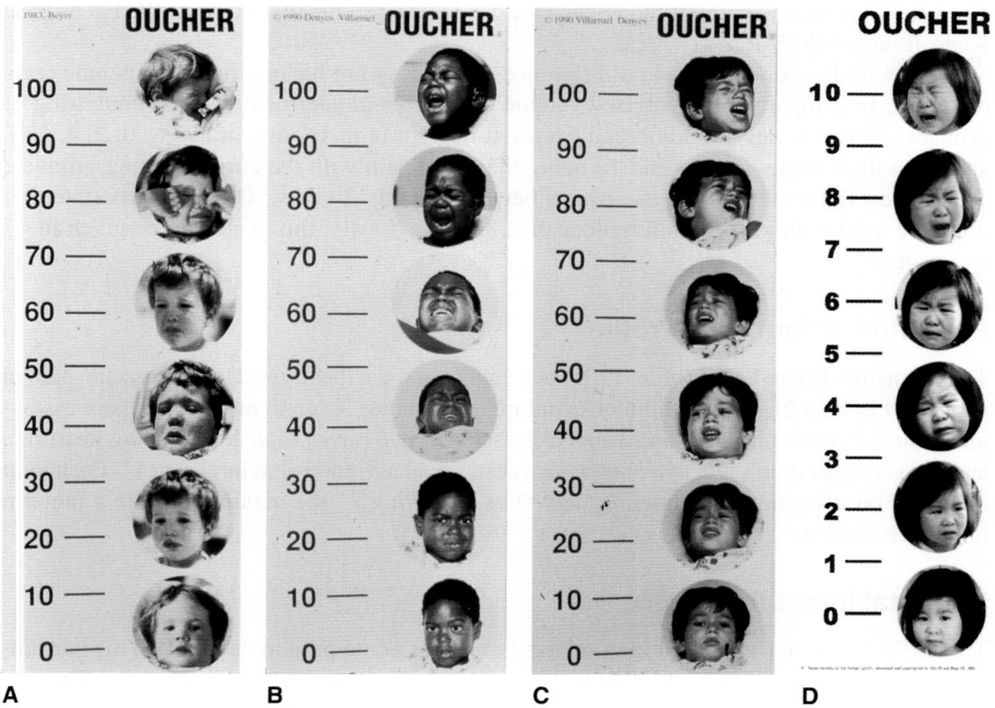

FIGURE 3.5 Example of Oucher Pain Scale.

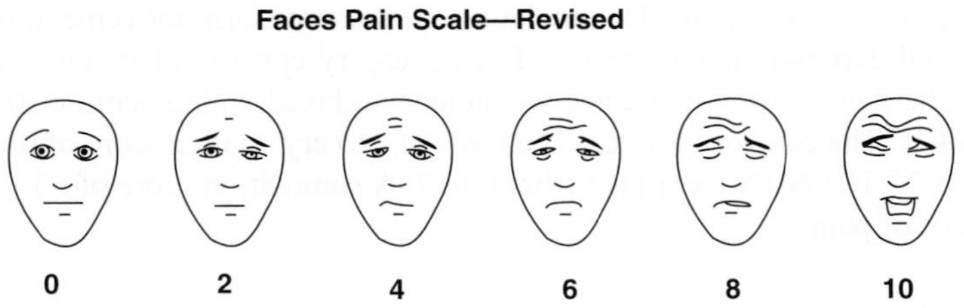

FIGURE 3.6 Example of Faces Pain Scale.

Pieces of Hurt Tool.[7] There have also been reports that the Oucher scale can detect alteration in pain post analgesic use in these patients.[7]

There are several limitations of the Oucher scale. Validity may not be strong when applied to younger children as old as 3-4 years old.[2] Numerical scales may be challenging for these groups. Furthermore, producing this scale may be expensive as making several versions of the Oucher scale with color photographs may not be economical.[7]

Faces Pain Scale

The Faces Pain Scale includes a horizontal scale of cartoon faces symbolizing pain intensity (Fig. 3.6). From left to right, the pain scale increases in magnitude.[2] This scale is for ages of 3-12 years, with this scale rating pain from 0 to 6. Zero means "no pain" to 6 meaning "most pain possible." This pain scale has its limitations, such as not being preferred by the pediatric population and the fact that that it was not scaled from 0 to 10.[2] Therefore, another version of the Faces Pain Scale was produced, known as the Faces Pain Scale-Revised (FPS-R).[2]

The revised version has several differences, including not having the scale include tears or smiles. In comparison, the revised version consists of gender-neutral faces consisting of grimaces.[2,8] The scales are numbered from left to right in increasing orders as 0, 2, 4, 6, 8, and 10, with 0 being no pain and 10 being the worst pain with the corresponding grimace. This scale can be used in the age groups between 4 and 12 years.[2] Other reports state that it can be used with most children older than 8 years.[9] Lastly, this scale can be given in 47 languages.[2]

Premature Infant Pain Profile

The Premature Infant Pain Profile (PIPP) is a validated scale that is used to assess acute pain in neonates (Table 3.2). The multidimensional model includes seven items used for pain assessment, three behavioral (including facial expressions), two physiological (including heart rate and oxygen saturation), and two contextual (gestational age and behavioral state).[10] Each item is graded on a 4-point scale ranging from 0 to 3, making 21 the maximum score a preterm infant can receive.

Neonatal Infant Pain Scale

The NIPS is another validated method used to assess acute pain in neonates. This particular method uses six different behavioral categories to gauge pain in neonates.[11] The criteria observed in the scale are facial expressions, cry, breathing patterns, arm movement, leg movement, and level of alertness. Indication of pain in an infant is any score of 3 or greater.

TABLE 3.2 EXAMPLE OF PIPP SCALE

	PIPP Scale			
Indicators	**0**	**1**	**2**	**3**
GA in Weeks	**≥36 wk**	**32-35 wk and 6 d**	**28-31 wk and 6 d**	**<28 wk**
Observe the NB for 15 s				
Alertness	Active	Quiet	Active	Quiet
	Awake	Awake	Sleep	Sleeping
	Opened eyes	Opened eyes	Opened eyes	Opened eyes
	Facial movements present	No facial movements	Facial movements present	No facial movements
Record HR and SpO_2				
Maximal HR	↑0 to 4 bpm	↑5 to 14 bpm	↑15 to 24 bpm	↑≥ 25 bpm
Minimal Saturation	↓0% to 2.4%	↓2.5% to 4.9%	↓5% to 7.4%	↓≥7.5%
Observe NB for 30 s				
Frowned forehead	Absent	Minimal	Moderate	Maximal
Eyes squeezed	Absent	Minimal	Moderate	Maximal
Nasolabial furrow	Absent	Minimal	Moderate	Maximal

Stevens B, Johnston C, Petryshen P, Taddio A. Premature Infant Pain Profile: development and initial validation. *Clin J Pain*. 1996;12(1):13-22. doi:10.1097/00002508-199603000-00004

Neonatal Facial Coding System

The Neonatal Facial Coding System (NFCS) relies solely on the presence or absence of facial expressions associated with pain in the infant patient. It is scored on a scale ranging from 0 to 8, with a score of 2 or greater indicating pain[12] (see Table 3.3).

TABLE 3.3 EXAMPLE OF NFCS

Facial Actions	0 Point	1 Point
Brow bulge	Absent	Present
Eye squeeze	Absent	Present
Deepening of nasolabial furrow	Absent	Present
Open lips	Absent	Present
Mouth stretch (horizontal or vertical)	Absent	Present
Tongue tautening	Absent	Present
Tongue protrusion	Absent	Present
Chin quiver	Absent	Present
Maximal score of 8 points, considering pain ≥3.		

Grunan RVE, Craig KD. Pain expression in neonates: facial action and cry. *Pain*. 1987;28:395-410.

TABLE 3.4 **EXAMPLE OF N-PASS**

	Nursing Recommendation for Therapy		
	Decrease	**No Change**	**Increase**
Pain: disagree (*n* = 40)			
N-PASS score <2 (*n*)	0	0	3
N-PASS score >2 (*n*)	0	37	0
Pain: agree (*n* = 178)			
N-PASS score <2 (*n*)	6	170	0
N-PASS score >2 (*n*)	0	0	2
Sedation: disagree (*n* = 33)			
N-PASS score <2 (*n*)	0	0	3
N-PASS score >2 (*n*)	1	29	0
Sedation: agree (*n* = 185)			
N-PASS score <2 (*n*)	2	182	0
N-PASS score >2 (*n*)	0	0	1

The Neonatal Pain, Agitation, and Sedation Scale (N-PASS) is a tool developed at Loyola University by Patricia Hummel, RNC, MA, APN/CNP, and Mary Puchalski, RNC, MS, APN/CNS.

Neonatal Pain, Agitation and Sedation Scale

The Neonatal Pain, Agitation and Sedation Scale (N-PASS) was developed to assess acute prolonged pain and sedation in all infants (Table 3.4). This scale relies on five behavioral and physiological criteria for pain assessment, including crying and irritability, behavior state, facial expression.[13] Each element is graded separately for pain (0, 1, 2) and sedation (0, −1, −2). The pain assessment portion is classified as "pain/agitation" as they are too difficult to differentiate clinically. A high pain score is indicative of intense behaviors, while a low sedation score is indicative of a deeper level of sedation. Preterm infants receive additional points depending on gestational age due to their limited ability to display and maintain behavioral manifestations of pain. A total score >3 suggests a moderate/severe level of pain, whereas a score <4 suggests a mild pain. The N-PASS is reliable in assessing pain for infants both post-surgically and in the event of ventilation.

CRIES

The CRIES uses a 10-point scale to assess postoperative pain in the neonatal patient population by measuring five different criteria; crying, the need for supplemental oxygen to maintain an SpO_2 of >95%, increased vital signs (specifically heart rate and blood pressure), facial expression, and sleeplessness[14] (Table 3.5). A score >4 suggests moderate to severe pain. In this event, patients may need additional analgesia.

Special Pediatric Populations: Nonverbal/ Cognitive Disability

r-FLACC

There are several observational pain assessment modalities for nonverbal or the cognitively impaired in the pediatric population. The revised Face, Legs, Activity, Cry, Consolability (r-FLACC) is one such tool (Table 3.6). This method was used to observe these patients in

TABLE 3.5 EXAMPLE OF CRIES SCALE

	0	1	2
Crying	No	High pitched	Inconsolable
Requires oxygen for saturation >95%	No	<30%	>30%
Increased vital signs	Heart rate and blood pressure less than or equal to preoperative state	Heart rate and blood pressure increase <20% of preoperative state	Heart rate and blood pressure increase >20% of preoperative state
Expression	None	Grimace	Grimace/grunt
Sleepless	No	Wakes at frequent intervals	Constantly awake

Krechel SW, Bildner J. CRIES: a new neonatal postoperative pain measurement score. Initial testing of validity and reliability. *Paediatr Anaesth*. 1995;5(1):53-61. doi:10.1111/j.1460-9592.1995.tb00242.x

TABLE 3.6 EXAMPLE OF r-FLACC SCALE

FLACC-REVISED (Revised descriptors for children with disabilities shown in brackets)			
Categories	**0**	**1**	**2**
Face	**No particular expression or smile**	**Occasional grimace or frown, withdrawn, disinterested** *[appears sad or worried]*	**Constant grimace or frown Frequent to constant quivering chin, clenched jaw** *[Distressed-looking face: Expression of fright or panic]*
Legs	**Normal position or relaxed**	**Uneasy, restless, tense** *[Occasional tremors]*	**Kicking or legs drawn up** *[Marked increase in spasticity, constant tremors or jerking]*
Activity	**Lying quietly, normal position moves easily**	**Squirming, shifting back and forth tense** *[Mildly agitated (eg, head back and forth, aggression); shallow, splinting, respirations, intermittent sighs]*	**Arched, rigid or jerking** *[Severe agitation head banging; Shivering (not rigors); Breath holding, gasping or sharp intake of breath; Severe splinting]*
Cry	**No cry (awake or asleep)**	**Moans or whimpers: occasional complaint** *[Occasional verbal outbursts or grunts]*	**Crying steadily, screams or sobs, frequent complaints** *[Repeated outbursts, constant grunting]*
Consolability	**Content, relaxed**	**Reassured by occasional touching, hugging, or being talked to, distractible**	**Difficulty to console or comfort** *[Pushing away caregiver, resisting care or comfort measures]*

Merkel S, et al. The FLACC: a behavioral scale for scoring postoperative pain in young children. *Pediatr Nurse*. 1997;23(3):293-297.

five categories, including face, legs, activity, cry, and consolability. Each category is assigned a score from 0 to 2 with a total max score of 10.[2] The revised version is different from the original as it allows one to add "open descriptors" for any deviation from the patients' usual activity.[2]

The revised version also includes improved descriptors aligned for patients with CI.[15] These changes were reportedly focused more on the activity and legs category—two categories that had lower agreements from previous observers on the original version.[15] Lastly, one can assess for any changes in pain behavior from baseline.[15] This test has positive reliability and validity in many groups with impairments.[2] It was reported that r-FLACC had a higher clinical utility compared to other assessment tools such as the Non-Communicating Children's Pain Checklist-Postoperative Version (NCCPC-PV) and the Nonverbal children and Nursing Assessment of Pain Intensity (NAPI).[16]

Non-Communicating Children's Pain Checklist–Postoperative Version

The Non-Communicating Children's Pain Checklist–Postoperative Version (NCCPC-PV) is another assessment tool for the nonverbal pediatric population. This pain assessment tool utilizes six categories. These categories include limbs, body, facial activity, social, and vocal.[2] These categories encompass 27 items altogether, with each item being assigned a number from 0 to 3. Zero means "not at all," and 3 meaning "very often." This test requires that the individual conducting the test observe the patient over a 10-minute period when scoring.[2] Reportedly, the highest validity was attributed to the vocal and facial sections. One possible disadvantage was that that there was questioning about its generalizability as this tool was tested among postoperative patients.[2]

Pediatric Pain Profile

The Pediatric Pain Profile (PPP) has shown to have positive reliability and validity among the pediatric population with cognitive impairment in the hospital and home setting (Table 3.7). This assessment follows a total of 20 categories involving mood, consolability, social, tone, expressions of the face, body, and body movement.[15] They are scored on a 4-point Likert scale with a total available score from 0 to 60. Scoring stems from the frequency of events through a 5-minute observation period.[2]

The PPP is used to assess pain on a reportedly "good" day and "bad day" in terms of pain. The information is utilized in addition to the patient's pain history to help establish a baseline of pain.[2] The disadvantage to the PPP is that the data in the acute setting are limited and likely need to be reassessed.[2] Furthermore, additional studies on its feasibility and difficulty on its use in practice should be conducted.[15] Notably, it may take some time investment to teach caregivers and parents how to utilize this pain assessment tool and conduct this modality with ongoing pain evaluations.[2]

Visual Analog Scale

The VAS can also be utilized in the pediatric population (Fig. 3.1). This scale may be appropriate for children over the age of eight.[2] It has been reported that the VAS shows positive validity and reliability for children older than 6 years of age (pain pdf chapter). Of note, prior studies have shown that children prefer the Faces Pain Scale over the VAS.[2]

TABLE 3.7 **EXAMPLE OF PPP**

In the last ______ Name ______	Not at all	A little	Quite a lot	A great deal	Unable to assess	Score
Was cheerful	3	2	1	0		
Was sociable or responsive	3	2	1	0		
Appeared withdrawn or depressed	0	1	2	3		
Cried/moaned/groaned/screamed or whimpered	0	1	2	3		
Was hard to console or comfort	0	1	2	3		
Self-harmed, eg, bit self or banged head	0	1	2	3		
Was reluctant to eat/difficult to feed	0	1	2	3		
Had disturbed sleep	0	1	2	3		
Grimaced/screwed up face/screwed up eyes	0	1	2	3		
Frowned/had furrowed brow/looked worried	0	1	2	3		
Looked frightened (with eyes wide open)	0	1	2	3		
Ground teeth or made mouthing movements	0	1	2	3		
Was restless/agitated or distressed	0	1	2	3		
Tensed/stiffened or spasmed	0	1	2	3		
Flexed inward or drew legs up toward chest	0	1	2	3		
Tended to touch or rub particular areas	0	1	2	3		
Resisted being moved	0	1	2	3		
Pulled away or flinched when touched	0	1	2	3		
Twisted and turned/tossed head/writhed or arched back	0	1	2	3		
Had involuntary or stereotypical movements/was jumpy/startled or had seizures	0	1	2	3		
Total						

Hunt A, Goldman A, Seers K, et al. Clinical validation of the paediatric pain profile. *Dev Med Child Neurol*. 2004;46(1): 9-18. doi:10.1017/s0012162204000039

Conclusion

There are several methods for pain assessment that have developed over decades and which provide the greatest benefits of clinical practice for each population. No perfect pain evaluation method is available. The clinician must appreciate each approach's relative strengths and weaknesses in clinical practice.

REFERENCES

1. Lazaridou A, Elbaridi N, Edwards RR, Berde CB. Chapter 5—Pain assessment. In: *Essentials of Pain Medicine*. 4th ed. Elsevier; 2018:39-46.e1.
2. Patel VB, DeZure CP. Ch 37: Measurement of Pain. In: Abd-Elsayed A, ed. *Pain: A Review Guide*. 1st ed. Springer; 2019:149.
3. Haefeli M, Elfering A. Pain assessment. *Eur Spine J*. 2006;15(Suppl 1):17-24.
4. Herr KA, Garand L. Assessment and measurement of pain in older adults. *Clin Geriatr Med*. 2001;17(3):457-478.
5. Poquet N, Lin C. The Brief Pain Inventory (BPI). *J Physiother*. 2016;62(1):52.
6. Cleeland C. *Brief Pain Inventory User Guide*. 2017:1-66.
7. Huguet A, Stinson JN, McGrath PJ. Measurement of self-reported pain intensity in children and adolescents. *J Psychosom Res*. 2010;68(4):329-336.
8. The Faces Pain Scale - Revised: What this means for patients [Internet]. TriHealth. 2014 [cited 2020 Mar 11]. https://www.trihealth.com/cancer/the-faces-pain-scale-revised-what-this-means-for-patients
9. IASP - International Association for the Study of Pain. *Faces Pain Scale Revised—Home [Internet]*. [cited 2020 Mar 11]. https://www.iasp-pain.org/Education/Content.aspx?ItemNumber=1519
10. Stevens BJ, Gibbins S, Yamada J, et al. The Premature Infant Pain Profile-Revised (PIPP-R): initial validation and feasibility. *Clin J Pain*. 2014;30(3):238-243.
11. Desai A, Aucott S, Frank K, Silbert-Flagg J. Comparing N-PASS and NIPS: improving pain measurement in the neonate. *Adv Neonatal Care*. 2018;18(4):260-266.
12. Peters JWB, Koot HM, Grunau RE, et al. Neonatal Facial Coding System for assessing postoperative pain in infants: item reduction is valid and feasible. *Clin J Pain*. 2003;19(6):353-363.
13. Hummel P, Puchalski M, Creech SD, Weiss MG. Clinical reliability and validity of the N-PASS: Neonatal Pain, Agitation and Sedation Scale with prolonged pain. *J Perinatol*. 2008;28(1):55-60.
14. Krechel SW, Bildner J. CRIES: a new neonatal postoperative pain measurement score. Initial testing of validity and reliability. *Paediatr Anaesth*. 1995;5(1):53-61.
15. Abu-Saad H. The assessment of pain in children. *Issues Compr Pediatr Nurs*. 1981;5(5-6):327-335.
16. Voepel-Lewis T, Malviya S, Tait AR, et al. A comparison of the clinical utility of pain assessment tools for children with cognitive impairment. *Anesth Analg*. 2008;106(1):72-78.

4

Epidemiology and Critical Factors in Inadequate Acute Pain Control and Effective Strategies for Treatment in Modern Medicine

Alan David Kaye, Chance M. Hebert, Katherine C. Babin, Winston Suh, Taylor Marie Boudreaux, Andrea E. Stoltz, and Elyse M. Cornett

Introduction

Pain is a phenomenon that affects many people. While many pain responses act as warning signs for various disease processes or harmful external stimuli impacting the body, uncontrolled pain can be debilitating and predispose individuals to other issues in the future. Despite ever-increasing knowledge regarding the pathophysiology of pain, current pain management standards often fall woefully short in providing patients with adequate relief.

With over 313 million individuals globally undergoing either inpatient or elective surgery as of 2012, this leaves a large population vulnerable to physical, social, and psychological dysfunction as the effects of untreated pain permeate all facets of life. Associations between inadequate acute pain management and increased morbidity, impaired quality of life, and elevated health care costs have been well documented.[1] The impacts of uncontrolled pain also trickle down to affect family members, friends, and coworkers of patients creating far-reaching consequences.[2] Over 80% of patients endorsed experiencing some degree of postoperative pain, with up to 60% progressing to suffer from chronic pain. Recognizing populations at the highest risk for the development of both severe postoperative pain and chronic pain is imperative to improving outcomes and decreasing the burden on the health care system overall. Such at-risk groups include women, racial minorities, children, and the elderly.[1]

Additionally, pain is a major contributory factor for emergency department (ED) visits in the United States. Emergency level visits for exacerbations of inadequately managed chronic pain also proliferate the rising costs of health care.[3] As of 2008, the combined annual cost of acute and chronic pain in the United States was estimated to be between $560 and $635 billion when considering the loss of productivity and disability in addition to direct health care costs. Major contributory disorders include arthritis, back pain, and headache, often resulting in permanent disability of many patients.[2] Promoting proper primary management of these issues could alleviate both undue patient suffering and stress on the already overburdened health system.

Traditionally, surgical pain was managed exclusively as a postoperative entity, with opioids as the primary treatment protocol. Current focus is shifting to an aggressive multidisciplinary approach involving preoperative antiinflammatories and nerve blocks in combination with opioids to target pathways even before the pain begins. Ultimately, this can allow for decreased perceived pain, improved quality outcomes, and shorter hospitalizations.[4]

Risk Factors of Inadequately Controlled Pain

Postoperative Pain

One study conducted a systemic review on the prevalence, consequences, and possible preventions of pain associated with surgical procedures. Specifically, a survey was conducted nationally in the United States to observe how many people who underwent surgery within the past 5 years, also experienced postoperative pain. Of the 300 adults included in the study, 86% experienced postoperative pain, and 75% of those patients experienced moderate to severe pain. Although the sample size of this specific study may be small, it accurately represents the population because, according to the U.S. Institute of Medicine, ~80% of patients who have surgical procedures will experience some postoperative pain.[1] Since there is such a high prevalence of pain related to inadequately controlled pain in patients, multiple studies have been done to determine if preoperative risk factors existed, which would create a greater chance of experiencing postoperative pain and the development of chronic pain also known as pain chronification. The studies collectively have found that aside from the analgesic/anesthetic involvement and type of procedure, other risk factors included preoperative pain, younger age, female sex, heightened anxiety, and incision size.[1] Related to statewide legislation throughout the country that limits acute pain management with opioids typically to 5-7 days, enhanced recovery after surgery techniques have blossomed. Some of these have included a variety of medications delivered perioperatively such as acetaminophen, gabapentinoid agents, nonsteroidal anti-inflammatory drugs, alpha-2 agonists, ketamine, and others that have been evaluated to reduce postoperative opioid consumption and reduced hospital time for patients as well as ultrasound-guided nerve blocks. In general, patients who have better acute pain management will have a better chance of not developing many of the issues related to chronic pain states. For all of these reasons, excellent manage of acute pain, which did not exist in previous decades, has significantly improved with many physiological benefits, improved patient satisfaction, and the potential for reduced likelihood of the development of chronic pain states and therefore reduced likelihood of opioids. Reduction in long-term use of opioids decreases the potential for addiction, physical dependence, overdose, and death.

Chronic Pain/Cancer

The care of patients with cancer or other diseases that cause chronic pain tends to come with a significant price tag and can overwhelm the patient with the burden of paying for the treatment. Many times, patients diagnosed with cancer will not be able to work, which can result in financial challenges, psychological issues, and stresses in family relationships. Cancer pain management has proven to be inadequate and challenging for many patients and has led to disparities in health care. One study revealed that 7% of the 511 patients reported a negative pain management index at primary and secondary care clinics. This index is calculated by analgesic potency minus the mean pain intensity. The majority of patients reporting a negative pain management index exposed the reality that the current pain management is inadequate.[5] A second study conducted in Amman, Jordan, was cross sectional in design in order to discover any risk factors in patients that correlated with a higher risk of inadequate pain control. From the total 800 patients surveyed, 56.4% of patients reported having a pain score higher than 4 out of 10 upon movement. Administration of preoperative medications and postoperative opioid/anesthetic significantly decreased the risk of the cancer patient experiencing poor pain control. Specifically, if medications are given solely intravenously, the patient will still have a high risk of inadequate pain control. However, if the medications are given orally and intravenously, the patient experiences a decreased risk of poor pain control.[6] Another issue that is still being evaluated clinically is the demonstrated effects of opioids causing dose-related inhibition of natural killer cells, which can theoretically increase propagation of cancer cells allowing for quicker spread of cancer. Therefore, best practice strategies for cancer patients are being studied to determine the best recipes for oncologic surgical procedures and consequent optimal outcomes and longevity from the cancer itself.

Acute Pain

Patients with acute pain often receive poor pain control or no treatment when they visit the ED. A 4-week prospective observational study of 3000 patients was conducted to determine the efficacy of pharmacological intervention on a variety of pain intensities. It was concluded that most patients found relief upon administration of analgesics, such as nonsteroidal anti-inflammatory drugs, opioids, or anesthetics. However, the reason for the constantly high prevalence of inadequate pain control is related to inaccuracy of pain reporting and understated pain intensity by nurses.[7] In this regard, unfortunately patients in ED settings are often questioned whether their acute pain is real and if the reason for coming in for care has more to do with drug dependency issues than real pain states.

Consequences of Inadequately Controlled Pain

Every year, millions of Americans seek treatment in ED for acute pain episodes. It is estimated that pain is the most frequently reported primary symptom, attributing to 45.4% of ED visits, and most patients rate their pain as moderate to severe.[8,9] Acute causes of pain can be generated by various sources, including trauma, illness, or postoperative pain.[10] With the advent of the increased use of surgical interventions, acute pain management is becoming increasingly important. However, it is questionable whether pain is being properly treated.[11] There are many barriers to proper pain management including lack of both physician and medical student training on the topic, lack of patient education, pain medication side effects, and the subjectivity of the pain measurement scale.[12] One study showed that pain prevalence in the ED was 70.7%, and only 32.5% of those patients were given pharmacological therapy to treat the pain.[7] Overall, this lack of pain control in the acute period can have detrimental long-term consequences for the patients.

Consequences of inadequate pain control extend beyond the pain itself.[13] One outcome of poorly controlled pain is reduced quality of life, which manifests in a variety of ways including impaired sleep, increased daytime drowsiness, and impaired physical functioning.[14] Another study showed that patients with pain classified as "severe" in the immediate postoperative period had up to 6 months of decreased mobility than those patients with less significant initial pain.[15] This change in quality of life can also alter the patient's psychological health, interfering with mood and enjoyment of life up to 6 months following the acute pain episode.[16]

Poor pain control can also affect the economy. Patients with poorly controlled pain at the forefront of their admission or immediately postoperatively tend to have increased length of hospital stay, time to discharge, readmission rates, and time before ambulation.[1] Upon readmission, pain is the primary complaint with an average cost of $1869 per visit. The annual cost to society of chronic pain conditions in the United States, of which many can be contributed to poorly controlled acute pain, is estimated at ~$560-635 billion dollars.[2]

There are also other consequences to the patient's health. Cardiac involvement including myocardial infarctions and coronary ischemia is more likely to occur in patients with poorly controlled pain. Hypoventilation, decreased functional vital capacity, and pulmonary infections are also widely known complications of poor pain control. Other effects can include reduced gastrointestinal motility and risk for ileus, increased urinary retention, clotting disorders, impaired immune function, and wound healing, which are important factors to have under control particularly in postoperative patients.[17]

Lastly, an important but poorly understood consequence of poorly controlled acute pain is chronic persistent surgical pain. This is defined as pain lasting longer than 3 months following a surgical procedure and is as high as 50% in those who undergo breast surgery.[18] The risk factors for this involve genetics, level of preoperative pain, type of surgery, and even preoperative anxiety.[19–22] Little is known about the mechanism of action of this chronic pain associated with poorly controlled acute pain, but it is well-accepted that it involves the peripheral and central sensitization of the nervous system from repetitive or prolonged noxious stimuli, like that of untreated acute pain.[17] For these reasons, multimodal analgesia and preemptive analgesia techniques have been popular, and many of the strategies have been codified as reliable components of enhanced recovery after surgery techniques.

Important Clinical Studies and Improvements for Inadequately Controlled Pain

Adequately controlling pain becomes especially difficult when dealing with patient opioid use and drug dependence. Raub et al. performed a case-based narrative review looking at acute pain management in hospitalized patients with opioid dependence, while Quinlan et al. look at acute pain management in patients with drug dependence syndrome.[23,24] Both did agree that treating acute pain in patients on opioids requires a series of steps, including providing adequate analgesia, preventing withdrawal, and conducting proper discharge planning. Both also looked at the management of acute pain in patients on medication-assisted therapies, especially with buprenorphine. However, as a partial opioid agonist, it creates a "ceiling effect" and thus limits the binding and maximal potential of full opioid agonists inadequately controlling pain.[1,2] So, while discontinuation of buprenorphine and starting a full opioid agonist have been previously considered as a favorable option, both stated the benefit of maintenance of buprenorphine with concomitant increased full opioid agonists dosing for adequate control of pain. Recent studies support this management path.[25]

Mura et al. also performed a 4-week prospective observational study in a second-level urban ED to assess the prevalence and intensity of pain (utilizing the numerical rating scale [NRS]) in such an environment along with causes and solutions to oligoanalgesia or undermanagement of pain.[7] The weakness in scales like the PMI (Pain Management Index) and the inability to consistently point toward inadequately controlled pain has been previously studied, but other studies have also shown that other scales like the visual analogical scale (VAS) and NRS can be used and are relatively reliable in the emergency setting.[26,27] In Mura's article, two key causes of inadequate treatment noted were that patients were simply not offered treatment or would leave before seeing a clinician due to poor evaluation of such pain and the perception that such pain was exaggerated.[7] In light of this, suggestions like utilization of the VAS/NRS at the moment of triage with the establishment of analgesia protocols and proper training of health professionals to improve assessment and attitude toward pain management have proven to be successful.[28] In summary, adequate control of pain begins at the preadmission point, requiring the clinician to reconcile medications and properly evaluate the patient and continues to discharge with proper plans for pain management.

Conclusion

Over 100 million Americans are living with chronic pain, and acute pain is the number one presenting symptom for hospital admission.[29] Compounding treatment of any patient with acute pain is history of chronic pain. Acute pain can herald a new diagnosis or worsening of a preexisting chronic pain state or disease process. As such, pain has been labeled as "the fifth vital sign" highlighting the importance of adequate recognition and treatment.[29] However, impending obstacles, including physician minimization of pain, lack of training, lack of holistic treatment approaches, medication dependence, and lack of standard classification, are barriers to treatment. These barriers have led to poor long-term patient outcomes and cost the health care system billions.[2]

This has sparked the development of evidence-based protocols, medication discoveries, research, and clinical practice guidelines. Studies by Raut et al. and Quinlan unanimously agree that treatment of pain, particularly in a patient with opioid addiction or drug dependence syndrome, requires a stepwise approach. They conclude that maintenance buprenorphine with a full opioid agonist (vs the previously accepted idea of discontinuation and initiation of a full opioid agonist) allows for better pain control in this population.[23,24] These studies highlight the importance of adequate pain control, especially since this patient population is often under treated.

Another study aimed to highlight the lack of standard classification using popular pain scales. For example, the PMI scale is constructed from scores categorized as 0 (no pain), 1 (1-4, mild pain), 2 (5-6, moderate pain), or 3 (7-10, severe pain) and then subtracted from the most potent level of prescribed analgesic drug scored as 0 (no analgesia), 1 (nonopioid), 2 (weak opioid), or 3 (strong opioid). A PMI ≥ 0 indicating adequate treatment.[30] Studies have shown that due to the highly subjective nature of the PMI, it has proved little benefit in practice.[26] Other studies, however, have highlighted the VAS and the NRS as reliable tools in measuring acute pain.[27] These studies highlight the importance of evaluating and categorizing pain.

Pain control is a major and complex problem that affects the patients, health care workers, and the health care system as a whole. To achieve optimal pain management, one must first recognize the barriers faced against effective control. Then, studies and research must be dedicated to disrupting these barriers. The findings then must be put into clinical practice. The key to successful pain management is thus ultimately education for doctors, nurses, patients, and executives. With continuing research and clinical studies, we hope to improve patient outcomes, health care costs, and better manage both acute and chronic pain.

REFERENCES

1. Gan TJ. Poorly controlled postoperative pain: prevalence, consequences, and prevention. *J Pain Res.* 2017;10:2287-2298.
2. Institute of Medicine (US) Committee on Advancing Pain Research Care, and Education. Pain as a Public Health Challenge. *Relieving Pain in America: A Blueprint for Transforming Prevention, Care, Education, and Research.* National Academies Press (US); 2011. https://www.ncbi.nlm.nih.gov/books/NBK92516/
3. Keating L, Smith S. Acute pain in the emergency department: the challenges. *Rev Pain.* 2011;5(3):13-17.
4. Johnson Q, Borsheski RR, Reeves-Viets JL. A review of management of acute pain. *Mo Med.* 2013;110(1):74-79.
5. Majedi H, Dehghani SS, Soleyman-Jahi S, et al. Assessment of factors predicting inadequate pain management in chronic pain patients. *Anesthesiol Pain Med.* 2019;9(6):e97229.
6. El-Aqoul A, Obaid A, Yacoub E, Al-Najar M, Ramadan M, Darawad M. Factors associated with inadequate pain control among postoperative patients with cancer. *Pain Manag Nurs.* 2018;19(2):130-138.
7. Mura P, Serra E, Marinangeli F, et al. Prospective study on prevalence, intensity, type, and therapy of acute pain in a second-level urban emergency department. *J Pain Res.* 2017;10:2781-2788.
8. Chang H-Y, Daubresse M, Kruszewski SP, Alexander GC. Prevalence and treatment of pain in EDs in the United States, 2000 to 2010. *Am J Emerg Med.* 2014;32(5):421-431.
9. Johnston CC, Gagnon AJ, Fullerton L, Common C, Ladores M, Forlini S. One-week survey of pain intensity on admission to and discharge from the emergency department: a pilot study. *J Emerg Med.* 1998;16(3):377-382.
10. Apfelbaum JL, Chen C, Mehta SS, Gan TJ. Postoperative pain experience: results from a national survey suggest postoperative pain continues to be undermanaged. *Anesth Analg.* 2003;97(2):534-540.
11. Guru V, Dubinsky I. The patient vs. caregiver perception of acute pain in the emergency department. *J Emerg Med.* 2000;18(1):7-12.
12. Sinatra R. Causes and consequences of inadequate management of acute pain. *Pain Med.* 2010;11(12):1859-1871.

13. Strassels SA, McNicol E, Wagner AK, et al. Persistent postoperative pain, health-related quality of life, and functioning 1 month after hospital discharge. *Acute Pain*. 2004;6:95–104. https://www.sciencedirect.com/science/article/pii/S1366007104000725
14. Pavlin DJ, Chen C, Penaloza DA, Buckley FP. A survey of pain and other symptoms that affect the recovery process after discharge from an ambulatory surgery unit. *J Clin Anesth*. 2004;16:200-206.
15. Morrison SR, Magaziner J, McLaughlin MA, et al. The impact of post-operative pain on outcomes following hip fracture. *Pain*. 2003;103(3):303-311.
16. VanDenKerkhof EG, Hopman WM, Reitsma ML, et al. Chronic pain, healthcare utilization, and quality of life following gastrointestinal surgery. *Can J Anaesth*. 2012;59(7):670-680.
17. Joshi GP, Ogunnaike BO. Consequences of inadequate postoperative pain relief and chronic persistent postoperative pain. *Anesthesiol Clin North Am*. 2005;23:21-36.
18. Kehlet H, Jensen TS, Woolf CJ. Persistent postsurgical pain: risk factors and prevention. *Lancet*. 2006;367(9522):1618-1625.
19. Hanley MA, Jensen MP, Ehde DM, Hoffman AJ, Patterson DR, Robinson LR. Psychosocial predictors of long-term adjustment to lower-limb amputation and phantom limb pain. *Disabil Rehabil*. 2004;26:882-893.
20. Katz J, Poleshuck EL, Andrus CH, et al. Risk factors for acute pain and its persistence following breast cancer surgery. *Pain*. 2005;119:16-25.
21. Tasmuth T, Estlanderb AM, Kalso E. Effect of present pain and mood on the memory of past postoperative pain in women treated surgically for breast cancer. *Pain*. 1996;68:343-347.
22. Diatchenko L, Slade GD, Nackley AG, et al. Genetic basis for individual variations in pain perception and the development of a chronic pain condition. *Hum Mol Genet*. 2005;14:135-143.
23. Raub JN, Vettese TE. Acute pain management in hospitalized adult patients with opioid dependence: a narrative review and guide for clinicians. *J Hosp Med*. 2017;12:375-379. https://www.journalofhospitalmedicine.com/jhospmed/article/136497/hospital-medicine/acute-pain-management-hospitalized-adult-patients-opioid
24. Quinlan J, Cox F. Acute pain management in patients with drug dependence syndrome. *Pain Rep*. 2017;2(4).
25. Macintyre PE, Russell RA, Usher KAN, Gaughwin M, Huxtable CA. Pain relief and opioid requirements in the first 24 hours after surgery in patients taking buprenorphine and methadone opioid substitution therapy. *Anaesth Intensive Care*. 2013;41(2):222-230.
26. Sakakibara N, Higashi T, Yamashita I, Yoshimoto T, Matoba M. Negative pain management index scores do not necessarily indicate inadequate pain management: a cross-sectional study. *BMC Palliat Care*. 2018;17:102.
27. Bijur PE, Latimer CT, Gallagher EJ. Validation of a verbally administered numerical rating scale of acute pain for use in the emergency department. *Acad Emerg Med*. 2003;10:390-392.
28. Stalnikowicz R, Mahamid R, Kaspi S, Brezis M. Undertreatment of acute pain in the emergency department: a challenge. *Int J Qual Health Care*. 2005;17(2):173-176.
29. Tompkins DA, Hobelmann JG, Compton P. Providing chronic pain management in the "Fifth Vital Sign" Era: historical and treatment perspectives on a modern-day medical dilemma. *Drug Alcohol Depend*. 2017;173(Suppl 1):S11-S21.
30. Mejin M, Keowmani T, Rahman SA, et al. Prevalence of pain and treatment outcomes among cancer patients in a Malaysian palliative care unit. *Pharm Pract*. 2019;17(1):1397.

5

Genetic Influences on Pain Perception and Management

Belal Alammar, Beth Ren, Blake Winston, Dev Vyas, Taylor Marie Boudreaux, Neil Kelkar, George Thomas, Elyse M. Cornett, and Alan David Kaye

Introduction

Recent advancements in molecular biology genome sequencing have revolutionized medicine and kindled the prospect of precise, personalized medical care. The complex interplay of pain response variability and pharmacogenomic diversity is a dynamic challenge to treating pain. Now with the completion of the Human Genome Mapping project in 2003 and the ongoing expansion of the Human Pain Genetics Database (HPGDB), the field's understanding of inter-individual pain response variability has expanded rapidly.

The HPGDB is a global inventory of genetic influences on pain perception and tolerance.[1] As of 2018, the HPGDB has incorporated 294 peer-reviewed studies reporting a total of 434 genetic variants associated with the pain experience.[1] This chapter will focus on genetic variants that have been widely recognized for their strong association to pain modulation (such as opioid receptor mu 1, catechol-O-methyltransferase [COMT], adenosine triphosphate binding cassette transporter B1 [ABCB1], and CYP2D6) and how an understanding of these genetic variants could be used to guide patient care.[2]

Pain is a complex and multivariable experience. A patient's pain phenotype is affected by both inherent genetic predisposition and intertwined environmental factors, including socioeconomic status, mental health, and medical comorbidities.[3] Pain phenotype heritability is estimated to be between 25% and 50%.[4] Rarely, pain conditions like hereditary sensory and autonomic neuropathy types I-V may adhere to classic mendelian inheritance (see Table 5.1).[5] However, for most genetic variants associated with pain, inheritance is considered non-mendelian.[5]

The International Association for the Study of Pain defines pain as "an aversive sensory and emotional experience typically caused by or resembling that caused by an actual or potential tissue injury."[6] Acute nociceptive pain is typically triggered from direct tissue injury and serves a physiological protective function to warn of potential harm.[7] As the damaged tissues heal, acute pain is expected to resolve; however, for a segment of the population, the pain persists and develops into a chronic pathological condition.[8]

In contrast to the physiologic protective function of acute pain, chronic pain is more of a pathological detrimental process. According to the Institute of Internal Medicine in 2011, chronic pain is a true public health epidemic, impacting 116 million Americans at an annual health care cost of $600 billion.[9] The pathophysiology of chronic pain involves a complex neuroplastic mechanism that takes place before and after injury.[10] Recent studies have focused on the intricate interplay of several factors implicated in the development of chronic pain: genetic predisposition, nerve growth factor modulation, microglial activation, and 5′ adenosine monophosphate–activated protein kinase regulation.[10] Therapy targeting these chronic pain mechanisms may prevent or alter this neuroplastic process.[10]

TABLE 5.1 HEREDITARY SENSORY AND AUTONOMIC NEUROPATHY TYPES I–V ADHERE TO MENDELIAN INHERITANCE

Hereditary Sensory and Autonomic Neuropathy	Genetic Variant	Inheritance
Type I	*SPTLC1*	Autosomal dominant
Type II	*HSN2*	Autosomal recessive
Type III	*IKBKAP*	Autosomal recessive
Type IV	*NTRK1*	Autosomal recessive
Type V	*trkA*	Autosomal recessive

From James S. Human pain and genetics: some basics. *Br J Pain*. 2013;7:171-178. https://doi.org/10.1177/2049463713506408

Pain Conditions Influenced by Genetic Factors

A current field of interest is genetic polymorphisms and how these variants can affect receptors, transporters, and enzymes that can cause alterations in pain sensitivity in chronic pain conditions. Nociception can be modulated at different anatomical sites at the cellular level, and differences in genomic variation that have an impact at these sites have been linked to differences in pain perception for several known conditions.[11-13] Four conditions observed for differences in pain sensitivity are catecholamine-induced musculoskeletal pain, low back pain (LBP), fibromyalgia, and chronic fatigue syndrome (CFS).[14]

Elevation of catecholamine hormones (eg, dopamine, epinephrine, norepinephrine) are associated with chronic musculoskeletal pain conditions. Notable differences in pain perception are linked with the COMT gene, which codes for COMT, the enzyme which is responsible for both peripheral and central catecholamine breakdown.[14-16] Patients with inhibited or downregulated COMT have been noted to have increased activation of both beta-2 and beta-3 adrenergic receptors, leading to increased expression of IL-6, which is proinflammatory.[16] These specific receptors cause reduced activity of catecholamines in other processes and lead to hyperalgesia and allodynia.[14]

Lower back pain is the number one cause of disability in the industrialized world.[14] Related to LBP's complex nature, it is implicated in psychological, mechanical, and pathological conditions.[14] One gene implicated in the pain response due to LBP is the IL-1 gene. Gene polymorphisms of IL-1 show differences in pain intensity and duration when controlled for age.[14,17-19] One specific cause of LBP that is of interest for studying genetic influences is intervertebral herniation (LDH). Several single-nucleotide polymorphisms in genes involved with pain transmission have been linked with disc herniation.[18,20,21] Studies show that specific polymorphisms might also play a role in the prognosis and resolution of symptoms.[12,18] Other biomarkers and gene variants that have been implicated with LBP and LDH are IL-6 and IL-1Ra (an inhibitor of IL-1).[14,19]

Patients who have fibromyalgia report aches and pain, irritability, and poor concentration. The underlying etiology is likely to be an abnormality in the central nervous system processing system.[5,22] Patients with fibromyalgia often report significant differences in their intensity of pain, familial history, and related conditions, suggesting an underlying genetic component.[23] Studies show that specific polymorphisms of COMT, dopamine-4, serotonin 5-HT, and a serotonin transporter have all been linked more frequently with patients who report fibromyalgia.[23]

Chronic fatigue syndrome is characterized as a debilitating pain disorder presenting with at least 6 months of severe fatigue, autonomic dysfunction, postexertional malaise, muscle/joint pain, cognitive difficulties, and sleep difficulty.[14,24] Patients with CFS may present with or without fibromyalgia.[14] It is accepted that CFS has a genetic predisposition due to the high rates of familial predisposition.[25,26] Two genes that could be involved in affecting the severity of this condition are TH2 and HTT. These two genes are responsible for tryptophan breakdown and serotonin synthesis and removing serotonin metabolites from cells, respectively.[27] Longer allelic variants of HTT were found in those with CFS than those without CFS, which affects the transcription efficiency of 5-HTT.[14]

Genetics and Opioid Therapy

The most common prescribed treatment for acute and chronic pain is opioid-based therapies. Misuse of opioids is prevalent in 21%-29% of patients prescribed opioids, with 9% of patients developing a substance use disorder. One hundred and twenty-eight patients a day die from opioid-related overdose in the United States. A large variance in the relief patients experience from opioids may play a role in the drug's overuse and subsequent overdose. Genetic differences account for 30%-76% of opioid response variance.[28]

Cytochrome P450 enzymes metabolize opioids, and variation in these enzymes are perhaps most studied in relation to opioid metabolism. CYP2D6 is the primary cytochrome P450 (CYP) enzyme that either activates opioids from prodrugs or breaks down the resulting substrates for elimination. Opioids that are prodrugs activated by CYP2D6 include codeine, oxycodone, hydrocodone, and tramadol. Opioids that are metabolized for excretion by CYP2D6 include pethidine, morphine, and methadone. CYP2D6 phenotypes include poor, intermediate, normal, and ultrarapid metabolizers. Poor and ultrarapid metabolizers of prodrugs lead to decreased efficacy and ultrarapid metabolizers lead to increased adverse effects. Poor metabolizers of drugs into its substrates for elimination lead to increased adverse effects, while ultrarapid metabolizers lead to decreased efficacy. CYP2D6 allele screening in patients and adjustment of the prescribed dosage can improve pain management. CYP3A4 and CYP3A5 enzymes similarly affect metabolism of certain opioids such as fentanyl, although studies show varying impact on efficacy that does not necessarily promote screening for alleles.[29]

Various other genes have been shown to affect the analgesic response to opioids. Opioid receptor mu 1 and opioid receptor delta 1 (OPRD1) are opioid receptors in human tissue. The A118G allele in ORM1 and T921C allele in OPRD1 reduces analgesic response to oxycodone by decreasing receptor expression. ABCB1, also known as multidrug resistance protein 1 (MDR1), functions as efflux receptors at the blood-brain barrier for clearance of opioids, most studied for morphine and oxycodone. The C3453T allele in ABCB1 leads to decreased efflux and increased adverse effects of opioids. COMT is an enzyme that metabolizes intracellular catecholamine neurotransmitters, such as dopamine, a neurotransmitter central to opioid addiction. The A158G allele in COMT decreases COMT activity and extracellular dopamine levels, leading to decreased opioid addiction.[30]

In the future, novel gene therapies and tools may offer alternatives to opioid therapies in pain treatment. RNA and DNA interference therapies can silence certain genes of pain. For example, silencing of voltage-gated sodium channel 1.7 (SCN9A) decreases pain in rodents with burns or bone cancer, although at the cost of inducing undesired immune responses. Antisense oligonucleotides can target SCN9A mRNA processing, although uptake by cells of these therapeutics are inconsistent. Clustered Regularly Interspaced Short Palindromic Repeats–Cas9 (CRISPR-Cas9) with a "dead" Cas9 can temporarily repress pain perception genes, although the vector of delivery and compressed packaging of the vector continue to be studied. Manufacturing costs and tedious drug approval processes continue to hinder rapid development of these promising gene therapies for pain management, but they may be the future of pain management.

Genetics and Nonopioid Therapy

Nonsteroidal Anti-inflammatory Drugs

Nonsteroidal anti-inflammatory drugs (NSAIDs) are the most used analgesics because of their lack of addictive sequelae. They can cause significant gastrointestinal bleeding as well as renal and cardiovascular negative effects. NSAIDs function by inhibiting prostaglandin synthesis via the cyclooxygenases 1 and 2 enzymes. NSAIDs are particularly associated with CYP2C9 polymorphisms, which modulate the clearance of these medications. CYP2C9 has been extensively studied, and 61 variant alleles have been discovered. They can be present across nearly all populations. The polymorphism with normal function is CYP2C9*1.[30] Those with decreased function are CYP2C9*2, (*5, *8, *11). Finally, the alleles that present with no function are CYP2C9*3 (*6, *13). Two alleles are inherited, and the enzyme function can vary depending on the combination present. Furthermore, the enzyme behaves in a substrate-dependent manner and must be studied with a variety of doses to fully understand. NSAIDs are mainly metabolized by the kidneys but are first hepatically transformed via cytochrome p450 into the isoforms CYP2C9, 1A2, and 3A4. The algorithm for the Clinical Pharmacogenetics Implementation Consortium indicates choosing NSAIDs not metabolized by CYP29 enzyme (eg, aspirin, ketorolac, naproxen, sulindac) or lowering the dose to avoid kidney damage in those with subpar enzyme function.[30]

Celecoxib, flurbiprofen, ibuprofen, and lornoxicam exhibit shorter half-lives in CYP2C9 normal regulators (NRs). Additionally, a meta-analysis of five studies showed that CYP2C9*1/*2 had no effect on celecoxib exposure. Current evidence suggests that normal and intermediate regulators with approved starting dose. Intermediate regulators with an activity score of at least 1.5 can metabolize comparable to normal regulators. Those with activity scores of 1 or less and nonregulators have significantly lower enzyme function and thus have prolonged half-lives and higher plasma concentrations of NSAIDs leading to greater risk of toxicity. Studies have shown an increase in celecoxib concentration by 60% and that of ibuprofen by 40%. Little is known about other medications, but it is recommended that intermediate regulators with an activity scale of less than one are recommended to start with a less than suggested dose and titrating up as clinically necessary. Such patients should be monitored for kidney and cardiac dysfunction. Poor regulators have been documented to have nearly a 400% increase in celecoxib concentration. For these patients, the FDA suggests initiating 25%-50% of the suggested dose. Furthermore, titration should not be started until a steady state has been achieved.[30]

Meloxicam has a longer half-life than both ibuprofen and celecoxib and as a result impaired CYP2C9 function causes much larger concentrations of meloxicam. Normal and intermediate regulators, those with an activity function of 1.5, are recommended to start with the lowest effective standard dose. Intermediate regulators with lower activity have an 80% increase of drug concentration. These individuals should begin therapy at half of the lowest suggested dose or consider alternatives. Poor regulators have a half-life of >100 hours and should start a clinically effective alternative.[31]

Piroxicam and tenoxicam have extremely long half-lives and any patient with lower than normal regulation ability, including intermediate regulators, should begin alternative therapy. Aceclofenac, aspirin, diclofenac, indomethacin, lumiracoxib, metamizole, nabumetone, and naproxen are not largely affected by CYP2C9 enzymes. Thus, the algorithm for the Clinical Pharmacogenetics Implementation Consortium indicates considering such medications for those who need alternative therapies.[31]

Ketamine

Ketamine is an *N*-methyl-D-aspartate receptor antagonist and does provide a portion of its analgesic effect through the μ and δ opioid receptors. In its pharmaceutically available state, ketamine is found in its R(–)- and S(+)-enantiomer forms, with the S(+)-enantiomer being more pharmacologically active. Both isomers of ketamine are hepatically transformed by the cytochrome P450, specifically using isoenzymes CYP2B6, CYP2C9, and CYP3A4.

Genetic variations of the CYP2B6, CYP2C9, and CYP3A4 have been implicated in variation of ketamine metabolism. CYP2B6*6 is a known mutation of the CYP2B6-encoded gene, which can diminish the metabolism of certain drugs. The CYP2B6*6 variant can result in a significantly lowered rate of steady-state metabolism, resulting in higher plasma concentrations.[32] It has also been associated with significantly increased drowsiness; however, increased rates of ketamine-induced psychedelic effects during emergence have not been found with this mutation.[33]

Lidocaine

Lidocaine belongs to a class of local anesthetics called aminoamides, and it can be used in a variety of applications, from topical anesthesia to peripheral nerve blocks, to epidural anesthesia. Aminoamides have a variety of molecular targets in the body but act predominately by reversibly blocking nerve conduction by way of blockade of sodium ion influx at voltage-gated sodium channels. Sodium channels themselves are made up of both alpha and beta subunits, and different subtypes of sodium channels are expressed in different tissues within the body. In theory, genetic variations that could have an impact on the efficacy of lidocaine could impact either the drug's duration of action, by way of a variation in protein binding at the sodium channel, or by way of its metabolism. Amides are metabolized by enzymatic biotransformation in the liver, primarily by the CYP1A2 enzyme, which is encoded by cytochrome P450 1A2 or CYP1A2 genes, and variations within these CYP1A2 genes could have significant implications in the pharmacokinetics of lidocaine. The implications for genetic variations having an impact on the efficacy of lidocaine are even more wide-ranging, however, with a 2005 study performed by Liem et al. that investigated an association between variations in the melanocortin-1-receptor (MC1R) and resistance to analgesia provided by subcutaneous lidocaine, with the results of their study demonstrating that subjects with red hair (MCR1 mutations) were both more sensitive to thermal pain and more resistant to the effects of subcutaneous lidocaine.[34]

Conclusion

The most common prescribed treatment for acute and chronic pain is opioid-based therapies. A large variance in the relief patients experience from opioids may play a role in the drug's overuse and subsequent overdose. Genetic differences account for 30%-76% of opioid response variance. Cytochrome P450 enzymes metabolize opioids and variation in these enzymes are perhaps most studied in relation to opioid metabolism. CYP3A4 and CYP3A5 enzymes similarly affect metabolism of certain opioids such as fentanyl, although studies show varying impact on efficacy that does not necessarily promote screening for alleles. Various other genes can affect the analgesic response to opioids. COMT is an enzyme that metabolizes intracellular catecholamine neurotransmitters, such as dopamine, a neurotransmitter central to opioid addiction. The A158G allele in COMT decreases COMT activity and extracellular dopamine levels, leading to decreased opioid addiction. In the future, novel gene therapies and tools may offer alternatives to opioid therapies in pain treatment. RNA and DNA interference therapies can silence certain genes of pain. Manufacturing costs and tedious drug approval processes continue to hinder rapid development of these promising gene therapies for pain management, but they may be the future of pain management. NSAIDs are one of the most used analgesics because of their lack of addictive sequelae. Celecoxib, flurbiprofen, ibuprofen, and lornoxicam exhibit shorter half-lives in CYP2C9 normal regulators (NRs). Meloxicam has a longer half-life than both ibuprofen and celecoxib and as a result impaired CYP2C9 function causes much larger concentrations of meloxicam. Piroxicam and tenoxicam have extremely long half-lives, and any patient with lower than normal regulation ability, including intermediate regulators, should begin alternative therapy. Ketamine is an *N*-methyl-D-aspartate receptor antagonist and does provide a portion of its analgesic effect through the μ and δ opioid receptors. Genetic variations of the CYP2B6, CYP2C9, and CYP3A4 have been implicated in the variation of ketamine metabolism. Lidocaine belongs to a class of local anesthetics called aminoamides, and it can be used in a variety of applications, from topical anesthesia to peripheral nerve blocks, to epidural anesthesia. In summary, pain is a multifaceted and complex sensation. A patient's pain phenotype is impacted by both hereditary predisposition and complicated environmental factors such as socioeconomic status, mental health, and medical comorbidities. Recent research suggests the intricate interplay of many processes involved in the development of chronic pain, including genetic predisposition, nerve growth factor regulation, microglial activation, and adenosine monophosphate–activated protein kinase regulation. Therapy targeting these chronic pain pathways may be able to halt or change this neuroplastic process.

REFERENCES

1. Meloto CB, Benavides R, Lichtenwalter RN, et al. Human pain genetics database: a resource dedicated to human pain genetics research. *Pain*. 2018;159(4):749-763. doi:10.1097/j.pain.0000000000001135
2. Fernandez Robles CR, Degnan M, Candiotti KA. Pain and genetics. *Curr Opin Anaesthesiol*. 2012;25(4): 444-449. doi:10.1097/ACO.0b013e3283556228.
3. Mogil JS. Pain genetics: past, present and future. *Trends Genet*. 2012;28:258-266.
4. Nielsen CS, Knudsen GP, Steingrimsdottir OA. Twin studies of pain. *Clin Genet*. 2012;82:331-340.
5. James S. Human pain and genetics: some basics. *Br J Pain*. 2013;7:171-178.
6. The International Association for the Study of Pain Definition of Pain Task Force. IASP. *Proposed New Definition of Pain*. 2019.
7. Crofford LJ. Chronic pain: where the body meets the brain. *Trans Am Clin Climatol Assoc*. 2015;126:167-183.
8. Mifflin KA, Kerr BJ. The transition from acute to chronic pain: understanding how different biological systems interact. *Can J Anesth*. 2014;61:112-122.
9. Institute of Medicine. Relieving pain in America: a blueprint for transforming prevention. *Care Educ Res*. 2011;181:397-399. https://doi.org/10.7205/MILMED-D-16-00012
10. Cohen I, Lema MJ. What's new in chronic pain pathophysiology. *Can J Pain*. 2020;4(4):13-18. doi:10.1080/24740527.2020.1752641
11. Meng W, Adams MJ, Reel P, et al. Genetic correlations between pain phenotypes and depression and neuroticism. *Eur J Hum Genet*. 2020;28(3):358-366. https://doi.org/10.1038/s41431-019-0530-2
12. Vehof J, Zavos HMS, Lachance G, Hammond CJ, Williams FMK. Shared genetic factors underlie chronic pain syndromes. *Pain*. 2014;155(8):1562-1568. https://doi.org/10.1016/j.pain.2014.05.002
13. Tsepilov YA, Freidin MB, Shadrina AS, et al. Analysis of genetically independent phenotypes identifies shared genetic factors associated with chronic musculoskeletal pain conditions. *Commun Biol*. 2020;3(1):329. https://doi.org/10.1038/s42003-020-1051-9
14. Fincke A. *Genetic Influences on Pain Perception and Treatment*. n.d. Retrieved April 29, 2021, from https://www.practicalpainmanagement.com/resources/genetic-influences-pain-perception-treatment
15. Diatchenko L, Slade GD, Nackley AG, et al. Genetic basis for individual variations in pain perception and the development of a chronic pain condition. *Hum Mol Genet*. 2005;14(1):135-143. https://doi.org/10.1093/hmg/ddi013
16. Nackley-Neely AG, Tan KS, Fecho K, et al. Catechol-O-methyltransferase inhibition increases pain sensitivity through activation of both β2 and β3 adrenergic receptors. *Pain*. 2007;128(3):199-208. https://doi.org/10.1016/j.pain.2006.09.022
17. Solovieva S, Leino-Arjas P, Saarela J, Luoma K, Raininko R, Riihimäki H. Possible association of interleukin 1 gene locus polymorphisms with low back pain. *Pain*. 2004;109(1):8-19. https://doi.org/10.1016/j.pain.2003.10.020

18. Tegeder I, Lötsch J. Current evidence for a modulation of low back pain by human genetic variants. *J Cell Mol Med.* 2009;13(8b):1605-1619. https://doi.org/10.1111/j.1582-4934.2009.00703.x
19. Bjorland S, Moen A, Schistad E, Gjerstad J, Røe C. Genes associated with persistent lumbar radicular pain: a systematic review. *BMC Musculoskelet Disord* 2016;17:500. https://doi.org/10.1186/s12891-016-1356-5
20. Margarit C, Roca R, Inda MDM, et al. Genetic contribution in low back pain: a prospective genetic association study. *Pain Pract.* 2019;19(8):836-847. https://doi.org/10.1111/papr.12816
21. Kurzawski M, Rut M, Dziedziejko V, et al. Common missense variant of SCN9A gene is associated with pain intensity in patients with chronic pain from disc herniation. *Pain Med Malden Mass.* 2018;19(5):1010-1014.
22. Chang PF, Arendt-Nielsen L, Graven-Nielsen T, Chen ACN. Psychophysical and EEG responses to repeated experimental muscle pain in humans: pain intensity encodes EEG activity. *Brain Res Bull.* 2003;59(6):533-543. https://doi.org/10.1016/s0361-9230(02)00950-4
23. Buskila D. Genetics of chronic pain states. *Best Pract Res Clin Rheumatol.* 2007;21(3):535-547. https://doi.org/10.1016/j.berh.2007.02.011
24. Sapra A, Bhandari P. Chronic fatigue syndrome. In: *StatPearls*. StatPearls Publishing; 2021. http://www.ncbi.nlm.nih.gov/books/NBK557676/
25. Hickie I, Bennett B, Lloyd A, Heath A, Martin N. Complex genetic and environmental relationships between psychological distress, fatigue and immune functioning: a twin study. *Psychol Med.* 1999;29(2):269-277. https://doi.org/10.1017/s0033291798007922
26. Hickie I, Kirk K, Martin N. Unique genetic and environmental determinants of prolonged fatigue: a twin study. *Psychol Med.* 1999;29(2):259-268. https://doi.org/10.1017/s0033291798007934
27. Narita M, Nishigami N, Narita N, et al. Association between serotonin transporter gene polymorphism and chronic fatigue syndrome. *Biochem Biophys Res Commun.* 2003;311(2):264-266. https://doi.org/10.1016/j.bbrc.2003.09.207
28. Vega-Loza A, Van C, Moreno AM, Aleman F. Gene therapies to reduce chronic pain: are we there yet? *Pain Manage.* 2020;10(4):209-212. https://doi.org/10.2217/pmt-2020-0021
29. Bugada D, Lorini LF, Fumagalli R, Allegri M. Genetics and opioids: towards more appropriate prescription in cancer pain. *Cancers.* 2020;12(7). https://doi.org/10.3390/cancers12071951
30. Singh A, Zai C, Mohiuddin AG, Kennedy JL. The pharmacogenetics of opioid treatment for pain management. *J Psychopharmacol.* 2020;34(11):1200-1209. https://doi.org/10.1177/0269881120944162
31. Theken KN, Lee CR, Gong L, et al. Clinical pharmacogenetics implementation consortium guideline (CPIC) for CYP2C9 and nonsteroidal anti-inflammatory drugs. *Clin Pharmacol Ther.* 2020;108(2):191-200. https://doi.org/10.1002/cpt.1830
32. Wang PF, Neiner A, Kharasch ED. Stereoselective ketamine metabolism by genetic variants of cytochrome P450 CYP2B6 and cytochrome P450 oxidoreductase. *Anesthesiology.* 2018;129(4):756-768. https://doi.org/10.1097/ALN.0000000000002371
33. Dinis-Oliveira RJ. Metabolism and metabolomics of ketamine: a toxicological approach. *Forensic Sci Res.* 2017;2(1):2-10. https://doi.org/10.1080/20961790.2017.1285219
34. Liem EB, Joiner TV, Tsueda K, Sessler DI. Increased sensitivity to thermal pain and reduced subcutaneous lidocaine efficacy in redheads. *Anesthesiology.* 2005;102(3):509-514.

6

Designing a Comprehensive Acute Pain Treatment Plan

Marian Sherman and Stephanie G. Vanterpool

Introduction

A comprehensive pain treatment plan for optimal pain management must address all causes of pain and functional limitation in a patient. In order to do so, the clinician should have a clear process for both identifying and addressing the underlying pain causes. As each patient is unique, the same treatment plan, dosing or approach, will likely not work similarly for all patients. While most clinicians today acknowledge that poorly controlled pain is a common and unresolved health outcome,[1,2] many physicians report inadequate knowledge of clinical pain management. Specifically, clinicians report that medical schools lack dedicated course structure to understanding and treating pain and that curricula underemphasize assessment of pain knowledge and related clinical competence.[3] It is imperative that future medical training expand and elevate the quality of pain management education to address the negative public health impact of poorly controlled pain. At this moment, to bridge this gap, we present a process by which clinicians can both identify the applicable causes of pain and functional limitation in their patients and develop a collaborative and comprehensive plan to address those causes.

First, we must delve into why accurately identifying all underlying causes of pain is critical to optimal pain treatment. A patient presenting with acute pain may have multiple causes at play. There may be physiologic causes, such as the sterile inflammation seen in a gout flare, or anatomic causes, such as the fractured bone in the case of musculoskeletal injury. Functional causes related to poor posture, body mechanics, or prolonged immobility may also contribute. Finally, we must also be cognizant of any psychosocial causes of pain that may contribute to pain perception, catastrophizing, and response to treatment.

If a patient with multiple pain etiologies presents for acute pain treatment, and all causes are not appropriately identified and addressed, that patient risks developing both prolonged suffering and mid to longer term disability. The development of a comprehensive treatment plan must therefore start with an understanding and accurate diagnosis of the underlying causes of pain. It is therefore our responsibility as clinicians to ensure that all causes of pain are accurately diagnosed and treated in a targeted fashion.

Pain States and Mechanisms

In their landmark article "Toward a Mechanism-Based Approach to Pain Diagnosis," Vardeh and colleagues highlight that understanding the underlying pathological processes associated with pain is key to improving patient management.[4] The more specific the identification of applicable pain states and mechanisms in a given patient, the more targeted the treatment plan that can be developed. A treatment plan that addresses only one pain state when more than one is present, or only targets one pain mechanism, or worse yet, is completely un-targeted in its approach, will likely result in suboptimal relief, and potentially produce additional, unintended consequences. Indeed, we have seen the result of this in the present opioid epidemic, as un-targeted opioid medications have been used to attempt to treat pain indiscriminately, irrespective of the underlying pain states and mechanisms, and often with unintended side effects and suboptimal overall relief.

Following is a brief discussion of pain states and mechanisms, which will be used to inform the treatment recommendations presented later in this chapter.

Pain States

The International Association for the Study of Pain recently updated the definition of pain as follows: "An unpleasant sensory and emotional experience associated with, or resembling that associated with, actual or potential tissue damage."[5] Different pain states are defined as result of the duration, etiology, or perception of the painful experience.[6] In this chapter, we will focus the discussion of pain states on the underlying etiology, understanding that these etiologies can be present in both acute and chronic pain presentations.

There are four broadly accepted general pain states: nociceptive pain, inflammatory pain, (sterile or infections), neuropathic pain, and central/dysfunctional pain.[4] The underlying clinical evidence, signs, and symptoms that allow identification of these pain states are highlighted in Table 6.1. While these criteria are not highly specific, as there is no gold standard for diagnosing these pain states, the signs and symptoms highlighted will often help the clinician discern the key characteristics on which to base further diagnostic efforts.

More often than not, more than one pain state can be present at the same time. For example, a patient with poorly controlled diabetes who presents with an acute lumbar disk herniation may be experiencing both nociceptive pain from the herniation and also chronic neuropathic pain from peripheral diabetic neuropathy. It is therefore important that one seeks to clarify all applicable pain states in a given patient.

Pain Mechanisms

Once the pain state is identified, the next step in determining appropriate targeted treatment is to identify the mechanism by which the pain is being transmitted and perceived. Understanding the pain mechanism is critical in guiding the selection of pharmacologic treatment options. By tailoring the selected pharmacologic treatment to the mechanism by which the pain is transmitted, clinicians can provide patients with more targeted and effective relief, while concurrently avoiding or minimizing nonspecific treatment options such as opioids.

The five pain mechanisms are as follows: nociceptive transduction, peripheral sensitization, ectopic activity, central sensitization, and central disinhibition.[4] Table 6.2 highlights the clinical

TABLE 6.1 PAIN STATES

Pain State	Pathology	Symptoms
Nociceptive	Evidence of noxious (mechanical, thermal, chemical) insult	Pain localized to area of stimulus/joint damage
Inflammatory	Evidence of inflammation (sterile or infectious)	Redness, warmth, swelling of affected area
Neuropathic	Evidence of sensory nerve damage	Burning, tingling or shocklike, spontaneous pain; paresthesias, dysesthesias
Dysfunctional/ centralized	Pain in the absence of detectable pathology	No identifiable noxious stimulus, inflammation or neural damage; evidence of increased amplification or reduced inhibition

Modified from Table 1 in Vardeh D, Mannion R, Woolf C. Toward a mechanism-based approach to pain diagnosis. *J Pain*. 2016;17(9):T50-T69. doi:10.1016/j.jpain.2016.03.001. Review (used with written permission).

TABLE 6.2 **GENERAL PAIN MECHANISMS AND SPECIFIC TREATMENT EXAMPLES**

Pain Mechanism	Clinical Diagnostic Criteria	Clinical Example	Specific Treatment Example
Nociceptive transduction	Proportionate pain in response to identifiable noxious stimulus	Mechanical nerve root compression	Remove mechanical stimulus
Peripheral sensitization	Primary hyperalgesia due to decreased transduction threshold of nociceptor terminal	Rheumatoid arthritis, cellulitis	Anti-inflammatory (eg, NSAID, COXIBs); immunosuppressant
Ectopic activity	Spontaneous pain in the absence of obvious trigger, relieved by local nerve block	Trigeminal neuralgia	Na channel blockers, Ca channel blockers
Central sensitization	Secondary hyperalgesia; temporal summation, allodynia	Complex regional pain syndrome (CRPS)	NMDA antagonists (eg, ketamine)
Central disinhibition	Secondary hyperalgesia, allodynia	Fibromyalgia	GABA-A subunit agonists Dual amine uptake inhibitors (eg, SNRI)

Adapted from Table 2 in Vardeh D, Mannion R, Woolf C. Toward a mechanism-based approach to pain diagnosis. *J Pain*. 2016;17(9):T50-T69. doi:10.1016/j.jpain.2016.03.001. Review (used with written permission).

diagnostic criteria and specific examples for each pain mechanism. As with pain states, the diagnostic criteria for pain mechanisms are not highly specific but are more of a guide to help the clinician discern what mechanisms are present. It is important to note that just like there can be multiple pain states present simultaneously, the same can be said for pain mechanisms.

Synthesizing the Comprehensive Pain Plan

In many acute pain settings, the primary cause of pain may be obvious—postsurgical pain, posttraumatic pain, etc. However, in those situations where the pain presentation is more complex or multifactorial, having a method to synthesize all the applicable information can be extremely valuable. One may consider a templated assessment that includes identification of underlying pain states, mechanisms, causes, and respective targeted treatments for each cause, to ensure that the plan is both comprehensive and effective. An example of one such assessment template is listed in Table 6.3.

Patient Education and Expectation Setting

A strong association has been shown between patient expectations for recovery and clinical outcomes. In particular, positive patient expectations are related to reduced pain after medical treatment.[7] As such, clinicians must educate patients about pain treatment plans and must set clear, positive expectations in order to optimize recovery and improve patient outcomes. Building a therapeutic relationship with the patient includes education of the causes of pain, brief explanation of medication management and/or procedural intervention, and importantly, a discussion of realistic expectations for pain relief and functional recovery. In order to set realistic patient expectations, the physician should lead a clear conversation about anticipated degree of pain relief and offer a qualitative description of the timeline and trajectory of pain relief.

A growing body of literature suggests that patients' pretreatment expectations predict a myriad of health outcomes across multiple medical disciplines.[8,9] Such correlation is similarly observed in pain management outcomes, where it is recognized that pretreatment patient expectations are predictors of analgesic treatment outcomes. Simple-to-apply cognitive interventions have been demonstrated to enhance the effectiveness of pain treatment. Specifically, verbal suggestion, conditioning, and mental imagery have been shown to induce patient

TABLE 6.3 COMPONENTS OF A COMPREHENSIVE PAIN ASSESSMENT TEMPLATE

Patient ID:	Patient descriptor (name, age, relevant clinical background).
Pain complaint:	Location and chronicity.
Pain state(s) present:	(Select all that apply): nociceptive, inflammatory, neuropathic, central/ dysfunctional.
Pain mechanism(s) present:	(Select all that apply): nociceptive transduction, peripheral sensitization, ectopic activity, central sensitization, central disinhibition.
Cause(s) of pain:	(Select all that apply): physiologic, anatomic, functional, psychosocial (specify and elaborate as needed)—eg, anatomic, postsurgical pain after total hip arthroplasty, or physiologic and anatomic pain due to disk herniation with radicular symptoms and ectopic activity of the nerve.
Rationale for treatment plan:	Address each cause, state, and mechanism with the comprehensive, multimodal treatment plan (M.I.P.S): • Medications (target the physiologic cause) • Interventions (target the anatomic cause) • Physical therapy (target the functional limitation) • Psychosocial treatment (target the psychosocial comorbidity)

expectations.[10] Through the use of verbal suggestion and verbal conditioning, clinicians can induce patient expectations of pain relief and, therefore, potentially optimize the effectiveness of pain treatment plan (Table 6.4 summarizes the authors' expectation interventions).

Chronic pain patients enrolled in multidisciplinary treatment programs also demonstrate that patient pretreatment expectations are strongly linked to treatment outcomes. In particular, patients who possess high positive expectations for successful pain relief and improvement in quality of life experience superior response to analgesic treatment.[11] The converse is also true, such that patients who expect to have pain often do have pain.[12] In order to optimize response to pain treatment, the clinician should discuss several points when collaborating with patients to set realistic expectations (summarized in Table 6.5).

Medications—Targeting the Physiologic Cause

As noted earlier in the chapter, pain management is multifaceted. A successful approach incorporates pharmacology, procedural intervention in select patients, detailed steps for physical recovery, and exploration of patient psychosocial resources. Beginning with pharmacology, choosing appropriate and effective pain medications depends upon understanding the physiology of pain. Acute pain is experienced by patients who undergo surgery, sustain traumatic injury, or become acutely ill. On a molecular level, the sensory experience of pain arises from activation of nociceptors (specialized receptors located at the site of injured tissue) that convert thermal, mechanical, and chemical stimuli into electrical signals. Following nociceptive

TABLE 6.4 EXPECTATION INTERVENTIONS

Brief expectation interventions can alleviate acute procedural pain
Accurate information about pain relief expectations.
Emphasize the positive *intended* outcomes of an analgesic intervention.
Emphasize the positive *expected* outcomes of an analgesic intervention.
Include discussion of possible negative side effects.

From Peerdeman KJ, van Laarhoven AIM, Keij SM, et al. Relieving patients' pain with expectation interventions. *Pain*. 2016;157(6):1179-1191. doi:10.1097/j.pain.0000000000000540

TABLE 6.5 DISCUSSION POINTS FOR ANALGESIC EXPECTATIONS

Clinician highlights for a brief discussion of analgesic expectations
Some pain tolerance will be necessary; it is unlikely to relieve pain completely.
Review medication and procedures that may be appropriate to relieve pain.
Provide suggestions for alternative methods to relieve pain.
Map out the anticipated trajectory of time for recovery.
Explore reentry to baseline or improved physical function.
Identify support systems.

transduction, the electrical signal is transmitted from the PNS, via A-delta fibers and C fibers, to the CNS where the signal is modulated and ultimately perceived as pain. Common mediators of nociceptive transduction include prostaglandins, substance P, bradykinin, and histamine; thus, medications that target these messengers will be most useful for signal interruption at the level of nociceptive transduction. Adjuvant medications that act as membrane stabilizers may also be used. Figure 6.1 illustrates physiologic pathways of pain and highlights complementary pharmacologic choices for designing a comprehensive pain management strategy.

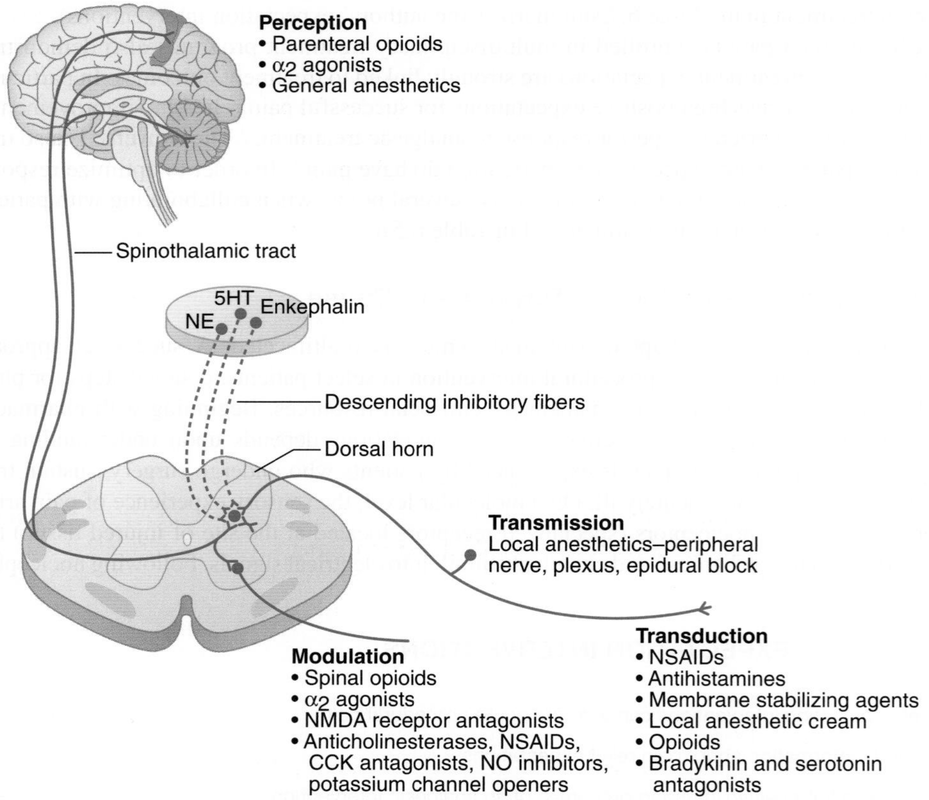

FIGURE 6.1 Pain—physiologic pathways and pharmacologic choices. Phys/pharm pain diagram copyright: from Anesthesia Key, referenced via https://www.google.com/search?q=neural+transduction+transmission+modulation+perception&rlz=1C1GCEB_enUS911US911&sxsrf=ALeKk03THZo6ISqATgPWPmQhb9HHLeyUAQ:1601826268725&source=lnms&tbm=isch&sa=X&ved=2ahUKEwiuwfTto5vsAhWwiOAKHcD-CLgQ_AUoAXoECBoQAw&biw=1222&bih=524#imgrc=n5YQ4skZe4A87M

A well-considered approach to acute pain management is a multimodal strategy that incorporates two or more drugs that act by different mechanisms to provide analgesia. These drugs may be administered by the same route or by different routes (ie, oral, intravenous systemic routes, peripheral or central nerve blockade, and transdermal). The American Society of Anesthesiologist's Practice Guidelines for Perioperative Acute Pain advises a multimodal analgesic plan begins with an around-the-clock regimen of COXIBs, NSAIDs, or acetaminophen unless contraindicated. Dosing regimens should be administered to optimize efficacy while minimizing the risk of adverse events. The choice of medication, dose, route, and duration of therapy should be individualized.[1] When nonopioids alone or in combination are insufficient, careful consideration of opioids is recommended to improve pain control. Opioids should be prescribed in oral formulation when possible, at lowest effective doses and for the shortest duration possible. Always it is prudent to discuss opioid-related side effects and complications, including the dangers of misuse and the development of tolerance and addiction. When considering treatment of new acute pain in patients with preexisting chronic pain conditions, it is necessary to target relief of acute pain, and at the same time, it is imperative to continue as usual all chronic pain medications. Table 6.2 highlights appropriate medication choices based on the diagnosed etiology of pain.

Interventions (Regional Nerve Blockade)—Targeting the Anatomic Cause

When acute pain is localized to a discrete anatomic region, it may be appropriate to consider regional nerve blockade to provide targeted pain relief. Typically, such clinical scenarios involve trauma or injury to a limb or to the thoracoabdominal region. Anesthesiologists and/or Pain Physicians may be consulted for placement of regional nerve blockade. Targeted nerve blocks can be performed as single injections with a limited duration of pain relief, or the specialist may elect instead to place a perineural catheter to extend the treatment duration. A valuable component of multimodal pain management, peripheral nerve blockade has been shown to reduce opioid use and offer superior pain relief when compared to opioid-predominant therapy.[13] In addition to the well-recognized advantages of reducing nausea, vomiting, constipation, and respiratory depression, opioid-sparing pain relief also reduces the level of patient sedation and preserves alertness and clarity of cognitive function. An alert patient is safer to navigate activities of daily living and is better able to participate in recovery activities such as physical therapy. Table 6.6 identifies anatomic regions for which targeted nerve blockade may provide relief of pain.

Physical Therapy—Targeting the Functional Cause

With medication administration and perhaps procedural intervention, the primary goal of clinical pain treatment is met, namely to reduce pain to a manageable level so that a patient may begin functional recovery. In other words, when the symptom of pain is sufficiently controlled, such that the patient is capable of actively participating in physical therapy, then functional restoration is initiated. Restoring physical function through rehabilitation is a necessary transition that improves the likelihood that pain control and physical function will be enduring. Physical therapy targets the functional limitations of pain. Having a clear understanding of the patient's previous functional baseline and limitations will help inform physical therapy as to goals and expectations. This can be accomplished through formal or informal functional assessments by clinicians, nursing or physical therapy. A Physical Therapist facilitates not only physical recovery but can also build emotional recovery and resilience. The specialist clearly identifies the goals of treatment; incorporates small,

TABLE 6.6 ANATOMIC LOCATION OF PAIN AND RELEVANT NERVE BLOCKADE

Anatomic Location of Pain	Targeted Peripheral Nerve Blockade
Upper extremity	Brachial plexus block
Lower extremity (anterior thigh, medial leg)	Femoral nerve block
Lower extremity (posterior thigh/leg, foot)	Sciatic nerve block (subgluteal, popliteal)
Hip, lower extremity (anterior, lateral thigh)	Fascia iliaca block
Thoracoabdominal analgesia, anterior/posterior chest cavity and wall	Thoracic paravertebral nerve block(s)
Hip, abdominal cavity and wall	Lumbar paravertebral nerve block(s)
Abdominal wall	Transversus abdominis plane block
Abdominal viscera and wall	Quadratus lumborum block

achievable intervals of increased activity level; and in doing so demonstrates adaptation and recovery.

Psychosocial Therapy—Targeting the Psychosocial Cause

Clearly not all patients will require formal psychological intervention as part of a rehabilitation plan; however, the clinician must consider psychological or psychosocial comorbidities as well as coping skills when designing an individualized pain treatment plan. Two extreme behavioral responses to coping with pain are confrontation and avoidance.[14] A patient's psychosocial framework can influence the success of the pain treatment plan. For example, a patient who trusts that acute pain can be treated and overcome and possesses a positive belief system is more likely to confront and achieve recovery. In contrast, a patient who exhibits cognitive and behavioral patterns consistent with pain catastrophizing (and rejects the possibility of pain relief) is more likely to perpetuate fear and persistence of functional impairment. Incorporating psychological and/or interdisciplinary care teams will benefit those patients whose successful treatment relies on formal psychosocial support.

Finally, evaluating patient risk factors associated with opioid misuse is another significant consideration when building a comprehensive pain plan. Opioids are commonly used in multimodal pain therapy, and in the context of the current opioid epidemic in the United States, it is both relevant and responsible to screen patients for characteristics associated with prolonged use of opioids.[15] In order to review medical and psychological comorbidities that may increase risk for prolonged opioid use and/or opioid misuse, clinicians can incorporate risk factors (identified in Table 6.7) into a series of screening questions.

Addressing these risks early, during formulation of a pain treatment plan, is useful for setting expectations for use of low-dose, short-term opioids. Communication and risk assessment can improve compliance with the overall treatment plan and yield better analgesic outcomes.

Conclusion

Designing a comprehensive pain treatment plan for optimal pain management necessitates proper diagnosis of the etiology of pain, assessment of the patient's functional limitation, and selection of multimodal treatment modalities including medications and procedural intervention. Successful implementation of the comprehensive plan requires setting realistic

TABLE 6.7 RISK FACTORS ASSOCIATED WITH PERSISTENT OPIOID USE

Risk factors associated with persistent new opioid use following surgery
Tobacco use
Alcohol and substance abuse disorders
Anxiety/depression
Mood disorders
Back pain/neck pain
Preoperative pain/centralized pain conditions

patient expectations, detailing an incremental recovery plan, and enlisting proper professionals to support physical and psychosocial needs. Because each patient is unique, the successful treatment plan must be individualized. This chapter presented a basic approach to building a pain treatment plan that may be used in caring for all patients who present with acute pain.

REFERENCES

1. Practice guidelines for acute pain management in the perioperative setting: an updated report by the American Society of Anesthesiologists Task Force on Acute Pain Management. *Anesthesiology.* 2012;116:248-273. https://doi.org/10.1097/ALN.0b013e31823c1030
2. Devin CJ, McGirt MJ. Best evidence in multimodal pain management in spine surgery and means of assessing postoperative pain and functional outcomes. *J Clin Neurosci.* 2015;22(6):930-938.
3. Shipton EE, Bate F, Garrick R, Steketee C, Shipton EA, Visser EJ. Systematic review of pain medicine content, teaching, and assessment in medical school curricula internationally. *Pain Ther.* 2018;7(2):139-161. doi:10.1007/s40122-018-0103-z
4. Vardeh D, Mannion R, Woolf C. Toward a mechanism-based approach to pain diagnosis. *J Pain.* 2016;17(9):T50-T69.
5. https://www.iasp-pain.org/PublicationsNews/NewsDetail.aspx?ItemNumber=10475
6. https://anesth.unboundmedicine.com/anesthesia/view/ClinicalAnesthesiaProcedures/728417/all/Definition_and_Terminology
7. Bishop FL, Yardley L, Prescott P, Cooper C, Little P, Lewith GT. Psychological covariates of longitudinal changes in back-related disability in patients undergoing acupuncture. *Clin J Pain.* 2015;31(3):254-264. doi:10.1097/AJP.0000000000000108
8. Mondloch MV, Cole DC, Frank JW. Does how you do depend on how you think you'll do? A systematic review of the evidence for a relation between patients' recovery expectations and health outcomes. *CMAJ.* 2001;165(2):174-179. http://proxygw.wrlc.org/login?url=https://www-proquest-com.proxygw.wrlc.org/docview/205003247?accountid=11243
9. Sohl SJ, Schnur JB, Montgomery GH. A meta-analysis of the relationship between response expectancies and cancer treatment-related side effects. *J Pain Symptom Manage.* 2009;38(5):775-784. doi:10.1016/j.jpainsymman.2009.01.008
10. Peerdeman KJ, van Laarhoven AIM, Keij SM, et al. Relieving patients' pain with expectation interventions. *Pain.* 2016;157(6):1179-1191. doi:10.1097/j.pain.0000000000000540
11. Cormier S, Lavigne GL, Choinière M, Rainville P. Expectations predict chronic pain treatment outcomes. *Pain.* 2016;157(2):329-338. doi:10.1097/j.pain.0000000000000379
12. Bayman EO, Parekh KR, Keech J, Larson N, Mark VW, Brennan TJ. Preoperative patient expectations of postoperative pain are associated with moderate to severe acute pain after VATS. *Pain Med.* 2019;20(3):543-554.
13. Kumar K, Kirksey MA, Duong S, Wu CL. A review of opioid-sparing modalities in perioperative pain management: methods to decrease opioid use postoperatively. *Anesth Analg.* 2017;125(5):1749-1760. doi:10.1213/ANE.0000000000002497.
14. Schofferman J. Restoration of function: the missing link in pain medicine? *Pain Med.* 2006;7(suppl_1):S159-S165. https://doi.org/10.1111/j.1526-4637.2006.00131.x
15. Brummett CM, Waljee JF, Goesling J, et al. New persistent opioid use after minor and major surgical procedures in US adults. *JAMA Surg.* 2017;152(6):e170504. doi:10.1001/jamasurg.2017.0504

7

Placebo and Nocebo, Understanding Their Role in Pain Medicine

Clifford Gevirtz

Introduction

Placebo, which is Latin for "I shall please," is a simulated medical intervention that could produce an actual or perceived improvement, which, in turn, is called the "placebo effect."

In medical research, placebos function as the control group in multiple designs of scientific experimental studies. They depend on the use of controlled and measured deception for their effect. Common forms of placebo include inert tablets, sham surgery, and the placement of random needles that convey false information to the patient.[1] Another example would be injecting saline or air into the epidural space. In a common placebo procedure, a patient is given an inert pill and told that it may improve his or her condition but not told that the pill is, in fact, inert. Such an intervention may cause the patient to believe that the treatment will change his or her condition, and this belief may in turn produce a subjective perception of a therapeutic effect, causing the patient to feel the condition has improved.

The placebo effect points to the importance of perception and how our central nervous system can produce a profound effect in the absence of any real external intervention. However, when used as treatment in clinical pain practice, the deception involved in the use of placebos creates a major dichotomy between the Hippocratic Oath and the honesty of the doctor-patient relationship.

The American Osteopathic Association[2] has published a position paper that specifically bans the use of placebo as part of therapy. Similarly, the United Kingdom Parliamentary Committee on Science and Technology[3] has stated that "… prescribing placebos… usually relies on some degree of patient deception" and "prescribing pure placebos is bad medicine. Their effect is unreliable and unpredictable and cannot form the sole basis of any treatment in the National Health Service."

The American Board of Anesthesiology Pain Management curriculum requires all pain practitioners to understand the role of placebo and nocebo in historical medical practice and their current use in clinical research.

History

The word *placebo* derives from a Latin translation of the Bible by St. Jerome,[4] in Psalm 114: "I shall please the Lord in the land of the living."

Placebos were first used in a medicinal context in the 18th century. In 1785, the *New Medical Dictionary* defined *placebo* as a "commonplace method or medicine." Placebos were widespread in medicine until the 20th century, and they were sometimes endorsed as necessary deceptions. In 1903, Richard Clarke Cabot, MD, a professor at Harvard Medical School, said that he was brought up to use placebos, but he ultimately concluded by saying, "I have not yet found any case in which a lie does not do more harm than good." From this point onward, the use of placebos as part of a regular regimen of medicine rapidly declined.

In a landmark article, "The Powerful Placebo," Henry Beecher, MD,[5] the founding chair of the Department of Anesthesiology at Massachusetts General Hospital and Harvard Medical School, reviewed the placebo effect and its clinically important effects. He documented several dramatic effects in clinical trials. This view was notably challenged when, in 2001, a more systematic review[6] of clinical trials concluded that there was no evidence of clinically important effects, except perhaps in the treatment of pain and some subjective outcomes. More recently, a Cochrane review on the use of placebos[7] reached similar conclusions. Most studies have attributed the difference from baseline until the end of the trial to a placebo effect, but the recent reviewers have sought to examine studies that had both placebo and untreated groups, in order to distinguish the placebo effect from the natural progression of the disease. However, while placebo effects may be short lived, even some brief measure of pain relief can have some benefit for the patient.

A Clinical Definition of Placebo

A *placebo* has been defined as "a substance or procedure … that is objectively without specific therapeutic activity for the condition being treated." Using this definition, a wide variety of things can be placebos and exhibit a placebo effect. Many substances administered through any means can act as placebos, including pills, lotions, creams, inhalants, and injections. Devices such as transcutaneous electrical nerve stimulation units and ultrasound machines can act as placebos, when placed in areas where no therapeutic effect is expected. Sham surgery and interventional procedures, sham intracranial electrodes, and sham acupuncture—either with sham needles or needles placed at nonacupuncture points—have all exhibited placebo effects. Even the presence of the physician, wearing a white coat within the patient's room, has been considered as a placebo. This has been demonstrated in a study of patient recovery, in which the patient's perceived recovery occurred sooner when the physician suggested that the patient "would be better in a few days." The study also demonstrated recovery to happen sooner when the patient is given treatment and the physician tells the patient that "the treatment will certainly make you better," rather than negative words such as "I am not sure that the treatment I am going to give you will have an effect."

Placebo Response: Mechanisms and Interpretation

This placebo response phenomenon is related to the perception and expectations of the patient; if the substance is viewed as helpful, it can heal, but if it is viewed as harmful, it can cause negative effects, which is known as the *nocebo* effect (vide infra). The basic mechanisms of placebo effects have been investigated since 1978, when it was demonstrated that the opioid antagonist naloxone could block placebo painkillers,[8] suggesting that the actions of endogenous opioids are involved.

Expectancy and Conditioning

Placebos exert an "expectancy" effect, whereby an inert substance that the patient thinks is a drug has effects similar to those of the actual drug. Placebos can act similarly through classical conditioning, where a placebo and an actual stimulus are used simultaneously until the placebo is associated with the effect from the stimulus. Both conditioning and expectations play roles in the placebo effect, and they make various types of contributions. Conditioning has a

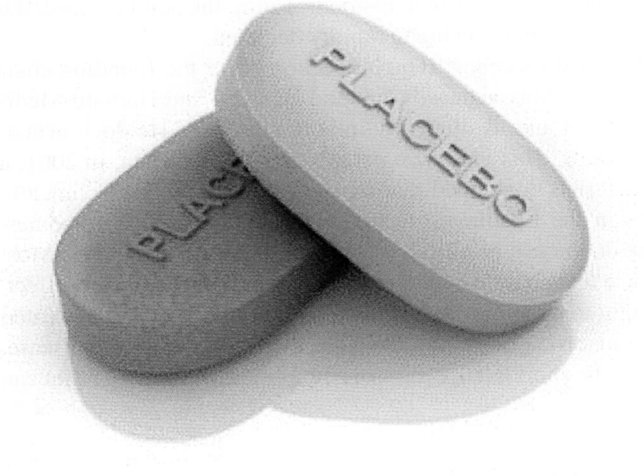

FIGURE 7.1 Placebo labeled pills.

longer-lasting effect, and it can influence earlier stages of information processing. The expectancy effect can be enhanced through factors such as the enthusiasm of the doctor, differences in size and color of placebo pills, or the use of other inventions such as injections. In a study,[9] the response to a placebo increased from 44% to 62% when the doctor treated patients with "warmth, attention, and confidence." Expectancy effects have been demonstrated to occur with a range of substances. Those who think that a treatment will work display a stronger placebo effect than those who do not, as evidenced in several studies of acupuncture.

Because the placebo effect is based on expectations and conditioning, the effect disappears if the patient is told that his or her expectations are unrealistic or that the placebo intervention is ineffective. A conditioned pain reduction can be totally removed when its existence is explained. For example, a placebo described as a muscle relaxant will cause muscle relaxation and, if described as the opposite, will result in increased muscle tension.

Because placebos are dependent upon perception and expectation, various factors that change the perception can increase the magnitude of the placebo response. For example, studies have demonstrated that the color and size of the placebo pill makes a difference, with "hot-colored" (eg, red, yellow) pills working better as stimulants, whereas "cool-colored" (eg, blue, purple) pills work better as depressants (Fig. 7.1). Capsules seem to be more effective than tablets, and size can make a difference. One group of researchers[10] has demonstrated that bigger pills increase the effect, whereas others[11] have argued that the effect is dependent upon cultural background. If the physician is of the same social group as the patient and with whom the patient may share a common bond, a larger effect maybe demonstrated. More pills, branding, past experience with similar pills, and a higher price increase the effect of placebo pills. Injection and acupuncture seem to have a larger effect than pills.

The placebo effect can work selectively. If an analgesic placebo cream is applied on one hand, it will reduce pain only in that hand and not elsewhere in the body. If a person is given a placebo under one name or nick name, and if he or she responds positively, the patient will respond in the same way on a later occasion to that placebo under that same name but not if another name is used.

The Placebo Effect and the Brain

Functional MRI has been used to study placebo analgesia and has revealed neuronal activation in the anterior cingulated, frontal, and insular cortices; the nucleus accumbens; the amygdala; and the periaqueductal gray matter. These higher cortical centers appear to project stimuli down the spinal cord in response to placebo. These placebo responses also show increased dopamine and mu opioid activity in the circuitry for reward responses and motivated behavior of the nucleus accumbens. Conversely, antianalgesic nocebo responses are associated with a lessening of activity in this part of the brain with decreased opioid and dopamine release. Analgesic placebo activation changes processing in the brainstem by enhancing the descending inhibition through the periaqueductal gray matter that acts on spinal nociceptive reflexes, whereas antianalgesic nocebos act in the opposite way.

In sum, functional imaging with placebo analgesia demonstrates that the placebo response is produced by a higher-to-lower cortical process dependent on frontal cortical areas that generate and maintain cognitive expectancies. The dopaminergic pathways may underlie these expectancies. Pathology that is not dependent on major "top-down" or cortically based regulation (eg, spinal cord injury or postherpetic neuralgia) may be less prone to placebo-related improvement.

Additional studies of the placebo effect, particularly placebo analgesia, have focused heavily on the endogenous opioid system. Placebo analgesic responses induced by manipulations of psychological mechanisms (conditioning and expectancies) are fully or partially reversible by the opioid antagonist naloxone,[12] indicating the involvement of the opioid system. Additional evidence[13] shows that nonopioid mechanisms and systems (such as serotonin, hormone secretion, and immune responses) are also involved.

It has recently been demonstrated that nocebo suggestions of increased pain can produce concurrent hyperalgesia and stimulation of the hypothalamic-pituitary-adrenal axis (HPA) responses[14] as reflected in increased plasma concentrations of adrenocorticotropic hormone and cortisol. Nocebo hyperalgesia and HPA hyperactivity are both antagonized by diazepam, suggesting that benzodiazepine treatable anxiety makes a major contribution to both responses. Administration of the mixed cholecystokinin (CCK) type-A/B receptor antagonist, proglumide, blocks nocebo hyperalgesia completely but has no effect on HPA hyperactivity, suggesting that there is selective involvement of CCK in the hyperalgesic, but not the anxiogenic, component of the nocebo effect.

It is important to note that neither diazepam nor proglumide have analgesic effects, that is, in the absence of nocebo-induced hyperalgesia. These findings suggest that there is a close relationship between anxiety and nocebo hyperalgesia, and they highlight the key role of CCKergic systems as a substrate of this relationship. When these facts are considered together, we can conclude that placebo analgesia and nocebo hyperalgesia rely upon, respectively, the activation of functionally opposing endogenous opioid and CCKergic systems.

The "Open-Hidden" Paradigm

The clinical application of the placebo is being reassessed in light of the knowledge we have gained from neurobiology and clinical imaging. The power of its clinical application has been clearly demonstrated in the open-hidden paradigm. In this paradigm, the patient may receive a treatment in the normal clinical "open" manner, in which the treatment is given by the clinician in full view of the patient, or in a "hidden" manner, with the patient unaware that the treatment is being administered. Open administration of a treatment is significantly more effective than hidden administration for pain.

The clinician should understand that the overall effect of drug administration is a combination of the pharmacologic action of the drug and the psychosocial context in which it is given. The open-hidden paradigm underscores the importance of expectation of receiving a treatment and the context in which it is given, which includes placebo mechanisms.

The power of expectation and the potential to exploit it clinically were dramatically demonstrated in a randomized trial of drug administration. Wager et al.[15] examined the effects of expectation on regional brain metabolic activity. This controlled study manipulated subjects' expectations so that one group of patients underwent open administration of a drug that they knew to be a stimulant, and the other group of patients received the same drug when they were expecting a placebo. Although both groups received the same dose of the same stimulant drug and had identical plasma concentrations of that drug, there were significant differences in regional brain metabolic activity demonstrated by functional MRI between those who expected a stimulant and those who expected a placebo. Shaping subjects' expectations not only altered regional brain metabolic activity, it also modified subjects' reported perceived "high" in response to the drug, again demonstrating the power of expectation in altering neurobiologic responses that may enhance response to drug treatment.

Many pain patients have a natural course of illness in which symptoms fluctuate, making it difficult to differentiate between a placebo or nocebo response and the natural course of illness at an individual patient level. Similarly, many "side effects" occur commonly with or without pharmacotherapies (eg, headache), making it often difficult to disentangle, at an individual patient level, between a treatment-emergent adverse event that is a nocebo response or one that has occurred independently of treatment.

Negative Consequences of Placebo

It is important to recognize that placebos can cause side effects associated with real treatment. For example, patients who have already been administered an opiate can then show respiratory depression when given a placebo.

Withdrawal symptoms can also occur after placebo treatment. This was demonstrated after the discontinuation of the Women's Health Initiative study[16] of hormone replacement therapy for treatment of menopausal symptoms. Women on the placebo arm had been enrolled for an average of 5.7 years. Moderate or severe withdrawal symptoms were reported by 40% of those taking placebo compared with 63% of participants receiving hormone replacement.

Placebos in Clinical Research

The informed consent form, particularly in crossover trials when participants are informed that they will receive placebo at some point in the trial, may influence both the adverse effects and therapeutic efficacy. Several types of trial designs may be particularly susceptible to confounding results because of placebo effects.

The crossover design has the advantage of using each patient as his or her own control, eliminating the problems created by variability among subjects. However, patients who receive active treatment in the first arm of the trial will have heightened placebo effects when the control intervention is given. This seems to be a conditioning effect that occurs despite the use of a washout period to eliminate continuing pharmacologic effects of a medication.

Rothman and Michels[17] have pointedly suggested, "The code of federal regulations under which the Federal Drug Administration operates is quite ambiguous about the acceptability of placebo controls." In one place, the agency suggests that they should be avoided. The regulations go on, however, to suggest including both placebo controls and active treatment controls in a study: "An active treatment study may include additional treatment groups, however, such as a placebo control...."[18]

In practice, FDA officials consider placebo controls the gold standard. In addition, guidelines for the clinical evaluation for many drugs, especially analgesics, require placebo groups.

The Code of Conduct for Research Involving Humans in Canada[19] states that use of placebos alone in clinical trials is ethically unacceptable when there are clearly effective therapies or interventions available. When proposing a placebo-controlled trial, it is necessary for the investigator to prove that no "clearly effective therapies" exist for the condition in question. Institutional research ethics boards need to verify these facts by consulting with outside experts and clinicians not involved in the study and the medical literature. Some studies are designed so that the placebo is used at first and then the effective medication is introduced, that is, there is a slight delay in providing effective treatment. In most pain conditions, a week's delay will not seriously harm the patient and will clarify the magnitude of the placebo effect.

Nocebo and the Nocebo Effect

In contrast to the placebo effect, inert substances also have the potential to cause negative effects via the "nocebo effect" (from the Latin nocebo meaning "I will harm"). In this effect, giving an inert substance has negative consequences.

A nocebo makes patients feel worse with many nonspecific symptoms. Common symptoms are sedation, headache, mild dizziness, malaise, and stomach discomfort. Many health professionals are unaware of nocebo; however, this adverse reaction can cause many patients to drop out of clinical trials, stop taking the medications they need, or end up using other medications that complicate their treatment.

The nocebo effect can result from conditioning, for example, when patients become nauseated upon reentering a room where they have previously received chemotherapy. Medications and the rooms where they are administered, and other environmental factors such as overly warm rooms, can take on symbolic features that have nocebo effects. The color red is associated with stimulation and blue with sedation; so, red and blue pills may produce those marked responses as unwanted side effects. Contagious and totally unfounded rumors are another source of nocebo responses. Many people, who have heard about allergies to various medications, wrongly think that they are allergic to these medications based on rumor and report reactions (eg, they are allergic to penicillin because it gave them an upset stomach).

Although anyone can experience a nocebo effect, it seems that a small segment of the population will respond strongly to both nocebos and placebos. In one experiment, subjects in three groups were asked to keep a hand in ice water for as long as they could.[20] One group was told that this could have beneficial effects for a period of up to 5 minutes (placebo instruction). The second group was told that it could be harmful, so the experiment would be stopped after, at most, 5 minutes as a precaution (a nocebo instruction). The third group was told only that their responses to cold were being tested (neutral instruction). People who indicated high anxiety about pain on a questionnaire before the experiment had the most pronounced responses as determined by the time they kept their hands in the cold water not only to the nocebo instruction but also with the opposite, the duration of time in the placebo.

Anyone with anxiety, depression, or hypochondriasis who starts therapy runs the risk of developing further symptoms in response to attempts at healing or comforting. In this case, the nocebo effect can be related to somatization. Somatoform disorders, identified by recurrent medically unexplained physical symptoms, have foundation in mood and personality disorders, as well as social circumstances. Somatoform reactions may also be reinforced and amplified by the perceived advantages of being treated as an invalid. This secondary gain should be regarded as another form of nocebo response.

Patients need help in understanding and tolerating, minimizing, or ignoring nocebo and other somatoform responses. These responses may be at work whenever the side effects of a medication or other treatment are vague and ambiguous, or the patient has been expecting it to cause problems. Patients can be asked about earlier disappointing experiences with medical procedures. If a patient says that he or she is especially sensitive to drugs, the physician might point out that anticipating bad effects can be a self-fulfilling prophecy. It may help to emphasize the limits of medicine and explain the close relationship between emotions and physical sensations, especially as it involves stress hormones. Above all, in prescribing any drug or other treatment, physicians must always act in a way that establishes trust and promotes the patient's participation and cooperation.

Conclusion

Placebo and nocebo are important factors in both clinical practice and in clinical research. Our understanding of the role of placebo has evolved from its deceitful use in medical practice more than 100 years ago to become a significant factor in adding to pain relief today. However, there is an unmet need to recognize its significant impact in everyday interactions with our patients. Just spending a few minutes encouraging and reinforcing our hopes and goals for our patients with pain can have dramatic effects.

REFERENCES

1. Colloca L, Barsky AJ. Placebo and nocebo effects. *N Engl J Med*. 2020;382(6):554-561.
2. Nichols KJ, Galluzzi KE, Bates B, et al. AOA's position against use of placebos for pain management in end-of-life care. *J Am Osteopath Assoc*. 2005;105:2-5.
3. UK Parliamentary Committee Science and Technology Committee. *Evidence Check 2: Homeopathy*. House of Commons London: The Stationery Office Limited; 2010.
4. Psalm 116:9. Vulgate version by Jerome, "Placebo Domino in regione vivorum," "I shall please."
5. Beecher HK. The powerful placebo. *J Am Med Assoc*. 1955;159:1602-1606.
6. Hróbjartsson A, Gøtzsche PC. Is the placebo powerless? An analysis of clinical trials comparing placebo with no treatment. *N Engl J Med*. 2001;344:1594-1602.
7. Laursen DRT, Hansen C, Paludan-Müller AS, Hróbjartsson A. Active placebo versus standard placebo control interventions in pharmacological randomised trials. *Cochrane Database Syst Rev*. 2020;(7):MR000055. doi:10.1002/14651858.MR000055
8. Benedetti F. The opposite effects of the opiate antagonist naloxone and the cholecystokinin antagonist proglumide on placebo analgesia. *Pain*. 1996;64:535-543.
9. Howe LC, Goyer JP, Crum AJ. Harnessing the placebo effect: exploring the influence of physician characteristics on placebo response. *Health Psychol*. 2017;36(11):1074.
10. Ongaro G, Kaptchuk TJ. Symptom perception, placebo effects, and the Bayesian brain. *Pain*. 2019;160(1):1-4. doi:10.1097/j.pain.0000000000001367
11. Wolf BB, Langley S. Cultural factors and the response to pain: a review. *Am Anthropol*. 2009;70:494-501.
12. Scott DJ, Stohler CS, Egnatuk CM, et al. Placebo and nocebo effects are defined by opposite opioid and dopaminergic responses. *Arch Gen Psychiatry*. 2008;65:220-231.
13. Lanotte M, Lopiano L, Torre E, et al. Expectation enhances autonomic responses to stimulation of the human subthalamic limbic region. *Brain Behav Immun*. 2005;19:500-509.
14. Oken BS. Placebo effects: clinical aspects and neurobiology. *Brain*. 2008;131:2812-2823.
15. Zunhammer M, Spisák T, Wager TD, Bingel U. Meta-analysis of neural systems underlying placebo analgesia from individual participant fMRI data. *Nat Commun*. 2021;12(1):1-11.
16. Ockene JK, Barad DH, Cochrane BB, et al. Symptom experience after discontinuing use of estrogen plus progestin. *JAMA*. 2005;294:183-193.
17. Rothman KJ, Michels KB. The continuing unethical use of placebo controls. *N Engl J Med*. 1994;331:394-398. http://www.nejm.org/toc/nejm/331/6/
18. U.S. Food and Drug Administration. Revised April 1, 2010. CFR– Code of Federal RegulationsTitle21. http://www.accessdata.fda.gov/scripts/cdrh/cfdocs/cfcfr/CFRSearch.cfm?fr=314.126
19. Canada Tri-Council Working Group on Ethics. *Code of Conduct for Research Involving Humans ("Final" Version)*. Minister of Supply and Services; 1997.
20. Staats P, Hekmat H, Staats A. Suggestion/placebo effects on pain: negative as well as positive. *J Pain Symptom Manage*. 1998;15:235-243.

8

Preemptive Analgesia and Surgical Pain

Islam Mohammad Shehata, Mahmoud Alkholany, Elyse M. Cornett, and Alan David Kaye

Introduction

Tissue injury from surgical incision is a noxious stimulus that leads to the formation of "inflammatory soup," resulting in the stimulation of nociceptors. Noxious stimuli provoke two types of alterations in the responsiveness of the nervous system based on its plasticity: peripheral and central sensitization. Peripheral sensitization occurs at the site of the ongoing inflammation, mediated by cytokines and chemokines released from the injured tissues and the immune cells to reduce the threshold of the nociceptor afferent peripheral terminal.[1] These mediators result in modified transduction and enhanced conduction of nociceptive impulses toward the central nervous system. The nociceptive barrage from the nociceptors at the site of injury travels through the small myelinated A and unmyelinated C fibers, increasing the excitability of nociceptive neurons within the central nervous system. This activity-dependent central sensitization (wind-up) amplifies the effects of peripheral inputs. It may cause central hyperexcitability, which accounts for the long-term persistence of pain beyond the offending stimulus.[2] Therefore, abolition of the initiating event should prevent secondary changes and thereby reduce the subsequent pain experience.

Definition

There is no agreed-upon definition of preemptive analgesia. However, preemptive analgesia can be defined broadly as an antinociceptive modality that has been given before an injury or noxious stimulus, including surgical incision, preventing establishment of the central sensitization and covering both periods of the surgery and the initial postoperative period.[3] Thereby, preemptive analgesia reduces acute surgical pain and potentially minimizes the risk of developing chronic postsurgical pain.[4]

This contrasts with preventive analgesia, where an analgesic has a preventive effect if its administration leads to a reduction in pain or analgesic consumption that extends beyond its expected duration of action (usually 5.5 half-lives).[5] Therefore, preventive analgesia refers to the effect of the intervention on the expected duration of analgesia regardless of the timing of the intervention related to the injury.

Mechanism of Preemptive Analgesia

Pathologic pain (surgery-evoked pain) is different from physiologic pain; it is of higher intensity and faster spread. Moreover, low-intensity stimuli can be activated due to the peripheral and central sensitization causing postsurgical allodynia and hyperalgesia.[6] A good understanding of the ascending and descending inhibitory pain pathways and neurotransmitters and receptors is important to understand the proposed mechanism of preemptive analgesia in preventing postoperative pain.[7] Preemptive analgesia may act by targeting these different levels before the incidence of the noxious stimuli. Consequently, it may preempt the injury-induced neurophysiological and biochemical modulation of the somatosensory system and reduce hyperexcitability and development of postoperative and chronic pain. This theory is supported by animal studies and *in vitro* and *in vivo* laboratory investigations.[8,9]

Underlying Physiology

There are four distinct processes in the sensory pathway: transduction, transmission, modulation, and perception. Each of these processes presents a potential target for analgesic therapy used in preemptive analgesia.[10]

Transduction

Chemical substances and enzymes called prostanoids (prostaglandins, leukotrienes, and hydroxy acids) are released from the damaged tissues, increasing the transduction of painful stimuli. Blocking the release of those mediators before surgical incision could potentially reduce the risk of perioperative pain and peripheral sensitization.[10]

Transmission in the Dorsal Horn

Several mediators are involved in the transmission of painful stimuli from A-delta and C fibers to secondary order neurons at Rexed laminae in the dorsal horn of the spinal cord. These mediators include substance P, the calcitonin gene–related peptide.[11,12] Substance P induces the release of excitatory amino acids, such as aspartate and glutamate, which act on the AMPA (2-amino-3-hydroxy-5-methyl-4-isoxazole-propionic acid) and NMDA (*N*-methyl-D-aspartate) receptors contributing to the development of the "wind-up" phenomenon—blocking the release/action of those mediators before surgical incision could decrease the risk of hyperexcitability, the development of central sensitization, and chronic pain.

Perception

The activation of supraspinal structures involved in sensory discrimination and the emotional-affective component of pain is mediated by EAAs, for example, glutamate.[13] However, the neurotransmitters involved in central processing of nociceptive information have not yet been elucidated, representing an area for future research and development.

Modulation

Modulation represents the interaction between excitatory and descending inhibitory pathways at the dorsal horn of the spinal cord, for example, periaqueductal gray. Neurotransmitters, including norepinephrine, serotonin, and opiate-like substances (endorphins), are involved in the brainstem inhibitory pathways that modulate pain in the spinal cord, hence the antinociceptive effect of antidepressants, which inhibit the reuptake of noradrenaline and serotonin and the effect of opiates.[14] Gamma-aminobutyric acid and glycine are two important inhibitory neurotransmitters that act at the dorsal horn. Blockade of spinal gamma-aminobutyric acid or glycine can result in allodynia by removing inhibitors that control NMDA receptors.[15]

Modalities of Preemptive Analgesia

Multimodal analgesia refers to the management of pain using a combination of analgesic drugs with differing pharmacological modes of action.[16] Combining pharmacological agents that act at one or more sites along the pain pathway (peripheral, spinal, or supraspinal sites) pose an additive effect with better pain relief and fewer side effects.[17,18] The different modalities of preemptive analgesia include nonopioids, opioids, and regional analgesia (Table 8.1).

TABLE 8.1 MODALITIES OF PREEMPTIVE ANALGESIA

Route	Drug	Mechanism of Action	Dose	Comments
Oral				
	Gabapentin	Structural analogues of γ-aminobutyric acid bind to α2δ subunit of voltage-dependent calcium channels and modify the action of a subset of *N*-methyl-D-aspartate–sensitive glutamate receptors, M-channel, neurexin-1α, and thrombospondin proteins	400 mg	Sedation, nausea, and vomiting especially in the elderly and renal impairment patients
	Pregabalin		150 mg	
	Celecoxib	Selective COX-2 inhibitors	200 mg	Increased cardiovascular risk in ischemic patients
Intravenous				
Nonopioid				
	Paracetamol	A centrally acting drug, which suppresses prostaglandin synthesis and cyclooxygenase (COX)	1 g	Well-tolerated drug
	NSAID	Inhibit both the COX-1 and COX-2 enzymes		• Platelet dysfunction • Renal dysfunction • Peptic ulcer
	Ketamine	*N*-methyl-D-aspartate receptor antagonist and binds to γ-aminobutyric acid, cholinergic, and voltage-gated sodium channel	0.15-0.5 mg/kg	Psychotomimetic side effects
	Magnesium sulphate	Antagonist of calcium channels and *N*-methyl-D-aspartate receptors	50 mg/kg	Reduction of requirement of propofol (induction and maintenance), neuromuscular blocking agents, and fentanyl

(Continued)

TABLE 8.1 MODALITIES OF PREEMPTIVE ANALGESIA (*Continued*)

Route	Drug	Mechanism of Action	Dose	Comments
Opioid	Opioid receptor agonist	Mu, kappa, and delta receptor agonist		• Postoperative respiratory depression • Urinary retention • Ileus • Nausea and vomiting • Shivering
Regional				
Intrathecal and epidural agents	Opioid receptor agents (diamorphine)			
Surgical wound infiltration	Bupivacaine, levobupivacaine, liposomal bupivacaine	Amide local anesthetics, which inactivate voltage-dependent sodium channels		• No significant risk of surgical wound infection • Local anesthetic systemic toxicity: central nervous system and cardiovascular system (cardiac arrest)
Peripheral nerve block				

Nonopioids

Paracetamol

Paracetamol, *N*-acetyl-*p*-aminophenol, is a centrally acting drug, which suppresses prostaglandin synthesis and cyclooxygenase (COX) similar to the nonsteroidal anti-inflammatory drug (NSAID) agents especially COX-2 selective inhibitors. Paracetamol is a common analgesic (for mild pain) and antipyretic drug with lesser peripheral anti-inflammatory properties and better tolerance than NSAID.[19] Many studies show promising results of preemptive paracetamol (1 g) for different types of surgery. Preemptive paracetamol decreased the pain score, thereby reducing the opioid consumption and the hospital length of stay.[20-22]

Nonsteroidal anti-inflammatory drugs

Nonsteroidal anti-inflammatory drugs act by inhibiting both the COX-1 and COX-2 enzymes. However, this nonselectivity leads to the inhibition of normal platelet function and gastrointestinal toxicity, which are unfavorable side effects.[23] The preemptive analgesic role of the NSAID is controversial, with a tendency toward no statistical significance of preincisional vs postincisional systemic intravenous NSAIDs.[24] However, many studies found that selective COX-2 inhibitors have more satisfactory results of the preemptive analgesia in decreasing the postoperative pain and opioid consumption, especially celecoxib (oral 200 mg).[25-27] Of notice, selective COX-2 inhibitors leave thromboxane A2 unaffected, which results in a prothrombotic state and vasoconstriction. Therefore, selective COX-2 inhibitors are proved to be associated with cardiac events, especially in patients with ischemic heart diseases.[28]

N-Methyl-D-Aspartate Receptor Antagonists

Ketamine

Ketamine has analgesic, anti-inflammatory, and antidepressant properties. Ketamine binds to diverse receptors; *N*-methyl-D-aspartate (which play an important role in preventing the wind-up phenomenon), γ-aminobutyric acid, cholinergic, and voltage-gated sodium channel, which provides a local anesthetic effect.[29] A meta-analysis of randomized controlled studies assessed the preemptive analgesic of ketamine, which failed to favor pretreatment.[24] However, recently many studies elicited the definitive role of preincisional ketamine in decreasing the early postoperative pain score and opioid consumption (dose range 0.15-0.5 mg/kg) without deleterious effects.[30-32]

Magnesium sulfate

Another well-recognized NMDA receptor antagonist is magnesium sulfate. Magnesium sulfate has many recognized roles in medicine as analgesic, anticonvulsant, and antiarrhythmic. These actions are attributed to interference with calcium channels and *N*-methyl-D-aspartate.[33] Additionally, magnesium has an α-adrenergic antagonistic feature and can inhibit catecholamine release, thus decreasing peripheral nociception. The preemptive analgesic role of magnesium sulfate (50 mg/kg) has been proved in many studies, which showed a lower pain score, decrease of opioid consumption, and prevention of chronic neuropathic pain.[34-36] However, in this dose, magnesium sulfate may reduce the anesthetic requirement and prolong the neuromuscular block with the nondepolarizing muscle relaxant agents.[37]

Gabapentinoids

Gabapentinoids, as structural analogs of γ-aminobutyric acid, possess an antiepileptic, anxiolytic, and antinociceptive properties by interacting with different binding sites. The main binding site is the α2δ subunit of voltage-dependent calcium channels. Additionally, gabapentin has been found recently that it can modify the action of a subset of *N*-methyl-D-aspartate–sensitive glutamate receptors, M-channel, neurexin-1α, and thrombospondin proteins by binding to α2δ-1.[38,39] Therefore, gabapentinoids are used as adjuvant therapy in many clinical indications involving neuropathic pain and chronic pain.

Different studies evaluated the efficacy of preoperative oral administration of gabapentin (300-1200 mg) and showed that it was effective for controlling acute postoperative pain as an opioid-sparing medication.[40] However, a prospective, randomized, placebo-controlled study showed that oral 400 mg of gabapentin may be the optimal dose without noticeable benefits of increasing the dose compared to 800 and 1200 mg.[41] Regarding pregabalin, an oral dose of 150 mg is efficient for preemptive analgesia, as proved by many studies.[42,43] Most of the studies recorded drowsiness, nausea, and vomiting as common adverse effects of gabapentinoid, especially in elderly frail patients and those with renal impairment.

Opioids

Despite the well-established role of opioid therapy in the management of moderate to severe pain, a systematic review of their preemptive analgesic role showed no improvement in postoperative pain control.[44] Moreover, opioid-induced hyperalgesia is a well-known phenomenon that has been related to the perioperative use of a potent and short-acting opioid such as remifentanil. Opioid-induced hyperalgesia may exaggerate the postoperative pain and cause excitatory neuroplasticity, which may theoretically result in chronic pain.[45] Therefore, the implementation of multimodal analgesia with its opioid-sparing effect can decrease the unfavorable effects of opioids. These side effects include postoperative respiratory depression, urinary retention, ileus, nausea and vomiting, and shivering.[46]

Regional Analgesia

Various studies confirmed the preemptive analgesic effects of different modalities of regional analgesia, including epidural (opioid, bupivacaine, and combination of both), nerve block, spinal, and local infiltration of the surgical site.[47] The studied surgeries were lower extremity, gynecology, thoracic, and abdominal surgery.

Surgical wound infiltration

One of the most promising modalities for preemptive analgesia is the preincisional surgical wound site infiltration with local anesthetics. Wound infiltration with local anesthetics is a well-established nonopioid component of multimodal analgesia. It is easy to perform, effective in decreasing postoperative pain scores and opioid consumption.[48] In addition, no studies proved that infiltration of the wound with local anesthetics is associated with an increased risk of surgical wound infection. Preincisional local anesthetic wound infiltration had been studied extensively, especially in major surgery such as abdominal surgery.[49,50] In many comparative studies, the control of postoperative pain was comparable to neuraxial techniques and intravenous opioids.[51,52] Combined pre- and postincisional local wound infiltration showed better results than each one alone.[53]

Neuraxial analgesia

Intrathecal and epidural opioids, especially diamorphine, showed a considerable role in controlling postoperative pain without an increase of adverse effects.[54,55] However, there is no solid evidence regarding its role in reducing central sensitization. Moreover, it is not supposed to hinder the inflammatory afferent input during the early postoperative period.[48] Therefore, combining the regional analgesia with antihyperalgesia drugs may improve the success of multimodal analgesia.

Conclusion

The theoretical aim of preemptive analgesia is to reduce postoperative pain, reduce analgesic consumption, and limit the pain-related pathological neuromodulation throughout the perioperative period (both from the incision and the subsequent inflammatory).[56] The clinical usefulness of preemptive analgesia has been found to be controversial. There is no clear evidence of its efficacy because of many reasons. These reasons include lack of consistency in research, differences in clinical trial design, difficulties in completely blocking nociceptive inputs, and the use of many different outcomes in clinical trials.[56,57]

Therefore, we should not focus on the timing of the analgesic intervention in relation to surgical insult but rather on its duration of effect and efficacy in controlling perioperative pain and preventing sensitization.[58] This introduces the broader concept of protective or preventive analgesia, which refers to the implementation of a multimodal analgesic plan (different mechanisms but synergistic action) that is capable of having an extended effect beyond the duration of action of the individual medications regardless of the timing in relation to surgical insult.[7,59] Therefore, the ideal analgesic plan should be personalized for every patient starting preemptively and with maintenance of the obtained effect thorough the perioperative period to prevent central sensitization and decrease the risk of developing chronic postsurgical pain.

REFERENCES

1. Silva RL, Lopes AH, Guimarães RM, Cunha TM. CXCL1/CXCR2 signaling in pathological pain: role in peripheral and central sensitization. *Neurobiol Dis*. 2017;105:109-116.
2. Neblett R. The central sensitization inventory: a user's manual. *J Appl Biobehav Res*. 2018;23(2):e12123.
3. Kissin I, Weiskopf RB. Preemptive analgesia. *J Am Soc Anesthesiol*. 2000;93(4):1138-1143.
4. Carroll I, Hah J, Mackey S, et al. Perioperative interventions to reduce chronic post-surgical pain. *J Reconstr Microsurg*. 2013;29(4):213-222.
5. Katz J, Clarke H, Seltzer ZE. Preventive analgesia: quo vadimus? *Anesth Analg*. 2011;113(5):1242-1253.
6. Kuner R. Central mechanisms of pathological pain. *Nat Med*. 2010;16(11):1258-1266.
7. Dahl JB, Møiniche S. Pre-emptive analgesia. *Br Med Bull*. 2005;71(1):13-27.
8. Kissin I, Lee SS, Bradley EL Jr. Effect of prolonged nerve block on inflammatory hyperalgesia in rats: prevention of late hyperalgesia. *Anesthesiology*. 1998;88:224-232.
9. Brennan TJ, Umali EF, Zahn PK. Comparison of pre- versus post-incision administration of intrathecal bupivacaine and intrathecal morphine in a rat model of postoperative pain. *Anesthesiology*. 1997;87:1517-1528.

10. Kelly DJ, Ahmad M, Brull SJ. Preemptive analgesia I: physiological pathways and pharmacological modalities. *Can J Anaesth*. 2001;48(10):1000-1010. doi:10.1007/BF03016591
11. Murase K, Randic M. Actions of substance P on rat spinal dorsal horn neurons. *J Physiol (Lond)*. 1984;346:203-217.
12. Skofitsch G, Jacobowitz DM. Calcitonin gene-related peptide coexists with substance P in capsaicin sensitive neurons and sensory ganglia of the rat. *Peptides*. 1985;6:747-754.
13. Jensen TS, Yaksh TL. Brainstem excitatory amino acid receptors in nociception: microinjection mapping and pharmacological characterization of glutamate-sensitive sites in the brainstem associated with algogenic behavior. *Neuroscience*. 1992;46:535-547.
14. Fields HL, Heinricher MM, Mason P. Neurotransmitters in nociceptive modulatory circuits. *Ann Rev Neurosci*. 1991;14:219-245.
15. Yaksh TL. Behavioral and autonomic correlates of the tactile evoked allodynia produced by spinal glycine inhibition: effects of modulatory receptor systems and excitatory amino acid antagonists. *Pain*. 1989;37:111-123.
16. Chaparro L, Wiffen PJ, Moore RA, et al. Combination pharmacotherapy for the treatment of neuropathic pain in adults. *Cochrane Database Syst Rev*. 2012;2012:CD008943.
17. Gilron I, Jensen TS, Dickeson AH. Combination pharmacotherapy for management of chronic pain: from bench to bedside. *Lancet Neurol*. 2013;12(11):1084-1095.
18. Remy C, Marret E, Bonnet F. Effects of acetaminophen on morphine side-effects and consumption after major surgery: meta-analysis of randomized controlled trials. *Br J Anaesth*. 2005;4:505-513.
19. Graham GG, Davies MJ, Day RO, Mohamudally A, Scott KF. The modern pharmacology of paracetamol: therapeutic actions, mechanism of action, metabolism, toxicity and recent pharmacological findings. *Inflammopharmacology*. 2013;21(3):201-232.
20. Arici S, Gurbet A, Türker G, Yavaşcaoğlu B, Sahin S. Preemptive analgesic effects of intravenous paracetamol in total abdominal hysterectomy. *Agri*. 2009;21(2):54-61.
21. Arslan M, Celep B, Çiçek R, Kalender HÜ, Yılmaz H. Comparing the efficacy of preemptive intravenous paracetamol on the reducing effect of opioid usage in cholecystectomy. *J Res Med Sci*. 2013;18(3):172.
22. Hassan HI. Perioperative analgesic effects of intravenous paracetamol: preemptive versus preventive analgesia in elective cesarean section. *Anesth Essays Res*. 2014;8(3):339.
23. Tacconelli S, Bruno A, Grande R, Ballerini P, Patrignani P. Nonsteroidal anti-inflammatory drugs and cardiovascular safety–translating pharmacological data into clinical readouts. *Expert Opin Drug Saf*. 2017;16(7):791-807.
24. Ong CK, Lirk P, Seymour RA, Jenkins BJ. The efficacy of preemptive analgesia for acute postoperative pain management: a meta-analysis. *Anesth Analg*. 2005;100(3):757-773.
25. Kashefi P, Honarmand A, Safavi M. Effects of preemptive analgesia with celecoxib or acetaminophen on postoperative pain relief following lower extremity orthopedic surgery. *Adv Biomed Res*. 2012;1:66.
26. Al-Sukhun J, Al-Sukhun S, Penttilä H, Ashammakhi N, Al-Sukhun R. Preemptive analgesic effect of low doses of celecoxib is superior to low doses of traditional nonsteroidal anti-inflammatory drugs. *J Craniofac Surg*. 2012;23(2):526-529.
27. Kaye AD, Baluch A, Kaye AJ, Ralf G, Lubarsky D. Pharmacology of cyclooxygenase-2 inhibitors and preemptive analgesia in acute pain management. *Curr Opin Anesthesiol*. 2008;21(4):439-445.
28. Martín Arias LH, Martín González A, Sanz Fadrique R, Vazquez ES. Cardiovascular risk of nonsteroidal anti-inflammatory drugs and classical and selective cyclooxygenase-2 inhibitors: a meta-analysis of observational studies. *J Clin Pharmacol*. 2019;59(1):55-73.
29. Zanos P, Moaddel R, Morris PJ, et al. Ketamine and ketamine metabolite pharmacology: insights into therapeutic mechanisms. *Pharmacol Rev*. 2018;70(3):621-660.
30. Lee J, Park HP, Jeong MH, Son JD, Kim HC. Efficacy of ketamine for postoperative pain following robotic thyroidectomy: a prospective randomised study. *J Int Med Res*. 2018;46(3):1109-1120.
31. Ye F, Wu Y, Zhou C. Effect of intravenous ketamine for postoperative analgesia in patients undergoing laparoscopic cholecystectomy: a meta-analysis. *Medicine*. 2017;96(51):e9147.
32. Yang L, Zhang J, Zhang Z, Zhang C, Zhao D, Li J. Preemptive analgesia effects of ketamine in patients undergoing surgery. A meta-analysis. *Acta Cir Bras*. 2014;29(12):819-825.
33. Verma VK, Kumar A, Prasad C, Hussain M. Effect of single-dose magnesium sulfate on total postoperative analgesic requirement in patients receiving balanced general anesthesia—a prospective, randomized, placebo controlled study. *Indian J Clin Anaesth*. 2019;6(1):148-151.
34. Kiran S, Gupta R, Verma D. Evaluation of a single-dose of intravenous magnesium sulphate for prevention of postoperative pain after inguinal surgery. *Indian J Anaesth*. 2011;55(1):31.
35. Omar H. Magnesium sulfate as a preemptive adjuvant to levobupivacaine for postoperative analgesia in lower abdominal and pelvic surgeries under epidural anesthesia (randomized controlled trial). *Anesth Essays Res*. 2018;12(1):256.

36. Ghezel-Ahmadi V, Ghezel-Ahmadi D, Schirren J, Tsapopiorgas C, Beck G, Bölükbas S. Perioperative systemic magnesium sulphate to minimize acute and chronic post-thoracotomy pain: a prospective observational study. *J Thorac Dis*. 2019;11(2):418.
37. Rodríguez-Rubio L, Nava E, Del Pozo JS, Jordán J. Influence of the perioperative administration of magnesium sulfate on the total dose of anesthetics during general anesthesia. A systematic review and meta-analysis. *J Clin Anesth*. 2017;39:129-138.
38. Taylor CP, Harris EW. Analgesia with gabapentin and pregabalin may involve *N*-methyl-D-aspartate receptors, neurexins, and thrombospondins. *J Pharmacol Exp Ther*. 2020;374(1):161-174.
39. Manville RW, Abbott GW. Gabapentin is a potent activator of KCNQ3 and KCNQ5 potassium channels. *Mol Pharmacol*. 2018;94(4):1155-1163.
40. Penprase B, Brunetto E, Dahmani E, Forthoffer JJ, Kapoor S. The efficacy of preemptive analgesia for postoperative pain control: a systematic review of the literature. *AORN J*. 2015;101(1):94-105.
41. Tomar GS, Singh F, Cherian G. Role of preemptive gabapentin on postoperative analgesia after infraumbilical surgeries under subarachnoid block—a randomized, placebo-controlled, double-blind study. *Am J Ther*. 2019;26(3):e350-e357.
42. Eman A, Bilir A, Beyaz SG. The effects of preoperative pregabalin on postoperative analgesia and morphine consumption after abdominal hysterectomy. *Acta Med Mediter*. 2014;2014(30):481.
43. Kim JH, Seo MY, Hong SD, et al. The efficacy of preemptive analgesia with pregabalin in septoplasty. *Clin Exp Otorhinolaryngol*. 2014;7(2):102.
44. Møiniche S, Kehlet H, Dahl JB. A qualitative and quantitative systematic review of preemptive analgesia for postoperative pain relief: the role of timing of analgesia. *Anesthesiology*. 2002;96(3):725-741.
45. Simonnet G. Preemptive antihyperalgesia to improve preemptive analgesia. *Anesthesiology*. 2008;108(3):352-354.
46. Lavand'homme P, Steyaert A. Opioid-free anesthesia opioid side effects: tolerance and hyperalgesia. *Best Pract Res Clin Anaesthesiol*. 2017;31(4):487-498.
47. Kelly DJ, Ahmad M, Brull SJ. Preemptive analgesia II: recent advances and current trends. *Can J Anesth*. 2001;48(11):1091.
48. Scott NB. Wound infiltration for surgery. *Anaesthesia*. 2010;65:67-75.
49. Kong M, Li X, Shen J, Ye M, Xiang H, Ma D. The effectiveness of preemptive analgesia for relieving postoperative pain after video-assisted thoracoscopic surgery (VATS): a prospective, non-randomized controlled trial. *J Thorac Dis*. 2020;12(9):4930.
50. Cantore F, Boni L, Di Giuseppe M, Giavarini L, Rovera F, Dionigi G. Pre-incision local infiltration with levobupivacaine reduces pain and analgesic consumption after laparoscopic cholecystectomy: a new device for day-case procedure. *Int J Surg*. 2008;6:S89-S92.
51. Wongyingsinn M, Kohmongkoludom P, Trakarnsanga A, Horthongkham N. Postoperative clinical outcomes and inflammatory markers after inguinal hernia repair using local, spinal, or general anesthesia: a randomized controlled trial. *PLoS One*. 2020;15(11):e0242925.
52. Relland LM, Tobias JD, Martin D, et al. Ultrasound-guided rectus sheath block, caudal analgesia, or surgical site infiltration for pediatric umbilical herniorrhaphy: a prospective, double-blinded, randomized comparison of three regional anesthetic techniques. *J Pain Res*. 2017;10:2629.
53. Fouladi RF, Navali N, Abbassi A. Pre-incisional, post-incisional and combined pre-and post-incisional local wound infiltrations with lidocaine in elective caesarean section delivery: a randomised clinical trial. *J Obstet Gynaecol*. 2013;33(1):54-59.
54. Wang Y, Guo X, Guo Z, Xu M. Preemptive analgesia with a single low dose of intrathecal morphine in multilevel posterior lumbar interbody fusion surgery: a double-blind, randomized, controlled trial. *Spine J*. 2020;20(7):989-997.
55. Aglio LS, Abd-El-Barr MM, Orhurhu V, et al. Preemptive analgesia for postoperative pain relief in thoracolumbosacral spine operations: a double-blind, placebo-controlled randomized trial. *J Neurosurg Spine*. 2018;29(6):647-653.
56. Gottschalk A, Smith DS. New concepts in acute pain therapy: preemptive analgesia. *Am Fam Physician*. 2001;63(10):1979.
57. Grape S, Tramèr MR. Do we need preemptive analgesia for the treatment of postoperative pain? *Best Pract Res Clin Anaesthesiol*. 2007;21(1):51-63.
58. Pogatzki-Zahn EM, Zahn PK. From preemptive to preventive analgesia. *Cur Opin Anesthesiol*. 2006;19(5):551-555.
59. Rosero EB, Joshi GP. Preemptive, preventive, multimodal analgesia: what do they really mean? *Plast Reconstr Surg*. 2014;134(4S-2):85S-93S.

9

Pain as a Subjective Multidimensional Experience

Yvonne Nguyen, Amy S. Aloysi, and Bryant W. Tran

Introduction

Regardless of culture, age, or life experience, pain is a feeling in which all people can relate. Scientific advances have shaped our understanding of pain, but its manifestations are not always predictable. Pain assessments are oversimplified with numerical scores, but in reality, the experience varies between each person, medical problem, and situation. In 1979, the International Association for the Study of Pain defined pain as "an unpleasant sensory and emotional experience associated with actual or potential tissue damage, or described in terms of such damage."[1] As our understanding of pain grows, many have questioned if this definition is still sufficient. Pain is now thought of as a subjective, multidimensional experience. An individual's perceptions mold their processing of experiences. This incorporates factors beyond sensory and emotional experiences as previously defined (Fig. 9.1).

Physiologic Processing of Pain

With advancements in technology, our understanding of pain has evolved. Previously, the brain and sensory processing of pain was believed to be a part of thalamic processing or solely sensory processing. However, anatomical studies including imaging studies such as functional magnetic resonance imaging and positron emission tomography have revealed several cortical areas involved in pain. Several studies agree the parietal, insular, and anterior cingulate cortices play major roles in acute pain perception and each likely process different aspects of pain.[2-4] This leads us to believe that pain should not be thought of as two distinct branches of physical sensory vs emotional behavior components. Rather, these elements interact with one another within neural networks resulting in multidimensional pain. These studies reveal multiple physiologic changes that occur in response to painful stimuli. For example, cerebral brain flow increases in specific regions in response to painful stimuli in humans and animals. Functional image studies reflect different responses when acute pain is introduced to a site of chronic pain vs acute pain to a pain-naive site.[5] These findings point to a complex physiologic processing of pain that is beyond the traditionally taught neurologic pain tracts (Fig. 9.2).

Individual Experience of Pain

The experience of pain, like many other medical conditions, varies between each patient. Looking at objective data from functional imaging studies, findings continue to support individual differences in pain perception.[6] Beyond physiologic differences, several factors alter the experience of pain including family history, cultures, gender, and psychology.

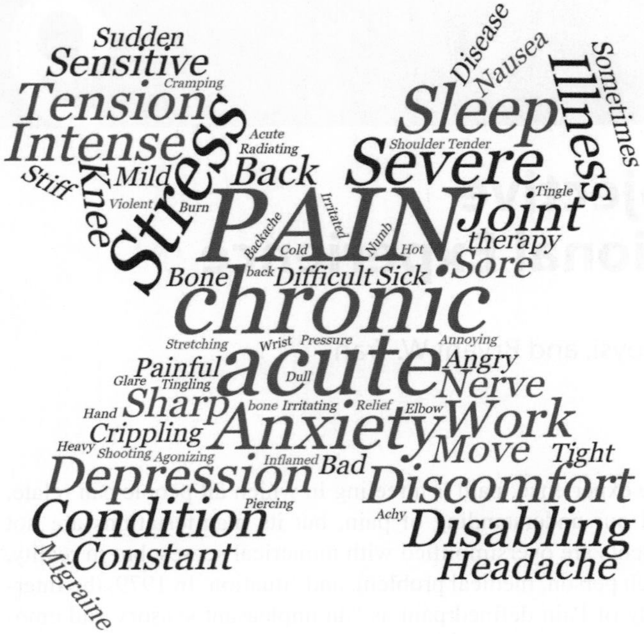

FIGURE 9.1 Sensory and emotional experiences associated with pain.

Studies have found that family history can shape an individual's experience of pain. Parental models affect an individual's response including reaction to pain and affect the frequency in which a patient may report pain. This is a reflection of coping mechanisms learned throughout childhood to stressors. Family history of pain may serve as a predictor to a patient's experience of pain and is an important area of focus when considering management especially in pediatric populations.[7,8] It may suggest a future direction of managing a family's pain and coping techniques rather than fixating on the individual level.

When looking at gender differences in the experience of pain, several studies have found women experience more chronic pain with higher incidences of migraines, fibromyalgia, and lower back pain. However, when looking at acute pain, such as the postoperative setting, there is minimal clinical difference between males and females.[9] In studies investigating the sex differences in pain perception, women tend to have stronger modulation to pain with increased inhibitory responses to repeated, painful stimuli. Women tend to have greater awareness of their pain, but this does not translate to a higher frequency of reported pain.[10] Many theories have been offered to explain the different pain thresholds and responses between men and women, but it is not yet fully understood.[9] Many argue that the socioeconomic and cultural factors may skew the data around genders differences to pain, given that most studies are focused on homogenous culture sample groups. This remains an important area of study, as women and men both respond to pain interventions differently. In order to optimize pain management in both the acute and chronic setting, additional research must be done to better understand the contribution of gender to multidimensional pain.

Genetics of pain medicine has been of greater interest in the past decade as the field of medicine has transitioned toward personalized treatment. In the past, cytochrome P-450 variants have been classically taught and discussed in the field in anesthesia as many medications undergo hepatic metabolism. For example, it is widely established that variants of CYP2D6, a cytochrome P-450 enzyme, affects a patient's response to codeine due to its role in metabolizing codeine to its active form, morphine.[11] Many have investigated the genetic elements of melanocortin 1 receptor, which is commonly associated with red hair, and its effect on analgesics and sedation. Recently, genetic studies have offered greater insight especially into chronic

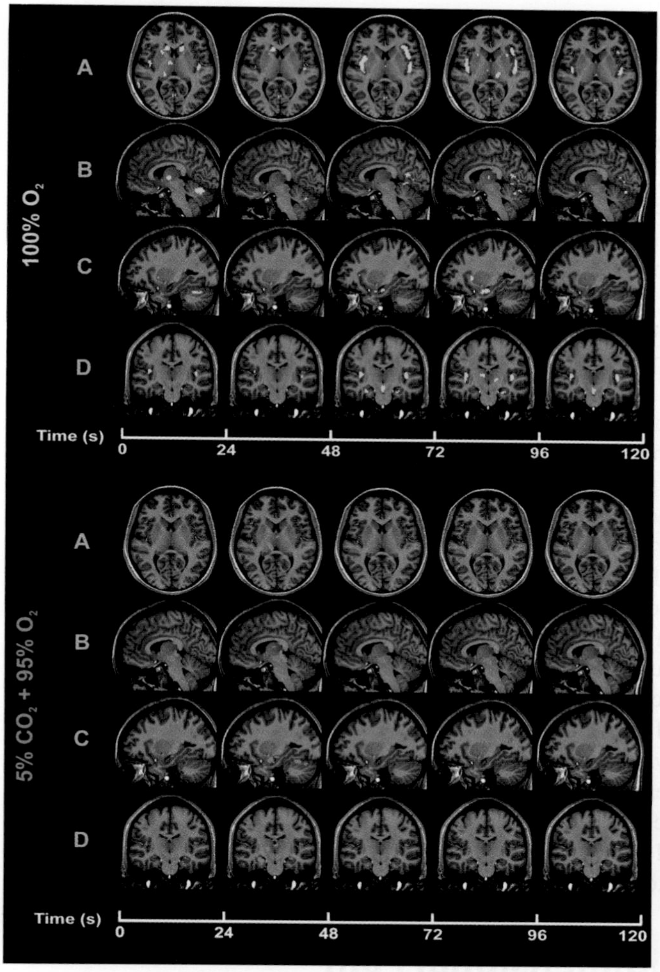

FIGURE 9.2 Functional MRI demonstrating pain processing. (Macey PM, Woo MA, Harper RM. Hyperoxic brain effects are normalized by addition of CO2. PLoS Med. 2007;4(5):e173. doi:10.1371/journal.pmed.0040173)

pain disorders and may be used in the future to predict postoperative pain needs. One of the most commonly studied genes is COMT, a gene associated with catechol-*O*-methyltransferase encoding, which plays a major role in adrenergic pathways. It is linked in several chronic pain disorders, and various polymorphisms have been linked with increased risk of chronic pain. Several other polymorphisms of genes such as ADRB2, HTR2A, SLC6A4, and SERPINA1 suggest an important genetic link between psychological disorders and predisposition to chronic pain.[12] These polymorphisms underline the physiologic impacts of psychological disorders. As research into the genetic elements of pain expands, it may shed more light on the clinical phenotypes associated with polymorphisms and guide patient response to pharmacologic agents with the potential for gene modulation of pain. This may lead to an era of individualized therapies with targeted pain modulation based on genetic data with greater pain control, minimal adverse effects, and improved integration of psychological disorder management.

Psychological Elements of Pain

Pain is a sensory experience that by definition is deeply intertwined with emotional experience. The Latin word "dolor," itself, is twofold in its dimensions, providing for corporeal as well as mental aspects of its meaning. The psychic aspect of *dolor* can be translated as: "a general designation of every painful, oppressive feeling (pain, distress, grief, tribulation, affliction, sorrow, anguish, trouble, vexation, mortification, chagrin)."[13]

The pain stimulus from the periphery is processed in brain regions intricately linked to emotional centers, resulting in feelings of anxiety, fear, sadness, and depression. The region where the emotional processing of nociception is thought to take place is the anterior insular cortex, where interoception, or conscious awareness of bodily state, occurs.[14] In particular, the rostral agranular insular cortex region has multiple connections to limbic cortices and mediates the affective aspects of pain.[14]

Pain is a uniquely subjective experience, and the individual patient's past experiences, personality, and expectations color the manifestation of symptoms. The psychological experience of pain drives a desire to escape or remove oneself from the noxious stimulus—sensation, emotion, and cognition are all involved.[14] A patient may feel unable to escape pain, thus trapped, increasingly focusing on it with associated rumination, depression, anxiety, and even suicidal ideation. Depression and anxiety are common comorbidities of chronic pain, affecting nearly 70% of chronic pain patients and are associated with higher rates of disability.[15]

A common cognitive distortion in the experience of pain is "catastrophizing," in which the worst outcomes are forecast, with accompanying amplification of distress. Pain catastrophizing is characterized by magnifying the threat of the pain stimulus, feelings of helplessness, and inability to stop thinking about the pain, before, during, or after the encounter.[16] Pain catastrophizing is associated with a number of negative outcomes, including higher pain scores, poorer adjustment, and even acute postoperative pain levels.[17]

Acute pain can evolve into chronic pain, defined as lasting for more than 3 months. The process of the chronification of pain may be associated with changes in the functional connectivity of the insular circuitry.[14] Early interventions in the first few months may be helpful in preventing distress and suffering in pain syndromes.[18] Factors associated with lower pain scores and better adjustment include self-efficacy, pain coping strategies, readiness to change, and acceptance.[18] Psychological interventions including cognitive-behavioral therapy can help provide these skills to patients to reduce the burden of disability from acute and chronic pain.

Approach to Multidimensional Pain

While research into pain is still underway to better understand the different elements that lead to the presentation of pain, it is important to consider these other facets to pain management. Mental health is a vital component of a person's well-being, but it is often overlooked in clinical evaluations. It plays a large role in a patient's clinical course and their experience of pain. However, pain is often looked at as a very objective, black and white marker. Usually, it is graded on a scale up to 10, but in reality, understanding a patient's pain often goes beyond a numerical value. This issue becomes very apparent in settings of palliative care, where pain is often the most common symptom, and the management of pain is the goal of their patient's well-being. Palliative care centers have put effort into developing pain assessment surveys to better elucidate the etiology of their patients' pain and its impact on their quality of life.[19] More descriptive pain assessments have been developed to understand a patient's pain outside of the palliative care setting in attempts to change the manner that pain is routinely assessed, and when compared to traditional pain scores, they were found to be better tools to guide multidimensional pain management.[20] Key components that these new assessments include are depression, anxiety, quality of life, and impact on life.

While it is difficult to offer "prophylaxis" for pain, it is possible to offer expectations for pain. When prescribed pain medication, patients may walk away not understanding the degree a medication may help or the significant side effects that may come with the medication. These are important conversations to incorporate into pain management. It allows a patient to weigh the risks and benefits of a treatment, and it creates a mental construct of their health and life after an intervention.

Pain is a field that continues to evolve. As it does, other dimensions of pain may be better understood and targeted for management. Until then, it is important to investigate each element of pain and understand a patient's mental health.

REFERENCES

1. Merskey H, Albe Fessard D, Bonica JJ, et al. Pain terms: a list with definitions and notes on usage. Recommended by the IASP subcommittee on taxonomy. *Pain*. 1979;6:249-252.
2. Talbot JD, Marrett S, Evans AC, et al. Multiple representations of pain in human cerebral cortex. *Science*. 1991;251:1355-1358.
3. Jones AKP, Derbyshire SWG. PET imaging of pain-related somatosensory cortical activity. In: Bromm B, Desmedt JE, eds. *Pain and the Brain: From Nociception to Cognition, Advances in Pain Research and Therapy*. Lippincott-Raven; 1995.
4. Derbyshire SWG, Jones AKP, Gyulai F, et al. Pain processing during three levels of noxious stimulation produces differential patterns of central activity. *Pain*. 1997;73:431-445.
5. Apkarian AV, Krauss BR, Fredrickson BE, et al. Imaging the pain of low back pain: functional magnetic resonance imaging in combination with monitoring subjective pain perception allows the study of clinical pain states. *Neurosci Lett*. 2001;299:57-60.
6. Peyron R, García-Larrea L, Grégoire MC, et al. Parietal and cingulate processes in central pain. A combined positron emission tomography (PET) and functional magnetic resonance imaging (fMRI) study of an unusual case. *Pain*. 2000;84(1):77-87.
7. Edwards PWB, Zeichner A, Kuczmierczyk AR, et al. Familial pain models: the relationship between family history of pain and current pain experience. *Pain*. 1985;21(4):379-384.
8. Schanberg LE, Anthony KK, Gil KM, et al. Family pain history predicts child health status in children with chronic rheumatic disease. *Pediatrics*. 2001;108(3):E47.
9. Fillingim RB, King CD, Ribeiro-Dasilva MC, et al. Sex, gender, and pain: a review of recent clinical and experimental findings. *J Pain*. 2009;10(5):447-485.
10. Koutantji M, Pearce SA, Oakley DAB. The relationship between gender and family history of pain with current pain experience and awareness of pain in others. *Pain*. 1998;77(1):25-31.
11. Ulrike MS, Lehnen K, Höthker F, et al. Impact of CYP2D6 genotype on postoperative tramadol analgesia. *Pain*. 2003;105(1):231-238.
12. Diatchenko L, Fillingim RB, Smith SB, et al. The phenotypic and genetic signatures of common musculoskeletal pain conditions. *Nat Rev Rheumatol*. 2013;9(6):340-350.
13. Lewis & Short: Latin-English Dictionary. Ed. Charles Short. 1879. Oxford University Press. https://www.latinitium.com/latin-dictionaries?t=lsn14669,do130,do157
14. Lu C, Yang T, Zhao H, et al. Insular cortex is critical for the perception, modulation, and chronification of pain. *Neurosci Bull*. 2016;32(2):191-201.
15. de Heer EW, Gerrits MM, Beekman AT, et al. The association of depression and anxiety with pain: a study from NESDA. *PLoS One*. 2014;9(12):e115077.
16. Quartana PJ, Campbell CM, Edwards RR. Pain catastrophizing: a critical review. *Expert Rev Neurother*. 2009;9(5):745-758.
17. Sobol-Kwapinska M, Bąbel P, Plotek W, Stelcer B. Psychological correlates of acute postsurgical pain: a systematic review and meta-analysis. *Eur J Pain*. 2016;20(10):1573-1586.
18. Keefe FJ, Rumble ME, Scipio CD, et al. Psychological aspects of persistent pain: current state of the science. *J Pain*. 2004;5(4):195-211.
19. Hølen JC, Hjermstad MJ, Loge JH, et al. Pain assessment tools: is the content appropriate for use in palliative care? *J Pain Symptom Manage*. 2006;32(6):567-580.
20. van Boekel RLM, Vissers KCP, van der Sande R, et al. Moving beyond pain scores: multidimensional pain assessment is essential for adequate pain management after surgery. *PLoS One*. 2017;12(5):e0177345.

10

Prediction and Prevention of Persistent Postsurgical Pain

Alan David Kaye, Nicole Rose Rueb, Lindsey K. Xiong, Stewart J. Lockett, Victoria L. Lassiegne, and Elyse M. Cornett

Introduction

Persistent postsurgical pain (PPSP) is chronic pain that lasts at least 3 months after surgery. The pain cannot be attributed to any other cause, such as infection or cancer, and must be distinctly characterized from any pain before the surgery.[1,2] PPSP can occur after a variety of procedures, including herniorrhaphy and cesarean sections, thoracotomies, radical mastectomies, and hysterectomies.[3] PPSP occurs in 10%-50% of patients. Severe PPSP affects as many as 2%-10% of all adults undergoing surgery. Possible etiologies of PPSP include persistent inflammation or damage to peripheral nerves resulting in neuropathic pain.

Inflammatory pain is defined as pain that occurs in response to tissue injury and inflammation. Inflammatory pain results from the release of inflammatory mediators leading to a lower threshold of nociceptors resulting in increased neuronal excitability. Neuropathic pain is caused by nerve injuries leading to aberrant transmission to the spinal cord and to the brain. Two of the most important determinants for the development of PPSP include iatrogenic nerve injury leading to neuropathic pain and the patient's severity of preoperative pain.[4] Severe preoperative pain is associated with sustained nociceptive input leading to changes in the central nervous system. The sustained nociceptive input may be enhanced by opioids leading to an exaggerated postoperative pain response.[5] Other risk factors for the development of PPSP include severity of postoperative pain, multiple surgeries, younger age, female, surgery site, and genetic and psychological influences.[2]

Predictors of the development of PPSP cannot be limited to one clear cause and is difficult to predict related to psychological, emotional, behavioral components, and genetic influences.[6] Methods to reduce the incidence of PPSP can take place preoperatively, perioperatively, and postoperatively. Preoperatively, patients with a high risk of developing PPSP should be identified and receive individualized pain management.[7] Perioperatively, techniques to avoid nerve damage should be implemented whenever possible. Postoperatively, acute pain management must be addressed since there is a correlation between a patient's intensity of acute postoperative pain and their predilection to develop PPSP.[4] Prior research on PPSP has focused on pharmacotherapy and drug modality, including patient-controlled analgesia and spinal delivery methods. However, PPSP is often inadequately treated. Research focus has shifted to evaluating patient individualized increased response to pain and patient inadequate response to analgesics. Methods of assessing preoperative pain include quantitative sensory testing (QST), which assesses quantifiable pain responses to mechanical, thermal, or electrical stimuli.[5] The QST measures pain thresholds to best quantify hyperalgesia.[8] QST may be a valuable source in predicting postoperative pain.[6]

Persistent postsurgical pain can lead to prolonged rehabilitation, poor surgical outcomes, and an increased risk of cardiovascular and pulmonary complications.[7] Proper preoperative screening for the susceptibility of PPSP and implementation of individualized therapies may lead to improvements in short-term and long-term morbidities caused by PPSP.[5] The following chapter explains risk factors for developing PPSP, prevention, and intervention.

Risk Factors of Persistent Postsurgical Pain

Risk factors for PPSP include genetic, demographic, psychosocial, pain, medical comorbidities, and surgical factors.[9]

Demographic Risk Factors

Younger age is associated with an increased risk of PPSP across multiple surgical types, including breast, cardiac, and hernia repair.[9-15] Few studies site female sex as a risk factor for postoperative pain.[9,16-18] However, more recent analyses show equivocal data on gender as a significant risk factor for PPSP, warranting further research.[9,13,15,19-21]

Genetic Risk Factors

The most extensively studied genetic target for PPSP is the COMT gene, which encodes catechol-*O*-methyltransferase enzyme and has been studied repeatedly in relation to experimental pain, chronic pain, and acute postoperative pain.[9,22-26] However, only a few studies have shown a significant association between COMT gene polymorphisms and PPSP, and this was only in the presence of another risk factor, pain catastrophizing.[25,27-29]

Medical Comorbidities

Preoperative medical comorbidities, their number, and severity may be important predictors of PPSP across multiple surgical types, with an emphasis on increased numbers especially important for predicting outcomes.[30-32]

Psychosocial Factors

Psychosocial factors, including depression, trait, and state anxiety; pain catastrophizing; and stress have often been implicated in the development of PPSP. However, meta-analyses have shown equivocal outcomes on the size of their effect.[33-38] Pain catastrophizing, as a key risk factor, is defined as the propensity to magnify the threat of pain and feel helpless in the context of painful stimuli.[32-34,39-42] In a meta-analysis, Theunissen and colleagues discerned that 55% of included studies found preoperative anxiety and pain catastrophizing as statistically significant predictors for PPSP, with no studies supporting a reversed effect and all studies with larger sample sizes indicating a positive correlation.[9,33] In conjunction with a more recent meta-analysis by Giusti and colleagues, researchers posit a weak, albeit statistically and clinically significant association between depression, state anxiety, trait anxiety, self-efficacy, and pain catastrophizing and PPSP.[33,35,37]

Pain as a Risk Factor

Pain has been repeatedly identified as the strongest predictor of PPSP across multiple surgery types. Preoperative pain, its duration, location, and intensity is a major risk factor for the development of acute postsurgical pain (APSP) and PPSP.[4,9,12,14,17,21,26,34,38,43] In multiple hernia repair studies, preoperative pain has been associated with an increased incidence of

PPSP.[12,44,45] Similar correlations were found in amputation populations with preamputation pain and postamputation phantom limb pain and in preoperative breast pain and phantom breast pain after mastectomy.[46-48] Furthermore, an emphasis on APSP and its relationship to PPSP across different surgical types has been reflected in the literature.[9,14,43,49,50] The connection between general preoperative pain, preoperative pain related to the surgical site, APSP, and PPSP is complex as preoperative pain may be attributable to multiple risk factors, including other medical comorbidities, and APSP may be due to increased pain susceptibility either as a consequence of poor pain management preoperatively or postoperatively.[9,34,36,49] Furthermore, Willingham and colleagues found that medical complications postoperatively were the strongest independent predictors of PPSP and associated with a twofold increase in risk of developing PPSP, further suggesting postoperative pain chronification into PPSP.[15]

Surgical Risk Factors

Surgical location and techniques, duration (lasting >3 hours), hospital surgical unit volume, intraoperative nerve handling, use of conventional vs laparoscopic approach, and tissue ischemia have been implicated in increasing risk of PPSP; however, studies also seem to be inconclusive on the size of effect of these risk factors.[9,14,36,44,51-56]

Prevention of Persistent Postsurgical Pain

Modification of Surgical Treatments

Surgical treatments should be used at physicians' discretion as the last step of management for mild disorders or highly symptomatic and potentially life-threatening events. The first preventative method of PPSP is to avoid surgery when possible. If surgery is indicated, several modifications can help avoid PPSP. One modification is decrease the number of nerves dissected and retracted in a surgery.[3] An increased number of nerves dissected and resected has a positive correlation with the severity of PPSP.[3] To decrease the number of neuropathies, minimally invasive surgeries should be implemented. Those surgical decisions include surgical approach (video vs open), type of incision (transverse vs midline), or type of movement (retraction or resection).[3] Additionally, less extensive surgeries should be utilized and include reducing time, less invasive wounds, and time under anesthesia.

Pharmacological Treatments

The anticonvulsants gabapentin and pregabalin are first-line treatments for neuropathic pain and have been studied as a possible treatment for PPSP.[3] Studies show that gabapentin and pregabalin provide a preventative analgesic effect.[3] Tricyclic and antidepressants and serotonin-norepinephrine reuptake inhibitors are used to treat chronic pain with the common association of depression with chronic pain but show no clinically significant effect with PPSP.[3] Nonsteroidal anti-inflammatory drugs and acetaminophen are beneficial to treat acute pain, but their prevention of PPSP has not been demonstrated. Steroids have anti-inflammatory effects and seem to have a positive effect in clinical trials, although there is still much controversy.[57]

Preventative and Perioperative Pain Intervention

Epidural and spinal opioids provide desensitization of nerve endings for a short time but are not completely effective.[58] Preoperative analgesic block significantly decreases acute pain postoperatively.[58] Regional analgesia techniques including peripheral sensitization, wound infiltration, and intercostal nerve blocks have been studied to treat PPSP.[3] However, although all of these are effective to treat acute pain, none of them show clinical significance to treat PPSP.[3]

Steroids have an effect on the hypothalamic-pituitary-adrenal axis, and evidence suggests that decreased hypothalamic-pituitary-adrenal axis activity is associated with poor outcomes after some surgeries.[57] Additionally, NDMA antagonists are associated with a clinically significant decrease in PPSP for up to 6 months, postoperatively. Alpha-2 agonists, such as clonidine, have been used perioperatively to treat acute pain. This is likely due to the antisensitizing and anti-inflammatory effects of these drugs. Furthermore, some evidence suggests that they have a preventative effect on PPSP.[3] Opioids are the analgesics of choice for intraoperative and postoperative pain control. Unfortunately, opioids have a strong correlation with the phenomenon known as "phantom pain." Phantom pain is pain that can radiate from a body part that is no longer there or currently does not have feeling or sensation. However, under the correct circumstances, opioids can be considered a preventative treatment as they are protective against severe postoperative pain, which is a risk factor for PPSP.[3]

Psychological Treatments

Presurgical psychological risk factors for PPSP have been consistently identified.[38] A 2009 systemic review by Kinrichs-Rocker found that depression, psychological vulnerability, stress, and a late return to work have a probable correlation with PPSP.[3] In an acceptance and commitment therapy (ACT), patients are taught a mindful way to respond to postsurgical pain that empowers them to overcome the negative cycle of pain, distress, and avoidance of opioid use to promote quality of life.[38] Clinical outcome data suggest that patients who received care from therapeutic pain specialist reduce their pain and opioid use, but those who also received ACT had a larger decrease in daily opioid use and report less pain and depression.[38] The ACT intervention consists of pain catastrophizing, pain education, redirecting pain, and relaxation with a prerecorded audio.[38] These studies show a promising correlation in psychological therapeutic methods and PPSP.

Significant Clinical Studies

Since sufficient pain control can improve outcomes and patient satisfaction, many studies have turned their attention to developing tools to predict which patients are at high risk for PPSP. One study aimed to test how accurately patients' performance in a tonic cold pain test could predict the development of postoperative pain using supervised machine learning techniques.[2] Nine hundred women were followed for 3 years after breast cancer surgery, and 763 were included in the final data analysis. Patients were required to submerge their hands in cold water (2-4 °C) for the maximum amount of time tolerated but not exceeding 90 seconds. The time to removal was recorded, and their pain was rated from 0 to 10 using a numerical rating scale. Surveys were sent out to the women at various time points for 3 years after their surgery, and the information from the surveys was collected and analyzed using a software package. 61 of 763 women reported PPSP, and the supervised machine learning–derived analysis calculated the negative predicted value (NPV) of this experimental pain predicting model to be 95%, suggesting that the test would be useful to exclude patients from developing persistent pain.[2] Thus, the researchers suggest the use of patient responses to cold-water immersion as a biomarker for the exclusion of the development of postoperative pain.[2] However, the positive predictive value of the test was 10%, indicating a high number of false positives, meaning that it would not be the best test to determine who will experience persistent pain after surgery.

The authors of the same study, who used supervised machine–derived analysis for the prediction of postsurgical pain, also used the software to develop a shorter questionnaire than those currently available to predict the development of postoperative pain. The current questionnaires that are used are very long and demand a significant amount of time and concentration of patients. These types of questionnaires are aimed at assessing certain psychological factors, which may act as modifiable markers of who will and will not develop sustained postsurgical pain.[3] Machine-learned predictors were first trained with several questionnaires containing psychological items, which have been known to correlate with pain and produced a 7-item combination form that performed just and a 69-question survey for predicting postsurgical pain.[3] This shorter survey proved to have a 95% NPV; thus, as the test discussed previously, it would be useful in excluding patients for developing lingering postsurgical pain.

Another study investigated a straightforward preoperative risk score for pain after breast cancer surgery. Four parameters were selected, including (1) preoperative pain at the surgical site, (2) history of depression, (3) age <50 years, and (4) expected pain of high intensity (>6/10).[4] A prospective observational study was then conducted to assess the predicative capacity of the risk score in 200 women undergoing surgery for breast cancer. Points for the score were based on the coefficients of the logistic regression model. A total score ≥2/5 forecasts a risk of developing pain at 4 months >30%.[4] The next step in prediction of postoperative pain would be to expand the research to include different surgery types and apply risk models for these patients. See Table 10.1.

Conclusion

Persistent postsurgical pain is pain that develops at least 3 months after a surgical procedure that is either a continuation of acute postoperative pain or follows an asymptomatic period. PPSP is located within the surgical field or within a dermatome that was affected during surgery. Finally, PPSP cannot be caused by an identifiable factor such as pain that was present preoperatively, cancer, or infection.[1,2] PPSP is difficult to treat despite advances in anesthesia and greatly reduces a patient's quality of life, causing both functional and psychological limitations. Acute postsurgical pain can lead to PPSP via central sensitization, which causes a reduction in nociceptor mechanical threshold. Exaggerated nociceptor responses to noxious stimuli lead to hyperalgesia and allodynia.[3,14]

Persistent postsurgical pain is difficult to treat, so the best treatment offered is symptom control rather than disease modification. Prevention is one of the best methods to reduce incidence of PPSP. Surgeons carry a great responsibility to avoid intraoperative nerve injury. They must have an increased awareness during dissections and retraction to decrease nerve damage. Surgeons must employ techniques to reduce inflammatory responses to nerve damage, which can result in chronic neuropathic pain. Minimally invasive techniques can also be employed to further reduce the risk of nerve damage. Minimally invasive techniques have proven to reduce incidences of PPSP. In a study by Fletcher, rates of PPSP in laparoscopic cholecystectomies is only 8.8% compared to 28% in open cholecystectomies.[59] Patients who are at a higher risk of developing PPSP have historically been inadequately identified.[4] Further analysis of preoperative patient parameters such as gender, age, preexisting conditions, cognitive, emotional, and culture aspects that contribute to pain variability will help future studies identify the most significant risk factors for developing PPSP. Perioperative risk factors such as duration and type of surgery, quantity of nerve damage, and severity and duration of acute postoperative pain should also be quantified to identify patients at risk. Until adequate identification and intervention become the standard for preventing PPSP, preoperative and postoperative pain control should be a priority as the severity of preoperative and postoperative pain often predicts a patient's susceptibility to developing PPSP.[2] Aggressive treatment of preoperative pain is essential due to neuroplasticity following an acute trauma, which can transform acute pain into chronic pain.[60]

TABLE 10.1 IMPORTANT CLINICAL STUDIES RELATED TO POSTSURGICAL PAIN

Author (Year)	Groups Studied and Intervention	Results and Findings	Conclusions
Ramsay (2000)[58]	This is a review that discusses the importance of proper postsurgical pain control in all surgical patients.	The paper suggests that if there is inadequate postsurgical pain control, this may lead to increased morbidity and mortality.	New surgical techniques, pharmacologic analgesia, and physician/nurse awareness are all key elements that should be taken advantage of to help reduce postsurgical pain.
Lotsch (2017)[61]	This was a study of 763 women who were tested to see how a tonic cold pain test correlated with postsurgical pain after breast cancer surgery. Patients immersed their hands in cold water (24 °C) and rated the pain on a scale from 0 to 10.	Data were analyzed using a machine-learned software package, and 61 women were found to have persistent postsurgical pain. The test had a 95% NPV, making it useful for exclusion of developing postoperative pain. The PPV was only 10%, meaning that there is also a high false-positive rate.	The tonic cold pain test may provide a way to exclude those who will not experience persistent postsurgical pain with 95% accuracy.
Lotsch (2018)[62]	Supervised machine learning was utilized to generate a short version of a questionnaire that would have the same predictive performance of pain persistence as full, long surveys in a cohort of 1000 women followed for 3 years after breast cancer surgery.	A 7-question set of the original psychological questions, provided the equivalent predictive performance parameters as the full questionnaires for the development of persistent postsurgical pain. The 7-item version offers a shorter and accurate identification of women in whom persistence of postsurgical pain is improbable (~95% NPV).	Using a machine-learning approach, a short list of seven items gathered from Beck Depression Inventory (BDI) and State-Trait Anxiety Inventory (STAI) is proposed as a foundation for a predictive tool for the persistence of pain after breast cancer surgery.
Dereu (2018)[63]	Prospective observational study that tested the predictive capacity of a 4-item score for persistent pain in 200 patients scheduled for breast cancer surgery. The four items included in the score were (1) preoperative pain at the surgical site, (2) history of depression, (3) age <50 years, and (4) expected pain of high intensity (>6/10).	Points for this score were based on the coefficients of the logistic regression model. A score ≥2/5 points forecasts a risk of developing clinically important pain at 4 months >30%, with an area under the curve-receiver operating characteristic of 0.81.	Known risk factors for persistent pain in patients scheduled for breast cancer surgery were studied, and they constructed a preoperative risk score simple enough to select high-risk patients in future prevention studies.

In summary, PPSP remains a problem for all involved, the patient, surgeons, pain management specialists, and anesthesiologists. Despite pharmacological advances, PPSP remains a problem. PPSP is difficult to treat, and treatments do not offer a cure rather they only offer symptom control at best. Aggressive pre- and postoperative pain intervention and research in quantifying parameters that can predict a patient's susceptibility to PPSP are methods that can be utilized to prevent incidences of PPSP.

REFERENCES

1. Werner MU, Kongsgaard UE. I. Defining persistent post-surgical pain: is an update required? *Br J Anaesth.* 2014;113(1):1-4.
2. Williams G, Howard RF, Liossi C. Persistent postsurgical pain in children and young people: prediction, prevention, and management. *Pain Rep.* 2017;2(5):e616.
3. Thapa P, Euasobhon P. Chronic postsurgical pain: current evidence for prevention and management. *Korean J Pain.* 2018;31(3):155-173.
4. Kehlet H, Jensen TS, Woolf CJ. Persistent postsurgical pain: risk factors and prevention. *Lancet.* 2006;367(9522):1618-1625.
5. Werner MU, Mjöbo HN, Nielsen PR, Rudin Å, Warner DS. Prediction of postoperative pain: a systematic review of predictive experimental pain studies. *Anesthesiology.* 2010;112(6):1494-1502.
6. Raja SN, Jensen TS. Predicting postoperative pain based on preoperative pain perception: are we doing better than the weatherman? *Anesthesiology.* 2010;112(6):1311-1312.
7. Abrishami A, Wong J. Preoperative pain sensitivity and its correlation with postoperative pain and analgesic consumption: a qualitative systematic review. *Anesthesiology.* 2011;114(2):445-457.
8. Martinez V, Fletcher D, Bouhassira D, Sessler DI, Chauvin M. The evolution of primary hyperalgesia in orthopedic surgery: quantitative sensory testing and clinical evaluation before and after total knee arthroplasty. *Anesth Analg.* 2007;105(3):815-821.
9. Schug SA, Bruce J. Risk stratification for the development of chronic postsurgical pain. *Pain Rep.* 2017;2(6):e627.
10. Kroman N, Jensen M-B, Wohlfahrt J, Mouridsen HT, Andersen PK, Melbye M. Factors influencing the effect of age on prognosis in breast cancer: population based study. *BMJ.* 2000;320(7233):474-479.
11. Poleshuck EL, Katz J, Andrus CH, et al. Risk factors for chronic pain following breast cancer surgery: a prospective study. *J Pain.* 2006;7(9):626-634.
12. Poobalan AS, Bruce J, King PM, Chambers WA, Krukowski ZH, Smith WCS. Chronic pain and quality of life following open inguinal hernia repair. *Br J Surg.* 2001;88(8):1122-1126.
13. Gjeilo KH, Klepstad P, Wahba A, Lydersen S, Stenseth R. Chronic pain after cardiac surgery: a prospective study. *Acta Anaesthesiol Scand.* 2010;54(1):70-78.
14. Bruce J, Quinlan J. Chronic post surgical pain. *Rev Pain.* 2011;5(3):23-29.
15. Willingham M, Rangrass G, Curcuru C, et al. Association between postoperative complications and lingering post-surgical pain: an observational cohort study. *Br J Anaesth.* 2020;124(2):214-221.
16. Thomas T, Robinson C, Champion D, McKell M, Pell M. Prediction and assessment of the severity of post-operative pain and of satisfaction with management. *Pain.* 1998;75(2-3):177-185.
17. Perkins FM, Kehlet H. Chronic pain as an outcome of surgery. *Anesthesiology.* 2000;93(4):1123-1133.
18. Kalkman JC, Visser K, Moen J, Bonsel JG, Grobbee ED, Moons MKG. Preoperative prediction of severe postoperative pain. *Pain.* 2003;105(3):415-423.
19. Caumo W, Schmidt AP, Schneider CN, et al. Preoperative predictors of moderate to intense acute postoperative pain in patients undergoing abdominal surgery. *Acta Anaesthesiol Scand.* 2002;46(10):1265-1271.
20. Taillefer M-C, Carrier M, Bélisle S, et al. Prevalence, characteristics, and predictors of chronic nonanginal postoperative pain after a cardiac operation: a cross-sectional study. *J Thorac Cardiovasc Surg.* 2006;131(6):1274-1280.
21. Johansen A, Schirmer H, Stubhaug A, Nielsen CS. Persistent post-surgical pain and experimental pain sensitivity in the Tromso study: comorbid pain matters. *Pain.* 2014;155(2):341-348.
22. Diatchenko L, Slade GD, Nackley AG, et al. Genetic basis for individual variations in pain perception and the development of a chronic pain condition. *Hum Mol Genet.* 2005;14(1):135-143.
23. Diatchenko L, Nackley AG, Slade GD, et al. Catechol-O-methyltransferase gene polymorphisms are associated with multiple pain-evoking stimuli. *Pain.* 2006;125(3):216-224.
24. Kambur O, Kaunisto MA, Tikkanen E, Leal SM, Ripatti S, Kalso EA. Effect of Catechol-o-methyltransferase-gene (COMT) variants on experimental and acute postoperative pain in 1,000 women undergoing surgery for breast cancer. *Anesthesiology.* 2013;119(6):1422-1433.

25. Hoofwijk DMN, van Reij RRI, Rutten BP, Kenis G, Buhre WF, Joosten EA. Genetic polymorphisms and their association with the prevalence and severity of chronic postsurgical pain: a systematic review. *Br J Anaesth.* 2016;117(6):708-719.
26. Montes A, Roca G, Sabate S, et al. Genetic and clinical factors associated with chronic postsurgical pain after hernia repair, hysterectomy, and thoracotomy: a two-year multicenter cohort study. *Anesthesiology.* 2015;122(5):1123-1141.
27. Rut M, Machoy-Mokrzyńska A, Ręcławowicz D, et al. Influence of variation in the catechol-O -methyltransferase gene on the clinical outcome after lumbar spine surgery for one-level symptomatic disc disease: a report on 176 cases. *Acta Neurochir (Wien).* 2014;156(2):245-252.
28. George SZ, Wallace MR, Wright TW, et al. Evidence for a biopsychosocial influence on shoulder pain: pain catastrophizing and catechol-O-methyltransferase (COMT) diplotype predict clinical pain ratings. *Pain.* 2008;136(1):53-61.
29. Hoofwijk DMN, van Reij RRI, Rutten BPF, et al. Genetic polymorphisms and prediction of chronic post-surgical pain after hysterectomy—a subgroup analysis of a multicenter cohort study. *Acta Anaesthesiol Scand.* 2019;63(8):1063-1073.
30. Peters ML, Sommer M, Kleef M, van Marcus MAE. Predictors of physical and emotional recovery 6 and 12 months after surgery. *Br J Surg.* 2010;97(10):1518-1527.
31. Gerbershagen HJ, Dagtekin O, Rothe T, et al. Risk factors for acute and chronic postoperative pain in patients with benign and malignant renal disease after nephrectomy. *Eur J Pain.* 2009;13(8):853-860.
32. Forsythe ME, Dunbar MJ, Hennigar AW, Sullivan MJ, Gross M. Prospective relation between catastrophizing and residual pain following knee arthroplasty: two-year follow-up. *Pain Res Manag.* 2008;13(4):335-341.
33. Theunissen M, Peters ML, Bruce J, Gramke H-F, Marcus MA. Preoperative anxiety and catastrophizing: a systematic review and meta-analysis of the association with chronic postsurgical pain. *Clin J Pain.* 2012;28(9):819-841.
34. Katz J, Seltzer Z. Transition from acute to chronic postsurgical pain: risk factors and protective factors. *Expert Rev Neurother.* 2009;9(5):723-744.
35. Hinrichs-Rocker A, Schulz K, Järvinen I, Lefering R, Simanski C, Neugebauer EAM. Psychosocial predictors and correlates for chronic post-surgical pain (PPSP)—a systematic review. *Eur J Pain.* 2009;13(7):719-730.
36. VanDenKerkhof EG, Peters ML, Bruce J. Chronic pain after surgery: time for standardization? A framework to establish core risk factor and outcome domains for epidemiological studies. *Clin J Pain.* 2013;29(1):2-8.
37. Giusti EM, Lacerenza M, Manzoni GM, Castelnuovo G. Psychological and psychosocial predictors of chronic postsurgical pain: a systematic review and meta-analysis. *Pain.* 2021;162(1):10-30.
38. Weinrib AZ, Azam MA, Birnie KA, Burns LC, Clarke H, Katz J. The psychology of chronic post-surgical pain: new frontiers in risk factor identification, prevention and management. *Br J Pain.* 2017;11(4):169-177.
39. Osman A, Barrios FX, Gutierrez PM, Kopper BA, Merrifield T, Grittmann L. The Pain Catastrophizing Scale: further psychometric evaluation with adult samples. *J Behav Med.* 2000;23(4):351-365.
40. Osman A, Barrios FX, Kopper BA, Hauptmann W, Jones J, O'Neill E. Factor structure, reliability, and validity of the Pain Catastrophizing Scale. *J Behav Med.* 1997;20(6):589-605.
41. Quartana PJ, Campbell CM, Edwards RR. Pain catastrophizing: a critical review. *Expert Rev Neurother.* 2009;9(5):745-758.
42. Sullivan MJL, Bishop SR, Pivik J. The Pain Catastrophizing Scale: development and validation. *Psychol Assess.* 1995;7(4):524-532.
43. Althaus A, Hinrichs-Rocker A, Chapman R, et al. Development of a risk index for the prediction of chronic post-surgical pain. *Eur J Pain.* 2012;16(6):901-910.
44. Liem SL, Van Duyn B, Van Der Graaf JMV, Van Vroonhoven JMV. Recurrences after conventional anterior and laparoscopic inguinal hernia repair: a randomized comparison. *Ann Surg.* 2003;237(1):136-141.
45. Wright D, Paterson C, Scott N, Hair A, O'Dwyer PJ. Five-year follow-up of patients undergoing laparoscopic or open groin hernia repair. *Ann Surg.* 2002;235(3):333-337.
46. Karanikolas M, Aretha D, Tsolakis I, et al. Optimized perioperative analgesia reduces chronic phantom limb pain intensity, prevalence, and frequency a prospective, randomized, clinical trial. *Anesthesiology.* 2011;114(5):1144-1154.
47. Krøner K, Knudsen UB, Lundby L, Hvid H. Long-term phantom breast syndrome after mastectomy. *Clin J Pain.* 1992;8(4):346-350.
48. Nikolajsen L, Ilkjaer S, Krøner K, Christensen JH, Jensen TS. The influence of preamputation pain on postamputation stump and phantom pain. *Pain.* 1997;72(3):393-405.
49. Gerbershagen HJ. Transition from acute to chronic postsurgical pain. *Schmerz.* 2013;27(1):81-96.
50. Roth RS, Qi J, Hamill JB, et al. Is chronic postsurgical pain surgery-induced? A study of persistent postoperative pain following breast reconstruction. *Breast.* 2018;37:119-125.
51. Fregoso G, Wang A, Tseng K, Wang J. Transition from acute to chronic pain: evaluating risk for chronic postsurgical pain. *Pain Physician.* 2019;22(5):479-488.
52. McGreevy K, Bottros MM, Raja SN. Preventing chronic pain following acute pain: risk factors, preventive strategies, and their efficacy. *Eur J Pain Suppl.* 2011;5(2):365-372.

53. Wildgaard K, Ravn J, Kehlet H. Chronic post-thoracotomy pain: a critical review of pathogenic mechanisms and strategies for prevention. *Eur J Cardiothorac Surg*. 2009;36(1):170-180.
54. Peters ML, Sommer M, de Rijke JM, et al. Somatic and psychologic predictors of long-term unfavorable outcome after surgical intervention. *Ann Surg*. 2007;245(3):487-494.
55. Cerfolio RJ, Price TN, Bryant AS, Sale Bass C, Bartolucci AA. Intracostal sutures decrease the pain of thoracotomy. *Ann Thorac Surg*. 2003;76(2):407-411; discussion 411-412.
56. Tasmuth T, Blomqvist C, Kalso E. Chronic post-treatment symptoms in patients with breast cancer operated in different surgical units. *Eur J Surg Oncol*. 1999;25(1):38-43.
57. Richebé P, Capdevila X, Rivat C. Persistent postsurgical pain: pathophysiology and preventative pharmacologic considerations. *Anesthesiology*. 2018;129(3):590-607.
58. Ramsay MA. Acute postoperative pain management. *Proc (Bayl Univ Med Cent)*. 2000;13:244-247.
59. Fletcher D, Stamer UM, Pogatzki-Zahn E, et al. Chronic postsurgical pain in Europe: an observational study. *Eur J Anaesthesiol*. 2015;32(10):725-734.
60. Kraychete DC, Sakata RK, Lannes L de OC, Bandeira ID, Sadatsune EJ. Postoperative persistent chronic pain: what do we know about prevention, risk factors, and treatment. *Braz J Anesthesiol*. 2016;66(5):505-512.
61. Lötsch J, Ultsch A, Kalso E. Prediction of persistent post-surgery pain by preoperative cold pain sensitivity: biomarker development with machine-learning-derived analysis. *Br J Anaesth*. 2017;119(4):821-829. doi:10.1093/bja/aex236
62. Lötsch J, Sipilä R, Tasmuth T, et al. Machine-learning-derived classifier predicts absence of persistent pain after breast cancer surgery with high accuracy. *Breast Cancer Res Treat*. 2018;171(2):399-411. doi:10.1007/s10549-018-4841-8
63. Dereu D, Savoldelli GL, Combescure C, Mathivon S, Rehberg B. Development of a simple preoperative risk score for persistent pain after breast cancer surgery: a prospective observational cohort study. *Clin J Pain*. 2018;34(6):559-565. doi:10.1097/AJP.0000000000000575

11

Running a Postoperative Pain Management Service

Alex D. Pham, Matthew R. Eng, Oscar A. Alam Mendez, Oren Cohen, Alan David Kaye, and Richard D. Urman

Introduction

Postoperative pain is a major problem. Up to 86% of patients experience postoperative pain with 75% of those reporting as moderate to severe in nature.[1] In fact, Tennant et al. reported that over half of patients reported inadequate pain management following their own cases.[2] Management of postoperative pain is tantamount for several reasons. Given that the opioid epidemic has nearly claimed 450 000 lives from overdose involving elicit and prescription opioids from 1999 to 2018, the role of opioids and attenuation of postoperative pain is crucial.[3] Excess opioid prescription is now recognized as an important factor of opioid abuse.[4] Furthermore, there are concerns that acute pain can become chronic pain.[4] Specific surgeries have been sighted to increase risk of acute postoperative pain becoming chronic pain including inguinal hernia repair, thoracotomy, and breast surgery.[5] Postoperative pain is one of the most common factors cited for unexpected admissions to the hospital as well as delayed discharge.[5] Given these factors and the fact that controlling postoperative pain can be challenging, it is necessary to establish an effective postoperative pain management service.

In this chapter, we will discuss and review (1) current postoperative pain management models, (2) general postoperative pain treatment strategies, (3) utility of pain specialist on site, (4) regular pain assessment measurement tools, (5) continued pain education of patient and team involved, (6) adopting analgesic guidelines such as the enhanced recovery after surgery (ERAS) guidelines, (7) documentation/follow-up plans, and (8) importance of maintaining communication among the team involved in the patient's care. It is our aim that we be able to review current guidelines and models to effectively run a postoperative pain management services to optimize postoperative pain control for our patients.

Current Postoperative Pain Management Models

Pain control in the perioperative setting has a direct influence in surgical outcomes. A patient experiencing unrelieved pain will have a decreased overall satisfaction and have difficulty engaging in rehabilitation sessions. This will lead to a prolonged recovery and an increase in morbidity, mortality, and the risk of developing persistent pain after surgery.[6-8] For this reason, an acute pain service (APS) is created as a multidisciplinary team focused on pain management and improving patient functional capacity in the preoperative, intraoperative, and postoperative phases.

An APS consists of a group of motivated medical providers who have knowledge in regional anesthesia and multimodal analgesia. These providers further elaborate an analgesic plan and perform peripheral or neuraxial blocks in the perioperative setting.[9,10] However, this group of providers could benefit from additional medical specialties who could help create a well-rounded approach to treating patients.

The evolution to a formalized service will involve the organization of a multidisciplinary team (anesthesiologist, nurses, surgeons, social workers, physical and occupational therapist) with well-defined goals in terms of analgesia and patient functional capacity.[11-13] This involves the allocation of financial, structural, and personnel resources to streamline patient care via specific protocols that result in low variability and effort, with high throughput patient care.[10]

Not every protocol can be strictly applied on every situation. In some instances, changes to the original plan must be made tailored to each patient. These circumstances could be the type of surgery, past medical history, medication history, and patient's desire. Adapting to these variations require depth knowledge in pain management, pharmacology, and multimodal analgesia (including interventional pain management such as neuraxial or peripheral nerve blocks) to select the most appropriate and safest plan.

Essential competencies of a modern APS were described in 2002 by N. Rawal in the Regional Anesthesia and Pain Medicine editorial, which remain the core goals of the discipline today.[14] (1) The APS must be available around the clock to provide consultation and interventions for severe acute pain; (2) Team leaders must round on the patients and assess pain severity and treatment efficacy; (3) The APS team must consist of communication between surgical teams, ward nurses, physical/occupational therapists, and pharmacologist in behalf of patient recovery; (4) The APS team must engage in continuing education for all medical providers, regarding safety and analgesia; (5) Continuous patient education on expectations and available treatments; (6) The APS team must undergo periodic audits and quality controls to ensure the best possible APS system.

Since the 1990s, the number ambulatory surgeries in the United States have increased more than 100%,[15,16] and the number of outpatient surgical procedures in the United States is expected to grow from ~129 million procedures in 2018 to ~144 million procedures by 2023. APS should provide optimal postoperative pain management to patients who receive outpatient procedures.

The complexity in this situation is being efficient with the utilization of time and resources in a high passed center. In a short period, the APS team should identify patients who are at risk for increased postoperative pain (chronic pain patients, history of substance abuse, and orthopedic surgeries) and develop an optimum pain control strategy for each patient who would prevent emergency room visits, delayed discharges, and unplanned re-admissions (by uncontrolled nausea, vomiting, or pain; over sedation with respiratory depression; or complications related to regional anesthesia).[5] For these reasons, it is imperative the implementation of multimodal analgesia (including regional techniques and peripheral nerve blocks catheters) to minimize opioids requirements. In the immediate postoperative period, nausea, vomiting, and pain should be treated aggressively with rescue medications. Effectiveness of nerve blocks and possible complications should be evaluated.

Upon discharge, instruction to continue nonopioids analgesic should be the first line. In cases when opioids are warranted, only short-acting opioids should be prescribed. In case of chronic pain patients, the medications should be individualized and early follow-up with the chronic pain clinic is advised.[5] In case of nerve catheter was used for outpatient pain control, the patient should receive specific clear instruction regarding nerve catheter maintenance and expectations upon catheter removal. The patient should be contacted over the phone daily by the APS personnel until the catheter is discontinued.

General Treatment Strategies

Pain is defined as an unpleasant sensory and emotional experience associated with actual or potential tissue damage.[17] The perception of pain can be complicated and can be dictated by several variables.[18] Good pain management in the perioperative period is not just humane, but also, poorly controlled pain has been related to increased morbidity and mortality[17,19-22] secondary to inability to participate in early rehabilitation, delaying discharge, prolonging recovery times,[19] and increased risk of persistent postsurgical pain[23] that contribute with the opioid crisis that we are facing.

Nociception is the process of a noxious stimulus as a result of four main processes: transduction, transmission, modulation, and perception. Transduction is the conversion of the stimulus to a signal or electrical impulse by a peripheral nociceptor. Transmission is the propagation of the impulse from the periphery to central nervous system. Modulation is the amplification or dampening of the signals by the release of excitatory or inhibitory neuropeptides in the dorsal horn of the spinal cord. Perception is processing of the signal by the sensory cortex.[24] Many medications to decrease pain target one or multiple areas of pain perception. Please refer to Table 11.1 for complete general treatment options.

Opioids are by far the mainstay treatment of moderate to severe nociceptive pain, especially in cancer-related situations. A retrospective study across 380 U.S. hospitals showed that about 95% of surgical patients were treated with opioids.[25]

The reason for their popularity is secondary to their effectiveness to decrease pain, multiple forms of administration and formulations (oral, intravascular, transdermal, sublingual, rectal, subcutaneous, intramuscular, transnasal, or neuraxial), they do not have ceiling effect, they have different modes of administration (scheduled, as needed, patient-controlled analgesia, or continuous infusion), and they have been widely studied drugs.

The main mechanism of action for analgesia is through opioid receptors agonism: μ, κ, and δ located in the peripheral and central nervous system. They are G protein coupled and, when activated, produce reduction of neuronal excitability by hyperpolarization on neurons capable of transduce, modulate, and perceive pain. This activation also explains their well-known side effects: respiratory depression, sedation, euphoria, and decreased gastrointestinal motility.[26] These side effects are responsible for increased morbidity, mortality, and length of stay[17,19,20] after surgery. This has generated the need for a shift in management when approaching postoperative analgesia.

Multimodal analgesia aims to reduce the of opioid dependency in the perioperative period by combining analgesic agents with different mechanism of actions, that work in conjunction to achieve a better analgesia, decreasing the opioid consumption, and consequently diminishing their associated side effects.[27] Commonly used drugs are nonsteroidal anti-inflammatory drugs (NSAIDs), acetaminophen, gabapentinoids, NMDA antagonist, and local anesthetics.

Nonsteroidal anti-inflammatory drugs like ketorolac, ibuprofen, or celecoxib interfere in the transmission and perception of pain. They exert their effect by inhibiting the enzyme cyclooxygenase 1 (COX-1) and/or cyclooxygenase 2 (COX-2) at the peripheral nociceptor

TABLE 11.1 GENERAL TREATMENT STRATEGIES SUMMARY[17-39]

1. Opioids (oral, intravascular, transdermal, sublingual, rectal, subcutaneous, intramuscular, transnasal, or neuraxial)
2. Multimodal analgesia
   i. NSAID
      - Ketorolac
      - Ibuprofen
      - Celecoxib
   ii. Acetaminophen
   iii. Gabapentinoids
      - Pregabalin
      - Gabapentin
   iv. Local anesthetics (epidural, spinal, perineural)
   v. Ketamine

and at the dorsal horn. As consequence, the production of prostaglandins from arachidonic acid is blocked, which decreases inflammation. NSAIDs have shown to reduce opioid requirements in mild to moderate pain and increased patient satisfaction.[28-30] Related side effects are a product of their own mechanism of action; by inhibiting COX-1, the decreasing production of prostaglandins E2 (PGE2) makes the gastric mucosa propene to gastric ulcers; decreasing PGE2 along with prostaglandin I2 (PGI2) impairs renal blood flow rising the risk of developing or worsening renal failure; blocking platelet's COX-1 decreases the formation of thromboxane A2 and interferes with platelet aggregation and bleeding. Selective COX-2 inhibitors like celecoxib have the advantage of not increasing the risk of bleeding or gastrointestinal ulceration; however, evidence shown a mild increased risk of cardiovascular events.[31]

Acetaminophen falls into the analgesics and antipyretic medications. Although its main mechanism of action is not well defined, it decreases prostaglandin production centrally in the brain (by blocking COX-1 and COX-2). Studies have also demonstrated the possibility of a variant form; COX-3.[32] Studies confirm its benefits in decreasing opioid requirements.[30] Unlike NSAIDs, acetaminophen lacks peripheral anti-inflammatory properties and can, therefore, be taken in combination with NSAIDs. This combination might be more effective than either NSAID or acetaminophen alone to decrease opioid consumption.[33] Although acetaminophen has a good safety profile, hepatotoxicity is a risk when daily doses surpass the 4000 mg.

Gabapentinoids (pregabalin and gabapentin) are involved in the pain modulation by inhibiting alpha-2-delta subunit of voltage-gated calcium channels in the dorsal horn.[31] Although off-label usage in the perioperative period, they have shown to have an opioid-sparing effect, reducing pain scores in the first 24 hours after surgery and improving neuropathic pain.[34] There is evidence of decreasing postoperative persistent pain by inhibiting central sensitization.[33] Increased sedation and visual impairments are some of the side effects.

Local anesthetics have been used extensively for thoracic and abdominal surgery via epidural, spinal, or peripheral nerve blocks. Local anesthetics interfere with transduction and transmission of painful stimulus by blocking sodium channels and preventing neuronal depolarization.

Epidural analgesia has shown improve surgical outcomes by decreasing surgical blood loss, incidence of thromboembolic events, postoperative pain, and improving pulmonary function,[23] although these findings have been challenged in by other authors.[35,36] When compared to patient-controlled analgesia, epidural analgesia has shown to achieve better pain control in the first 72 hours postoperative in multiple randomized controlled trials.[19] Common complications from epidural catheter placement include hypotension, urinary retention, and inadequate analgesia, which can happen in 27% of patients after lumbar and 32% after thoracic epidural.[19] Main indication for epidural analgesia is extensive surgery in a high-risk patient, whereas in minimal invasive surgery, its benefit is more controversial.

Perineural local anesthetic injections are highly effective and are superior to intravenous opioid analgesia. Multiple randomized controlled trials showed that regional anesthesia techniques may prevent persistent pain postoperative following thoracotomy and breast cancer surgery and reduce the associated postoperative nausea, vomiting, and sedation related to opioid usage.[17] But despite this strong evidence, regional anesthesia has poor utilization.[37]

Ketamine is making resurgence in the management of postoperative period in subanesthetic doses. Its mechanism of action is complex, involving NMDA receptor antagonism, μ-opioid receptors, muscarinic receptors, monoaminergic receptors, and γ-aminobutyric acid receptors.[38] It has shown to decrease morphine consumption, pain scores, and postoperative nausea in major abdominal surgeries when given as a bolus during surgery and continuing as an infusion for 48 hours postoperatively.[38,39] The main challenge with this treatment are the psychotomimetic side effects.

Utility of Pain Specialist on Site (Acute Pain/Regional Specialist)

An effective APS may benefit the hospital resource utilization, hospital economics, and most importantly the patient experience and satisfaction.[40] Whether a patient is a surgical patient or experiencing acute pain during their hospitalization, a pain specialist driven service can be beneficial. Cost-effectiveness and a reduction of hospital length of stay have been demonstrated in several patient populations.[40-42] Complications that arise from patients with poor control include postoperative ileus, constipation, nausea/vomiting, pruritus, respiratory depression, and delirium.[43] Anesthetic/pain medication-induced nausea and vomiting is an even greater threat to the patient than pain itself.[44] Expert-guided treatment of pain can reduce hospital length of stay, improve pain control, improve patient satisfaction, and reduce complications of pain medication therapeutics.

Regional anesthesia pain procedures also have a large role in running a pain service.[43,45] Performance of targeted regional pain procedures can reduce the patient's need for opioid medication. Orthopedic surgical patients may benefit from upper extremity or lower extremity blocks. Upper extremity blocks include interscalene nerve block, supraclavicular nerve block, infraclavicular nerve block, or axillary nerve block. Lower extremity nerve blocks include femoral nerve block, saphenous nerve block, iPACK block, PENG block, or popliteal sciatic nerve block. Abdominal pain can be treated with a variety of nerve blocks including the transversus abdominis plane block, rectus sheath block, quadratus lumborum block, or erector spinae block. Regional nerve blocks may be performed as either single-shot procedures with pain relief ranging from hours to days or as continuous catheters that may provide relief through an infusion pump. Neuraxial blockade may also be beneficial to patients to reduce lower extremity pain or abdominal pain. Please refer to Figure 11.1 for benefits of having pain specialist on site.

Patients on chronic opioids pose a challenging issue for admitting physicians.[46,47] The risk of undertreating the patient's pain or overdosing a patient is a constant threat.

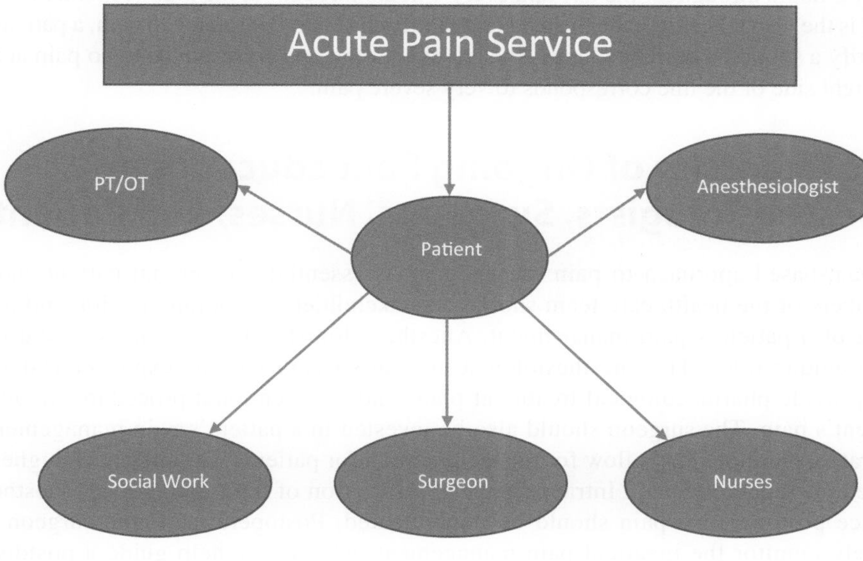

*PT/OT = Physical Therapy/Occupational Therapy

FIGURE 11.1 Benefits of acute pain specialist.[40-47]

A pain service specialist who has more experience provides treatment plans that are safe and effective. Additionally, ethical, psychological, and physiologic negative consequences may result from mismanaged pain. Often, a multimodal approach of regional anesthetic techniques, NSAIDs, anticonvulsants, and other non–opioid-based pain medications is employed.

Regular Pain Assessment of Patients/Rounding/ Pain Assessment Tools

An APS team depends on effective patient educators and accurate assessment of pain.[40] An effective patient educator equips the patient to be informed of different treatment options, side effects, and expectations. Patients need to be presented with an understanding of what pain medications have been prescribed, the frequency, and their expected benefit. A schedule of routine pain medications and PRN pain medications according to pain severity should be well explained. Many institutions implement a communication board with pain scales and pain management plans to facilitate education. Patients should also be educated in regard to side effects and potential complications of taking pain medications. An effective educator should inform the patient of the risks in both overtreating and undertreating pain. Finally, a patient's expectations of what medications or interventional pain procedures should be explained. For instance, many medications or interventional regional nerve blocks may not provide complete pain relief. Matching a patient's expectations with the expected result of a therapeutic improves patient trust and satisfaction with pain management.

Accurate assessment of pain is critical to proper treatment of pain.[48-50] Patients have historically struggled to communicate or quantify the amount of pain they are experiencing. Nurse charting tools should be utilized on a regular basis to track patient pain levels. These tools include the numerical rating scale (NRS), the four P's (presence, pain, position, and personal needs). The 11-point NRS ranges from 0 (no pain) to 10 (worst pain imaginable). Qualitative descriptions of the NRS may be translated as 0-3 mild pain, 46 moderate pain, and 7-10 severe pain. Regular intervals of assessment by nurses improves the diagnosis and treatment of pain, every 2 hours throughout the day and every 4 hours throughout the night. Another commonly used is the visual analog scale. Instead of quantifying a number related to pain, a patient would identify a spot on a horizontal line. The left side of the line corresponds to no pain at all, and the right side of the line corresponds to very severe pain.

The Necessity of Ongoing Pain Education to Anesthesiologists, Surgeons, Nurses, and Patients

A team-based approach to pain management is essential for optimal patient care.[51] All members of the health care team should be stakeholders in communication and management of a patient's pain management. Anesthesiologists, surgeons, nurses, and patients have unique roles. The anesthesiologist or pain specialist is the expert consultant who can provide pharmacological treatment plans and interventional procedures to address a patient's pain. The surgeon should also be invested in a patient's pain management. Preoperative planning may allow for the team to plan for patients who may have higher anticipated postoperative pain. Intraoperatively, infiltration of long-acting local anesthetics to reduce postoperative pain should be implemented. Postoperatively, the surgeon should closely monitor the inpatient pain management, which may help guide a postdischarge pain management plan. Nurses are critical to an acute pain management team. Nurses provide education on pain management expectations, pain assessment tools, and available therapies that the physician has ordered.

Developing and Adopting Analgesic Guidelines: Enhanced Recovery After Surgery (ERAS) Guidelines

Enhanced recovery after surgery protocols are evidence-based guidelines aimed to decrease the time of recovery after a surgical procedure by focusing in preoperative counseling, infection prevention, nutrition, multimodal analgesia, postoperative nausea/vomiting prevention, blood conservative strategies, and early mobilization.

Enhanced recovery after surgery represents an important paradigm shift in the perioperative care that requires the coordination of multiple disciplines like preanesthetic clinic, nurses, physiotherapists, anesthetists, and surgeons.

In the preoperative office visit, patients and their families should be educated on their active role in the recovery process and the upcoming perioperative experiences and expectations; this improves patient anxiety and pain perception leading to a decreased anxiolytic medication and better postoperative pain management.[52] The patients should receive instruction on fasting guidelines, which include 6 hours for solids and a liquid carbohydrate load 2 hours before surgery[52,53]; anemia should be recognized and corrected; tobacco and alcohol cessation should be recommended to improve metabolic state and possible respiratory complications.[53-55]

The day of surgery and the use of anxiolytics should be reserved only for clear cases of patient distress or in preprocedural situations, that is, epidural or peripheral nerve block. When sedation is indicated, long-acting opioids or benzodiazepines should be avoided due to their increased risk of prolonging length of stay.[56] The use of forced-air warming should start in preoperative ward 30-60 minutes before the induction to promote euthermia during surgery. Hypothermia increases the risk of infection, increased blood loss, and increased oxygen requirements.[57]

The use of opioids, especially long-acting ones, carries many side effects like respiratory depression, sedation, urinary retention, and constipation that increase morbidity and mortality.[6,30,52,53] For this reason, it is imperative to decrease the opioid requirements by implementing a multimodal approach to achieve analgesia throughout the perioperative period, with the use of regional anesthesia, gabapentinoids, NSAIDs, acetaminophen, NMDA receptors antagonist, and alpha-2 agonist.[19,30,55]

During the operative period, special attention should be given to the prevention of hypothermia with the continuation of forced air warming; thromboembolic events by administering mechanical and pharmacological such as intermittent pneumatic compression and unfractionated or low molecular heparin, respectively; fluid overload with a goal-directed therapy strategy when possible; and perioperative nausea, vomiting, and infection prevention.

In the postoperative period, ileus has been found to be an independent and major factor for a prolonged discharge.[58-60] It is a consequence of a release of inflammatory mediation secondary to surgical stress,[61] opioids use, and fluid overload. To prevent this from happening, laparoscopic surgery should be used when possible, and the provider should schedule daily postoperative mobilization goals. Furthermore, the use of midthoracic epidural, gum chewing, and fluid overload prevention[62] are all important components of ERAS protocols.

Enhanced recovery after surgery represent a challenge to traditional patient perioperative care,[53,63] and as such, their adherence has been a slow process. It involves a committed multidisciplinary team that must overcome the institutional, financial, staff, and patient-related barriers, to develop and apply proper standardized protocols.[61]

Despite the significant evidence indicating that ERAS protocols improve outcomes such as decreasing patient length of stay, improving patient analgesia and satisfaction, shortening the return to bowel function, and decreasing overall complication and readmissions[52,53,55,56,62]; their success is in a direct relationship with protocol compliance.[53,64-66] This emphasizes the importance of having a cohesive ERAS team focused on continuous education to design and audit protocols and their compliance.[67]

The Importance of Documentation About the Daily Inpatient/Outpatient Follow-up and Plan

An often overlooked and underappreciated aspect of effective patient postoperative pain management is the daily inpatient/outpatient follow-up and plan. Oftentimes, failure of sufficient pain management can be due to poor documentation of the initial and subsequent pain assessments (and, thus, an accurate depiction of the improvement of pain over time), accurate evaluation of pain type and location, efficacy and response to medications already administered, and an accurate and concise plan moving forward. This can be broken up into three categories: (1) quality of rounding/follow-up, (2) accurate documentation of pain management efficacy, and (3) a clear/concise plan moving forward. Effective implementation of this into the postoperative pain management process can drastically reduce overuse of narcotics and readmission rates, increase patient satisfaction, and optimize early mobilization—thus, faster recovery. Overall, these simple implementations lead to decreased complications, such as pulmonary and cardiac complications, DVT, development of chronic pain, opioid dependence, and subsequent addiction. Particularly, in the inpatient setting, this leads to reduced cost of care and faster discharge times.[20]

Quality rounding and follow-up of a postoperative patient in the setting of pain management provides a fundamental foundation for improved pain control and satisfaction. The nationally accepted assessment tool for evaluation of pain is the 10-point pain scale, where 1 is minimal pain and 10 is maximal pain. The obvious limitation to this tool is the subjective nature of the patient's response and the timing of the response relative to the patient's most recent medication dose, meal, or sleep. Thus, an objective portion to the tool can be implemented by evaluating the patient's clinical improvement such as comfort of breathing, mobilization, appetite, and overall mood.[20] As these characteristics are largely dependent on the time of the patient's last medication dose, introducing a standardized protocol that utilizes an interdisciplinary approach with nurses, respiratory therapists, and physical therapists to intermittently document a subjective and objective pain assessment can offer a valuable trend of patient pain that would otherwise not be assessed with daily provider rounding. A study analyzing 720 nursing records for the documentation of pain management in postoperative patients found that nurse's documentation of pain management presented major limitations, including vague subjective statements that oftentimes left out the nature, location, or duration of pain (n = 430, 60%). It was found that nearly half of the records offered a goal of care that did not give any measurable data and rarely implemented a pain score. When pain scores were implemented, they were not consistently reported in relation to the administration of analgesic medications and thus did not offer useful data for tailoring pain management.[68] While this study focused on nurses, quality documentation should be an interdisciplinary effort. Implementing a standardized protocol that utilizes subjective and objective data can offer significant improvements in patient outcomes and satisfaction.

Considerable research has been made in the utilization of self-reported pain diaries in the setting of outpatient pain management and follow-up planning. While effective, there were two major limitations that have historically been identified—(1) patient compliance and (2) provider-led regimen changes based on feedback. With EMR now becoming commonplace, a study by Marceau et al. utilizing electronic pain diaries as opposed to previously accepted paper diaries showed that patients reported more frequently that a provider suggested changes in medication regimen based on patient entries ($P < .05$), and patients were more understanding of their condition, their symptoms, and their overall improvement.[69] Much of the research in electronic pain diaries is focused on chronic pain, and thus, its effectiveness in the acute pain setting is not yet understood.

The Importance of Maintaining Communication and Organization Between APS: Inpatient Pain Service, Surgeons, Preoperative/Intraoperative Personnel, Postoperative Personnel, Patient Safety, and Efficient Usage of Resources (Human, Medications, and Time) as Priority

As discussed above, the importance of interdisciplinary documentation provides a cornerstone for effective acute pain management in a postoperative patient that leads to significantly improved outcomes and decreased complications. Similarly, interdisciplinary communication in the preoperative, intraoperative, and postoperative setting has also been shown to improve overall outcomes.

A study analyzed preoperative communication with the patient regarding the evolution of pain throughout the recovery process, the use of endorphins as natural analgesia, the efficacy of nonopioid medications, and the negative effects of opioids. The experimental group received pre-op education, while the control did not. It was found that 90% of the experimental group declined postoperative opioid prescriptions, while 100% of the control group filled their prescriptions. The control group reported significantly greater average pain scores ($P < .05$) and significantly longer duration of pain ($P < .005$).[70]

Proper communication between inpatient pain services and surgeons can significantly improve post-op pain and, thus, decrease post-op complications. Such communication can include discussing available options for pre-op nerve blocks, limitations of opioid analgesia, options for post-op nerve blocks, and much more. Multidisciplinary communication is a mainstay in the implementation of a successful APS. An effective APS implements organized and structured nursing guidelines and pain treatment protocols that offer closure in the knowledge gaps that would otherwise limit postoperative pain management.[71] An interventional study about the implementation of an APS noted a significant reduction in VAS (visual analog scale) pain scores among 671 surgical patients ($P < .001$).[71] This study focused on the development of a quality manual over a 3-year period that was distributed to surgical ward personnel, surgeons, and anesthesiologists, and demarcated responsibilities among the hierarchy of staff that a patient will encounter throughout their stay. The model standardized the facility's perioperative pain management and allowed for improved communication among surgeons, anesthesiologists, and nurses.

The Importance of Having Multiple Channels of Communications: Being Able to Be Reached by Multiple Services, Answering Consults, and Have Inpatient/Outpatient Follow-up

In 2001, the Joint Commission suggested the implementation of pain as the fifth vital sign. More than ever, the effectiveness of pain management in the inpatient setting had been popularized as a marked enhancement in positive patient outcomes. An effective APS provides a multidisciplinary interdepartmental service that a hospital can rely on to decrease opioid dependence, decrease overall recovery time, and increase patient satisfaction. We have seen a rapid evolution of the role of acute pain management—starting as a perioperative service and becoming a hospital-wide consultant service. These changes have led to the implementation of other specialties into the APS model, such as addiction medicine, psychiatry, PM&R, and chronic pain medicine.[72] The ultimate goal of such a service is to address and discuss the risks and benefits of interventional vs pharmacological pain control and offer a treatment that reduces further suffering and morbidity. In 2005, Rawal discussed the basic requirements that make the implementation of an APS an effective hospital resource. One of these requirements calls for the use of an around-the-clock pain management specialist as a consultant.[10] These shifts in the APS model offer an expansion of the service from a perioperative specialty to a hospital-wide pain management consulting service.

Conclusion

Postoperative pain control is challenging. Given the opioid epidemic claiming thousands of lives and the fact that acute pain can convert to chronic pain especially given high-risk surgeries, control of postoperative pain is tantamount.[3,5] Postoperative pain has led to delayed discharged and hospital admission.[5] Severe postoperative pain is also associated with pulmonary and cardiovascular complications.[5] Given these factors, is necessary that an efficient and effective postoperative pain management be presents for these patients to optimize postoperative pain control.

REFERENCES

1. Ismail S, Siddiqui AS, Rehman A. Postoperative pain management practices and their effectiveness after major gynecological surgery: an observational study in a tertiary care hospital. *J Anaesthesiol Clin Pharmacol.* 2018;34:478-484.
2. Tennant F, Ciccone TG. New guidelines for post-op pain management. *Pract Pain Manag.* 2016. https://www.practicalpainmanagement.com/resources/news-and-research/new-guidelines-post-op-pain-management
3. Understanding the Epidemic [Internet]. Centers for Disease Control and Prevention. https://www.cdc.gov/drugoverdose/epidemic/index.html
4. The Lancet. Best practice in managing postoperative pain. *Lancet.* 2019;393(10180):1478. http://dx.doi.org/10.1016/S0140-6736(19)30813-X
5. Vadivelu N, Kai AM, Kodumudi V, Berger JM. Challenges of pain control and the role of the ambulatory pain specialist in the outpatient surgery setting. *J Pain Res.* 2016;9:425-435.
6. Rodgers A, Walker N, Schug S, et al. Reduction of postoperative mortality and morbidity with epidural or spinal anaesthesia: results from overview of randomised trials. *BMJ.* 2000;321:1493-1497.
7. Kehlet H, Holte K. Effect of postoperative analgesia reduces on surgical outcome. *Br J Anaesth.* 2001;87:62-72.
8. Beattie WS, Badner NH, Choi P. Epidural analgesia reduces postoperative myocardial infarction: a meta-analysis. *Anesth Analg.* 2001;93:853-858.
9. Le-Wendling L, Glick W, Tighe P. Goals and objectives to optimize the value of an acute pain service in perioperative pain management. *Tech Orthop.* 2017;32:200-208.
10. Rawal N. Organization, function, and implementation of acute pain service. *Anesthesiol Clin North Am.* 2005;23:211-255.
11. Cronin AJ, Keifer JC, Davies MF, et al. Postoperative sleep disturbance: influences of opioids and pain in humans. *Sleep.* 2001;24(1):39-44.
12. Wu CL, Richman JM. Postoperative pain and quality of recovery. *Curr Opin Anaesthesiol.* 2004;17(5):455-460.
13. Taylor RS, Ullrich K, Regan S, et al. The impact of early postoperative pain on health-related quality of life. *Pain Pract.* 2013;13(7):515-523.
14. Rawal N. Acute pain services revisited—good from far, far from good? *Reg Anesth Pain Med.* 2002;27:117-121.
15. Rapp SE, Ready LB, Nessly ML. Acute pain management in patients with prior opioid consumption: a case-controlled retrospective review. *Pain.* 1995;61(2):195-201.
16. US Outpatient Surgical Procedures Market by Surgical Procedure Type, Patient Care Setting - US Forecast to 2023. https://www.researchandmarkets.com/research/tfnm9z/united_states?w=5
17. Rawal N. Current issues in postoperative pain management. *Eur J Anaesthesiol.* 2016;33(3):160-171.
18. Hanoch Kumar K, Elavarasi P. Definition of pain and classification of pain disorders. *J Adv Clin Res Insight.* 2016;3:87-90. doi:10.15713/ins.jcri.112
19. Lee B, Schug SA, Joshi GP, Kehlet H; PROSPECT Working Group. Procedure-specific pain management (PROSPECT)—An update. *Best Pract Res Clin Anaesthesiol.* 2018;32:101-111.

20. Ramsay MA. Acute postoperative pain management. *Proc (Bayl Univ Med Cent)*. 2000;13:244-247.
21. Sharrock NE, Cazan MG, Hargett MJ, Williams-Russo P, Wilson PD Jr. Changes in mortality after total hip and knee arthroplasty over a ten-year period. *Anesth Analg*. 1995;80:242-248.
22. Katz J, Jackson M, Kavanagh BP, Sandler AN. Acute pain after thoracic surgery predicts long-term post-thoracotomy pain. *Clin J Pain*. 1996;12:50-55.
23. Garimella V, Cellini C. Postoperative pain control. *Clin Colon Rectal Surg*. 2013;26:191-196.
24. Levy BF, Tilney HS, Dowson HM, Rockall TA. A systematic review of postoperative analgesia following laparoscopic colorectal surgery. *Colorectal Dis*. 2010;12(1):5-15.
25. Oderda G, Gan T. Effect of opioid-related adverse events on outcomes in selected surgical patients. *J Pain Palliat Care Pharmacother*. 2013;27:62-70.
26. Minami M, Satch M. Molecular biology of the opioid receptors: structures, functions and distributions. *Neurosci Res*. 1995;23:121-145.
27. Savarese JJ, Tabler NG Jr. Multimodal analgesia as an alternative to the risks of opioid monotherapy in surgical pain management. *J Healthc Risk Manag*.. 2017;37(1):24-30.
28. Hu G, Huang K, Hu Y, et al. Single-cell RNA-seq reveals distinct injury responses in different types of DRG sensory neurons. *Sci Rep*. 2016;6:31851.
29. Djouhri L, Lawson SN. A beta-fiber nociceptive primary afferent neurons: a review of incidence and properties in relation to other afferent A-fiber neurons in mammals. *Brain Res Brain Res Rev*. 2004;46(2):131-145.
30. Gupta A, Bah M. NSAIDs in the treatment of postoperative pain. *Curr Pain Headache Rep*. 2016;20(11):62.
31. Obeng OA, Hamadeh I, Smith M. Review of opioid pharmacogenetics and considerations for pain management. *Pharmacotherapy*. 2017;37(9):1105-1121.
32. Osterweis M, Kleinman A, Mechanic D, eds. *Pain and Disability: Clinical, Behavioral, and Public Policy Perspectives*. National Academies Press; 1987:204.
33. Mishriky BM, Waldron NH, Habib AS. Impact of pregabalin on acute and persistent postoperative pain: a systematic review and meta-analysis. *Br J Anaesth*. 2015;114(1):10-31.
34. Marret E, Kurdi O, Zufferey P, et al. Effects of nonsteroidal antiinflammatory drugs on patient-controlled analgesia morphine side effects: meta-analysis of randomized controlled trials. *Anesthesiology*. 2005;102(6):1249-1260.
35. Pöpping DM, Elia N, Van Aken HK, et al. Impact of epidural analgesia on mortality and morbidity after surgery. Systematic review and meta-analysis of randomized controlled trials. *Ann Surg*. 2014;259:1056-1067.
36. Leslie K, Myles P, Devereaux P, et al. Neuraxial block, death and serious cardiovascular morbidity in the POISE trial. *Br J Anaesth*. 2013;111:382-390.
37. Chandrasekharan NV, Dai H, Turepu KL, et al. COX-3, a cyclooxygenase-1 variant inhibited by acetaminophen and other analgesic/antipyretic drugs: cloning, structure, and expression. *Proc Natl Acad Sci U S A*. 2002;99:13926-13931.
38. Schwenk ES, Viscusi ER, Buvanendran A, et al. Consensus guidelines on the use of intravenous ketamine infusions for acute pain management from the American Society of Regional Anesthesia and Pain Medicine, the American Academy of Pain Medicine, and the American Society of Anesthesiologists. *Reg Anesth Pain Med*. 2018;43:456-466.
39. Radvansky BM, Shah K, Parikh A. Role of ketamine in acute postoperative pain management: a narrative review. *Biomed Res Int*. 2015;2015.
40. Werner MU, Nielsen PR. The acute pain service: present and future role. *Curr Anaesth Crit Care*. 2007;18:135-139. doi:10.1016/j.cacc.2007.03.017
41. Lee A, Chan SKC, Ping Chen P, Gin T, Lau ASC, Hung Chiu C. The costs and benefits of extending the role of the acute pain service on clinical outcomes after major elective surgery. *Anesth Analg*. 2010;111:1042-1050. doi:10.1213/ANE.0b013e3181ed1317
42. Watcha MF, White PF. Economics of anesthetic practice. *Anesthesiology*. 1997;86:1170-1196. doi:10.1097/00000542-199705000-00021
43. Hopkins PM. Does regional anaesthesia improve outcome? *Br J Anaesth*. 2015;115:ii26-ii33. doi:10.1093/bja/aev377
44. Cao X, White PF, Ma H. An update on the management of postoperative nausea and vomiting. *J Anesth*. 2017;31:617-626. doi:10.1007/s00540-017-2363-x
45. Herrick MD, Liu H, Davis M, Bell JE, Sites BD. Regional anesthesia decreases complications and resource utilization in shoulder arthroplasty patients. *Acta Anaesthesiol Scand*. 2018;62:540-547. doi:10.1111/aas.13063
46. Salama-Hanna J, Chen G. Patients with chronic pain. *Med Clin North Am*. 2013;97:1201-1215. doi:10.1016/j.mcna.2013.07.005
47. Moseley GL. A pain neuromatrix approach to patients with chronic pain. *Man Ther*. 2003;8:130-140. doi:10.1016/S1356-689X(03)00051-1
48. Williamson A, Hoggart B. Pain: a review of three commonly used pain rating scales. *J Clin Nurs*. 2005;14:798-804. doi:10.1111/j.1365-2702.2005.01121.x
49. Herr K, Coyne PJ, Key T, et al. Pain assessment in the nonverbal patient: position statement with clinical practice recommendations. *Pain Manag Nurs*. 2006;7:44-52. doi:10.1016/j.pmn.2006.02.003

50. Song W, Eaton LH, Gordon DB, Hoyle C, Doorenbos AZ. Evaluation of evidence-based nursing pain management practice. *Pain Manag Nurs*. 2015;16:456-463. doi:10.1016/j.pmn.2014.09.001
51. Chou R, Gordon DB, De Leon-Casasola OA, et al. Management of postoperative pain: A clinical practice guideline from the American pain society, the American society of regional anesthesia and pain medicine, and the American society of anesthesiologists' committee on regional anesthesia, executive committee, and administrative council. *J Pain*. 2016;17:131-157. doi:10.1016/j.jpain.2015.12.008
52. Lassen K, Soop M, Nygren J, et al.; Enhanced Recovery After Surgery (ERAS) Group. Consensus review of optimal perioperative care in colorectal surgery: Enhanced Recovery After Surgery (ERAS) Group recommendations. *Arch Surg*. 2009;144(10):961-969.
53. Pędziwiatr M, Mavrikis J, Witowski J, Adamos A, Major P, Nowakowski M. Current status of Enhanced Recovery After Surgery (ERAS) protocol in gastrointestinal surgery. *Med Oncol*. 2018;35:95.
54. Ljungqvist O. To fast or not to fast before surgical stress. *Nutrition*. 2005;21:885-886.
55. Kahokehr A, Sammour T, Zargar-Shoshtari K, et al. Implementation of ERAS and how to overcome the barriers. *Int J Surg*. 2009;7:16-19.
56. Fearon KC, Ljungqvist O, Von Meyenfeldt M, et al. Enhanced recovery after surgery: a consensus review of clinical care for patients undergoing colonic resection. *Clin Nutr*. 2005;24(3):466-477.
57. de Brito Poveda V, Clark AM, Galvão CM.: A systematic review on the effectiveness of prewarming to prevent perioperative hypothermia. *J Clin Nurs*. 2013;22:906-918.
58. Hoffmann H, Kettelhack C. Fast-track surgery—conditions and challenges in postsurgical treatment: a review of elements of translational research in enhanced recovery after surgery. *Eur Surg Res*. 2012;49:24-34.
59. Hah JM, Bateman BT, Ratliff J, et al. Chronic opioid use after surgery: implications for perioperative management in the face of the opioid epidemic. *Anesth Analg*. 2017;125(5):1733-1740.
60. Brat GA, Agniel D, Beam A, et al. Postsurgical prescriptions for opioid naive patients and association with overdose and misuse: retrospective cohort study. *BMJ*. 2018;360:j5790.
61. Luckey A, Wang L, Jamieson PM, Basa NR, Million M, Czimmer J. Corticotropin-releasing factor receptor 1-deficient mice do not develop postoperative gastric ileus. *Gastroenterology*. 2003;125:654-659.
62. Marret E, Remy C, Bonnet F. Meta-analysis of epidural analgesia versus parenteral opioid analgesia after colorectal surgery. *Br J Surg*. 2007;94:665-673.
63. Pearsall EA, Meghji Z, Pitzul KB, et al. A qualitative study to understand the barriers and enablers in implementing an enhanced recovery after surgery program. *Ann Surg*. 2015;261:92-96.
64. Segerdahl M, Warren-Stomberg M, Rawal N, et al. Clinical practice and routines for day surgery in Sweden: results of a nation-wide survey. *Acta Anaesthesiol Scand*. 2008;52:117-124.
65. Wind J, Polle SW, Fung Kon Jin PHP, et al. Systematic review of enhanced recovery programmes in colonic surgery. *Br J Surg*. 2006;93:800-809.
66. Spanjersberg WR, Reurings J, Keus F, van Laarhoven CJ. Fast track surgery versus conventional recovery strategies for colorectal surgery. *Cochrane Database Syst Rev*. 2011;(2):CD007635.
67. Nadler A, Pearsall EA, Victor JC, Aarts M-A, Okrainec A, McLeod RS. Understanding surgical residents' postoperative practices and barriers and enablers to the implementation of an Enhanced Recovery After Surgery (ERAS) Guideline. *J Surg Educ*. 2014;71:632-638.
68. Shoqirat N, Mahasneh D, Dardas L, et al. Nursing documentation of postoperative pain management: a documentary analysis. *J Nurs Care Qual*. 2019;34(3):279-284.
69. Marceau LD, Link C, Jamison RN, Carolan S. Electronic diaries as a tool to improve pain management: is there any evidence? *Pain Med*. 2007;8(suppl_3):S101-S109. https://doi.org/10.1111/j.1526-4637.2007.00374.x
70. Sugai DY, Deptula PL, Parsa AA, et al. The importance of communication in the management of postoperative pain." *Hawaii J Med Public Health*. 2013;72(6):180-184.
71. Bardiau FM, Taviaux NF, Albert A, Boogaerts JG, Stadler M. An intervention study to enhance postoperative pain management. *Anesth Analg*. 2003;96(1):179-185. doi: 10.1213/00000539-200301000-00038
72. Upp J, Kent M, Tighe PJ. The evolution and practice of acute pain medicine. *Pain Med*. 2013;14(1):124-144. https://doi.org/10.1111/pme.12015

12

The Role of Patient and Family Education

Ahmad Elsharydah and Maria Michaelis

Postoperative pain continues to be a significant issue in health care, with a considerable proportion of patients experiencing severe pain after surgery and finding pain management at home challenging. There are several barriers to effective pain management, involving both patients and health care professionals.[1] Patient education is a useful way to overcome many of these barriers. Addressing postoperative pain and how structured patient education, from admission to discharge, is important for patient experience and recovery. Patient education about postoperative pain, provided by skilled health care professionals, may improve postoperative recovery, potentially improving patient outcomes. In this chapter, we will explore the importance of patient and family education regarding acute pain management and its effect on outcomes, patient and family responsibilities for better pain control, realistic expectations from pain control, and patient/family engagement in recovery activities. Also, we added a section looking into special considerations for the pediatric patient.

Significance of Patient and Family Education for Acute Pain Management

Patient and family education regarding the management of acute pain after injury or surgery plays an important role in the successful pain control and expedition of recovery. Timely and appropriate education also decreases patient anxiety and worries about postoperative pain. One patient survey had shown that more than half of the patients surveyed were concerned about experiencing pain after surgery and that this caused some of them even to postpone surgery.[2] The emphasis on the patient and family education is not new. In 1992, the Department of Health and Human Services published the Acute Pain Clinical Practice Guideline,[3] which stressed the significance of patient and family education for acute pain management. The essential elements of pain education (shown in Fig. 12.1), as stated in these guidelines, include telling the patient the following:

- Preventing and controlling pain is important to your care.
- There are many interventions available to manage pain; analgesics (opioid and nonopioid) are the most effective in managing acute pain.
- Some people are afraid of using opioids because of the side effects and risk of addiction. Side effects can be managed effectively with medication. The risk of addiction when using opioids to control acute pain is extremely low.
- Your responsibility in achieving good pain control is to tell us when you are experiencing pain or when the nature or level of pain changes.
- Complete pain relief usually is not achievable; however, we will work with you to keep pain at a level that allows you to engage in activities necessary to recover and return home.

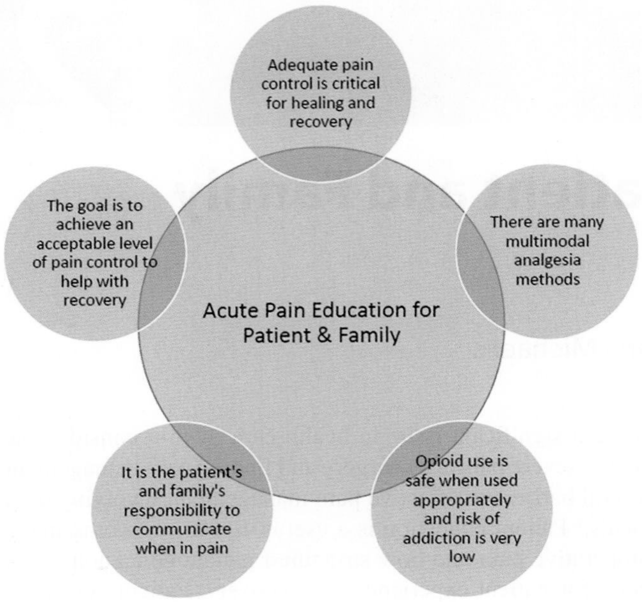

FIGURE 12.1 The essential elements of patient and family education regarding the management of acute pain.

It is good to set up goals for pain management during the hospitalization and after discharge. These goals are centered around the functional requirements during the recovery period after surgery or injury. Examples of the functional requirements are ambulation, physical therapy, and deep breathing. These activities promote recovery and improve outcomes. These goals are best established with coordination between physicians, nursing staff, patient, family member, and other health care providers involved in the patient treatments and recovery.[4] One dimension of the plan is to establish a tolerable and acceptable pain level during these activities such as physical therapy or dressing changes. Knowledge of the patient pain history is critical to create effective pain management plan for the current hospitalization or home recovery period.

Patient Realistic Expectations for Acute Pain Management

Patient expectations can be a difficult concept to quantify—but setting appropriate expectations plays an important role in patient outcomes, especially overall patient satisfaction with their overall surgical experience and pain control. Furthermore, the nature of patient expectations can sometimes be challenging to define but typically involves the patient's anticipation of an event—such as an increase in joint function after surgery.[5] Moreover, a gap in expectations often exist between the physician and the patient. Acknowledgment of this gap upfront, prior to surgery, may minimize the negative consequences of unmet expectations. Several factors such as age, gender, and health status can also influence a patient's expectation for recovery after surgery.[6] Health care provider awareness of these factors may also decrease may expedite and smooth the recovery leading to better overall patient satisfaction.

The Expectation Gap Between the Patient and Health Care Providers

Discrepancies between what patients and their doctors expect from medical treatment are well-documented in the medical literature. Even on the basic understanding of what constitutes "quality of life," doctor and patient perceptions may significantly diverge. If quality of life issues and the potentially divergent perspectives are not acknowledged and integrated into the patient's assessment, it can result in a lack of understanding about the efficacy of treatment or even lack of compliance.[7] One study examined the expectation gap among joint replacement patients to understand its nature: 168 patients undergoing either a total hip or total knee replacement filled out a questionnaire regarding their expectations of how surgery would affect pain levels, function, and overall well-being. At the same time, their surgeons filled out an identical questionnaire about their own expectations for their patients. The study revealed a substantial gap between the expectations of these two groups, with 52.5% of the patients having expectations that exceeded that of their surgeon.[5] One way to minimize this gap is a frank discussion between the surgeon and the patient ahead of the surgery including a thorough risk-benefit analysis of the procedure. During this meeting, the patient and the physician can collaboratively make an informed decision about whether surgery is the best choice for their individual needs. This process is time consuming but can help patients to create realistic expectations and decrease the risk of dissatisfaction after surgery.[8] Other ways may help to decrease the expectation gap is to use psychological interventions. In one study, patients undergoing cardiac surgery underwent a psychology-based, presurgical intervention to help manage their expectations of surgery. Compared to the control group who did not undergo a presurgical intervention, these patients showed an increased recovery from their disability, an increased ability to return to work, and an increased mental quality of life.[9]

Patient and Family Responsibilities

There are many things that family members/caregivers bring to the table when it comes to acute pain management. Often times, these people know the patient best. They know what kind of coping mechanisms the patient already possesses, and likewise, they know where there are some gaps in being able to cope with postoperative pain. One important aspect to educate patient and family about is that communication regarding uncontrolled pain or changes in pain characteristics are essential to address before it hinders recovery and rehabilitation. Furthermore, patient and family need to know that uncontrolled pain may lead to postoperative persistent pain and sometime to a difficult to manage chronic pain.

Moreover, it is imperative that patients and their families be fully engaged in the recovery process. Nonpharmacological methods including the improvement of knowledge of patients and his/her family members in the management and control of pain can reduce patients' experiences of pain. A study aimed to investigate the effects of family-oriented educational intervention on postoperative pain after orthopedic surgery showed decrease in pain severity and the use of opioids for the cohort of patients who received preoperative and postoperative educational intervention with the attendance of family members, compared to a control group.[5]

Methods for Patient and Family Pain Control Education

Effective pain management education may begin as early as the planning for surgery in the surgical clinic or in the anesthesia preoperative clinic. There are three stages of the education process. First, the health care provider has to assess the patient's educational needs and potential barriers to learning. Next, reasonable and achievable educational objectives need to be set up before the next step of education and teaching begins. Finally, the patient's understanding should be periodically assessed. There are several methods for patient and family education on pain management. Teaching ranges from in-person instruction during the preoperative surgical and anesthesia visits to the use of written or visual educational materials, such as brochures or videos. The health care team to decide about the method to use depends on the set up of their practices, the availability of these methods, and the patients' specific needs. For example, for minor ambulatory surgeries, most of the education can be established by phone the day before of the surgery and a brief reminder by the discharging nurse.

Opioids Use and Risks Education

Increase patient awareness about the importance and methods of proper medication disposal have significant effect on patient behavior and willingness for the appropriate disposal unused opioids after injury or surgery and may enhance drug take-back programs that may promote and incentivize more patients to utilize the services.[10] Participants who received counseling on opioid disposal were more likely to have disposed of unused opioid medications.[11] Dissemination of the educational brochure improved disposal of unused opioids after surgery. This low-cost, easily implemented intervention can improve disposal of unused opioids and ultimately decrease the amount of excess opioids circulating in our communities.[12]

Some patients are afraid of using opioids for acute pain control because of their fear of side effects and addiction. Therefore, part of patient and family education is to assure them that opioids are still an essential part of their pain management, especially after extensive and painful surgical procedures and major trauma. The side effects of opioids can be managed successfully, and the risk of addiction is extremely low if the opioid is used appropriately. Opioid use education has positive behavioral consequences, which may lower the risk of abuse[13] and improve the disposal of unused opioids.[14] Furthermore, patient education regarding the concept of multimodal analgesia increases the utilization of nonopioid analgesics and decreases the need of opioids.

Acute Pain Management for the Pediatric Patient

The American Society of Anesthesiologists (ASA) Task Force on Acute Pain Management[15] believes that optimal care for infants and children (including adolescents) requires special attention to the biopsychosocial nature of pain. This specific patient population presents developmental differences in their experience and expression of pain and suffering, and their response to analgesic pharmacotherapy. Caregivers in both the home and hospital may have misperceptions regarding the importance of analgesia as well as its risks and benefits. In the absence of a clear source of pain or obvious pain behavior, caregivers may assume that pain is not present and defer treatment. Safe methods for providing analgesia are underused in pediatric patients for fear of opioid-induced respiratory depression. The emotional component of pain is particularly strong in infants and children. Absence of parents, security objects, and familiar surroundings may cause as much suffering as the surgical incision. Children's fear of injections makes intramuscular or other invasive routes of drug delivery aversive. Even the valuable technique of topical analgesia before injections may not lessen this fear. A variety of techniques may be effective in providing analgesia in pediatric patients. Many are the same as for adults, although some (eg, caudal analgesia) are more commonly used in children.

Aggressive and proactive pain management is necessary to overcome the historic under treatment of pain in children. Perioperative care for children undergoing painful procedures or surgery requires developmentally appropriate pain assessment and therapy. Analgesic therapy should depend upon age, weight, and comorbidity. Unless contraindicated, analgesic therapy should involve a multimodal approach. Behavioral techniques, especially important in addressing the emotional component of pain, should be applied whenever feasible.

Education of the caregivers about special consideration for optimal perioperative analgesia for their little ones and the methods available to provide good pain relief is critical. Older children who understand the instructions should be included in the pain management discussion from the start.

In summary, patient and family education regarding the significance of pain control after surgery or injury, the available pain therapies, their responsibilities during the recovery period in regard to pain management, and their engagement in the recovery activities have a critical role to reach safe and acceptable pain management. This eventually leads to higher patient satisfaction and better outcomes. Special considerations for the management of acute pain of the pediatric patient should be recognized by the health care provider as well. As health care providers, our overall goal for patients of all ages should be full recovery and optimal pain control to get there.

REFERENCES

1. Ingadótti B, Zoëga S. Role of patient education in postoperative pain management. *Nurs Stand*. 2017;32:50-63.
2. Apfelbaum JL, Chen C, Mehta SS, Gan TJ. Postoperative pain experience: results from a national survey suggest postoperative pain continues to be undermanaged. *Anesth Analg*. 2003;97:534-540.
3. Carr DR, Jacox AK, Chapman CR, et al. *Acute Pain Management: Operative or Medical Procedures and Trauma, No 1*. U.S. Dept. of Health and Human Services; 1992. AHCPR Pub No 92-0032; Public Health Service.
4. Gittell JH, Fairfield KM, Bierbaum B, et al. Impact of relational coordination on quality of care, postoperative pain and functioning, and length of stay: a nine-hospital study of surgical patients. *Med Care*. 2000;38:807-819.
5. Ghomlawi HM, Fernando NF, Mandl LA, et al. How often are patient and surgeon recovery expectations for total knee arthroplasty aligned? Results of a pilot study. *HSS J*. 2011;7:229-234.
6. Achaval MS, Kallen MA, Amick B, et al. Patent expectations about total knee arthroplasty outcomes. *Health Expect*. 2015;19:299-308.
7. Janse AJ, Gemke RJ, Viterwaal CS, van der Turl I, Kimpen JL, Sinnema G. Quality of life: patients and doctors don't always agree: a meta-analysis. *J Clin Epidemiol*. 2004;87:653-661.
8. Choi YJ, Ra HJ. Patient satisfaction after total knee arthroplasty. *Knee Surg Relat Res*. 2016;28:1-15.
9. Rief W, Shedden-Mora MC, Laferton JA, et al. Preoperative optimization of patient expectations improves long-term outcome in heart surgery patients: results of the randomized controlled PSY-HEART trial. *BMC Med*. 2017;15:4.
10. Buffington DE, Lozicki A, Alfieri T, Bond TC. Understanding factors that contribute to the disposal of unused opioid medication. *J Pain Res*. 2019;12:725-732.
11. Varisco TJ, Fleming ML, Bapat SS, Wanat MA, Thornton D. Health care practitioner counseling encourages disposal of unused opioid medications. *J Am Pharm Assoc (2003)*. 2019;59:809-815.
12. Hasak JM, Roth Bettlach CL, Santosa KB, Larson EL, Stroud J, Mackinnon SE. Empowering post-surgical patients to improve opioid disposal: a before and after quality improvement study. *J Am Coll Surg*. 2018;226:235-240.
13. Hero JO, McMurtry C, Benson J, Blendon R. Discussing opioid risks with patients to reduce misuse and abuse: evidence from 2 surveys. *Ann Fam Med*. 2016;14:575-577.
14. Lewis ET, Cucciare MA, Trafton JA. What do patients do with unused opioid medications? *Clin J Pain*. 2014;30:654-662.
15. American Society of Anesthesiologists Task Force on Acute Pain Management. Practice guidelines for acute pain management in the perioperative setting: an updated report by the American Society of Anesthesiologists Task Force on Acute Pain Management. *Anesthesiology*. 2012;117:248-273.

SECTION II

Organ Systems

13

Acute Cardiac Related Pain and Differential Diagnoses

Kunal Mandavawala, Stuart M. Sacks, and Kheng Sze Chan

Medical Cardiac Pain

Ischemic Heart Disease

One of the most common presentations of acute pain that is of cardiac origin falls into the category of ischemic heart disease, which includes stable angina pectoris as well as the acute coronary syndromes (ACS). The pain that ensues is due to a narrowing or complete occlusion of one of the coronary arteries or its branches, which leads to an imbalance between blood supply and oxygen demand and thus inadequate perfusion of the myocardial tissue. The four major factors that determine oxygen demand include heart rate, systolic blood pressure (afterload), myocardial wall tension or stress (preload), and myocardial contractility. Myocardial oxygen supply is influenced by the diameter of the coronary arteries, coronary perfusion pressure, and heart rate. Heart rate is relevant as coronary artery flow occurs primary in diastole, which shortens with increasing heart rates.[1]

Coronary Artery Anatomy

Blood supply to myocardial tissue arises from the coronary arteries, which branch off of the aorta as the left and right coronary arteries. The left coronary artery further branches into the left anterior descending artery and the left circumflex artery (LCX). The right coronary artery gives rise to the posterior descending artery (PDA), which provides blood supply to the posterior and inferior wall of the left ventricle, in 70%-80% of the population, who are referred to as having a right dominant coronary circulation. Five percent to ten percent of the population are left heart dominant, with the PDA originating from the LCX, and 10%-20% are codominant, with the PDA being supplied by both the LCX and right coronary artery.[2] This becomes relevant, as the PDA gives off branches, which supply the atrioventricular node.

Stable Angina

Diagnosis

Stable angina pectoris is a result of fixed atherosclerotic lesions that cause narrowing of one or more coronary arteries. Patients with stable angina pectoris tend to experience a pain or pressure sensation in the substernal area, which can radiate to the left arm, shoulder, or jaw, by the mechanism of referred pain.[3] Pain associated with this condition is typically not present at rest but occurs predictably with physical activity or emotional stress. Pain and other associated symptoms, which can include exertional dyspnea, fatigue, and/or nausea (termed "anginal equivalents"), remit with rest or nitroglycerin.[4] Typically, the patient will have difficulty localizing the pain to a specific location.

Should symptoms be present for at least 2 months with no change in severity, character, or triggering factors, then the patient is defined as having chronic stable angina.[5]

Diagnosis of stable angina is typically by history and physical examination, as well as ECG and laboratory studies. History most often will illustrate chest pain or other anginal equivalents, which arise with activity or stress and remit with rest or nitroglycerin. If an ECG is obtained during the time of anginal symptoms, it will often show ST segment depression, but an ECG may be normal when a patient is asymptomatic. Thus, stress testing is often performed in patients who are asymptomatic at the time of initial evaluation.[6]

In terms of laboratory studies, cardiac biomarkers (eg, troponin, CK-MB) may also be helpful. However, in a patient with true stable angina pectoris, these markers tend to be negative, as increased biomarkers tend to indicate myocardial injury and thus a diagnosis of ACS.[7]

Treatment

Medical treatment of the pain associated with stable angina pectoris has two components: (1) prevention of anginal symptoms and (2) acute symptom management.

There are multiple medications that are commonly utilized as antianginal therapy and include beta-blockers, calcium channel blockers, nitrates, and the newer medication, ranolazine. They may be used as monotherapy, but combination therapy is often needed for optimal symptom control.

Beta-blockers tend to be used as first-line treatment, as the resulting decrease in heart rate both leads to an increase in supply (longer diastolic time) and decrease in demand. The decrease in demand can also be attributed to a decrease in myocardial contractility.

Should patients be unable to tolerate a beta-blocker, other therapies such as long-acting nitrates or calcium channel blockers may be used.

Calcium channel blockers can be used as monotherapy or combination therapy, and their mechanism of pain relief is a result of coronary and peripheral vasodilation and reduction in contractility.

Long-acting nitrates reduce time to onset of angina and improve exercise tolerance.

Combination therapy may also be useful,[8] and ranolazine, a sodium channel blocker, can be added should other therapies fail.

The cornerstone of treatment for acute anginal symptoms is the use of short-acting nitrates, which is administered sublingually. Should nitrates fail to relieve pain, concern for progression to an ACS arises.

Revascularization

Revascularization via percutaneous coronary intervention (PCI) is often indicated for patients who fail medical therapy or do not tolerate medical therapy. For patients who do not have symptom control with medical therapy, PCI often improves symptoms.[9] Other interventions such as coronary artery bypass grafting (CABG) may also be indicated depending on the severity and location of coronary lesions; however, such guidelines are beyond the scope of this book.

Other treatment modalities

Thoracic epidural

Cardiac sympathetic blockade via the use of thoracic epidural anesthesia has been shown to dilate coronary arteries and has been used for pain control in patients with unstable angina. It has shown to be effective, as perceived pain from myocardial ischemia is mediated by sympathetic afferent nerves.[9] Thoracic epidural anesthesia has also been effectively utilized for patients with refractory angina with significant improvement in quality of life.[10]

Enhanced external counterpulsation

Enhanced external counterpulsation is a noninvasive FDA-approved therapy for refractory angina. The mechanism of action is similar to that of an intra-aortic balloon pump in that a vigorous pressure pulse is applied during diastole to allow for improved coronary perfusion. Unlike an intra-aortic balloon pump, however, this is accomplished by external blood pressure cuffs, rather than an internal device. Studies have shown that enhanced external counterpulsation likely results in an improved quality of life as a result of improved anginal symptoms. There is class IIb evidence to support its use.[11]

Transmyocardial laser revascularization

Transmyocardial laser revascularization is a treatment utilized for refractory angina when CABG or PCI is not indicated. The proposed mechanism is that transmyocardial laser revascularization stimulates angiogenesis, which results in reduction of anginal symptoms. It has been shown to lower angina scores, increase exercise tolerance time, and improve patients' perceptions of quality of life.[12]

Spinal cord stimulation

Investigation into other treatment modalities for refractory angina pectoris is underway. This includes the use of spinal cord stimulation, which was first described as a therapy for chronic refractory angina in 1987.[13] This is a therapy that stimulates the spinal cord to relieve pain via a low-voltage current. The proposed mechanism is via the "gate control" theory of pain, and it is proposed that the electrical stimulation "closes the gate" and inhibits the conduction of pain signals to the brain from the initial source.[14] Currently, the use of spinal cord stimulation remains a class IIb recommendation with a level of evidence of B and C.[15]

Acute Coronary Syndromes

Diagnosis

The three presentations of ACS include unstable angina (UA), acute non–ST-elevation myocardial infarction (NSTEMI), and acute ST-elevation myocardial infarction (STEMI). In patients who have known angina, there are various presentations that should raise concern for an ACS: angina at rest for more than 20 minutes, new-onset angina that significantly limits activity, and increasing angina that is more frequent, longer, or occurs with less exertion than previous episodes.

Unstable angina is diagnosed in patients who present with any of the above presentations, with or without changes on ECG, and who do NOT have detectable cardiac biomarkers such as troponin.

Non–ST-elevation myocardial infarction is clinically difficult to differentiate from UA but presents with elevated troponins as the differentiating factor.

ST-elevation myocardial infarction presents with symptoms of myocardial ischemia in addition to ST elevation or a new left bundle-branch block on ECG as well as elevated cardiac biomarkers.[16]

The mechanism of pain associated with ACS is identical to that of stable angina, but the pain associated with ACS is persistent.

Treatment

Management of these patients is a combination of medical management, which includes pain relief, +/– revascularization. Medications administered to patients suspected of having ACS include 325-mg aspirin, sublingual +/– IV nitroglycerin, beta-blockade (if the patient does not have signs of heart failure or bradycardia), morphine (for pain), heparin, and atorvastatin.

For patients with a diagnosis of STEMI, revascularization is at the core of treatment. Primary PCI is the strongly preferred treatment, but fibrinolysis may be utilized if PCI is not available, and fibrinolysis is not contraindicated. All patients should additionally receive dual antiplatelet therapy and anticoagulation (regardless of whether fibrinolysis is used).[17]

Surgical intervention is infrequently performed in patients with STEMI and is typically seen following a failed or complicated PCI, patients in cardiogenic shock, or patients with mechanical complications of MI.

For patients with a diagnosis of UA or NSTEMI, all patients should receive dual antiplatelet therapy and anticoagulation regardless of whether PCI is performed.[18] Should these patients receive revascularization, PCI is typical, though in patients with multivessel disease, CABG is often preferred.[19]

Should ACS be associated with cocaine use, one must be sure to avoid the use of beta-blockade, and benzodiazepines may be used to relieve symptoms.

Vasospastic angina

Vasospastic angina is an alternative condition, which is a result of vasospasm in patients who may or may not have obstructive coronary lesions. It clinically presents with rest angina associated with ST elevation or ST depression on ECG, and pain typically promptly responds to sublingual nitrates. Diagnosis has three components: nitrate responsiveness, transient ischemic ECG changes with no obvious cause, and angiographic evidence of coronary artery spasm. Risk factors and triggers include certain drugs such as cocaine.

Chronic treatment focuses on prevention of recurrence and typically includes the use of calcium channel blockers. Long-acting nitrates are second line for chronic treatment. Nonselective beta-blockers should be avoided due to the possibility of unopposed alpha stimulation of the coronary vessels.[20]

Acute pericarditis/myocarditis

The pericardium is a fibroelastic sac that surrounds the heart composed of two layers: an outer fibrous layer and an inner serous layer. Pericardial fluid is contained between these two layers.

Acute pericarditis is the result of inflammation of the pericardial sac. Patients with acute pericarditis tend to present with chest pain of sudden onset that can be described as sharp and pleuritic (worsened with cough or inspiration), and it improves with sitting up and leaning forward. Sitting up and leaning forward relieves pain via a reduction of pressure on the parietal pericardium. Pain associated with this condition may also radiate to the trapezius ridge. Radiation of pain is due to referred pain.[21]

In developed countries, the most common cause is presumed to be viral in origin, and pericarditis often follows a flulike or gastrointestinal syndrome. In developing countries, tuberculosis is the most common cause. Other causes include autoimmune diseases such as systemic lupus erythematosus, hypothyroidism, radiation, cancer, and postcardiac injury syndrome, which can manifest after procedures such as PCI, pacemaker insertion, or transcatheter aortic valve replacement. However, often a cause is not found, and most cases are classified as idiopathic.

Diagnosis involves a combination of history, physical examination, laboratory, and imaging studies. History involves chest pain with characteristics described above. On physical examination, patients may have a pericardial friction rub that can be heard with the patient leaning forward as a result of friction caused by inflammation between the layers of the pericardium. ECG findings classically show diffuse ST elevation and PR depression.

Should patients have involvement of the myocardium, troponin may be elevated but does not indicate prognosis in these patients.[22] If there is severe involvement of the myocardium, LV wall motion may be severely depressed. Inflammatory markers, such as ESR, and CRP are elevated in most cases but are not specific for this condition. Studies have shown, however, that high-sensitivity CRP identifies patients who have a higher risk of recurrence.[23]

Imaging also aids in diagnosis, and often echocardiography is all that is needed. Imaging can help identify complications such as tamponade and constrictive pericarditis as well as to identify and quantify any associated pericardial effusion. It can also be used to assess myocardial function in the setting of possible myocardial involvement.[24]

Anti-inflammatory medication is the primary treatment for acute pericarditis and its associated pain. Nonsteroidal anti-inflammatory drugs (NSAIDs) are the first-line treatment in these patients. Options include ibuprofen, indomethacin, and ketorolac (if patients cannot take oral medications). If patients have concomitant coronary artery disease, aspirin is preferred to NSAIDs. Colchicine, a microtubule inhibitor, should also be added as it has been shown to reduce "incessant and recurrent pericarditis."[25] Steroids have been used as second- or third-line treatments, with low-dose steroids being superior to high-dose steroids, with low-dose steroids having a lower rate of treatment failure and recurrence.[26] Trials investigating other anti-inflammatory agents, such as IL-1 inhibitors, are underway.

Invasive interventions are indicated for patients who develop tamponade or constrictive pericarditis. In the case of cardiac tamponade, pericardiocentesis or a surgical pericardial window is indicated. Should a patient have constrictive pericarditis with active inflammation, anti-inflammatory therapy is attempted first, and pericardiectomy is performed in refractory cases. Should constrictive pericarditis be present without active inflammation, pericardiectomy is the first-line treatment.

Aortic dissection

Aortic dissection is a rare clinical condition that presents acutely with severe chest or back pain and acute hemodynamic instability. Most commonly, aortic dissections result from an intimal tear leading to a "dissection" of blood that courses along the tunica media and separates the tissues along its course. Dissections can course as far as the iliac arteries or even further.

There are various complications associated with aortic dissection, which may include rupture into the pericardium leading to tamponade, acute dissection of the aortic valvular annulus leading to acute aortic regurgitation, dissection extension into the coronary arteries leading to myocardial infarction, and renal or other end-organ failure due to obstruction of branches such as the renal arteries or carotid arteries.

There are two anatomical classifications to aortic dissection, the Debakey and Stanford classifications, but the Stanford (Daily) system is more widely used. Dissections involving the ascending aorta are classified as type A dissections, while those that involve sites distal to the ascending aorta are classified as type B dissections.

Risk factors for aortic dissection include hypertension (the most important factor), cocaine use (leads to an abrupt change in blood pressure), connective tissue disorders such as Marfan or Ehlers-Danlos syndromes, preexisting aortic aneurysm, bicuspid aortic valve, aortic instrumentation or surgery, coarctation of the aorta, Turner syndrome, and vasculitides such as Takayasu and giant cell arteritis.[27,28]

Patients with acute aortic dissection can have variable symptoms depending on the extent of dissection and the structures affected. Pain associated with this condition is most commonly abrupt, knifelike, and is located in the chest or back. Patients describe this as pain they have never experienced before. Type A dissections tend to be associated with more pain in the anterior chest, while type B dissections tend to be associated with more pain in the back. Pain can radiate anywhere in the thorax or the abdomen. Syncope, heart failure, or stroke may be other presenting symptoms, though painless dissection is relatively uncommon.

Other symptoms that may be noted include pulse differential between extremities due to extension to the subclavian artery in some cases. In addition, lower extremity pulses may be affected if the dissection extends to the iliac vessels. Patients may also have focal neurological deficits as well as acute aortic valve regurgitation.

Diagnosis of aortic dissection is often a combination of history, physical examination, and imaging studies. CT angiography is the most common imaging study used for diagnosis if the patient is hemodynamically stable, but TEE can also be used. In fact, TEE is typically recommended for diagnosis if the patient is hemodynamically unstable, as this suggests involvement of the ascending aorta.[29]

Management varies depending if the patient has a type A or type B aortic dissection. In general, type A dissections require emergent surgery, whereas type B should be medically managed. Early management focuses on pain control and limiting propagation of the dissection via "impulse control" therapy. Typically, this involves controlling blood pressure by keeping systolic blood pressure between 100 and 120 mm Hg and heart rate <60 beats per minute. Common medications used for this purpose include esmolol or labetalol as well as vasodilators such as nitroprusside or nicardipine. Care must be taken that vasodilators are not begun until after beta-blockade is established, as vasodilators can lead to a reflex tachycardia. In terms of pain control, IV opioids are preferred.[30]

As stated above, a type A aortic dissection is a surgical emergency. A type B dissection that shows evidence of malperfusion is treated with aortic stent-grafting or surgery, but a type B dissection without malperfusion can be managed medically with impulse control and serial imaging.

Surgical Cardiac Pain

Anatomy

General anatomical considerations

A median sternotomy is the most common incision for open heart surgeries, as it affords the best access to the mediastinum and provides for easier exposure of every chamber and valve of the heart, with the exception of the posterior-lying left atrium.[31] A median sternotomy involves a longitudinal incision through the sternum, which is composed of three parts: the manubrium, body, and xiphoid process. In broad terms, the anterior thoracic wall is innervated by the intercostal nerves, which are formed by the anterior rami of the T1-T11 spinal nerves.[32] After exiting the intervertebral foramina, these nerves travel anteriorly in between the innermost and internal intercostal muscles. As they pass the internal mammary artery, they rise anteriorly and become the anterior cutaneous branch of the intercostal nerves.[3] More specifically, the anterior thoracic wall is innervated by the anterior cutaneous branches of the 2nd-6th intercostal nerves, while the posterior and lateral walls are innervated by the 2nd-11th intercostal nerves. Each thoracic nerve provides innervation to a striplike dermatome of the chest wall, with the exception of T1, which typically supplies only a small portion of the back and most of the medial forearm.[32] The area overlying the manubrium and superior-most aspects of the sternal body is innervated by the supraclavicular nerve, which arises from the C3 and C4 nerve roots. A dermatomal map is illustrated in Figure 13.1.

If full mediastinal access is not required, a variety of thoracotomy incisions can be made instead of full sternotomy. The specific location of the incision is dependent on the surgery being performed. A right-sided anterolateral thoracotomy can be used for tricuspid, mitral, and aortic valve surgeries, while left anterolateral thoracotomy can be used for transapical aortic valve replacement as well as for select coronary artery bypass operations.[37] The relevant anatomy for thoracotomy is similar to that of sternotomy, as innervation is via the intercostal nerves. However, the lateral cutaneous branches, which pierce through the external intercostal and serratus anterior muscles, are most relevant here.[38] The innervation of the lateral thoracic wall is more dense than that of the anterior wall. As such, while the incision for a thoracotomy is typically smaller than full sternotomy, the former tends to be more painful.[39]

Additional sources of incisional pain in traditional cardiac surgery involve cannulation sites for cardiopulmonary bypass. While typical central cannulation sites (ie, the ascending aorta and right atrium) can be accessed via sternotomy, there are a number of instances in which peripheral cannulation sites may be desired. The most common peripheral cannulation sites are the axillary and femoral vessels. Surgical access to the axillary artery occurs via an incision just below the clavicle. This area is innervated by both the second intercostal nerve

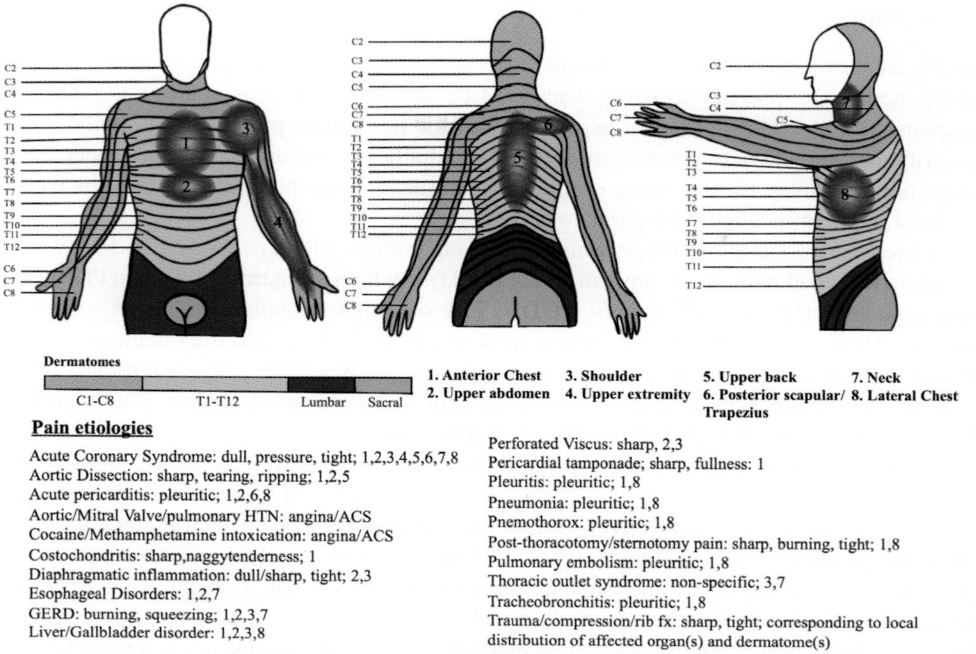
Dermatomes
C1-C8
T1-T12
Lumbar
Sacral
1. Anterior Chest
2. Upper abdomen
3. Shoulder
4. Upper extremity
5. Upper back
6. Posterior scapular/ Trapezius
7. Neck
8. Lateral Chest
Pain etiologies
Acute Coronary Syndrome: dull, pressure, tight; 1,2,3,4,5,6,7,8
Aortic Dissection: sharp, tearing, ripping; 1,2,5
Acute pericarditis: pleuritic; 1,2,6,8
Aortic/Mitral Valve/pulmonary HTN: angina/ACS
Cocaine/Methamphetamine intoxication: angina/ACS
Costochondritis: sharp,naggytenderness; 1
Diaphragmatic inflammation: dull/sharp, tight; 2,3
Esophageal Disorders: 1,2,7
GERD: burning, squeezing; 1,2,3,7
Liver/Gallbladder disorder: 1,2,3,8
Perforated Viscus: sharp, 2,3
Pericardial tamponade; sharp, fullness: 1
Pleuritis: pleuritic; 1,8
Pneumonia: pleuritic; 1,8
Pnemothorox: pleuritic; 1,8
Post-thoracotomy/sternotomy pain: sharp, burning, tight; 1,8
Pulmonary embolism: pleuritic; 1,8
Thoracic outlet syndrome: non-specific; 3,7
Tracheobronchitis: pleuritic; 1,8
Trauma/compression/rib fx: sharp, tight; corresponding to local distribution of affected organ(s) and dermatome(s)

FIGURE 13.1 Relative dermatomal pain distribution by etiologies. (From Klineberg E, Mazanec D, Orr D, Demicco R, Bell G, McLain R. Masquerade: medical causes of back pain. *Cleve Clin J Med*. 2007;74(12):905-913; Netterimages.com. Visceral Referred Pain. 2020. Accessed August 23, 2020. https://www.netterimages.com/visceral-referred-pain-labeled-reynolds-2e-rehabilitation-frank-h-netter-73698.html; McConaghy J, Oza R. Outpatient diagnosis of acute chest pain in adults. 2020. Accessed August 23, 2020. https://www.aafp.org/afp/2013/0201/p177.html; Hollander J, Chase M. Uptodate. Uptodate.com. 2020. Accessed September 7, 2020. https://www.uptodate.com/contents/evaluation-of-the-adult-with-chest-pain-in-the-emergency-department/contributors, Ref.[33-36])

and by the third and fourth cervical roots. Incision for the femoral vessels occurs inferior to the inguinal ligament, which is innervated by the ilioinguinal and genitofemoral nerves.[32,38]

Procedure-specific anatomical considerations

Coronary artery bypass grafting

Coronary artery bypass grafting is the most commonly performed cardiac surgery in the world.[40] The grafting component of the procedure lends it additional anatomical considerations for pain that are not relevant in other cardiac surgeries. The left internal mammary artery (LIMA) is considered to be the bypass vessel of choice, especially for disease of the left anterior descending coronary artery. LIMA harvest often requires additional sternal retraction forces and has been shown to increase the intensity of postoperative pain as well as cause greater pain inferior and lateral to the left nipple.[41] In instances where the LIMA either cannot be harvested or is insufficient, either radial artery or saphenous vein harvest is typically performed. Open radial artery harvest requires a large incision, typically extending the length of the forearm, whereas endoscopic harvest requires a smaller 3-cm incision proximal to the wrist.[42] Great saphenous vein harvest can also be done in either an open or endoscopic manner, with the former requiring a much larger incision.[43]

Percutaneous techniques

Femoral access, as described above as a peripheral cannulation site for cardiopulmonary bypass, is also relevant for percutaneous valve repairs and replacements. Mitral valve repairs are typically done via accessing the femoral vein, whereas transcatheter aortic valve replacements are done via the femoral artery.[38]

Prevalence and Location of Acute Postsurgical Cardiac Pain

As the anatomy discussed earlier would suggest, acute pain after cardiac surgery has many components. The primary incision, whether it be sternotomy or thoracotomy, is often only responsible for a portion of pain experienced in the immediate postoperative period. Other contributors include tissue retraction, visceral manipulation and dissection, the placement of large-bore cannulas, drains, and prolonged immobilization on the operating table as well as bed rest in the immediate postoperative period.

A prospective study of 200 patients undergoing cardiac surgery reported 86.5% of extubated patients had pain on postoperative day (POD) 1, which increased to 90% on POD 2 and remained similar through POD 3. By POD 7, 77% of patients continued to report some level of pain. They also reported that pain was most severe on POD 2, and only decreased by 1.3 points on a 10-point scale by POD 7.[44] A prospective study of 705 patients reported similar findings, with patients experiencing significant pain with even simple activities through POD 6, including moving in bed, deep breathing, and even at rest.[45]

The most common sites of pain in the immediate postoperative period are the sternum, epigastric area, and left breast, with 68%, 31.5%, and 15.5% of patients experiencing pain at those sites on POD 1, respectively. Other notable sites for POD 1 pain include the upper back, left shoulder, and right breast. By POD 7, the sternum is still the most common site of pain, but both shoulders become a much more common complaint. This change is likely due to the removal of drains in the lateral chest wall and epigastric area, while muscle aches and bone pain from prolonged immobilization and bed rest begin to become more apparent. In this study, lower extremity pain was seen exclusively in patients with saphenous vein harvest and remained less prevalent or intense than sternal and shoulder pain.[44]

Treatment Modalities

Opioids

Opioids remain a mainstay for the treatment of acute surgical cardiac pain, likely due to their efficacy, relative hemodynamic stability, and the limited concern for postoperative respiratory depression and sedation in this population, as the vast majority are brought to the ICU intubated and sedated. Historically, high doses of morphine (up to 3 mg/kg) were used for induction of general anesthesia in cardiac surgical patients. However, the rising popularity of fast track cardiac anesthesia has caused this technique to fall out of favor, as the large doses of morphine caused significant postoperative respiratory depression.[46] In the late 1970s, the use of high-dose fentanyl (25 μg/kg) was proven to be adequate for induction of maintenance of anesthesia while being superior to morphine in terms of hemodynamic stability and time to extubation.[46] Sufentanil and remifentanil have also become increasingly popular in cardiac surgery, with their increased potency and shorter context-sensitive half times.

Another popular trend in cardiac surgery is the reduction in intraoperative opioid dosing. This has gained popularity due to mounting evidence of dose-dependent opioid-induced hyperalgesia as well as the national spotlight on reducing opioid use. A recent meta-analysis of 18 trials with 1400 patients compared high- and low-dose opioid regimens on ICU length of stay and a myriad of secondary outcomes. The cutoff dose for fentanyl was 20 μg/kg, 2 μg/kg for sufentanil, 2 mg/kg for morphine, and either a total dose of 1.7 mg or infusion rate of 0.1 μg/kg/min for remifentanil. Their analysis showed no difference in ICU or hospital length of stay, time to extubation, vasopressor requirement, myocardial infarction, or stroke rate.[47] While they did not comment specifically on pain, the doses used in these studies are effective for analgesia during cardiac surgery. This may be of particular importance in the case of remifentanil, which has shown to increase opioid requirements in the immediate postoperative period when compared to fentanyl and sufentanil.[48,49]

The use of intraoperative methadone has also recently been investigated. A 2015 double-blinded RCT of 156 patients undergoing cardiac surgery with median sternotomy compared the intraoperative use of methadone 0.3 mg/kg with fentanyl 12 μg/kg. The use of a single dose of methadone significantly reduced morphine requirements for the first 24 hours after surgery, including the 12 hours after extubation, while pain scores in the methadone group continued to remain lower for the entirety of the 72-hour study design.[50] A follow-up study showed that those patients who received intraoperative methadone had fewer episodes of pain per week at 1 month than their counterparts who received fentanyl.[51]

Once patients arrive in the intensive care unit, opioids continue to be used for pain control. A great source of debate has been the role of patient-controlled analgesia (PCA) as opposed to the more traditional nurse-controlled analgesia in this patient population. While PCA is not typically possible in the immediate postoperative cardiac surgery patient due to sedation and mechanical ventilation, the popularity of fast track cardiac anesthesia has increased its relevance. The use of PCA has been examined extensively; a meta-analysis of 10 RCTs of over 600 patients concluded that while patients with a PCA used more morphine equivalents in the 48 hours after surgery, they had significant improvement in pain scores. Interestingly, however, this study did not find improvement in pain scores at 24 hours.[52] This finding, in conjunction with the increased opioid utilization in the PCA groups, suggests that nurse-controlled analgesia may be as effective in the early postoperative period when nursing care is typically more closely monitored than when patients are further out from surgery. Research regarding the optimal opioid for PCA has been done but is limited in scope. One study compared morphine, fentanyl, and remifentanil PCA initiated at the end of surgery after standardized anesthesia with intraoperative fentanyl boluses. They found that while patients in all three groups had similar pain scores for 24 hours after extubation, the remifentanil group had less nausea and pruritus than the morphine and fentanyl groups, respectively.[53] However, this study is limited in that it only examined patients undergoing off-pump CABG.

Multimodal analgesia

The relatively common and concerning side effects of opioids have increased interest in multimodal opioid-sparing regimens after surgery. Many centers now have "enhanced recovery after cardiac surgery" protocols, which often include acetaminophen, gabapentinoids, and NSAIDs. These medications are sometimes administered preoperatively and then re-dosed in the intra- and postoperative settings with the hope that the use of analgesics with different mechanisms of action will have a synergistic effect.

There is some evidence that multimodal analgesia is effective in cardiac surgery. An RCT of 180 patients undergoing cardiac surgery with median sternotomy compared a multimodal regimen of ketorolac, paracetamol, gabapentin, and dexamethasone to morphine and paracetamol. Both regimens were started at the time of extubation and continued for 4 days after. They found that the multimodal group had significantly lower pain scores as well as a lower incidence of nausea and vomiting. They quoted no safety issues with the multimodal regimen but did note a trend in rising creatinine levels in some patients in the multimodal group.[54] While insignificant in this study, the risk of renal injury does appear to be significant with the use of NSAIDs after cardiac surgery. Another RCT of 180 patients compared ibuprofen to oxycodone after cardiac surgery and found that while there was no difference in mortality between the two groups, there was a significant increase in the rate of acute kidney injury, which resolved after ibuprofen discontinuation.[55]

Ketamine is a potent anesthetic and analgesic known for its sympathomimetic effects. While the mechanism is debated, studies have suggested that ketamine is actually a direct myocardial depressant and exerts its sympathomimetic effects indirectly via the release of endogenous catecholamines. As such, the use of ketamine can cause significant tachycardia and has been shown to increase myocardial oxygen demand by as much as 50% in an animal model. A study examining ketamine in cardiac surgery noted significant tachycardia with induction but overall stable hemodynamics.[56] There are very limited data on the use of ketamine for analgesia after cardiac surgery. One study compared ketamine to a placebo and found improvement in pain scores and decreased opioid consumption, while another found that the use of ketamine either by itself or when combined with a gabapentinoid significantly improved pain control 24 hours after cardiac surgery.[56,57] The paucity of data concerning the use of ketamine in this setting is likely due in part to the sympathomimetic effects outlined earlier; in fact, the Consensus Guidelines on the Use of IV Ketamine for Acute Pain Management seems to discourage its use in these patients, citing grade C evidence and stating that "ketamine should be avoided in individuals with poorly controlled cardiovascular disease."[58]

Epidurals

Thoracic epidurals have long been known to have many advantages in patients undergoing cardiac surgery. The placement of an epidural in the high thoracic levels, in addition to anesthetizing the thoracic nerves that give rise to the intercostal nerves, can cause a sympathectomy of the T1-T4 cardiac accelerator fibers. This can prevent tachycardia and catecholamine release, decreasing myocardial oxygen demand. Additionally, nociceptive blockade at the spinal level has been shown to attenuate the surgical stress response as well as improve coronary blood flow and ventricular function.[59,60]

However, thoracic epidurals are not widely used in this patient population, likely due to fears regarding the possibility of epidural hematoma. A meta-analysis examined the placement of over 88 000 epidurals in patients undergoing cardiac surgery and determined the risk of epidural hematoma to be 1:3352.[61] While low, this risk is likely as high as three times the risk in the general population. This increase is most likely attributable to the systemic heparinization needed for cardiopulmonary bypass. For this reason, the most recent ASRA guidelines continue to state that the risk of epidural anesthesia in patients appears to be too great for the perceived benefits. Their recommendations to reduce the risks further are to avoid heparinization at least 60 minutes after placement and to delay surgery for at least 24 hours in the event of a traumatic tap.[62] These recommendations would suggest that patients should be admitted the day before surgery for epidural placement, which is typically not feasible in today's health care environment.

Nevertheless, thoracic epidurals are sometimes used in patients undergoing cardiac surgery and appear to be effective at controlling postoperative pain. A recent Cochrane review found that when compared to systemic analgesics, epidurals reduced pain for 72 hours after surgery. More specifically, they cited 10 studies that found a 1.35 point reduction in pain on a 10-point scale in the 6- to 8-hour period after surgery. There was insufficient evidence to make any conclusions about epidural analgesia compared to peripheral nerve blocks.[63]

Regional nerve blocks

The concerns mentioned above with thoracic epidurals, as well as the rising popularity of ultrasound-guided peripheral nerve blocks in other populations, have led to the adaptation of these techniques for patients undergoing cardiac surgery. Techniques used in this patient population include blocks of the erector spinae plane, transversus thoracic plane, paravertebral space, parasternal intercostals, and pectoral nerve. Overall, these techniques confer an improved safety profile, analgesic efficacy, and decreased concerns for hemodynamic instability. Each technique has unique considerations, which are summarized in Table 13.1. Figure 13.2 outlines the typical distribution of each block.

Overall, these techniques are effective, but there are limited data comparing the techniques to each other. A recent meta-analysis of 17 studies was unable to comment on the relative superiority of one technique over another but did state that each regional technique described above was at least as effective as conventional analgesic techniques in controlling pain after cardiac surgery.[68]

TABLE 13.1 **CONSIDERATIONS FOR VARIOUS TRUNCAL REGIONAL BLOCKS**

Block	Benefits	Risks	Location
Paravertebral	• Easily reproducible • Improved safety profile • Hemodynamic stability • Comparable analgesic benefits as epidural • Decreased nausea and urinary retention compared to epidural	• Risk of epidural, subdural, subarachnoid, vertebral artery LA injection • Nerve injury including SLN, RLN, PN, cervical sympathetic chain (Horner syndrome) • LAST	• Injected into paravertebral space close to vertebral body where the SN emerges from IF • Dense ipsilateral somatic and sympathetic blockade along consecutive dermatomes above and below LA deposition
Pectoralis	• Decreased coughing • Opioid sparing • Hemodynamic stability • Improved safety profile	• Bilateral blocks (increase time and amount of LA) • LAST • Thoracoacromial artery injury • Long thoracic nerve injury • Pneumothorax	• PEC1 block: injected between pectoralis major and pectoralis minor muscles, 2nd-3rd rib level. Blocks medial and lateral pectoral nerves • PEC2 block: injected between pectoralis minor and serratus anterior muscles, 3rd-4th rib level. • Blocks lateral cutaneous branches of intercostal nerves T2-T6 including intercostobrachial nerve, long thoracic nerve, and intercostal nerves
Erector Spinae Plane	• Decreased coughing • Opioid sparing • Hemodynamic stability • Improved safety profile	• Bilateral blocks (increase time and amount of LA) • LAST • Pneumothorax	• LA deposited ventrally to the ESP muscle and superficial to the transverse processes, T5 level. Blocks spinal nerve dorsal and ventral rami (T2-T9 level)
Serratus anterior plane	• Decreased coughing • Opioid sparing • Hemodynamic stability • Improved safety profile	• Bilateral blocks (increase time and amount of LA) • LAST • Thoracoacromial artery injury • Long thoracic nerve injury • Pneumothorax	• Injected above or below the serratus anterior muscle, 4th-6th rib level. Blocks lateral cutaneous branches of intercostal nerves (~T3-T9) including intercostobrachial nerve, long thoracic nerve, thoracodorsal nerve
Parasternal	• Opioid sparing • Hemodynamic stability • Improved safety profile 'Technically easier than the TTP since transversus thoracic muscle can be difficult to visualize on ultrasound if it is small	• Bilateral blocks (increase time and amount of LA) • LAST • Pneumothorax • Nerve injury	• Injected between the pectoralis major and external intercostal muscles. Blocks anterior branches of the intercostal nerves (~T2-T7)

(Continued)

TABLE 13.1 **CONSIDERATIONS FOR VARIOUS TRUNCAL REGIONAL BLOCKS *(CONTINUED)***

Block	Benefits	Risks	Location
Transversus thoracic plane	• Opioid sparing • Hemodynamic stability • Improved safety profile	• Bilateral blocks (increase time and amount of LA) • LAST • Pneumothorax • Nerve injury • Bleeding/hematoma Potentially challenging, close proximity to pleura and IMA	• Injected between internal intercostal and transversus thoracic muscle, 3rd-5th rib level. Blocks anterior cutaneous branches of intercostal nerves (~T2-T7)

IF, intervertebral foramen; IMA, internal mammary artery; LA, local anesthesia; LAST, local anesthesia systemic toxicity; PN, phrenic nerve; RLN, recurrent laryngeal nerve; SLN, superior laryngeal nerve; SN, spinal nerve.
From Chakravarthy M. Regional analgesia in cardiothoracic surgery: a changing paradigm toward opioid-free anesthesia? *Ann Cardiac Anaesth*. 2018;21(3):225; Liu H, Emelife P, Prabhakar A, et al. Regional anesthesia considerations for cardiac surgery. *Best Pract Res Clin Anaesthesiol*. 2019;33(4):387-406; Mittnacht A, Shariat A, Weiner M, et al. Regional techniques for cardiac and cardiac-related procedures. *J Cardiothorac Vasc Anesth*. 2019;33(2):532-546; Kelava M, Alfirevic A, Bustamante S, Hargrave J, Marciniak D. Regional anesthesia in cardiac surgery: an overview of fascial plane chest wall blocks. *Anesth Analg*. 2020;131(1):127-135, Ref.[64-67]

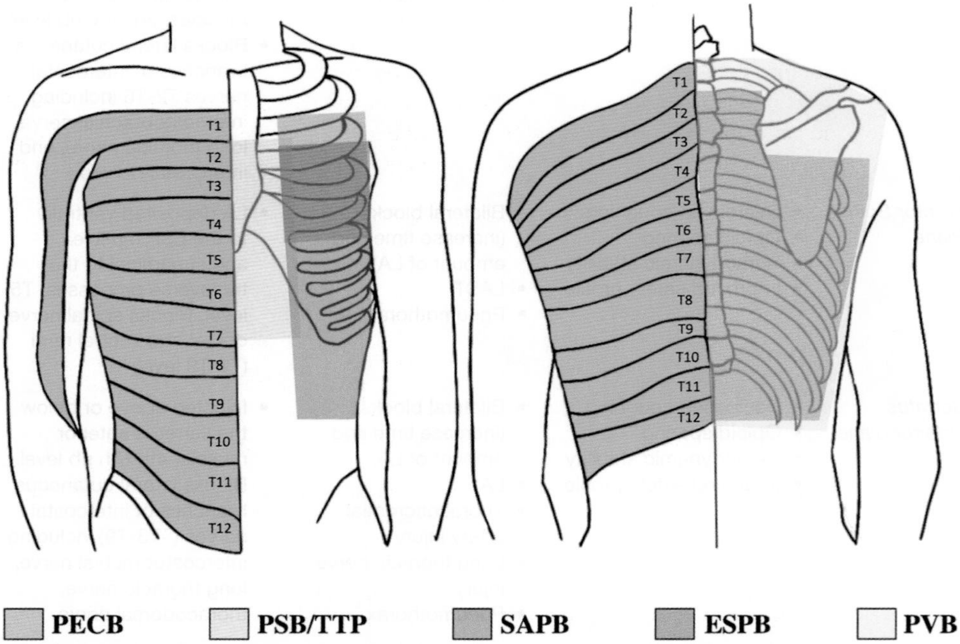

FIGURE 13.2 Chest wall anatomical diagram with expected dermatomal sensory blockade distribution of respective regional block techniques. ESPB, erector spinae plane block; PECB, pectoralis block (PEC1 and II); PSB, parasternal block; PVB, paravertebral block; SAPB, serratus anterior plane block; TTPB, transversus thoracic plane block. (From Chakravarthy M. Regional analgesia in cardiothoracic surgery: a changing paradigm toward opioid-free anesthesia? *Ann Cardiac Anaesth*. 2018;21(3):225; Liu H, Emelife P, Prabhakar A, et al. Regional anesthesia considerations for cardiac surgery. *Best Pract Res Clin Anaesthesiol*. 2019;33(4):387-406; Mittnacht A, Shariat A, Weiner M, et al. Regional techniques for cardiac and cardiac-related procedures. *J Cardiothorac Vasc Anesth*. 2019;33(2):532-546; Kelava M, Alfirevic A, Bustamante S, Hargrave J, Marciniak D. Regional anesthesia in cardiac surgery: an overview of fascial plane chest wall blocks. *Anesth Analg*. 2020;131(1):127-135, Ref.[64-67])

Differential Diagnoses

There are various other medical conditions that may mimic cardiac chest pain. Such conditions include those of pulmonary/pleural, gastrointestinal, musculoskeletal, and psychiatric etiologies.

Respiratory infections such as pneumonia or bronchitis can often be associated with a cough and chest discomfort, and patients having asthma exacerbations can present with symptoms of chest tightness. Treatment for the pain associated with these underlying conditions is often to simply treat the condition itself.

Gastrointestinal causes include gastroesophageal reflux disease, esophageal spasm, Boerhaave syndrome, and pancreatitis. Gastroesophageal reflux disease pain can be substernal in nature, thus mimicking anginal symptoms. It is often treated with a proton pump inhibitor or H2 blocker. Antacid medications may also help. Esophageal spasm is a condition that can be mistaken for angina, as symptoms may respond to nitroglycerin or calcium channel blockers, just as angina pectoris does. However, these patients also tend to present with symptoms of dysphagia for solids and liquids.[69,70]

Psychiatric causes of chest discomfort should also be considered, as patients experiencing panic attacks may feel heaviness or pressure in their chest along with a sense of doom. Treatment varies, but SSRIs and benzodiazepines have demonstrated efficacy.

Musculoskeletal causes of chest pain include costochondritis, intercostal muscle strains, and rib contusions/fractures following trauma. For isolated musculoskeletal chest pain, nonpharmacologic measures can be tried first, such as application of cold and heat. If pharmacologic management is needed, management is usually with acetaminophen or an NSAID at low doses. For moderate pain, stronger oral NSAIDs may be used.

Fibromyalgia, rheumatoid arthritis, and spondyloarthritis can also cause chest wall pain. Neoplasms and acute chest syndrome, which is associated with sickle cell disease, can also be musculoskeletal presentations of chest pain. Treatment of pain associated with these conditions is specific to the condition itself.

REFERENCES

1. Crossman DC. The pathophysiology of myocardial ischaemia. *Heart*. 2004;90(5):576-580. doi:10.1136/hrt.2003.029017
2. Gorlin R. Coronary anatomy. *Major Probl Intern Med*. 1976;11:40-58.
3. Foreman RD. Neurological mechanisms of chest pain and cardiac disease. *Cleve Clin J Med*. 2007;74:S30-S33.
4. Garratt KN. Stable angina pectoris. *Curr Treat Options Cardiovasc Med*. 2000;2(2):161-172.
5. Kaski J, Arrebola-Moreno A, Dungu J. Treatment strategies for chronic stable angina. *Expert Opin Pharmacother*. 2011;12:2833-2844.
6. Sylvén C, Beermann B, Jonzon B, Brandt R. Angina pectoris-like pain provoked by intravenous adenosine in healthy volunteers. *Br Med J (Clin Res Ed)*. 1986;293(6541):227-230. https://doi.org/10.1136/bmj.293.6541.227
7. Fihn SD, Blankenship JC, Alexander KP, et al. 2014 ACC/AHA/AATS/PCNA/SCAI/STS focused update of the guideline for the diagnosis and management of patients with stable ischemic heart disease: a report of the American College of Cardiology/American Heart Association Task Force on Practice Guidelines, and the American Association for Thoracic Surgery, Preventive Cardiovascular Nurses Association, Society for Cardiovascular Angiography and Interventions, and Society of Thoracic Surgeons. *J Am Coll Cardiol*. 2014;64(18):1929-1949. https://doi.org/10.1016/j.jacc.2014.07.017
8. Emanuelsson H, Egstrup K, Nikus K, et al. Antianginal efficacy of the combination of felodipine-metoprolol 10/100 mg compared with each drug alone in patients with stable effort-induced angina pectoris: a multicenter parallel group study. The TRAFFIC Study Group. *Am Heart J*. 1999;137(5):854-862. https://doi.org/10.1016/s0002-8703(99)70409-6
9. Bishop VS, Malliani A, Thorén P. Cardiac mechanoreceptors. In: Shepherd JT, Abboud FM, eds. *Handbook of Physiology: The Cardiovascular System, III*. Lippincott Williams & Williams; 1983:497-555.

10. Richter A, Cederholm I, Fredrikson M, Mucchiano C, Träff S, Janerot-Sjoberg B. Effect of long-term thoracic epidural analgesia on refractory angina pectoris: a 10-year experience. *J Cardiothorac Vasc Anesth.* 2012;26(5):822-828.
11. Jan R, Khan A, Zahid S, et al. The effect of enhanced external counterpulsation (EECP) on quality of life in patient with coronary artery disease not amenable to PCI or CABG. *Cureus.* 2020;12(5):e7987. https://doi.org/10.7759/cureus.7987
12. Burkhoff D, Schmidt S, Schulman SP, et al. Transmyocardial laser revascularisation compared with continued medical therapy for treatment of refractory angina pectoris: a prospective randomised trial. *Lancet.* 1999;354(9182):885-890.
13. Murphy DF, Giles KE. Dorsal column stimulation for pain relief from intractable angina pectoris. *Pain.* 1987;28:365-368.
14. Melzack R, Wall PD. Pain mechanisms: a new theory. *Science.* 1965;150:971-979.
15. Fihn SD, Gardin JM, Abrams J, et al.; American College of Cardiology Foundation/American Heart Association Task Force. 2012 ACCF/AHA/ACP/AATS/PCNA/SCAI/STS guideline for the diagnosis and management of patients with stable ischemic heart disease: a report of the American College of Cardiology Foundation/American Heart Association task force on practice guidelines, and the American College of Physicians, American Association for Thoracic Surgery, Preventive Cardiovascular Nurses Association, Society for Cardiovascular Angiography and Interventions, and Society of Thoracic Surgeons. *Circulation.* 2012;126:354-471. http://dx.doi.org/10.1161/CIR.0b013e318277d6a0
16. Thygesen K, Alpert JS, Jaffe AS, et al. Fourth universal definition of myocardial infarction (2018). *J Am Coll Cardiol.* 2018;72:2231.
17. O'Gara PT, Kushner FG, Ascheim DD. ACCF/AHA guideline for the management of ST-elevation myocardial infarction: a report of the American College of Cardiology Foundation/American Heart Association Task Force on Practice Guidelines. *J Am Coll Cardiol.* 2013;61(4):e78-e140.
18. Amsterdam EA, Wenger NK, Brindis RG, et al. 2014 AHA/ACC guideline for the management of patients with non-ST-elevation acute coronary syndromes: a report of the American College of Cardiology/American Heart Association Task Force on Practice Guidelines. *J Am Coll Cardiol.* 2014;64(24):e139-e228.
19. Eagle KA, Guyton RA, Davidoff R, et al. ACC/AHA 2004 guideline update for coronary artery bypass graft surgery: a report of the American College of Cardiology/American Heart Association Task Force on Practice Guidelines (Committee to Update the 1999 Guidelines for Coronary Artery Bypass Graft Surgery). *Circulation.* 2004;110(14):e340-e437.
20. Beltrame JF, Crea F, Kaski JC, et al. International standardization of diagnostic criteria for vasospastic angina. *Eur Heart J.* 2017;38:2565-2568.
21. Chiabrando JG, Bonaventura A, Vecchié A, et al. Management of acute and recurrent pericarditis: JACC state-of-the-art review. *J Am Coll Cardiol.* 2020;75:76.
22. Bonnefoy E, Godon P, Kirkorian G, Fatemi M, Chevalier P, Touboul P. Serum cardiac troponin I and ST-segment elevation in patients with acute pericarditis. *Eur Heart J.* 2000;21:832-836.
23. Imazio M, Brucato A, Maestroni S, et al. Prevalence of C-reactive protein elevation and time course of normalization in acute pericarditis: implications for the diagnosis, therapy, and prognosis of pericarditis. *Circulation.* 2011;123:1092-1097.
24. Klein AL, Abbara S, Agler DA, et al. American Society of Echocardiography clinical recommendations for multimodality cardiovascular imaging of patients with pericardial disease: endorsed by the Society for Cardiovascular Magnetic Resonance and Society of Cardiovascular Computed Tomography. *J Am Soc Echocardiogr.* 2013;26:965-1012.e15.
25. Imazio M, Brucato A, Cemin R, et al. A randomized trial of colchicine for acute pericarditis. *N Engl J Med.* 2013;369:1522-1528.
26. Imazio M, Brucato A, Cumetti D, et al. Corticosteroids for recurrent pericarditis: high versus low doses: a nonrandomized observation. *Circulation.* 2008;118:667-671.
27. Pape LA, Awais M, Woznicki EM, et al. Presentation, diagnosis, and outcomes of acute aortic dissection: 17-year trends from the international registry of acute aortic dissection. *J Am Coll Cardiol.* 2015;66(4):350-358. doi:10.1016/j.jacc.2015.05.029
28. Nienaber CA, Eagle KA. Aortic dissection: new frontiers in diagnosis and management: Part I: from etiology to diagnostic strategies. *Circulation.* 2003;108(5):628-635. doi:10.1161/01.CIR.0000087009.16755.E4
29. Nienaber CA, von Kodolitsch Y, Nicolas V, et al. The diagnosis of thoracic aortic dissection by noninvasive imaging procedures. *N Engl J Med.* 1993;328(1):1-9. doi:10.1056/NEJM199301073280101
30. Hiratzka LF, Bakris GL, Beckman JA, et al. 2010 ACCF/AHA/AATS/ACR/ASA/SCA/SCAI/SIR/STS/SVM guidelines for the diagnosis and management of patients with Thoracic Aortic Disease: a report of the American College of Cardiology Foundation/American Heart Association Task Force on Practice Guidelines, American Association for Thoracic Surgery, American College of Radiology, American Stroke Association, Society of Cardiovascular Anesthesiologists, Society for Cardiovascular Angiography and Interventions, Society of Interventional Radiology, Society of Thoracic Surgeons, and Society for Vascular Medicine

[published correction appears in Circulation. 2010 Jul 27;122(4):e410]. *Circulation*. 2010;121(13):e266-e369. doi:10.1161/CIR.0b013e3181d4739e

31. Zhu X. *Surgical Atlas of Cardiac Anatomy*. Springer Netherlands; 2015.
32. Moore K. *Clinically Oriented Anatomy*. 6th ed. Wolters Kluwer Health; 2009.
33. Klineberg E, Mazanec D, Orr D, Demicco R, Bell G, McLain R. Masquerade: medical causes of back pain. *Cleve Clin J Med*. 2007;74(12):905-913.
34. Netterimages.com. Visceral Referred Pain. 2020. Accessed August 23, 2020. https://www.netterimages.com/visceral-referred-pain-labeled-reynolds-2e-rehabilitation-frank-h-netter-73698.html
35. McConaghy J, Oza R. Outpatient diagnosis of acute chest pain in adults. 2020. Accessed August 23, 2020. https://www.aafp.org/afp/2013/0201/p177.html
36. Hollander J, Chase M. Uptodate. Uptodate.com. 2020. Accessed September 7, 2020. https://www.uptodate.com/contents/evaluation-of-the-adult-with-chest-pain-in-the-emergency-department/contributors
37. Sellke F, Ruel M. *Atlas of Cardiac Surgical Techniques*. 2nd ed. Elsevier; 2018.
38. Netter F. *Atlas of Human Anatomy*. 7th ed. Elsevier; 2019.
39. Ball M, Falkson SR, Adigun OO. Anatomy, angle of Louis. [Updated 2021 Jul 31]. In: *StatPearls* [Internet]. StatPearls Publishing.
40. Eisenberg E, Pultorak Y, Pud D, Bar-El Y. Prevalence and characteristics of post coronary artery bypass graft surgery pain (PCP). *Pain*. 2001;92:11-17.
41. Mueller XM, Tinguely F, Tevaearai HT, Revelly JP, Chioléro R, von Segesser LK. Pain pattern and left internal mammary artery grafting. *Ann Thorac Surg*. 2000;70(6):2045-2049. doi:10.1016/s0003-4975(00)01947-0
42. Blitz A, Osterday RM, Brodman RF. Harvesting the radial artery. *Ann Cardiothorac Surg*. 2013;2(4):533-542. doi:10.3978/j.issn.2225-319X.2013.07.10
43. Altshuler P, Welle NJ. Saphenous vein grafts. [Updated 2021 Feb 13]. In: *StatPearls* [Internet]. StatPearls Publishing.
44. Mueller XM, Tinguely F, Tevaearai HT, Revelly JP, Chioléro R, von Segesser LK. Pain location, distribution, and intensity after cardiac surgery. *Chest*. 2000;118(2):391-396. doi:10.1378/chest.118.2.391
45. Milgrom LB, Brooks JA, Qi R, Bunnell K, Wuestfeld S, Beckman D. Pain levels experienced with activities after cardiac surgery. *Am J Crit Care*. 2004;13(2):116-125.
46. Kwanten LE, O'Brien B, Anwar S. Opioid-based anesthesia and analgesia for adult cardiac surgery: history and narrative review of the literature. *J Cardiothorac Vasc Anesth*. 2019;33(3):808-816. doi:10.1053/j.jvca.2018.05.053
47. Rong LQ, Kamel MK, Rahouma M, et al. High-dose versus low-dose opioid anesthesia in adult cardiac surgery: a meta-analysis. *J Clin Anesth*. 2019;57:57-62. doi:10.1016/j.jclinane.2019.03.009
48. de Hoogd S, Ahlers SJGM, van Dongen EPA, et al. Randomized controlled trial on the influence of intraoperative remifentanil versus fentanyl on acute and chronic pain after cardiac surgery. *Pain Pract*. 2018;18(4):443-451. doi:10.1111/papr.12615
49. Zakhary WZA, Turton EW, Flo Forner A, von Aspern K, Borger MA, Ender JK. A comparison of sufentanil vs. remifentanil in fast-track cardiac surgery patients. *Anaesthesia*. 2019;74(5):602-608. doi:10.1111/anae.14572
50. Murphy GS, Szokol JW, Avram MJ, et al. Intraoperative methadone for the prevention of postoperative pain: a randomized, double-blinded clinical trial in cardiac surgical patients. *Anesthesiology*. 2015;122(5):1112-1122.
51. Murphy GS, Avram MJ, Greenberg SB, et al. Postoperative pain and analgesic requirements in the first year after intraoperative methadone for complex spine and cardiac surgery. *Anesthesiology*. 2020;132(2):330-342. doi:10.1097/ALN.0000000000003025
52. Bainbridge D, Martin JE, Cheng DC. Patient-controlled*versus* nurse-controlled analgesia after cardiac surgery—a meta-analysis. *Can J Anesth*. 2006;53:492.
53. Gurbert A, Goren S, Sahin S, Uckunkaya N, Korfali G. Comparison of analgesic effects of morphine, fentanyl, and remifentanil with intravenous patient-controlled analgesia after cardiac surgery. *J Cardiothorac Vasc Anesth*. 2005;18:755-758.
54. Rafiq S, Steinbrüchel DA, Wanscher MJ, et al. Multimodal analgesia versus traditional opiate based analgesia after cardiac surgery, a randomized controlled trial. *J Cardiothorac Surg*. 2014;9:52. doi:10.1186/1749-8090-9-52
55. Qazi SM, Sindby EJ, Nørgaard MA. Ibuprofen—a safe analgesic during cardiac surgery recovery? a randomized controlled trial. *J Cardiovasc Thorac Res*. 2015;7(4):141-148. doi:10.15171/jcvtr.2015.31
56. Mazzeffi M, Johnson K, Paciullo C. Ketamine in adult cardiac surgery and the cardiac surgery Intensive Care Unit: an evidence-based clinical review. *Ann Card Anaesth*. 2015;18:202-209.
57. Anwar S, Cooper J, Rahman J, Sharma C, Langford R. Prolonged perioperative use of pregabalin and ketamine to prevent persistent pain after cardiac surgery. *Anesthesiology*. 2019;131(1):119-131. doi:10.1097/ALN.0000000000002751
58. Schwenk E, Viscusi E, Buvanendran A, et al. Consensus guidelines on the use of intravenous ketamine infusions for acute pain management from the American Society of Regional Anesthesia and Pain Medicine, the American Academy of Pain Medicine, and the American Society of Anesthesiologists. *Reg Anesth Pain Med*. 2018;43(5):456-466. doi:10.1097/AAP.0000000000000806

59. Kirnö K, Friberg P, Grzegorczyk A, Milocco I, Ricksten SE, Lundin S. Thoracic epidural anesthesia during coronary artery bypass surgery: effects on cardiac sympathetic activity, myocardial blood flow and metabolism, and central hemodynamics. *Anesth Analg*. 1994;79(6):1075-1081.
60. Hutchenson J, Sonntag H, Hill E, et al. High thoracic epidural anesthesia's effect on myocardial blood flow, oxygen consumption, myocardial work and markers of ischemia during coronary artery bypass grafting: a randomised controlled trial. *Anesth Analg*. 2006;102:SCA-13.
61. Landoni G, Isella F, Greco M, Zangrillo A, Royse CF. Benefits and risks of epidural analgesia in cardiac surgery. *Br J Anaesth*. 2015;115(1):25-32.
62. Horlocker T, Vandermeuelen E, Kopp S, Gogarten W, Leffert L, Benzon H. Regional anesthesia in the patient receiving antithrombotic or thrombolytic therapy: American Society of Regional anesthesia and pain medicine evidence-based guidelines (fourth edition). *Reg Anesth Pain Med*. 2018;43(3):263-309. doi:10.1097/AAP.0000000000000763
63. Guay J, Kopp S. Epidural analgesia for adults undergoing cardiac surgery with or without cardiopulmonary bypass. *Cochrane Database Syst Rev*. 2019;(3):CD006715. doi:10.1002/14651858.CD006715.pub3.
64. Chakravarthy M. Regional analgesia in cardiothoracic surgery: a changing paradigm toward opioid-free anesthesia? *Ann Card Anaesth*. 2018;21(3):225.
65. Liu H, Emelife P, Prabhakar A, et al. Regional anesthesia considerations for cardiac surgery. *Best Pract Res Clin Anaesthesiol*. 2019;33(4):387-406.
66. Mittnacht A, Shariat A, Weiner M, et al. Regional techniques for cardiac and cardiac-related procedures. *J Cardiothorac Vasc Anesth*. 2019;33(2):532-546.
67. Kelava M, Alfirevic A, Bustamante S, Hargrave J, Marciniak D. Regional anesthesia in cardiac surgery: an overview of fascial plane chest wall blocks. *Anesth Analg*. 2020;131(1):127-135.
68. Kar P, Ramachandran G. Pain relief following sternotomy in conventional cardiac surgery: A review of non neuraxial regional nerve blocks. *Ann Card Anaesth*. 2020;23:200-208.
69. Drenth JP, Bos LP, Engels LG. Efficacy of diltiazem in the treatment of diffuse oesophageal spasm. *Aliment Pharmacol Ther*. 1990;4:411.
70. Orlando RC, Bozymski EM. Clinical and manometric effects of nitroglycerin in diffuse esophageal spasm. *N Engl J Med* 1973;289:23.

14

Acute Vascular- and Hematologic-Related Pain and Differential Diagnosis

Gopal Kodumudi, Vijay Kata, Islam Mohammad Shehata, and Alan David Kaye

Introduction

Acute vascular-related pain has a diverse array of etiologies, including peripheral arterial disease, large and small vessel vasculitides, thrombosis, and avascular necrosis (AVN). Hematologic-related pain includes complications of sickle cell disease (SCD) such as acute chest syndrome (ACS) and priapism. The pain that is encountered in these disease processes can be a combination of multiple mechanisms (nociceptive, inflammatory, neuropathic). The clinical features, diagnostic features, and treatment are discussed for each of these etiologies of vascular- and hematologic-related pain states.

Peripheral Arterial Disease

Peripheral arterial disease (PAD) is a common disease that involves atherosclerosis and partial or complete occlusion of arteries of the lower extremities. It is believed that 10%-15% of the population and ~200 million people around the globe suffer from this condition. Risk factors for PAD include smoking (strongest association) and diabetes.[1] Of all patients with PAD, only 10%-30% actually experience the symptoms of intermittent claudication. Atherosclerosis causes arterial stenosis that can eventually completely occlude the artery. When compensatory mechanisms such as vasodilation and collateral vessels, fail, ischemia will eventually occur. Severity of the ischemia depends on how extensive the occlusion is. Intermittent claudication specifically occurs when blood flow to the lower extremities is significantly diminished during physical exertion but is sufficient at rest. Critical ischemia is the terminal stage of the inadequate blood flow—diminished tissue perfusion causes pain at rest with eventual gangrene.

Current treatment options for PAD include antiplatelet therapy, some oral anticoagulants such as rivaroxaban (but not warfarin, which has failed to show treatment benefit), risk factor reduction (eg, controlling hypertension and hypercholesterolemia with ACEi/ARBs and statins), medications (eg, cilostazol, naftidrofuryl, carnitine, buflomedil, inositol), and finally revascularization.

Neurogenic Claudication

Spinal stenosis occurs when central canal and neural foramina are narrowed by degenerative arthritis. Other possible causes that narrow these spaces include facet join arthropathy, loss of disk height, and hypertrophy of the ligamentum flavum. The most common regions in descending order of frequency are L4-L5, L5-S1, and L3-L4.[2] People over the age of 60 years are more commonly affected by this condition. Direct compression of the nerve roots and ischemia results in the neurologic claudication. Possible symptoms include pain, discomfort, weakness, numbness, or paresthesias in the lower back, buttocks, and legs. Symptoms are exacerbated by standing with the spine extended (walking, standing). Severe symptoms can include bladder incontinence. The pain is relieved with lumbar flexion to 20°-40° (bending over, sitting). Treatment options include physical therapy, epidural steroid injections, and surgery.

Osteoarthritis

Osteoarthritis is a degenerative joint disease that is the most frequent cause of chronic debility in elders. The hyaline cartilage between joints degenerates due to overuse. Symptoms include aching pain that worsens with use, decreased range of motion, and stiffness. Common locations in the lower extremities include the knees and hips.

Giant Cell Arteritis

Large vessel vasculitis such as giant cell arteritis and Takayasu arteritis are conditions where granulomatous inflammation of blood vessel wall occurs especially in the aorta and aortic branches.

Giant cell arteritis occurs in the older population, more commonly with women, with a mean age of diagnosis of age 72. Granulomatous inflammation most often presents in the extracranial arteries of the head, coming off from the second to fifth order aortic branches.

There is a higher incidence in people of northern European descent.[3] All layers of the arterial wall can be affected by the granulomatous infiltrates of multinucleated giant cells and histiocytes. The adventitia of the blood vessels is a critical site in GCA.[4]

Diagnosis

Giant cell arteritis is most commonly diagnosed by superficial temporal artery biopsy in the temple region. Other arteries included are the ophthalmic, vertebral posterior ciliary arteries, central retinal arteries, and the external and internal carotid arteries. The symptoms of GCA include headaches that can be sharp, dull, or throbbing in quality. A serious complication and ophthalmic emergency is vision loss of the affected ophthalmic artery. A fleeting blurring of vision with exercise or heat or posture is called amaurosis fugax, and it may lead to complete blindness if not treated emergently.

Another manifestation of GCA is jaw claudication caused by decreased blood flow to extracranial branches of the carotid artery to the temporalis or masseter muscles. GCA can also manifest as fevers and chills of unknown origin. Temporal artery biopsy is the confirmatory diagnostic procedure. Carotid, axillary subclavian, and femoral arteritis along with aortitis are other forms of large vessel arteritis seen in GCA.

Laboratory Abnormalities

A high erythrocyte sedimentation rate is seen in most patients with GCA. C-reactive protein is also a useful laboratory marker. Elevated platelet counts elevated alkaline phosphatase and hypochromic or normochromic anemia can be other laboratory abnormalities.

Treatment of GCA

Glucocorticoids have been extremely effective in decreasing the rate of blindness associated with GCA causing relief usually within 48 hours.[5]

Takayasu Arteritis

Takayasu arteritis is a rare disease that occurs predominantly in women. Aortic wall dilatation and aortic aneurysm occurs in TA when the smooth muscle is replaced by fibrous tissue due to granulomatous polyarteritis in large elastic arteries. In TA, a major component of the infiltrates is CD8 T cells that cause cytolytic tissue injury.

The initial manifestations of TA include malaise, night sweats, fever loss of appetite, abdominal pain, and weight loss. Vasoocclusive disease and ischemic changes of the vertebral and carotid arteries can lead to symptoms such as headache and stroke ophthalmologic symptoms.[6] Blood pressure changes, pulselessness, and arm claudication can occur with occlusions of the subclavian and brachiocephalic arteries. Aortitis of the aorta can lead to arrhythmia, congestive heart failure, ischemic heart disease, and aortic dilatation.

The diagnosis of TA with symptoms of vasoocclusion and systemic inflammation is done by vascular imaging of conventional angiography. Long-term immunosuppressive treatment with glucocorticoids is the treatment of choice of doses of 40-60 mg of prednisone and is needed for progressive or relapsing disease.[7] Antiplatelet agents such as aspirin are also recommended to complement treatment with glucocorticoids. TA is considered a devastating disease. Surgical management such as bypass grafts in addition to immunosuppressive treatment with glucocorticoids can lead to better prognosis.

Polyarteritis Nodosa

Polyarteritis nodosa is inflammation in the small- to medium-sized arteries and spares large-sized arteries. Polyarteritis nodosa affects the arteries of the kidney in over 70% of the cases, with the GI tract being in involved in about 50% of the cases. Laboratory tests are nonspecific.

Nerve conduction abnormalities may be confirmed with nerve conduction velocities and electromyography. Full-thickness skin biopsy confirms the diagnosis. Along with treatment with glucocorticoids, a simultaneous treatment of plasma exchange over 6 weeks has been done followed by antiviral therapy.[3]

Buerger Disease (Thromboangiitis Obliterans)

Buerger disease (thromboangiitis obliterans [TAO]) affects the upper and lower extremities as a segmental, inflammatory disease of the small- and medium-sized arteries. It often presents with a systemic inflammatory response.[8]

Presentation of TAO can occur as pain or claudication of extremities followed by ischemic rest pain and is associated with ulcerations in fingers and toes. Smoking cessation is strictly advised. TAO is nonatherosclerotic where the media and intima are involved. In TAO, all three layers of the arterial wall are infiltration of round cells. There are no specific laboratory tests for TAO. Small collateral arteries around occlusion in arteriography may be seen described as "cockscrewing" or "pig-tailing" around occlusions. Management involves cessation of smoking. For symptoms, treatment with vasodilators such as calcium channel blockers and prostaglandin analogs have been used.[9]

Avascular Necrosis

Avascular necrosis is also known as ischemic bone necrosis, aseptic necrosis, or osteonecrosis. It involves compromise of subchondral blood supply that can lead to death of bone cells. Weight-bearing joints can collapse when the epiphysis of long bones in these joints get affected. The hip is the most common joint involved and is often associated with glucocorticoid use.[10]

Other common sites for AVN include the femoral head, humerus head, knee, and talus. Prognosis of AVN is poor, and many progress to total failure requiring surgical interventions such as arthroplasty. Postoperative complications of prosthesis malfunction, neurovascular compromise, and surgical site infections are an added challenge.[11]

Ischemic Embolisms

Deep vein thrombosis (DVT) involves thrombi in the leg veins, renal veins, or axillary subclavian veins. Pulmonary embolisms occur when those thrombi dislodge and travel to the lungs. Following myocardial infarction and stroke, pulmonary embolism is the third most common cardiovascular diagnosis. Pulmonary embolism is frequently underdiagnosed.[12] The thrombi embolize to the pulmonary vascular bed and increase right ventricular afterload and can result in hypotension and cardiac arrest.[13]

Incidence of thromboembolism can be increased by active cancer, immobility, recent major surgery, cardiopulmonary conditions such as congestive heart failure, and chronic obstructive pulmonary disease. Symptoms of acute PE include sudden dyspnea syncope, tachycardia, tachypnea, hypotension pleuritic chest pain, and hemoptysis. Nonspecific laboratory markers exist for PE. Ventilation perfusion scan (VQ scan) and chest CTA are useful to rule out PE. Ultrasonography is a powerful tool in the diagnosis of DVT. Anticoagulation reduces mortality in DVT and PE. Early anticoagulation is associated with reduced mortality for acute pulmonary embolism.[14]

Entrapment Neuropathies

The most common peripheral neuropathies are radiculopathies and carpal tunnel syndrome. Irritation or compression of peripheral nerves causes peripheral neuropathies, the most common of which is carpal tunnel syndrome. Other common entrapment neuropathies are cubital tunnel syndrome and sciatica where compression by a herniated disc or nerve root irritation occurs. Risk factors contributing to entrapment neuropathies include ischemia, fibrosis, systemic diseases, demyelination, and central nervous system contributions. Demyelination can be induced by prolonged ischemia.[15] Reduction of action potential in nerve damage in entrapments leads to loss of function.[16]

Neuroinflammation can lead to neuropathic pain by activation of immune cells where axon cells are damages. Physiotherapy, pharmacological interventions with local steroid injections, and surgical decompression such as carpel tunnel decompression and lumbar microdiscectomy for sciatica have been performed with varying success.

Sickle Cell Disease Pain Syndromes

Sickle cell disease is a group of red blood cell disorders caused by a point mutation in the beta chain of a hemoglobin molecule that alters a red blood cell's ability to transport oxygen. In SCD, red blood cells become sickle shaped and cause vascular complications. Some of the most common reasons for hospitalizations in SCD patients are ACS and priapism.

Acute Chest Syndrome

Pathophysiology

Acute chest syndrome is an acute or chronic pulmonary insult resulting in clumping of sickled red blood cells causing a cycle of lung inflammation leading to vasoocclusive crises. The pathophysiology also includes increased levels of vascular cell adhesion molecule-1, which is an endothelial adhesion receptor, and decreased levels of nitric oxide.[17] ACS is a painful condition that is associated with multiple risk factors, which include infection, bronchial hyperreaction, hypoxia, genotype inheritance, and opioid use.[18]

Clinical Diagnosis

A clinical diagnosis for ACS generally involves the presentation of a fever and respiratory symptoms such as chest pain, cough, tachypnea, and hypoxemia. A patient's chest X-ray displaying a segmental pulmonary infiltrate without atelectasis along with respiratory symptoms. Clinical presentations in children and adults can vary with differing complications and presenting factors. In cases of ACS, children typically present with cough, fever, laborious breathing, and wheezing, while adults are more prone to clinical presentations of dyspnea, chest pain, and a possible vasoocclusive crisis.[19] Pediatric patients also showed lower hemoglobin levels and oxygen tension fraction within the arterial blood at the time of diagnosis.

Treatment

The goal of any ACS event is supportive care with antibiotics, pain control, hydration, and ventilation.[19] Advantages of earlier treatment include lower mortality rates, shorter hospital stays, and less chance of recurrence. The use of an incentive spirometry device to prevent atelectasis and chest physiotherapy can help maintain adequate ventilation. A third-generation cephalosporin should be used to prevent against pneumococcal infection with possible vancomycin for MRSA infection.[17] Pain medications have been important in the management of ACS episodes in SCD patients. The goal of pain medication is to achieve analgesia while preventing respiratory depression leading to hypoventilation. One example of a medication used for ACS in SCD patients includes a monoclonal antibody called crizanlizumab that binds P-selectin. In a sample of 198 patients, it was found that pain crises with high-dose crizanlizumab averaged around 1.63 crises per year, while those who were given a placebo had median rates of 2.98 crises per year.[20] Additionally, the use of crizanlizumab decreased the average days spent in the hospital and increased the median time until the first ACS pain crisis episode. These results are significant and indicate a safe and effective medicine that increases the quality of life of ACS patients.

Priapism

Another complication of SCD is priapism. Priapism is a condition that results in a persistent penile erection not stemming from sexual arousal or desire but as a result of vascular complication.[21] Priapism was first correlated with SCD and pain in 1934, and over time research has shown that it affects approximately one-quarter to one-third of males throughout their lifetime.

Pathophysiology

Priapism in SCD occurs due to a chronic problem of diminished availability of nitric oxide from endothelium. The decreased availability of nitric oxide results from hemolyzed hemoglobin binding free nitric oxide causing a decreased nitric oxide level.[22] Arginase, an enzyme that breaks up L-arginine, is released during the ongoing hemolysis and further disrupts nitric oxide formation from L-arginine). The chronic decrease in nitric oxide production in the endothelium causes a decrease in cGMP and phosphodiesterase 5 (PDE5), expression that promotes priapism due to failure of cGMP to relax the corpus cavernosum.[22]

Clinical Diagnosis

A complete blood count taken in a SCD patient shows low hemoglobin levels and increased white blood cells, platelets, reticulocytes, mean corpuscular volume, bilirubin, and mean corpuscular hemoglobin that help characterize the severity of the priapism event.[23] The length of priapism episodes, which mainly occur at nighttime, and degree of pain vary with each patient. Furthermore, there exists a limited diagnosis of priapism in SCD because of underreporting by patients, a lack of physician awareness, and insufficient prospective studies.[21] Other diagnostic measures of priapism include a blood gas measurement to distinguish between ischemic and nonischemic priapism, imaging studies, laboratory tests, and a physical examination.

Identifying the subtype of priapism present can help create a more targeted treatment plan. The different types of priapism include ischemic (low-flow), nonischemic (high-flow), and stuttering (recurrent and intermittent) priapism. Ischemic priapism is the most common and is due to a defect in venous blood outflow. Ischemic priapism can be diagnosed by measuring venous blood in the corpora cavernosa showing $PO_2 < 30$ mm Hg, a $PCO_2 > 60$ mm Hg, and a $pH < 7.25$ along with clinical suspicion and complete blood count analysis.[24] Nonischemic priapism is due to increased arterial blood flow into the corpora cavernosa. Nonischemic priapism can be diagnosed by presence of a perineal compression sign from arteriocorporal fistulas due to compromised blood supply in addition to physical examination and blood gas analysis revealing normal arterial PO_2, PCO_2, and pH. Stuttering priapism is the most common type in SCD patients. This occurs due to low PDE5 levels due to decreased expression of nitric oxide leading to defects in corpora cavernosal relaxation.[24]

In a research study that sampled patients throughout the United States, it was found that 89% of individuals experience a priapism episode before 20 years of age.[25] The average age of the first episode was 12 years, with the mean number of episodes equaling 15.7 and the length of each episode typically lasting 125 minutes.[25] Through a better understanding of the pathophysiology of the disease, physicians can implement medications and treatments that utilize evidence-based strategies that increases positive outcomes for SCD patients.

Treatment

Priapism can last for hours so effective management techniques such as corporal aspiration, corporal injection of sympathomimetics, pharmacotherapy, hormone therapy, distal shunting, penile aspiration/drainage, and penile prosthesis have all displayed promising results for SCD patients.[24] Sympathomimetics cause vasoconstriction mediated by alpha-adrenergic receptors and cause contraction of the corpora cavernosa smooth muscle leading to cessation of the erection.[22] PDE5 inhibitors reestablish a baseline level of cGMP in the corpora cavernosa that fixes the nitric oxide dysfunction caused by hemolysis and vascular endothelium compromise in SCD. Hormone therapy such as antiandrogen therapy, estrogen receptor agonists, and GnRH antagonists is useful in preventing the proerectile state.[22] Other treatment options include intravenous fluids, opioids, alkalization, hydroxyurea, and exchange transfusion.[26] Hydroxyurea reacts with hemoglobin to make nitric oxide and restore the nitric oxide deficit created from the hemolysis occurring in SCD patients. Common therapeutic methods sought by patients for priapism-induced pain include warm showers, ejaculation, over the counter analgesics, and physical exercise.

REFERENCES

1. Essa H, Torella F, Lip GYH. Current and emerging drug treatment strategies for peripheral arterial disease. *Expert Opin Pharmacother*. 2020;21:1603-1616.
2. Munakomi S, Foris LA, Varacallo M. Spinal stenosis and neurogenic claudication. In: *StatPearls* [Internet]. StatPearls Publishing; 2020. https://www.ncbi.nlm.nih.gov/books/NBK430872/
3. Weyand CM, Goronzy JJ. Vasculitides. *Primer Rheum Dis*. 2008:398-450.
4. Weyand CM, Goronzy JJ. The immune response of GCA leans towards a T cell mediated immune pathology. Medium- and large-vessel vasculitis. *N Engl J Med*. 2003;349:160-169.
5. Hayreh SS, Zimmerman B, Kardon RH. Visual improvement with corticosteroid therapy in giant cell arteritis. Report of a large study and review of literature. *Acta Ophthalmol Scand*. 2002;80(4):355-367.
6. Arnaud L, Haroche J, Mathian A, Gorochov G, Amoura Z. Pathogenesis of Takayasu's arteritis: a 2011 update. *Autoimmun Rev*. 2011;11(1):61-67.
7. Liang P, Hoffman GS. Advances in the medical and surgical treatment of Takayasu arteritis. *Curr Opin Rheumatol*. 2005;17(1):16-24.
8. Olin JW. Thromboangiitis obliterans: 110 years old and little progress made. *J Am Heart Assoc*. 2018;7(23):e011214.
9. Fazeli B, Dadgar Moghadam M, Niroumand S. How to treat a patient with thromboangiitis obliterans: a systematic review. *Ann Vasc Surg*. 2018;49:219-228.
10. Weinstein RS. Glucocorticoid-induced osteonecrosis. *Endocrine*. 2012;41:183-190.
11. Franceschi F, Franceschetti E, Paciotti M, et al. Surgical management of osteonecrosis of the humeral head: a systematic review. *Knee Surg Sports Traumatol Arthrosc*. 2017;25(10):3270-3278.
12. Weinberg AW, Jaff MR, Tapson VF. Pulmonary embolism: an international crisis. *Endovasc Today*. 2019:3-4.
13. Piazza G, Goldhaber SZ. Acute pulmonary embolism: part I: epidemiology and diagnosis. *Circulation*. 2006;114(2):e28-e32.
14. Smith SB, Geske JB, Maguire JM, Zane NA, Carter RE, Morgenthaler TI. Early anticoagulation is associated with reduced mortality for acute pulmonary embolism. *Chest*. 2010;137(6):1382-1390.
15. Gupta R, Rowshan K, Chao T, Mozaffar T, Steward O. Chronic nerve compression induces local demyelination and remyelination in a rat model of carpal tunnel syndrome. *Exp Neurol*. 2004;187:500-508.
16. Tampin B, Vollert J, Schmid AB. Sensory profiles are comparable in patients with distal and proximal entrapment neuropathies, while the pain experience differs. *Curr Med Res Opin*. 2018;34:1899-1906.
17. Jain S, Bakshi N, Krishnamurti L. Acute chest syndrome in children with sickle cell disease. *Pediatric Allergy Immunol Pulmonol*. 2017;30(4):191-201.
18. Farooq S, Omar MA, Salzman GA. Acute chest syndrome in sickle cell disease. *Hosp Pract*. 2018;46(3):144-151.
19. Friend A, Girzadas D. Acute chest syndrome. In: *StatPearls* [Internet]. StatPearls Publishing; 2020. https://www.ncbi.nlm.nih.gov/books/NBK441872/
20. Ataga KI, Kutlar A, Kanter J, et al. Crizanlizumab for the prevention of pain crises in sickle cell disease. *N Engl J Med*. 2017;376(5):429-439.
21. Arduini GA, Marqui AB. Prevalence and characteristics of priapism in sickle cell disease. *Hemoglobin*. 2018;42(2):73-77.
22. Anele UA, Morrison BF, Burnett AL. Molecular pathophysiology of priapism: emerging targets. *Curr Drug Targets*. 2015;16(5):474-483.
23. Alkindi S, Almufargi SS, Pathare A. Clinical and laboratory parameters, risk factors predisposing to the development of priapism in sickle cell patients. *Exp Biol Med*. 2019;245(1):79-83.
24. Shigehara K, Namiki M. Clinical management of priapism: a review. *World J Mens Health*. 2016;34(1):1-8. doi:10.5534/wjmh.2016.34.1.1.
25. Mantadakis E, Cavender JD, Rogers ZR, Ewalt DH, Buchanan GR. Prevalence of priapism in children and adolescents with sickle cell anemia. *J Pediatr Hematol Oncol*. 1999;21:518-522.
26. Kato GJ. Priapism in sickle-cell disease: a hematologist's perspective. *J Sex Med*. 2012;9(1):70-78.

15

Acute Pleuritic- and Thoracic-Related Pain: Clinical Considerations

Benjamin Cole Miller, Megan A. Boudreaux, Erica V. Chemtob, G. Jason Huang, Elyse M. Cornett, and Alan David Kaye

Introduction

Pleuritic pain is a type of chest pain that is linked to problems with lung membranes called the pleura. It is often characterized by a sudden sharp, stabbing, or burning pain in the chest when inhaling or exhaling.[1] The lung itself is insensitive to pain so the discomfort associated with respiratory disease must arise from the pleura, tracheobronchial tree, or chest wall.[2] It is because of this that pleuritic pain can often mimic cardiac, pericardial, abdominal, and musculoskeletal disease.[2] Thus, patients with any type of chest pain should be worked up with a broad differential as to localize the location of the pain.

Overall, chest pain encompasses ~1% of primary care visits every year.[3] This percent is even higher in settings like the emergency room.[2] Despite the large number of cases, most are relatively benign with the most common causes being chest wall pain, reflux esophagitis, and costochondritis.[3] However, related to severity of the more serious causes of chest pain including pulmonary embolism, myocardial infarction, pericarditis, pneumonia, aortic dissection, and pneumothorax, a workup must focus on ruling these out before a clinician considers more benign causes.[4] In patients with general chest pain, acute coronary syndrome (ACS), which is a term used to describe a range of conditions associated with reduced flow to the heart such as myocardial infarction and angina, is the most common life-threatening condition seen.[5] Pulmonary embolisms are another common life-threatening condition that present mostly as pleuritic pain but can also present as chest wall pain depending on the location of the embolism.[6]

Cardiac disease is currently the leading cause of death in the United States, making it all the more vital for physicians to not miss the signs when patients present to them. However, with such a wide differential associated with pleuritic and thoracic pain as well as roughly only 1.5% of the patients presenting to a primary care office with chest pain related to life-threatening causes, it can be difficult for physicians to differentiate serious causes vs more benign causes.[3] It is thus important for physicians to quickly as well as accurately take and perform a good history and physical exam.[7] The time course of the onset of symptoms is the most useful information in the history for narrowing the differential diagnosis as often the most lethal causes of chest pain typically have the most acute onset.[1] During the course of the history and physical, it is vital to be able to identify patients with signs of life-threatening conditions who will need further workup including electrocardiogram (ECG), echocardiography, or urgent transfer to the catheterization laboratory.[5]

Acute pleuritic and thoracic pain are very common forms of pain and can be associated with life-threatening conditions if not recognized and treated appropriately. This type of pain encompasses a wide array of differential diagnoses, making recognition and treatment more difficult.[7] It is because of this that any type of chest pain should be assessed with a high degree of suspicion that focuses to rule out the life-threatening causes first and foremost while working up the more benign causes after.[2]

Etiology Epidemiology Risk Factors Pathophysiology

Etiology and Epidemiology

There are many different causes for chest pain, with each separate etiology requiring different diagnostic studies and treatments. Throughout the course of evaluating a patient with acute chest pain, it is important to first differentiate between emergent and nonemergent causes. Immediately, life-threatening causes of chest pain include myocardial ischemia, thoracic aortic dissection, tension pneumothorax, or pulmonary embolism.[8]

In addition to keeping in mind which diagnoses are the most dangerous, it is important to remember the most common causes of chest pain. It is estimated chest pain is the chief complaint for 5% of all emergency department presentations. Therefore, being able to quickly evaluate a patient and develop a plan is of the utmost importance. The most common causes of emergency department visits for chest pain include ACS, gastrointestinal reflux, and musculoskeletal causes.[9]

According to one study conducted by Freurfaard and colleagues, ACS was the most common cause of emergency department visits where the chief complaint was chest pain. Approximately 31% of all emergency department visits for acute-onset chest pain were related to ACS. Aortic aneurysms, another cardiovascular pathology, accounted for ~1% of all emergency department visits. Gastrointestinal reflux disease and musculoskeletal pathologies accounted for 30% and 28% of chest pain cases, respectively. In terms of lung pathologies, pulmonary embolism accounted for 2% of presentations and pneumonia/pleuritis also accounted for 2% of emergency department visits.[10]

Pathophysiology and Risk Factors

The pathophysiology and various risk factors associated with the differentials for chest pain are important to understand. Obtaining a thorough history to evaluate the patient for risk factors associated with the various etiologies of chest pain will guide the clinician in the quest for a diagnosis. Once the physician determines the diagnosis, understanding the pathophysiology behind the diagnosis will further guide treatment and intervention.

The most common, life-threatening cause of chest pain is ACS. ACS is an umbrella term that is comprised of unstable angina, non–ST-segment elevation myocardial infarction, and ST-segment elevation myocardial infarction (STEMI). The key difference between unstable angina and myocardial infarction is based on the presence or absence of cardiac biomarkers in a patient's serum. Because the ischemic events are transient in angina, cardiac biomarkers such as troponin will not be markedly elevated. However, in myocardial infarction, biomarkers will be elevated, indicating myocardial necrosis has occurred.[11] Key risk factors associated with ACS include diabetes, hypertension, hyperlipidemia, and a prior history of MI.[9]

Musculoskeletal causes of chest wall pain are also quite common. The key diagnostic feature of musculoskeletal causes of chest pain is that the pain is reproducible upon palpation. One of the most common causes of musculoskeletal chest pain includes costochondritis, which is inflammation of the costal cartilages. Costochondritis is a self-limited condition that is usually not associated with an identifiable trigger. It is thought that repetitive exercises and activities can contribute to the development of costochondritis. Because of the nonspecific nature of this condition, it is imperative that costochondritis only be included as a diagnosis of exclusion after other, more life-threatening causes of acute chest pain have been ruled out[12] (Table 15.1).

TABLE 15.1 COMMON CAUSES OF ACUTE CHEST PAIN

Organ System	Diagnosis	Pathophysiology	Risk Factors
Cardiac	Acute coronary syndrome	Acute rupture of an atherosclerotic plaque in a coronary artery with subsequent thrombus formation[11]	Diabetes History of myocardial infarction Family history of heart disease Hypertension Hyperlipidemia[9]
	Thoracic aortic dissection	Inflammation of the aortic wall leading to vessel damage via degeneration of the tunica media and apoptosis of smooth muscle cells, which in turn leads to separation of and blood flow in between the layers of the aortic wall[13]	African American race Male gender Increasing age (peak incidence between 50 and 65 years old) History of connective tissue disorders (Marfan syndrome)[13]
	Myocarditis	Inflammation of the myocardium with subsequent necrosis of myocytes related to an infectious or cardiotoxic agent[14]	**In the United States:** common infectious causes include parvovirus B19 and human herpes virus 6 **In developing nations:** common infectious causes include rheumatic heart disease secondary to untreated *Streptococcus* infections or Chagas disease Commonly encountered cardiotoxic agents include alcohol, cocaine, and various pharmaceuticals[14]
Pulmonary	Pneumonia	Infection of the lung tissue secondary to viral, fungal, or bacterial causes[15]	Recent upper respiratory infection Hospitalization Endotracheal intubation and ventilation Comatose patients (impaired cough reflex) Increased susceptibility in immunodeficiency (HIV and organ transplant recipients) Decreased mucociliary clearance (smokers and Kartagener syndrome)[15]
	Pneumothorax	Most often associated with rupture of bullae or blebs Iatrogenic/trauma-related causes[16]	Smoking Tall, thin body habitus Pregnancy Marfan syndrome COPD Asthma TB CF Iatrogenic causes (pleural biopsy, positive pressure ventilation) Trauma[16]

Organ System	Diagnosis	Pathophysiology	Risk Factors
	Pulmonary embolism	Interference of blood flow in the pulmonary artery and/or its branches secondary to a thrombus that began at another origin (deep veins of the legs)[17]	History of deep venous thrombosis or pulmonary embolism Hormone usage (oral contraceptives) Recent surgery Malignancy Prolonged nonambulatory status[9]
Gastrointestinal	Gastrointestinal reflux disease	Decreased tone of the lower esophageal sphincter (LES)[18]	Older age Obesity Smoking Anxiety/depression Less physical activity[18]
	Peptic ulcer disease	Increased acidity of the stomach leading to destruction of the lining of the stomach extending into the submucosa/muscularis propria[19]	*H pylori* infection NSAID use Zollinger-Ellison syndrome Malignancy Stress African American/Hispanic race[20]
	Esophageal rupture	Full-thickness tear in the esophageal wall leading to leakage of gastric contents and saliva into the thoracic cavity[21]	History of traumatic injury Foreign body Iatrogenic causes Retching (Boerhaave syndrome)[21]
Musculoskeletal	Costochondritis	Inflammation of costal cartilages[12]	Often idiopathic May be secondary to repetitive exercises Higher frequency in female and Hispanic patients[22]
	Fibromyalgia	Nonspecific diagnosis of exclusion with diffuse musculoskeletal pain and tenderness not explained by another pathological process[23]	Female gender Increased incidence in patients with comorbid rheumatic disease Anxiety/depression[24]

Evaluation and Diagnosis

Rapidly and accurately identifying the life-threatening causes of acute chest pain is a challenging and critical task of physicians. The evaluation and diagnosis of patients with acute chest pain can be improved by implementing a systematic approach. The first step in risk stratification is taking a careful medical history and physical. Early diagnostic tests, including cardiac biomarkers, D-dimer, EKG, and echocardiography, can further narrow down the differential.

History and Physical Exam

The timing and onset of symptoms is crucial in identifying life-threatening diagnoses. Lethal etiologies typically present with an acute onset over minutes, whereas more benign etiologies progressively worsen over days to weeks. The characterization, radiation, and location of pain are clues to further narrow the differential. "Sharp" or "stabbing" pain is more characteristic of noncardiac etiologies, whereas "pressurelike" pain points toward acute myocardial infarction (AMI).[1] Pain that radiates to the back is associated with aortic dissection, and pain radiating to the shoulders can point toward AMI.[2] Pain that lessens when the patient is upright and leaning forward is typical of pericarditis. A targeted physical exam can further narrow the differential. Tachycardia or tachypnea is typical of pulmonary embolism or AMI. Hypotension or markedly widened pulse pressure should prompt evaluation for aortic dissection. Pneumonia leads to decreased breath sounds, while pneumothorax leads to hyperresonance. Other important history and physical exam findings are detailed in Table 15.2.

TABLE 15.2 LIFE-THREATENING ETIOLOGIES OF CHEST PAIN

Diagnosis	History	Physical Exam	Imaging	Tests and Calculators
Acute myocardial infarction	Pressurelike pain, nausea/vomiting, pain radiating to arm or shoulder	Diaphoresis, third heart sound, hypotension	CXR normal	Cardiac troponin levels, ECG with STEMI
Pulmonary embolism	Dyspnea, history of recent plane ride, OCP's, previous DVT, or malignancy	Sinus tachycardia, tachypnea, hypoxia	CTA = filling defect CXR	D-dimer ECG with right heart strain
Aortic dissection	Tearing sensation, pain radiates to back or abdomen	Blood pressure/radial pulse discrepancy, aortic regurgitation murmur	CTA	D-dimer
Pneumothorax	Dyspnea	Hyperresonance on percussion, decreased breath sounds, hypotension, tracheal deviation	CXR = air in pleural space	
Pneumonia	Cough, fever, productive or foul-smelling sputum	Egophony, pleural rub, rhonchi	CXR or CT = consolidation	CBC
Malignant pleural effusion	History of malignancy, older age, constitutional symptoms (night sweats, weight loss)	Decreased breath sounds, dullness on percussion	CXR = fluid in pleural space	Pleural fluid cytology, light criteria for thoracentesis fluid
Pericarditis	Sharp pain, recent or current viral infection	Pleuritic chest pain that worsens with sitting up	CXR = cardiomegaly	ECG = diffuse concave upward ST segments, PR segment depression without T wave inversion
Esophageal rupture	Dysphagia, hematemesis, neck swelling	Subcutaneous emphysema, hypotension, pneumothorax/persistent air leak from thoracostomy tube	CXR = mediastinal or free peritoneal air CT = mediastinal widening, extraesophageal air	Gastrografin (water soluble contrast) esophagram

From Overview of Acute Coronary Syndromes (ACS)—Cardiovascular Disorders [Internet]. Merck Manuals Professional Edition. [cited 2021 May 2]. https://www.merckmanuals.com/professional/cardiovascular-disorders/coronary-artery-disease/overview-of-acute-coronary-syndromes-acs

Diagnostic Testing and Imaging

Cardiac Etiology

Early diagnostic tests to rule in or out ACS include cardiac biomarkers, EKG, and echocardiography. High-sensitivity cardiac troponin (hs-cTn) testing is highly accurate in detecting cardiac injury, with a precise quantification of injury around the 99th percentile and should be done within 60 minutes.[3] ECG should be performed and interpreted within the first 10 minutes of arrival.[4] Transthoracic echocardiography is indicated in patients with ACP and high suspicion of ACS or acute aortic syndromes, myocarditis, or pericarditis; hemodynamic instability; acute heart failure; or underlying cardiac disease.[5] When aortic dissection is suspected, transesophageal echocardiography is the first-line test and most sensitive imaging modality.[6] Exercise ECG or noninvasive stress testing is used for low-risk patients prior to discharge from the ED.[7]

Noncardiac Etiology

Computed tomography angiography (CTA) is used to noninvasively examine the coronary or pulmonary arteries and is highly accurate. CTA of the aorta is the preferred first-line imaging when suspecting aortic dissection and pulmonary CTA is first line if suspecting high-risk PE (with associated shock, hypotension).[8] Chest X-ray should be performed within 30 minutes for patients with a high suspicion of acute life-threatening conditions such as pericardial effusion, pneumonia, PE, pneumothorax, or aortic dissection.[9] Lung ultrasonography is also used to detect pneumothorax or pleural effusion and has a higher sensitivity and specificity (>90%) for fluid or air compared to chest X-ray.[10] Abdominal ultrasound or CT is used to investigate gastrointestinal causes of acute chest pain, such as pancreatitis, cholecystitis, or biliary colic.

Treatment/Management

The management and treatment of acute pulmonary and thoracic pain is heavily dependent on the suspected underlying etiology. There are many clinical tools such as the Marburg Heart Score,[25] laboratory findings, and imaging that can be done to aid in developing the differential diagnoses, which are discussed in greater detail in the previous section. Additional considerations for pain management may include individual pharmacogenomics impact[26] and drug allergies.[27] Ketamine is not routinely used in the treatment of acute pulmonary and thoracic pain and will not be discussed here.

Opioids

Opioids are also routinely given for control of acute pain. Morphine is one of the most studied drugs and has long been a staple for pain control as evidenced by the oft taught mnemonic MONA.[28]

Although proven for pain control, there is some controversy in the routine use of morphine for pain control in cardiovascular ischemic patients. The 2005 CRUSADE study found that patients who suffered from myocardial infarction had worse outcomes with larger infarct size and suboptimal reperfusion success when they were treated with morphine compared to those who were not.[29] This association appears to have been replicated in other studies as well.[30] The proposed biological mechanism is related to morphine's effect in delaying and attenuating actions of antiplatelet medications such as ticagrelor.[31,32] However, there are conflicting studies as well that found no effect of morphine treatment on ST-elevation myocardial infarction outcomes.[33,34]

NSAIDs and Corticosteroids

Nonsteroidal anti-inflammatory drugs (NSAIDs) and corticosteroids have long been used for their anti-inflammatory effects and pain control. Indomethacin has been well studied for the control of pleural pain,[35,36] and the class-effect has been generalized and routinely given for viral or nonspecific pleuritic chest pain.[36,37]

It should be noted, however, that for NSAIDs, particularly naproxen, an associate has been found with increased risk for AMI.[38] There are some questions regarding whether COX-2 selectivity plays a role in increased cardiovascular risk for NSAIDs; Gunter et al. found that rofecoxib skewed the data for cardiovascular risk for the COX-2 selective group.[39] It is also well known to be irritating the gastric mucosa and can contribute to gastritis and peptic ulcers.[40]

Because of the significant side effects associated with corticosteroids, there has been a decrease in its use for pain control. It is, however, still used in cases that NSAIDs may not be tolerated and for tuberculous pleurisy as it can also reduce effusions and related symptoms.[37,41]

An alternative being explored is colchicine. Deftereos et al have found possible potential benefit but need report requiring additional study as it was not sufficiently powered to reach statistical significance.[42]

Antacids and the "GI Cocktail"

The "GI cocktail" is a popular therapeutic given at many acute care and emergency centers. It is often given for immediate relief acute thoracic pain caused by dyspepsia and heartburn. There is some variability in ingredients, but most recipes include an antacid and local anesthetic. Some recipes include an anticholinergic such as dicyclomine or Donnatal as well.

The GI cocktail increased in popularity and usage as early studies such as that by Kagan et al. found the addition of dicyclomine effective in significantly earlier and better pain relief vs antacids only for heartburn and nausea.[43] They also later found that dicyclomine alone was just as effective as dicyclomine with an antacid.[44] These studies were, however, done in the outpatient setting over a period of weeks. Even at the time, the results were controversial as Stephens et al did not find such benefit.[45]

Local anesthetics were added to antacids and anticholinergics as part of the GI cocktail when it was found that Mylanta II alone was inferior to Mylanta II with 2% viscous lidocaine.[46] Local anesthetics such as benzocaine was tested and found to be noninferior to viscous lidocaine when replaced to the Maalox and Donnatal cocktail.[47] However, Berman et al. question the use of the GI cocktail entirely as they found no significant difference between liquid antacid and the addition of either lidocaine or Donnatal or both.[48]

One particular concern is use of the GI cocktail to aid in diagnosis. This may not be wise as it has been shown to improve accuracy of differential diagnosis and cannot reliably exclude ischemia[49] moreover, there are reported cases of GI cocktail masking ischemic pain.[50]

Oxygen and Nitroglycerin

Oxygen has also become a staple for helping to relieve pain associated with ischemia.[28,51] Like morphine, however, there are studies that are challenging its routine use for myocardial infarction patients in the absence of demonstrated hypoxia or hypoxemia. Hofmann et al found that oxygen use in suspected AMI with $PO_2 > 90\%$ did not reduce 1-year all mortality. Ranchord et al. and Abuzaid et al. found no evidence of benefit or harm for oxygen use in STEMI.[52,53] Of concern, however, are studies that have found associations suggesting possible harm. While Cabello et al. did not find associations to reach level of statistical significance, it was noted.[51] Rawles et al. noted no evidence of benefit with increased frequency of sinus tachycardia in oxygen group as well as reported cerebral, renal, and retinal vasoconstriction along with reduced coronary blood flow after inhalation of high concentrations of oxygen.[54]

Of concern, Stub et al. found increase in the rate of recurrent myocardial infarction in the oxygen group compared with the no oxygen group, increase in frequency of cardiac arrhythmia, and also increase of myocardial infarct size.[55]

Nitroglycerin demonstrated to improve angina pectoris pain[56] and has also become a mainstay of pain control in cardiovascular ischemia.[28] Early nitroglycerin treatment was associated with a lower incidence of infarct complications within the first 10 days defined as CHF, infarct extension, or cardiac death. Mortality at 3 months was lower in group treated early.[57] It also reduces pulmonary capillary wedge pressure and improves pulmonary edema resistant to diuretic therapy in CHF following MI.[58]

Conclusion

Pleuritic and thoracic pain are common presenting complaints to a wide range of medical specialties. Most of these presentations are related to benign causes; however, they often present similarly to the more severe pathologies. These severe pathologies can often be life threatening and require a quick, concise workup and management to prevent negative outcomes. This type of pain is a commonly seen complaint, which can be life threatening, and presents to all medical fields. It is thus vital that physicians and health care team members of all types are made aware of the different presentations and how to accurately work it up to potentially save the life of these patients.

The lung being insensitive to pain causes the pain to be felt in adjacent systems including the pleura, tracheobronchial tree, and chest wall. This can result in the presentation to overlap with other pathologies. When assessing an individual with chest pain, it is important to begin with a large differential with an emphasis on ruling out the life-threatening causes first. Chest pain can be caused by multiple systems including cardiac, pericardial, pleural, abdominal, and musculoskeletal. To begin narrowing down the cause in a timely manner, it is essential to obtain a thorough history and physical. The acuity of the onset of symptoms can often indicate the severity of the underlying pathology. Sever symptoms that arise over minutes is a more ominous indication of a life-threatening pathology than symptoms that arise over weeks to months. Other key determinates that can guide management is characterization, radiation, and location of the pain, as etiologies will present slightly different depending on the underlying cause. Through characterizing the type of pain, a medical specialist will be able to better identify pathology that requires a more in-depth workup.

The history and physical will direct the course of diagnostic testing and imaging that need to be done. In patients with warning signs of acute life-threatening cardiac-related chest pain, diagnostic imaging must be done in a timely manner. Initial testing for chest pain with severe symptoms includes EKG, troponin, and chest X-ray. The results of these tests will further determine the course of action to be taken next. For noncardiac-related pain, chest X-ray and CTA are usually used to initially guide treatment. It is vital that medical specialists are able to use the information gained from the history and physical to guide them in getting the necessary diagnostic imaging. Once imaging is performed, the medical specialist must then know how to treat the underlying condition. Treatment varies according to the etiology. As pleuritic pain can often overlap with other etiologies, the workup in determining the cause will help provide the appropriate treatment.

Pleuritic and thoracic pain are common causes of patients seeking medical help. Related to the similarity in presentation, it can be difficult to differentiate severe etiologies from benign. It is because of this that it falls in the hands of medical specialists to approach pleuritic and thoracic pain in a systematic way that aims to rule out life-threatening causes first. In attaining a thorough history and physical with the knowledge of what to look out for, medical specialists will be able to determine the necessary diagnostic imaging and thus treatment a patient requires.

REFERENCES

1. Reamy BV, Williams PM, Odom MR. Pleuritic chest pain: sorting through the differential diagnosis. *Am Fam Physician*. 2017;96(5):306-312.
2. Jones K, Raghuram A. Investigation and management of patients with pleuritic chest pain presenting to the accident and emergency department. *J Accid Emerg Med*. 1999;16(1):55-59.
3. McConaghy JR. Outpatient diagnosis of acute chest pain in adults. *Am Fam Physician*. 2013;87(3):6.
4. Johnson K, Ghassemzadeh S. Chest pain. In: *StatPearls* [Internet]. StatPearls Publishing; 2021 [cited 2021 Apr 14]. http://www.ncbi.nlm.nih.gov/books/NBK470557/
5. Stepinska J, Lettino M, Ahrens I, et al. Diagnosis and risk stratification of chest pain patients in the emergency department: focus on acute coronary syndromes. A position paper of the Acute Cardiovascular Care Association. *Eur Heart J*. 2020;9(1):76-89.
6. Kass SM, Williams PM, Reamy BV. Pleurisy. *Am Fam Physician*. 2007;75(9):1357-1364.
7. Jackson M, Lee R, Hodgson L, Adams N. Problem based review: pleuritic chest pain. *Acute Med*. 2012;11:172-182.
8. Chest Pain—Cardiovascular Disorders [Internet]. Merck Manuals Professional Edition. [cited 2021 Apr 30]. https://www.merckmanuals.com/professional/cardiovascular-disorders/symptoms-of-cardiovascular-disorders/chest-pain
9. Johnson K, Ghassemzadeh S. Chest pain. In: *StatPearls* [Internet]. StatPearls Publishing; 2021 [cited 2021 May 2]. http://www.ncbi.nlm.nih.gov/books/NBK470557/
10. Fruergaard P, Launbjerg J, Hesse B, et al. The diagnoses of patients admitted with acute chest pain but without myocardial infarction. *Eur Heart J*. 1996;17(7):1028-1034.
11. Overview of Acute Coronary Syndromes (ACS)—Cardiovascular Disorders [Internet]. Merck Manuals Professional Edition. [cited 2021 May 2]. https://www.merckmanuals.com/professional/cardiovascular-disorders/coronary-artery-disease/overview-of-acute-coronary-syndromes-acs
12. Schumann JA, Sood T, Parente JJ. Costochondritis. In: *StatPearls* [Internet]. StatPearls Publishing; 2021 [cited 2021 May 2]. http://www.ncbi.nlm.nih.gov/books/NBK532931/
13. Aortic Dissection—Cardiovascular Disorders [Internet]. Merck Manuals Professional Edition. [cited 2021 May 2]. https://www.merckmanuals.com/professional/cardiovascular-disorders/diseases-of-the-aorta-and-its-branches/aortic-dissection
14. Myocarditis—Cardiovascular Disorders [Internet]. Merck Manuals Professional Edition. [cited 2021 May 2]. https://www.merckmanuals.com/professional/cardiovascular-disorders/myocarditis-and-pericarditis/myocarditis
15. Jain V, Vashisht R, Yilmaz G, Bhardwaj A. Pneumonia pathology. In: *StatPearls* [Internet]. StatPearls Publishing; 2021 [cited 2021 May 2]. http://www.ncbi.nlm.nih.gov/books/NBK526116/
16. McKnight CL, Burns B. Pneumothorax. In: *StatPearls* [Internet]. StatPearls Publishing; 2021 [cited 2021 May 2]. http://www.ncbi.nlm.nih.gov/books/NBK441885/
17. Vyas V, Goyal A. Acute pulmonary embolism. In: *StatPearls* [Internet]. StatPearls Publishing; 2021 [cited 2021 May 2]. http://www.ncbi.nlm.nih.gov/books/NBK560551/
18. Clarrett DM, Hachem C. Gastroesophageal reflux disease (GERD). *Mo Med*. 2018;115(3):214-218.
19. Narayanan M, Reddy KM, Marsicano E. Peptic ulcer disease and *Helicobacter pylori* infection. *Mo Med*. 2018;115(3):219-224.
20. Malik TF, Gnanapandithan K, Singh K. Peptic ulcer disease. In: *StatPearls* [Internet]. StatPearls Publishing; 2021 [cited 2021 May 2]. http://www.ncbi.nlm.nih.gov/books/NBK534792/
21. Kassem MM, Wallen JM. Esophageal perforation and tears. In: *StatPearls* [Internet]. StatPearls Publishing; 2021 [cited 2021 May 2]. http://www.ncbi.nlm.nih.gov/books/NBK532298/
22. Disla E, Rhim HR, Reddy A, Karten I, Taranta A. Costochondritis. A prospective analysis in an emergency department setting. *Arch Intern Med*. 1994;154(21):2466-2469.
23. Practitioners TRAC of G. RACGP—Musculoskeletal chest wall pain [Internet]. [cited 2021 May 2]. https://www.racgp.org.au/afp/2015/august/musculoskeletal-chest-wall-pain/
24. Bhargava J, Hurley JA. Fibromyalgia. In: *StatPearls* [Internet]. StatPearls Publishing; 2021 [cited 2021 May 2]. http://www.ncbi.nlm.nih.gov/books/NBK540974/
25. Harskamp RE, Laeven SC, Himmelreich JC, Lucassen WAM, van Weert HCPM. Chest pain in general practice: a systematic review of prediction rules. *BMJ Open*. 2019;9(2):e027081.
26. Cornett EM, Carroll Turpin MA, Pinner A, et al. Pharmacogenomics of pain management: the impact of specific biological polymorphisms on drugs and metabolism. *Curr Oncol Rep*. 2020;22(2):18.
27. Patil SS, Sun L, Fox CJ, et al. Multiple drug allergies: recommendations for perioperative management. *Best Pract Res Clin Anaesthesiol*. 2020;34(2):325-344.
28. American Heart Association. Part 7: the era of reperfusion. *Circulation*. 2000;102(suppl_1):I-172.
29. Meine TJ, Roe MT, Chen AY, et al. Association of intravenous morphine use and outcomes in acute coronary syndromes: Results from the CRUSADE Quality Improvement Initiative. *Am Heart J*. 2005;149(6):1043-1049.
30. de Waha S, Eitel I, Desch S, et al. Intravenous morphine administration and reperfusion success in ST-elevation myocardial infarction: insights from cardiac magnetic resonance imaging. *Clin Res Cardiol*. 2015;104(9):727-734.

31. Kubica J, Adamski P, Ostrowska M, et al. Morphine delays and attenuates ticagrelor exposure and action in patients with myocardial infarction: the randomized, double-blind, placebo-controlled IMPRESSION trial. *Eur Heart J.* 2016;37(3):245-252.
32. Lapostolle F, Van't Hof AW, Hamm CW, et al. Morphine and ticagrelor interaction in primary percutaneous coronary intervention in ST-segment elevation myocardial infarction: ATLANTIC-Morphine. *Am J Cardiovasc Drugs*. 2019;19(2):173-183.
33. Bonin M, Mewton N, Roubille F, et al. Effect and safety of morphine use in acute anterior ST-segment elevation myocardial infarction. *J Am Heart Assoc*. 2018;7(4):e006833. https://www.ahajournals.org/doi/10.1161/JAHA.117.006833
34. Gwag HB, Park TK, Song YB, et al. Morphine does not affect myocardial salvage in ST-segment elevation myocardial infarction. *PLoS One*. 2017;12(1):e0170115.
35. Klein RC. Effects of indomethacin on pleural pain. *South Med J.* 1984;77(10):1253-1254.
36. Sacks PV, Kanarek D. Treatment of acute pleuritic pain. *Am Rev Respir Dis.* 1973;108(3):666-669.
37. Reamy BV, Williams PM, Odom MR. Pleuritic chest pain: sorting through the differential diagnosis. *Am Fam Physician.* 2017;96(5):7.
38. Bally M, Dendukuri N, Rich B, et al. Risk of acute myocardial infarction with NSAIDs in real world use: bayesian meta-analysis of individual patient data. *BMJ.* 2017;357:j1909.
39. Gunter BR, Butler KA, Wallace RL, Smith SM, Harirforoosh S. Non-steroidal anti-inflammatory drug-induced cardiovascular adverse events: a meta-analysis. *J Clin Pharm Ther.* 2017;42(1):27-38.
40. Hawkey CJ. Healing and prevention of NSAID-induced peptic ulcers. *Scand J Gastroenterol Suppl.* 1994;201:42-44.
41. Ryan H, Yoo J, Darsini P. Corticosteroids for tuberculous pleurisy. *Cochrane Database Syst Rev.* 2017;3(3):CD001876. http://doi.wiley.com/10.1002/14651858.CD001876.pub3
42. Deftereos S, Giannopoulos G, Angelidis C, et al. Anti-inflammatory treatment with colchicine in acute myocardial infarction: a pilot study. *Circulation.* 2015;132(15):1395-1403.
43. Kagan G, Rose R. A comparison of an antacid plus antispasmodic combination and aluminium hydroxide in dyspepsia. *Curr Med Res Opin.* 1977;5(2):200-203.
44. Kagan G, Huddlestone L, Wolstencroft P. Comparison of dicyclomine with antacid and without antacid in dyspepsia. *J Int Med Res.* 1984;12(3):174-178.
45. Stephens C, Lever L, Hoare A. Dicyclomine for idiopathic dyspepsia. *Lancet.* 1988;1:1004.
46. Welling LR, Watson WA. The emergency department treatment of dyspepsia with antacids and oral lidocaine. *Ann Emerg Med.* 1990;19(7):785-788.
47. Vilke GM, Jin A, Davis DP, Chan TC. Prospective randomized study of viscous Lidocaine versus Benzocaine in a GI cocktail for dyspepsia. *J Emerg Med.* 2004;27(1):7-9.
48. Berman DA, Porter RS, Graber M. The GI Cocktail is no more effective than plain liquid antacid: a randomized, double blind clinical trial. *J Emerg Med.* 2003;25(3):239-244.
49. Chan S, Maurice AP, Davies SR, Walters DL. The use of gastrointestinal cocktail for differentiating gastro-oesophageal reflux disease and acute coronary syndrome in the emergency setting: a systematic review. *Heart Lung Circ.* 2014;23(10):913-923.
50. Dickinson MW. The "GI Cocktail" in the evaluation of chest pain in the emergency department. *J Emerg Med.* 1996;14(2):245-246.
51. Cabello JB, Burls A, Emparanza JI, Bayliss S, Quinn T. Oxygen therapy for acute myocardial infarction. *Cochrane Database Syst Rev.* 2016;(12):CD007160.
52. Abuzaid A, Fabrizio C, Felpel K, et al. Oxygen therapy in patients with acute myocardial infarction: a systemic review and meta-analysis. *Am J Med.* 2018;131(6):693-701.
53. Ranchord AM, Argyle R, Beynon R, et al. High-concentration versus titrated oxygen therapy in ST-elevation myocardial infarction: a pilot randomized controlled trial. *Am Heart J.* 2012;163(2):168-175.
54. Rawles JM, Kenmure AC. Controlled trial of oxygen in uncomplicated myocardial infarction. *BMJ.* 1976;1(6018):1121-1123.
55. Stub D, Smith K, Bernard S, et al. Air versus oxygen in ST-segment–elevation myocardial infarction. *Circulation.* 2015;131:2143-2150.
56. Copelan HW. Nitroglycerin for angina pectoris. *JAMA.* 1978;239(22):2340.
57. Flaherty JT, Weiss JL, Silverman KJ, Weisfeldt ML. A randomized prospective trial of intravenous nitroglycerin in patients with acute myocardial infarction. *Circulation.* 1983;68(3):13.
58. Gold HK, Leinbach RC, Sanders CA. Use of Sublingual nitroglycerin in congestive failure following acute myocardial infarction. *Circulation.* 1972;46(5):839-845.

16

Acute Orthopedic (eg, Bone Fracture, Disc Herniation, Arthritis) and Differential Diagnosis Related Pain

Chikezie N. Okeagu, Meredith K. Shaw, Devin S. Reed, and Justin Y. Yan

Introduction

Acute orthopedic pain, or pain of the musculoskeletal system, is perhaps the most common of any of the manifestations of acute pain. The musculoskeletal system is large, consisting of all muscles, bones, joints, and associated tissues such as tendons and ligaments, presenting ample locations from which pain can emanate. Unlike other pain conditions that preferentially affect people of certain ages or genders, musculoskeletal pain does not have a predilection for any specific demographic. It is likely that every person on earth has experienced some form of acute pain involving their musculoskeletal system. As such, proper prevention, identification, and treatment are exceedingly important.

Acute orthopedic pain typically arises from one of two mechanisms: injury or surgery. Musculoskeletal injuries are common, with nearly a third of emergency department visits resulting from injury or trauma.[1] This encompasses a variety of etiologies including bone fractures, disc herniation, and sprains, strains, or tears of muscles, ligaments, and tendons. Of these, the most common injuries are those of the back and spine. Next most frequent are sprains, dislocations, and fractures that, when combined with the aforementioned back and spine injuries, account for almost 50% of all musculoskeletal injuries.[2] Acute pain after orthopedic surgery is also a significant consideration as orthopedic procedures are regarded as some of the most intensely painful surgeries. This is because the periosteum has the lowest pain threshold of the deep somatic structures, and as a result, bone injury inflicted during surgery is more painful than injury to other tissues. As the number of orthopedic procedures performed every year continues to climb, their contribution to the total burden of acute musculoskeletal pain will become increasingly substantial. Kurtz et al. projected that between 2005 and 2030, total knee arthroplasties, one of the most commonly performed orthopedic procedures, will increase by 673% to nearly 3.5 million yearly. This trend is also predicted to be seen in total hip arthroplasties with an expected increase of 174% over this time frame.[3]

In addition to the increasing number of orthopedic procedures, the recent shift toward more ambulatory surgeries and earlier discharge after surgery has transformed the appearance of postoperative pain management. Once largely an inpatient endeavor relegated to house officers and floor nurses, decreased lengths of stay have forced surgeons and anesthesiologists to devise new strategies to deliver pain relief while allowing patients to leave the hospital. Coupled with this increase in outpatient procedures has been a realization that poor postsurgical pain management predisposes patients to the development of postoperative complications such as venous thromboembolism, myocardial ischemia, pulmonary complications, and poor wound healing.[4,5] Furthermore, poorly managed acute pain often allows for the progression to chronic pain.[2,4] This chapter will present a comprehensive overview of approaches to assessment and management of patients with acute orthopedic pain related to injury or surgery.

Assessment and Patient Education

A thorough history and physical is indispensable in the evaluation of acute musculoskeletal pain complaints. Pain perception is complex, involving not only nociception but also social, emotional, and psychological elements. As a result, pain is a highly subjective experience making it very challenging to accurately assay a patient's level of discomfort. In fact, across several studies, no association has been found between the severity of musculoskeletal injuries such as ankle sprains and fractures and the intensity of pain reported by patients.[6] Because of this, many tools have been developed to aide in the assessment of patients' pain. While the formats of these tools differ, they all have the same aim; namely, to help quantify pain in order to inform proper treatment.

History and Physical

It is important to collect information regarding onset, position, quality, radiation, severity, aggravating/alleviating factors, and associated symptoms or activities. This will help differentiate orthopedic pain that is related to injury from acute pain resulting from other etiologies such as gout or septic arthritis. The etiology of pain will dictate treatment. While most causes of acute musculoskeletal pain are managed similarly, there are some outliers. Septic arthritis, for example, is a surgical emergency and therefore must be identified quickly. Likewise, while patients with gout may experience some benefit from the analgesic approaches taken with other causes of musculoskeletal pain, it is also important for them to prevent further episodes with lifestyle modifications and prophylactic medications.

Single Rating Pain Scales

Single rating pain scales are widely used. Included in this category are such scales as the Numerical Rating Scale (NRS), the Verbal Rating Scale (VRS), the Visual Analog Scale (VAS), and face rating scales (Fig. 16.1). An essential component of these pain scales is the inclusion of anchor points such as "no pain" and "worst pain imaginable" at either end.[4] This allows the patient to weigh their current symptoms in relation to these reference points.

Due to its convenience, the NRS is one of the most commonly used scales in medicine. Application of the scale involves asking patients to rank their pain on a numerical scale, usually 0-10 with 0 corresponding to no pain and 10 to the worst pain imaginable. The validity of this scale has been demonstrated in studies, and its simplicity allows it to be administered quickly. Furthermore, since only numerical values are used, the scale can be applied widely without the need for translation. Despite the many positive aspects of the scale, it does have some shortcomings. The scale only evaluates pain intensity and does not provide a way to assess the several other dimensions of pain (eg, emotional, psychological). Intervals between numbers are not necessarily equal; that is, the difference between a 1 and 2 on the scale is likely not the same as the difference between a 9 and a 10. Additionally, patients are typically asked to rate their current pain or worst level of pain in the preceding 24 hours. Use of the scale in this way fails to properly account for fluctuations in pain symptoms.[4,7]

The VRS differs from the NRS in that descriptive adjectives such as "mild," "moderate," or "severe" are used in lieu of number for pain rating. Just as in the NRS, end points such as "no pain at all" and "extreme pain" are used as references. Like the NRS, the VRS has been demonstrated to be a reliable assessment tool. Since words instead of numbers are used, it may

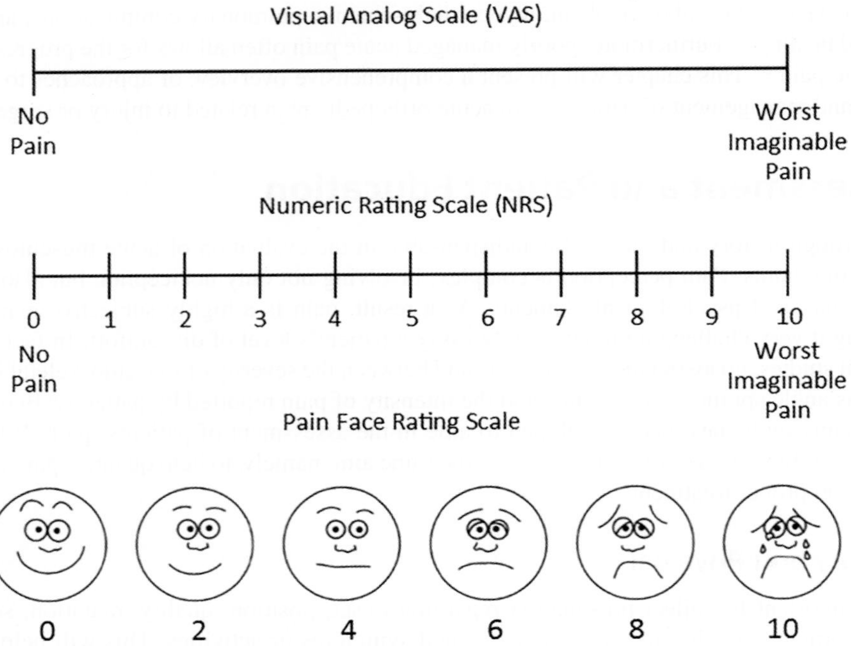

FIGURE 16.1 Pain assessment tools.

take more time to administer since patients must read all possible responses before choosing one. Similarly, this may present obstacles when treating patients who are not familiar with the language in which the scale is written. As the response choices are limited, patients may find it difficult to select which adjective best fits their pain. Lastly, just as with the NRS, the difference between mild and moderate pain, for example, is not necessarily the same as the difference between moderate and severe.[4,7]

The VAS is one of the most widely used instruments for pain assessment. It consists of a straight line with the end points denoting the extremes of pain (ie, 0 or "no pain" and 10 or "worst pain imaginable"). Patients are asked to mark the line at a point that corresponds to their pain level. The distance between the left side of the scale and the mark indicates the patient's level of pain. Variations of the VAS include the mechanical VAS in which patients use a slider on a linear scale rather than drawing a mark and computer-based models of the VAS. Descriptive terms or numerical scales are sometimes added to the VAS. In these instances, the scale is known as a Graphic Rating Scale. Like other single rating scales, VAS and Graphic Rating Scale have been found to be valid tools for assessing pain. Additionally, differences in pain intensity measured with the VAS are representative of the difference in magnitude of pain experienced by the patient. Among the single rating scales, this is unique to the VAS and presents its major advantage of other tools. The VAS is more difficult for some patients to understand making it more susceptible to errors when completing.[4,7]

Lastly, pain face rating scales have been found to correlate positively with other assessments of pain intensity. Patents are asked to choose from a selection of facial expressions, which represent a level of pain. Similar to the NRS, this scale is advantageous as there is no need for patients to be literate to complete the assessment.[4]

Pain Assessment Questionnaires

The use of questionnaires allows for a more thorough evaluation of the various dimensions of pain. The McGill Pain Questionnaire is the most commonly used assessments in this category. The first part of the questionnaire consists of an outline of a human on which patients mark the location of their pain. The second part allows patients to report the intensity of their current pain on a 1-5 scale. The third part consists of 78 words across 20 sections that are related to pain. Different sections are associated with different components of pain, namely affective, sensory, evaluative, and miscellaneous. Each word is assigned a point value, and patients mark as many words as necessary to best describe their pain. A pain rating index is derived by tallying the total number of points. Administration of the McGill Pain Questionnaire can be time consuming and cumbersome. As such, a short-form McGill Pain Questionnaire that can be completed much more quickly is more commonly used.[4,7,8]

Postoperative Pain Assessment

In the postoperative period, serial assessments should be conducted as a single measurement presents only a "snapshot" and may not appropriately represent a patient's level of pain. A sensible time interval should be chosen based on the individual situation. Any of the aforementioned tools can be utilized in order to evaluate a patients' pain symptoms. Subsequent measurements should be compared to monitor progression of pain and efficacy of pain interventions.[4]

Managing Patient Expectations

Regardless of the method used to assess pain, it is vital to provide patients with proper education regarding their condition and what they can expect from treatment. Patients and health care providers often have differing understandings of what qualifies as successful treatment. A study conducted by Ghomrawi et al. revealed that more than 50% of total joint arthroplasty patients had higher expectations than their surgeons in regard to postoperative pain relief, function, and well-being.[9] When treating acute pain, it is important to make patients aware that it may not be safe or even possible to completely eliminate their pain. Schutte et al. conducted a study in which they surveyed patients scheduled to undergo surgery regarding the level of postoperative pain that would be considered satisfactory. Initially, 41% indicated that "no pain" would be the appropriate level of postoperative pain. After educating patients as to what amount of pain control could realistically be achieved postoperatively, >80% were willing to accept a higher level of pain.[10] Lastly, it is important to maintain a dialogue with the patient throughout the postoperative period or course of treatment of acute musculoskeletal pain. Recovery can take weeks to months, during which time the patient may experience fluctuating pain symptoms. Physicians should continue to provide education including the most updated information regarding expected outcomes of treatment.

Treatments

The treatment of acute pain from orthopedic injuries is best accomplished by using a multimodal analgesia regimen. 7.7% of opiate prescriptions are from orthopedic surgeons despite the fact that they only represent 2.5% of all physicians.[1] A better understanding of pain management of orthopedic injuries can help the patient population combat the opioid epidemic. These include but are not limited to oral analgesics, peripheral blocks, neuraxial blocks, and local infiltrations. Additional therapy such as psychosocial support has also been shown to improve outcomes.[1] The combination of opioid analgesia with other treatment modalities such as nonsteroidal anti-inflammatory drugs (NSAIDs) has resulted in better pain outcomes than opioid monotherapy.[1,2] Opioids prescribed specifically by a single provider and at the lowest effective dose for the shortest effective time is important in order to decrease opiate use.

Oral Analgesics

Before escalating to opioid prescriptions, nonopioid oral analgesics provide a good option for acute orthopedic pain management. Inpatient nonopioid regimens following major orthopedic injury include ketorolac followed by ibuprofen, gabapentin, and scheduled acetaminophen. Postdischarge regimens include a combination of ibuprofen, gabapentin, and scheduled acetaminophen. Studies have shown that NSAIDs can provide equivalent analgesia in comparison to opioids.[2] NSAIDs inhibit the enzyme cyclooxygenase (COX) to prevent formation of downstream inflammatory and pain mediators. The mechanisms of action for gabapentin and acetaminophen for analgesia remain more unclear. Gabapentin is thought to bind to the alpha2-delta subunit of the dorsal horn neuron's voltage-dependent calcium channels to decrease calcium entry and inhibiting nerve function. Acetaminophen works in theory through decreasing CNS nociception.[3] The relation between NSAID use and impaired fracture healing has been brought into question in recent decades.[2] Studies with human participants supporting the notion of NSAIDs correlating to decreased fracture healing have largely been underpowered.[1,2]

Opioid Analgesics

Opioids are the most frequently prescribed medications for severe orthopedic injuries. The dangers of opioids have been well documented. Drug overdoses have tripled in the last 15 years with opioids involving 61% of overdose deaths.[4] Recommendations and guidelines have been put in place for safe prescription of opiates. These include prescribing immediate-release opioids vs extended-release, having a single prescriber per patient, and providing multimodal pain regimens vs opioid monotherapy.[1,4] Adherence to these guidelines decreases occurrence of addiction, abuse, and diversion. Inpatient medication regimens following major orthopedic injury frequently include combinations of oxycodone/acetaminophen and hydromorphone. Postdischarge regimens include a combination of oxycodone/acetaminophen, hydrocodone/acetaminophen, and tramadol. Opioids mainly exert their function by binding endogenous opioid receptors. These receptors are all G-protein–coupled receptors, which inhibit neuronal pain signaling.[4,5] Guidelines for dosing of opioid prescriptions is based on daily morphine equivalent dose per day (MEQ/d). The upper dosage limits of opioid prescriptions are 50 mg MEQ/d for general practitioners and 90 mg MEQ/d for specialists.[4] Prescriptions over 100 mg MEQ/d have been linked to many fold increases in opioid overdose risk.[4]

Regional Anesthesia

Regional anesthesia such as peripheral nerve and neuraxial blocks are good adjuncts to oral analgesic regimens. Regional nerve blocks work by injecting analgesic medication around a targeted nerve, which blocks pain transmission from any downstream nerve fibers. Incorporating regional blocks have been shown to decrease postoperative pain scores as well as decrease overall opioid usage.[4,6] Options include single shot regional blocks, indwelling catheters, regional blocks, and field blocks. A single-shot nerve block is a one-time injection, while an indwelling catheter provides analgesia to the patient in a continuous fashion. Single-shot blocks have been shown to decrease pain scores for up to 8 hours after surgery. Indwelling catheter blocks in comparison have been shown to decrease pain scores for up to 72 hours after surgery.[6] Regional anesthesia, however, is associated with rebound and breakthrough pain, which can severely reduce effectiveness of pain reduction. Rebound pain is defined as hyperalgesia usually 8-24 hours after a regional block has worn off.[6] Breakthrough pain is a sudden spike in pain when on a pain regimen that has previously controlled the pain well. Rebound and breakthrough pain can be mitigated with multimodal strategies of pain control. These include using opioid analgesia before a block is expected to wear off, using steroidal and NSAID options concurrently with blocks, using continuous blocks, and using adjuvant solutions that lengthen the effects of the block.

Local infiltration is another analgesic technique used in treatment of acute orthopedic pain. Local infiltration produces loss of sensation to a superficial, localized part of the body.

Local infiltration has been shown to be equally effective in reducing postoperative pain scores compared to other treatment modalities. One option is a liposomal bupivacaine suspension, considered advantageous for a single-shot block or local infiltration lasting up to 72 hours similar to indwelling catheters but allowing decreased inpatient orthopedic stays. Use of liposomal bupivacaine, however, only produces a modest decrease in opioid consumption accompanied with nonsignificant increase in pain scores for hip and knee procedures, suggesting limited utility after orthopedic operations.[7]

Patient-Controlled Analgesia

Patient-controlled analgesia (PCA) is a method of pain control that allows the patient to control delivery of pain medications on their own. Often, a computerized pump is utilized that contains a set amount of medication prescribed by a provider, which can either provide the patient with a continuous basal rate of infusion of the medication or may allow the patient to self-administer additional pain doses of the pain medication simply by pressing a button.[11,12] PCA pumps can deliver medications intravenously or can provide medication dosing through epidural or other catheters inserted by an anesthesia provider. While PCA pumps have built-in safety features limiting the total amount of analgesic medication that the patient can administer at any one given time or over the period of the pump's usage, there is still concern about operator or technical issues that can result in programming mistakes resulting in excessive sedation, respiratory depression, and even death. PCA pump usage should be monitored by a provider with detailed training.

Proper use of the PCA pump in pain management is imperative for a patient's recovery, as ineffective pain management in the postoperative period may prolong a patient's recovery period by causing increased pain intensity causing neuroendocrine and metabolic catabolism, which can result in poor wound healing. Poor wound healing can require the patient to undergo further procedures and delay postoperative therapy sessions and thus postoperative mobility, potentially contributing to other postoperative complications such as pneumonia and deep vein thrombosis.[11]

Transcutaneous Electrical Nerve Stimulation

Transcutaneous electrical nerve stimulation (TENS) is a common nonpharmacologic and noninvasive adjunctive treatment for pain. TENS attempts to modulate pain through the delivery of low-voltage electric currents through electrode pads placed on the skin from a small portable machine that the patient is able to control. TENS is thought to work in reducing pain perceived by the patient by activating opioid, serotonin, and muscarinic receptors centrally and opioid and α-2 noradrenergic receptors peripherally through an endogenous descending inhibitory pathway when the unit stimulates large diameter peripheral afferent nerve fibers.[6,13] Patients who have an implanted pacemaker or defibrillator have an open wound at the site where pads would be applied, or lymphedema should not be prescribed a TENS unit.

A meta-analysis of TENS and an adjunct to other pain relief methodology found that TENS (vs a placebo TENS unit) around the surgical wound significantly reduced postoperative analgesic consumption by 26.5% (range –6% to 51%). However, they found that the effectiveness may be dependent on the amplitude of the current the TENS unit is delivering, which is patient controlled.[6,14] Patients must be educated about the differences between low intensity, where the patient feels a strong sensation but no motor contraction occurs, and high intensity, where nonpainful motor contraction occurs.[13] Several studies involving the TENS unit postoperatively have determined that TENS unit use decreased postoperative pain and thereby opioid analgesic requirements in the postoperative period.[6,15-17]

Cryotherapy

Cryotherapy, or the controlled therapeutic application of an external cold source such as ice bags, gels packs, submersion in ice baths, or gaseous cryotherapy with or without pneumatic compression, is used to reduce tissue temperature. This reduction in temperature has been shown to provide multi-factorial reduction in painful stimuli. This increases the patient's tolerance to pain by decreasing tissue edema, decreasing inflammatory mediators, decreasing blood flood secondary to vasoconstriction, and overall decreasing the metabolic demand of the surgically impacted tissues.[6,18-22] Studies have demonstrated conflicting results when comparing cryotherapy to placebo in regard to pain control and pain medicine consumption in the postoperative period; however, the studies tend to favor that cryotherapy is beneficial for patients in both regards.[6,23,24] Additionally, inconclusive results have arisen when comparing cryotherapy modalities—so no one therapy is preferred.[6] However, patients and pain practitioners must be educated on the proper techniques of each modality as complications including nerve palsies and frostbite can occur.[25,26]

Treatment Approaches/Concepts in Treatment

Multimodal Approach

Multimodal analgesia is a method of pain management, which utilizes multiple classes of analgesics with varying mechanisms of action for improved pain relief.[27] This can include the use of local anesthetics, opioid and nonopioid medications, as well as nonpharmacologic therapies. By using a multimodal approach, high-dose requirements of any one drug are avoided, thereby mitigating dose-dependent adverse effects and preventing toxicity associated with the use of one agent.[28] Importantly, this type of approach can reduce opioid requirements.[27] Research also indicates that a multimodal approach can improve the effects of analgesia due to additive and synergizing effects.[29] This type of pain management approach can be personalized, selecting appropriate treatments based on patient history and individualized requirements.

Pain Services

Acute pain management services have become common in both the hospital and ambulatory setting. Pain services are made up of caregivers that are specifically trained to manage pain; they are generally composed of a multidisciplinary team of surgeons, pharmacists, and nurses. Pain levels and treatment considerations vary based on individual characteristics, medical history, and the type of injury or surgical insult. Therefore, a patient-tailored plan is ideal for optimal pain management. Pain services work with patients and their families to design a personalized treatment plan as well as facilitate patient education. These services gauge pain control perioperatively, assure quality of care, and manage orders for IV PCA, regional blocks, and oral medications.[28]

Preemptive Analgesia

Preemptive analgesia is the administration of analgesic treatment prior to any tissue injury in order to reduce postoperative pain. This can include preoperative administration of opioids, NSAIDs, or local blocks.[28] Preventative treatment blocks the detection of a painful or injurious stimulus by sensory neurons, including the surgical insult as well as stimuli produced by inflammatory mediators due to damaged tissue.[30] Though clinical research provides mixed results, there are studies that have found that preemptive analgesia can delay the first request for pain medication in recovery and minimize the severity of persistent pain syndromes.[28,31,32]

Conclusion

As discussed, orthopedic pain arising from injury or surgery can be treated using a multitude of methods. The manner best for each patient must be decided upon by the anesthesiology provider in an individualized basis, as patients with similar injuries may demonstrate different pain levels and may be able to be controlled through different measures with equal effectiveness. Additionally, as discussed above, several techniques have limited success depending upon many patient factors including but not limited to patient age, medical history, manner of injury, location of pain, and many others. In addition, the shift toward more outpatient surgical procedures, for patient comfort and to prevent postoperative complications, has forced the anesthesiologist to think about pain control in a different way in order to prevent and treat patient pain more successfully. This often includes utilizing a multimodal approach in order to prevent pain from the onset and to utilize different pain receptors to maximize efficacy. Utilizing multiple methods require the anesthesiologist to be proficient and knowledgeable in all aspects of all pain control modalities in order to provide the best care to their patients as possible. Optimizing pain control is imperative in all surgical fields; however, it is vitally important especially in a field where early bone and musculoskeletal manipulation through use after surgery, often through physical and occupational therapy, is required to establish a successful long-term recovery.

REFERENCES

1. Todd KH, Ducharme J, Choiniere M, et al. Pain in the emergency department: results of the pain and emergency medicine initiative (PEMI) multicenter study. *J Pain*. 2007;8(6):460-466.
2. Ekman EF, Koman LA. Acute pain following musculoskeletal injuries and orthopaedic surgery: mechanisms and management. *J Bone Joint Surg Am*. 2004;86(6):1316-1327.
3. Kurtz S, Ong K, Lau E, Mowat F, Halpern M. Projections of primary and revision hip and knee arthroplasty in the United States from 2005 to 2030. *J Bone Joint Surg Am*. 2007;89(4):780-785.
4. Jadon A, Hospital TM. Chapter-114 Pain Management in Orthopedic Patient. 2017;(January 2016).
5. Tetzlaff JE. Treatment of acute pain in the orthopedic patient. *Pract Pain Manag*. 2020;4(4). https://www.practicalpainmanagement.com/treatments/pharmacological/treatment-acute-pain-orthopedic-patient
6. Hsu JR, Mir H, Wally MK, Seymour RB. Clinical practice guidelines for pain management in acute musculoskeletal injury. *J Orthop Trauma*. 2019;33(5):e158-e182.
7. Haefeli M, Elfering A. Pain assessment. *Eur Spine J*. 2006;10:S17.
8. Waldman SD. Pain assessment tools for adults. In: *Pain Review*. Elsevier; 2009:375-380.
9. Ghomrawi HMK, Ferrando NF, Mandl LA, Do H, Noor N, Gonzalez Della Valle A. How often are patient and surgeon recovery expectations for total joint arthroplasty aligned? Results of a pilot study. *HSS J*. 2011;7(3):229-234.
10. Schutte SS, Le-Wendling LT. When expectations outpace reality: a survey of patient knowledge gaps in postoperative pain management. *J Clin Anesth*. 2020;66:109942.
11. Miaskowski C. Patient-controlled modalities for acute postoperative pain management. *J Perianesth Nurs*. 2005;20(4):255-267.
12. Viscusi ER. Emerging techniques for postoperative analgesia in orthopedic surgery. *Am J Orthop*. 2004;33:13-16.
13. DeSantana JM, Walsh DM, Vance C, Rakel BA, Sluka KA. Effectiveness of transcutaneous electrical nerve stimulation for treatment of hyperalgesia and pain. *Curr Rheumatol Rep*. 2008;10:492-499.
14. Bjordal JM, Johnson MI, Ljunggreen AE. Transcutaneous electrical nerve stimulation (TENS) can reduce postoperative analgesic consumption. A meta-analysis with assessment of optimal treatment parameters for postoperative pain. *Eur J Pain*. 2003;7(2):181-188.
15. Tedesco D, Gori D, Desai KR, et al. Drug-free interventions to reduce pain OR opioid consumption after total knee arthroplasty a systematic review and meta-analysis. *JAMA Surg*. 2017;152(10):e172872.
16. Rakel BA, Zimmerman MB, Geasland K, et al. Transcutaneous electrical nerve stimulation for the control of pain during rehabilitation after total knee arthroplasty: a randomized, blinded, placebo-controlled trial. *Pain*. 2014;155(12):2599-2611.
17. Mahure SA, Rokito AS, Kwon YW. Transcutaneous electrical nerve stimulation for postoperative pain relief after arthroscopic rotator cuff repair: a prospective double-blinded randomized trial. *J Shoulder Elbow Surg*. 2017;26(9):1508-1513.

18. Algafly AA, George KP. The effect of cryotherapy on nerve conduction velocity, pain threshold and pain tolerance. *Br J Sports Med.* 2007;41(6):365-369.
19. White GE, Wells GD. Cold-water immersion and other forms of cryotherapy: physiological changes potentially affecting recovery from high-intensity exercise. *Extrem Physiol Med.* 2013;2:26.
20. Adie S, Kwan A, Naylor JM, Harris IA, Mittal R. Cryotherapy following total knee replacement. *Cochrane Database Syst Rev.* 2012;(9):CD007911.
21. Nadler SF, Weingand K, Kruse RJ. The physiologic basis and clinical applications of cryotherapy and thermotherapy for the pain practitioner. *Pain Physician.* 2004;7(3):395-399.
22. Ho SSW, Coel MN, Kagawa R, Richardson AB. The effects of ice on blood flow and bone metabolism in knees. *Am J Sports Med.* 1994;22(4):537-540.
23. Wittig-Wells D, Johnson I, Samms-McPherson J, et al. Does the use of a brief cryotherapy intervention with analgesic administration improve pain management after total knee arthroplasty? *Orthop Nurs.* 2015;34(3):148-153.
24. Kuyucu E, Bülbül M, Kara A, Koçyiğit F, Erdil M. Is cold therapy really efficient after knee arthroplasty? *Ann Med Surg.* 2015;4(4):475-478.
25. Bassett FH, Kirkpatrick JS, Engelhardt DL, Malone TR, Grana W. Cryotherapy-induced nerve injury. *Am J Sports Med.* 1992;20:516-518.
26. Brown WC, Hahn DB. Frostbite of the feet after cryotherapy: a report of two cases. *J Foot Ankle Surg.* 2009;48(5):577-580.
27. Beaussier M, Sciard D, Sautet A. New modalities of pain treatment after outpatient orthopaedic surgery. *Orthop Traumatol Surg Res.* 2016;102:S121-S124.
28. Sinatra RS, Torres J, Bustos AM. Pain management after major orthopaedic surgery: current strategies and new concepts. *J Am Acad Orthop Surg.* 2002;10:117-129.
29. Raffa RB, Pergolizzi JV, Tallarida RJ. The determination and application of fixed-dose analgesic combinations for treating multimodal pain. *J Pain.* 2010;11:701-709.
30. Kissin I. Preemptive analgesia. *Anesthesiology.* 2000;93:1138-1143.
31. McQuay HJ, Carroll D, Moore RA. Postoperative orthopaedic pain—the effect of opiate premedication and local anaesthetic blocks. *Pain.* 1988;33:291-295.
32. Brull SJ, Lieponis JV, Murphy MJ, Garcia R, Silverman DG. Acute and long-term benefits of iliac crest donor site perfusion with local anesthetics. *Anesth Analg.* 1992;74:145-147.

17

Acute Nervous System Related Pain

Madelyn K. Craig, Gopal Kodumudi, Devin S. Reed, William C. Bidwell, and Alan David Kaye

Introduction

Acute nervous system pain can be broadly divided into central nervous system pain and peripheral nervous system acute pain. Central nervous system acute pain can be further divided into central nervous system pain caused by primary and secondary etiologies. The peripheral nervous system acute pain classification is more dependent on the etiologies of acute pain in the peripheral nervous system.

In this chapter, we review the diverse etiologies and treatments of acute nervous system related pain. In this chapter, we discuss primary and secondary causes of central nervous system pain, the wide variety of etiologies of pain, and pain caused by pathology of the peripheral nervous system. Clinical features and treatments are reviewed for both central and peripheral nervous system acute pain.

Central Nervous System Related Acute Pain

Headaches are a common medical complaint; it is estimated that up to one in seven Americans are diagnosed with migraines.[1] Migraine, cluster, and tension-type headaches are the most commonly experienced primary central nervous system acute pain.

Migraine headache can be moderate to severe intensity, is usually unilateral, and is often associated with sensitivity to light and sound. Migraine without aura headache usually lasts for 3-72 hours while migraine with aura typically lasts minutes with unilateral, sensory visual, language, and speech symptoms systems, followed by headache and migraine symptoms. Chronic migraine lasts for more than 15 days in a month for more than 3 months, with features of migraine on a minimum of 8 days in a month.

Cluster Headaches

Cluster headaches are a form of primary headaches that are rare but severe. The headache is unilateral with at least one autonomic ipsilateral symptom. The headaches occur daily for weeks to months with remission periods extending to months and years. The headache can occur several times a day or every other day. A link between pain attack and vasodilatation in cluster headache seems to exist.

Tension-Type Headache

Tension-type headache, also called as muscle contraction headache, is usually bilateral, does not worsen, can last for minutes or weeks, and describes as of a tightening or pressing quality. Photophobia may be present, but nausea or vomiting are typically not seen.

TABLE 17.1 FEATURES OF DIFFERENT TYPES OF HEADACHES

	Migraine	Tension-Type	Cluster
Location	Adults: Unilateral in 60%-70%, bifrontal or global in 30% Children and adolescents: Bilateral in majority	Bilateral	Always unilateral, usually begins around the eye or temple
Characteristics	Gradual in onset, crescendo pattern; pulsating; moderate or severe intensity; aggravated by routine physical activity	Pressure or tightness, which waxes and wanes	Pain begins quickly, reaches a crescendo within minutes; pain is deep, continuous, excruciating, and explosive in quality
Patient appearance	Patient prefers to rest in a dark, quiet room	Patient may remain active or may need to rest	Patient remains active
Duration	4-72 hours	30 minutes to 7 days	15 minutes to 3 hours
Associated symptoms	Nausea, vomiting, photophobia, phonophobia; may have aura (usually visual but can involve other senses or cause speech or motor deficits)	None	Ipsilateral lacrimation and redness of the eye; stuffy nose; rhinorrhea; pallor; sweating; Horner syndrome; restlessness or agitation; focal neurologic symptoms rare; sensitivity to alcohol

Acute primary headaches can be distinguished by several factors; in Table 17.1, features of each of these primary headaches are explained including location, characteristics, duration, and associated symptoms.

Treatments

Migraine and Tension Type

Nonsteroidal anti-inflammatory drugs (NSAIDs) and acetaminophen have long been the treatment of choice for migraines and tension-type headaches but there are other treatment options available including, triptans, antiemetics, dihydroergotamine, and peripheral nerve blocks. Newer treatments include neuromodulation, calcitonin gene–related peptide (CGRP) antagonists, and lasmiditan. Table 17.2 shows the level of evidence for various pharmacologic treatments. It should be noted that opioids are generally avoided.

Selecting a treatment should be determined by onset, progression, side effects, and duration. A large number of migraines occur in the morning with progression during sleep and are hard to treat by the time they are diagnosed so consider aggressive treatment. Non-oral treatment should be considered for rapidly progressing headaches, long-duration headaches, or headaches associated with nausea and vomiting. Often, the same patient may have variability in their attacks.[2] A stepwise approach is not recommended for initiation of therapy, rather stratified care showed better outcomes.

TABLE 17.2 **LEVEL OF EVIDENCE FOR VARIOUS PHARMACOLOGIC TREATMENTS**

Level A	Level B	Level C	Level U	Others
Analgesic Acetaminophen 1000 mg (for nonincapacitating attacks)	Antiemetics Chlorpromazine IV 12.5 mg Droperidol IV 2.75 mg Metoclopramide IV 10 mg Prochlorperazine IV/IM 10 mg; PR 25 mg	Antiepileptic Valproate IV 400-1000 mg	NSAIDs Celecoxib 400 mg	Level B negative other Octreotide SC 100 µg
Ergots DHE Nasal spray 2 mg Pulmonary inhaler 1 mg	Ergots DHE IV, IM, SC 1 mg Ergotamine/caffeine 1/100 mg	Ergots Ergotamine 1-2 mg	Others Lidocaine IV Hydrocortisone IV 50 mg	Level C negative antiemetics Chlorpromazine IM 1 mg/kg Granisetron IV 40-80 µg/kg
NSAIDs Aspirin 500 mg Diclofenac 50, 100 mg Ibuprofen 200, 400 mg Naproxen 500, 550 mg	NSAIDs Flurbiprofen 100 mg Ketoprofen 100 mg Ketorolac IV/IM 30-60 mg	NSAIDs Phenazone 1000 mg		NSAIDs Ketorolac tromethamine nasal spray
Opioids Butorphanol nasal spray 1 mg		Opioids Butorphanol IM 2 mg Codeine 30 mg PO Meperidine IM 75 mg Methadone IM 10 mg Tramadol IV 100 mg		Analgesic Acetaminophen IV 1000 mg

(Continued)

TABLE 17.2 LEVEL OF EVIDENCE FOR VARIOUS PHARMACOLOGIC TREATMENTS (*Continued*)

Level A	Level B	Level C	Level U	Others
Triptans Almotriptan 12.5 mg Eletriptan 20, 40, 80 mg Frovatriptan 2.5 mg Naratriptan 1, 2.5 mg Rizatriptan 5, 10 mg Sumatriptan Oral 25, 50, 100 mg Nasal spray 10, 20 mg Patch 6.5 mg SC 4, 6 mg Zolmitriptan nasal spray 2.5, 5 mg Oral 2.5, 5 mg	Others $MgSO_4$ IV (migraine with aura) 1-2 g Isometheptene 65 mg	Steroid Dexamethasone IV 4-16 mg		
Combinations AAC 500/500/130 mg Sumatriptan/naproxen 85/500 mg	Combinations Codeine/acetaminophen 25/400 mg Tramadol/acetaminophen 75/650 mg	Others Butalbital 50 mg Lidocaine intranasal		
		Drug combinations Butalbital/acetaminophen/ caffeine/codeine 50/325/40/30 mg Butalbital/acetaminophen/ caffeine 50/325/40 mg		

Modified from Marmura MJ, Silberstein SD, Schwedt TJ. The acute treatment of migraine in adults: the American headache society evidence assessment of migraine pharmacotherapies. *Headache*. 2015;55(1):3-20.

A nonpharmacologic approach to treatment may be chosen for patients with a poor response, a contraindication to pharmacologic treatment, or because the patient requests an alternate treatment. These options include neuromodulation and peripheral nerve blocks.

External trigeminal neurostimulation/transcutaneous supraorbital neurostimulation stimulates the supraorbital and supratrochlear nerves, and in the acute setting, is used for 60 minutes to alleviate pain. Migraine prevention requires 20 minutes of stimulation nightly. Single pulse transcranial stimulation uses magnetic pulses to the occiput. These pulses may stop spreading depolarizations and inhibit thalamocortical pain pathways. The magnet is pulsed several times for acute pain relief and 4 pulses twice daily as preventative with a max of 17 pulses per day. Vagal nerve stimulation uses a handheld device that inhibits vagal afferents. This inhibits cortical spreading depolarization and thalamocortical pathways. Two cycles of 2 minutes each are used repeated again 15 minutes later if pain persists.[3] It should be noted that data for neuromodulation were drawn from small randomized controlled trials, and while neuromodulation is FDA approved for migraines, it does meet the same standards as pharmacologic treatments.

Peripheral nerve blocks that are used for migraine treatment include occipital and sphenopalatine ganglion blocks. The occipital nerve block can be achieved by injecting 5 mL of 0.5% bupivacaine or ropivacaine near the greater and lesser occipital nerve. The sphenopalatine ganglion block is performed by using cotton-tipped pledgets that are soaked in 4% lidocaine. These pledgets are inserted along the superior border of the middle turbinate until it reaches the mucosa.[4]

Some newer therapies include lasmiditan and CGRP antagonists. Lasmiditan is a selective serotonin 1F receptor agonist. It was FDA approved in 2019 for the acute treatment of migraines. Initial dosing of 50 mg is recommended. On subsequent attacks, dose may be increased to 100-200 mg with no more than 1 dose in 24 hours. Lasmiditan does have many adverse effects including dizziness, fatigue, and nausea.[5] CGRP antagonists (ubrogepant and rimegepant) modulate trigeminovascular pain. Rimegepant is given as a single 75 mg/d dose, and ubrogepant is 50-100 mg with a maximum dose of 200 mg/d.[6]

Cluster headaches are typically unilateral, escalate rapidly, and are associated with autonomic symptoms as outline in Table 17.1. Treatment of cluster headaches begins with oxygen and a triptan (if intranasal, then administered contralateral to headache) as early as possible. Treatment can vary widely and can include many of the therapies for migraines as it is based mainly on empirical data.

Secondary Headache

Any headache with an underlying condition as the cause is termed as secondary headache. The treatment of any secondary headache is aimed primarily at treating the underlying cause.

The most common presenting symptom of giant cell arteritis is headache. It is treated by decreasing the vascular inflammation with prednisone usually 40-60 mg/d (or equivalent steroid) for 2-4 weeks followed by reducing the dose by 10 mg every 2 weeks to 20 mg, then by 2.5 mg every 2-4 weeks to 10 mg, then by 1 mg every 1-2 months if no relapse has occurred.[7]

Headaches secondary to a space-occupying lesion usually resolve with resection or resolution of the lesion and are usually due to vasogenic, intracellular, osmotic edema, or less commonly a mass effect. Strategies to control edema include osmotic therapy (mannitol), diuretics, glucocorticoids, hypothermia, hyperventilation, fluid restriction, and elevation of the head of the bed. Dexamethasone is the preferred steroid with 4-6 mg every 6-8 hours being the most common dose. If headaches still persist, then conventional headache treatments may be used including opioids.[8]

Subarachnoid hemorrhage usually presents with a sudden and severe headache and often is described as the worst headache of the patient's life. Pain control of the headache is usually achieved with a short-acting opioid such as morphine. Other conventional therapies can be used; however, aspirin is usually avoided until after the aneurysm is secured. Nimodipine 60 mg every 4 hours is used to treat vasospasm. The mechanism of benefit is unknown but has shown improved outcomes.[9]

Idiopathic intracranial hypertension typically displays a pattern of progressive headaches that are severe, are poorly defined, and often are associated with horizontal diplopia. It is seen mainly in young obese females. Treatment consists of weight loss, carbonic anhydrase inhibitors, and topiramate. Serial lumbar punctures can relieve headache and are an option during avoidance of medical therapy or pregnancy but are generally not recommended. Conventional migraine headache treatment is used if above treatments are ineffective.[10]

Headache related to central nervous system infection is treated primarily by controlling infection. Conventional migraine treatment may be used as support. Headache related to central venous thrombosis is estimated to require bed rest of hospital admission in 14% of patients with central venous thrombosis.[11] For patients with elevated intracranial pressure, acute treatment to control intracranial pressure is similar to the treatment outlined in the section on subarachnoid hemorrhage. Severe headache treatment can include topiramate, therapeutic lumbar puncture or even lumboperitoneal shunt.[12]

Withdrawal headaches can occur from the overuse of many medications but most commonly analgesics. This overuse can be due to treatment of headaches or other therapy. The treatment is rapid withdrawal of the overused medication. The exception to this is with the use of barbiturates, benzodiazepines, opioids, and any medication with a contraindication to sudden discontinuation. These medications must be tapered off. Bridge/withdrawal therapy is usually provided and includes many of the conventional migraine treatment. Choice of bridge therapy must be determined based on the medication to be discontinued usually to avoid the same class of medication.[12]

Causes of Acute Peripheral Neuropathy

The causes of acute peripheral neuropathy include inflammatory: hereditary, infectious, metabolic, infectious, traumatic, and toxic.

Acute Diabetic Peripheral Neuropathy

Painful diabetic peripheral neuropathy is a common painful neuropathy.[13] Painful diabetic neuropathy can be seen in about 90% of patients with both type I and type II diabetes.[14] Foot ulceration, nephropathy, and retinopathy are often associated with painful diabetic neuropathy.[15] The acute painful neuropathy is mainly by exclusion, and treatment involves tight glycemic control prophylactically and also by medications for pain. These medications include first-line anticonvulsant treatment with gabapentin or pregabalin and antidepressants such as duloxetine and venlafaxine, which prevent the uptake of noradrenaline and serotonin. Opioids have also been used to treat painful diabetic neuropathy with some clinical evidence.[16]

Medication such as topical medication such as the lidocaine patch and capsaicin has also been used and has reported efficacy data. The pathophysiological mechanisms for painful diabetic neuropathy or diabetic neuropathic pain are not completely understood. A relationship with hyperglycemia has been noted.[17]

Presence of allodynia or pain to touch suggests that central nervous system can also be affected by DPN. Painful allodynia, mood changes, and depression can cause decreased quality of life and make the management of this condition even more challenging.[14]

Herpes Zoster, Postherpetic Neuralgia Acute Peripheral Neuropathy

Acute pain related to nerve involvement can occur in herpes zoster and in postherpetic neuralgia. Herpes zoster occurs annually in about one million persons in the United States with 10%-15% developing postherpetic neuralgia. There is a lifetime prevalence of one in three people getting shingles and that is why getting a vaccine is so important to minimize the likelihood of having this painful disease. Herpes zoster is more common in patients who are immunocompromised from diseases such as leukemia, Hodgkin disease, systemic lupus erythematosus, rheumatoid arthritis, and organ transplants.[18]

Primary sensory neurons are affected by the varicella-zoster infection. They have ectopic pacemaker sites, which are hyper excitable. These ectopic hyper excitable sites can cause pain in both herpes zoster and in postherpetic neuralgia. The central nervous system can exacerbate the peripheral input that is maintained by ectopic activity.[19] Herpes zoster is a reactivation of the virus causing the infection with varicella-zoster. A complication of herpes zoster infection is postherpetic neuralgia (10%-15% incidence, eg, 100 000-150 000 new cases in the United States per year). Treatment with analgesics and antiviral drugs within first 72 hours is helpful to decease the severity and complications in both herpes zoster and postherpetic neuralgia.[19]

Medications for treatment of pain in herpes zoster and postherpetic neuralgia include anticonvulsant medications such as gabapentin and pregabalin; tricyclic antidepressants topical analgesics such as capsaicin, tramadol, and opioids; and oral analgesics.[20] Postherpetic neuralgia occurs because of reactivation of latent varicella-zoster. There are now extended-release formulations of gabapentin (eg, Gralise) and pregabalin, which reduce the likelihood of sedation and dizziness.

Cancer Pain

Cancer pain, despite the several effective treatments available, is still inadequately controlled in about 50% of cancer patients.[21] Cancer pain by surgical injury postoperatively can be controlled by short-acting opioid, NSAID, local anesthetic, and paracetamol. When using opioids, it is essential to minimize side effects and optimizing analgesia. There are also several routes by which opioids are utilized and could be used on a case-by-case basis as most appropriate. For example, morphine can be given by oral liquid, intravenous, suppository, subcutaneous, immediate-release drug, or slow modified-release long-acting formulations that can be given once or twice daily. Fentanyl can be given via formulations transnasally and transdermally. Other opioids used for cancer pain in multiple formulations include oxycodone, oxymorphone, hydrocodone, and hydromorphone. Moderate to severe cancer pain has also been treated with tapentadol or tramadol, which binds to mu receptors but also blocks the monoamine uptake. Opioid abuse is often treated with buprenorphine or methadone, and these agents, in addition to treating opioid addiction, can also be used for treatment of pain. Use of adjuvant analgesics, dose titration, and follow-up protocols are all necessary to provide optimum and safe analgesia to patients with cancer pain.[22] Methadone is another opioid that can be considered in patients with cancer pain. It has no active metabolites with a long half-life of ~24 hours and can be used via several routes such as sublingual, oral, intravenous, rectal, and subcutaneous routes and have a role in opioid rotation.

Guillain-Barré Syndrome

Guillain-Barré syndrome (GBS) is an immune-related, usually postinfectious, neuropathy and is one of the common causes for acute and flaccid neuromuscular paralysis. Respiratory illnesses as well as gastrointestinal infections have been known to be associated with this disease.[23] Ascending weakness, proximal and distal weakness, and sensory dysesthesias in hands and feet can be seen.[24] Pain is a common complaint in patients with GBS. The relationship between the disability that occurs in patients with GBS and pain is not clear, and up to about 80% of patients with GBS can suffer from pain.[25] Several types of pain are seen in patients with GBS, suggesting that the origin of pain can be neuropathic and nociceptive. These types of pain include visceral pain, arthralgia, paresthesia, muscle pain, sciatic and back pain, paresthesia, dysesthesia and meningeal signs.[26] The drugs that have been used for the treatment of pain in GBS have been morphine, dexamethasone, and remifentanil.[27]

Vasculitis Toxicity

Inflammation of blood vessels due to several causes can cause more than 30 pathologies of blood vessels.[28] When the cause of vasculitis is primary, it is called primary systemic vasculitides. The etiology of vasculitis is unknown and includes conditions such as Takayasu disease; Behçet disease; Kawasaki disease, a disease occurring in young children; and giant cell arteritis, which is seen in the elderly. There are a wide array of symptoms affecting multiple systems in vasculitis including diplopia, bilateral vision loss, purpura, hematuria, pulmonary infiltrates, ischemic events, glomerulonephritis, sinusitis, and GBS.

Guillain-Barré syndrome is an immune-mediated inflammatory disease of the peripheral nervous system that is potentially fatal and often triggered by infections. Sensory and motor weakness in the legs, arms, and cranial muscles can be seen. Autonomic system involvement can lead to hemodynamic changes of blood pressure instability and arrhythmias of the heart. Respiratory failure is seen in a significant percentage (20%) of patients. Management of complications and associated sequelae is critical.

Critical disease polyneuropathy is a syndrome that is most often associated with patients with failure to wean from mechanical ventilation. Muscle weakness and atrophy, more distal than proximal, with sparing of musculature of face can be seen. The polyneuropathy is more motor than sensory as evidenced by electrophysiology.[29]

Complex regional pain syndrome (CRPS) is a painful condition that can occur after a nerve injury or trauma. It usually affects the extremities and is often associated with psychological comorbidities of isolation and depression. Other terms used to describe the condition include reflex sympathetic dystrophy, causalgia, and chronic pain. CRPS is further divided into CRPS I (previously known as reflex sympathetic dystrophy), which is not associated with nerve injury, and CRPS II (previously called as causalgia), which is associated with a nerve injury.

Chronic CRPS can lead to structural changes in the central nervous system as well. A variety of treatments have been tried with varying successes. These include treatment with medication such as anti-inflammatory medications such as NSAIDs, bisphosphonates, and steroids as well as more invasive treatments such as sympathetic blocks and spinal cord stimulation.[22,30]

Entrapment or compression neuropathies can occur with the compression of peripheral nerves. Edema and ischemia occur in the initial stages after peripheral nerve compression followed by Wallerian axonal degeneration if nerve compression is prolonged. Carpal tunnel syndrome (occurring with the entrapment of median nerve at the wrist), ulnar neuropathy, and radial neuropathies are examples of entrapment neuropathies by chronic compression. The compression of the purely sensory lateral femoral cutaneous nerve can lead to pain, paresthesia, and numbness and is called meralgia paresthetica. Tarsal tunnel syndrome is a rare syndrome compression of the tibial nerve at the tarsal tunnel. Compression of the tibial nerve by Baker cyst at the knee level leading to proximal tibial neuropathy has been described. Predisposing medical conditions for entrapment neuropathies include diabetes, acromegaly, obesity, chronic kidney disease, and hypothyroidism.

HIV Sensory Neuropathy

One of the most common neurological complications of HIV seen in about 50% of patients is distal symmetric polyneuropathy. Decreased distal extremities sensation, including pain and paresthesias, in a stocking-glove distribution and decreased deep tendon reflexes are seen. Several medications for relief of pain include anticonvulsants such as pregabalin, lamotrigine, and gabapentin; antidepressants such as duloxetine and amitriptyline; and topical agents such as lidocaine and capsaicin patches have been used. The use of combination antiretroviral therapy cART has increased the survival length of patients with HIV infection.[31]

Neuropathic Cancer Pain

Neuropathic cancer pain occurs by direct nerve damage by cancer tumors. It can occur due to compression of nerve by tumor and tumor treatments such as radiation, surgery, and chemotherapy. One nerve or more nerves may be involved leading to neuropathies and plexopathies. The involvement of nerves includes infiltration, strangulation by fibrosis, or compression. The pain is often described as electrical or burning. Manifestations of decreased sensation and muscle weakness can also be present. Treatments include pharmacological therapy by anticonvulsants, antidepressants, opioids, topical agents such as capsaicin and lidocaine, and surgery.[32]

Nutritional Deficiency Related Neuropathies

Nutrition deficiency can occur because of malabsorption; malnutrition; drugs, which inhibit nutrition and autoimmune conditions such a pernicious anemia; alcohol abuse; bariatric surgery, eventually leading to malabsorption; and increased loss such as in diarrhea. Most nutritional deficiency related neuropathies are sensory neuropathies and dependent on the length of exposure. The essential nutrient thiamine is needed as a coenzyme for several enzymes involved in the metabolism of amino acids and carbohydrates and muscle strength reflex. Deficiency of thiamine can cause dry beriberi, which can lead to neuropathies in the peripheral nervous system or wet beriberi affecting the cardiovascular system. Some nutrients in excess can cause neuropathies. In general, essential nutrients when deficient or in excess can lead to neuropathies.

Cobalamin, a vitamin, is a cofactor important in methylation, and deficiency can lead to demyelination of the lateral, dorsal columns and optic and peripheral nerves.[33]

Central Neuropathic Pain

Compressive Myelopathy

Compressive myelopathy results from compression of the spinal cord. There are numerous etiologies that may lead to compression, only a few are discussed here.

Cervical spondylotic myelopathy

Cervical spondylotic myelopathy is a progressive degenerative disorder of the vertebral bodies and intervertebral discs causing narrowing of the spinal canal and neuroforamina. Disc protrusion, osteophytes, ligamentous thickening, and vertebral instability can all lead to narrowing of the canal. Several risk factors for developing spondylosis have been identified and include congenital narrowing, genetic factors, repetitive manual labor, and smoking. Men are often affected more than women. It is the leading cause of myelopathy in patients over 55 years of age. The majority of patients with spondylosis do not develop symptoms. However, those who develop symptoms may experience radicular features (upper extremity pain/weakness/paresthesia/numbness), "Lhermitte phenomenon" with neck flexion (eg, worsening of existing paresthesia, electric shock sensation into the extremities), gait disturbance/unsteadiness, and sphincter dysfunction (a late finding). Nurick grading scale for myelopathy is shown in Table 17.3.

Patients with Nurick grade 0 myelopathy may be treated with conservative therapies including anti-inflammatories, antispasmodics, and hard collar. Unfortunately, half of these patients' symptoms worsen requiring surgical intervention. The goal of treatment is to prevent worsening of neurologic function.

Ossified posterior longitudinal ligament

Ossification of the posterior longitudinal ligament results from calcification of the posterior longitudinal ligament. Ossified posterior longitudinal ligament can involve any spinal segment but is more common in the cervical and thoracic regions. It is more commonly seen in Asian populations and is associated with certain conditions such as rheumatoid arthritis. Surgical intervention is almost always needed as ossification progresses. The number of levels involved determines whether an anterior or posterior approach is used. Corpectomy may also be performed.

Neoplastic spinal cord compression

The spine is one of the more common sites for neoplasm metastasis especially for breast, lung, prostate, and kidney cancer. Extradural compression in the thoracic spine is most common. Treatment options include hormonal, chemotherapy, radiotherapy, steroids, or surgical intervention. Several factors must be taken into consideration when deciding each patient's treatment options. High-dose steroids effectively treat vertebral pain secondary to metastatic spinal cord compression. Radiotherapy is an option when compression results from metastasis in epidural soft tissue, stable vertebral lesions, or if surgical intervention is contraindicated. Surgical intervention is considered when the patient has a life expectancy of more than 6 months. Other indications for surgery include pain, instability, and neurological deficit. Schwannomas, neurofibroma, and meningiomas may be surgically resected via laminectomy, which may be curative. Stereotactic linac radiotherapy may be performed for patients unable to undergo

TABLE 17.3 NURICK GRADING SCALE FOR MYELOPATHY

0	Signs/symptoms of nerve root involvement without evidence of spinal cord disease
1	Signs of spinal cord disease without difficulty walking
2	Slight difficulty in walking that did not prevent full-time employment
3	Difficulty walking that prevents full-time employment or ability to complete housework but does not require assistance with walking
4	Only able to walk with assistance of walker or another person
5	Chair bound or bed ridden

surgery, in cases of recurrence, or malignant transformation. Intramedullary intradural lesions including ependymomas, astrocytomas, hemangioblastomas, lipomas, cavernomas, and epidermoid/dermoids are typically treated with surgical resection. Radiation treatment is controversial but may be considered for high-grade astrocytomas, residual tumor after resection, or tumor recurrence.

Spinal infection

Epidural abscess is a rare potentially devastating infection that can expand, compressing the spinal cord resulting in severe symptoms, permanent neurologic deficits, or even death. Symptoms include fever, malaise, back pain, midline tenderness, and neurologic deficits. Biopsy or aspiration to determine a causative organism is an essential component in the treatment plan. Conservative treatment consists of intravenous antibiotics, usually for at least 6-8 weeks, possibly followed by a duration of oral antibiotics. Indications for surgical decompression include neurologic deficits, spinal instability, sepsis, ring-enhancing lesions, and failure of antibiotic therapy. Elderly and immunocompromised patients, MRSA infections, and diabetic comorbidity are also indications for surgery. Antibiotics alone may also be chosen for patients who refuse surgery or who are medically unstable for surgery.[34]

HIV Myelopathy

Myelopathy is less common in HIV patients than peripheral nervous system disorders. HIV-associated myelopathy, also known as vacuolar myelopathy (VM), can occur at any time but is more common in uncontrolled disease. Due to the lack of symptoms or underdiagnosis, there is not reliable data on incidence and prevalence of HIV myelopathy. In one study, 46% of patients with AIDS showed VM at autopsy. Vacuolation of myelin in the dorsal and lateral thoracic spinal cord columns produces pathology similar to subacute combined degeneration from vitamin B_{12} deficiency. Unfortunately, cobalamin levels are usually normal in patient with VM, and vitamin supplementation does not affect disease progression. Bilateral lower extremity weakness with spasticity, bowel and bladder dysfunction, erectile dysfunction, gait ataxia, and variable sensory disturbances typically develop over weeks to months. At this time, treatment is supportive and focuses on managing symptoms with antispasticity agents and physical therapy.[35]

Multiple Sclerosis–Related Pain

Pain is a very common compliant in patients with multiple sclerosis with a prevalence estimated around 60%. Headache, peripheral neuropathic pain, back pain, Lhermitte phenomenon, painful spasms, and trigeminal neuralgia are the more commonly reported pain syndromes.[36,37] Pain in MS can be categorized into nociceptive and neuropathic pain.

Nociceptive pain includes low back pain, pain from muscle spasticity, and optic neuritis. Treatment of low back pain includes NSAIDs, acetaminophen, antidepressants, and opioids. Gabapentin is first-line treatment for spasticity followed by oral baclofen and cannabinoids. Intrathecal baclofen is reserved for patients with severe spasticity not responsive to oral medications. High-dose steroids have been successful in alleviating pain secondary to optic neuritis. Gabapentin, pregabalin, lamotrigine, intravenous lidocaine, and oral mexiletine have been used to treat painful tonic spasms. Since IV lidocaine has been successful in treating tonic spasms, it is suggested patients may benefit from carbamazepine and oxcarbazepine as both are oral medications that also inhibit sodium channels.

Neuropathic pain in MS is typically categorized as either paroxysmal (trigeminal neuralgia, Lhermitte sign, or "MS hug") or persistent (dysesthetic extremity pain). Trigeminal neuralgia is characterized as recurring episodes of sudden, brief, electric-shock–like pain in certain facial areas. First-line therapy for trigeminal neuralgia is sodium channel blockers, carbamazepine or oxcarbazepine. In the majority of cases, treatment failure is due to adverse side effects of these medications. In patients who cannot tolerate therapeutic dosage of carbamazepine or oxcarbazepine, combination therapy with lamotrigine, baclofen, or pregabalin/gabapentin may be tried. Any of these medications may also be used as an alternative to carbamazepine/oxcarbazepine if patients do not respond. For those patients who fail medical therapy, surgical intervention may be warranted. Microvascular decompression has been shown to provide the longest duration of pain relief compared with other surgical interventions. Other surgical options include rhizotomy via chemical (glycerol blockade), mechanical (balloon compression), or thermal (radiofrequency thermocoagulation) mechanisms.[38]

Lhermitte phenomenon is characterized as a transient electric shock sensation radiating down the spine or limbs often caused by flexion of the neck. Although it is not specific to MS, it is frequently associated with MS. Symptoms of Lhermitte phenomenon usually resolves spontaneously without treatment. However, treatment options for recurrent episodes include gabapentin, pregabalin, carbamazepine, or oxcarbazepine. Sodium channel blockers (lidocaine and mexiletine) have also been associated with improvement in pain.[39]

"MS hug" or "Anaconda sign" is a pressurelike sensation in the thoracic and abdominal regions that feel as if being gripped or squeezed that may cause respiratory limitation or pain with breathing. It is thought to be related to neuropathic pain from the spinal cord or spasticity of thoracic or abdominal musculature. Treatment options for neuropathic origin include amitriptyline, gabapentin, pregabalin, or topicals containing neuropathic pain medication, NSAID, or local anesthetic. If related to spasticity, baclofen, tizanidine, or gabapentin could be used.

Persistent neuropathic pain is most commonly described as a constant, burning pain in bilateral lower extremities. First-line therapy includes calcium channel blockers, gabapentin and pregabalin; TCAs; and SNRIs, duloxetine and venlafaxine. Cannabinoids have been shown to relieve neuropathic pain in several studies; however, due to results in long-term studies showing high rates of discontinuation and risk of causing psychosis in high-risk individuals, they have been classified as second-line therapy and their use recommended only if all other treatments fail.

Parkinson Disease–Related Pain

Musculoskeletal pain is the most commonly reported type of pain in patients with Parkinson disease, followed by dystonic pain. Other less common types of pain noted in patients with Parkinson's are both neuropathic types of pain (radicular and central pain). Musculoskeletal pain is described as aching or cramping. This type of pain is typically due to muscle rigidity and severe bradykinesia, although impaired mobility and abnormal postures may also play a role. Dystonic pain is caused by prolonged, forceful muscle contractions resulting in twisted postures and deformities. Central pain is described as unexplained stabbing, burning, or scalding sensations without a radicular origin. The first step in treating PD-related pain is optimizing their dopaminergic or other antiparkinsonian medications. The RECOVER study showed improvement in pain with the treatment of rotigotine therapy. Rotigotine is recommended for all three types of PD-related pain (musculoskeletal, dystonic, and neuropathic). Apomorphine is recommended for musculoskeletal and dystonic pain. Acetaminophen is first-line treatment for the majority of PD-related pain. Opioids are second-line treatment options. Gabapentin or pregabalin may be used for radicular pain. Duloxetine is recommended for central neuropathic pain. In patients with dystonic pain that did not respond to dopaminergic treatment optimization, botulinum toxin injections have been used. Surgical options include deep brain stimulation, pallidotomy, and spinal cord stimulation. Subthalamic deep brain stimulation is used for several pain types in PD with complete improvement in dystonic pain in the majority of patients. Dystonic pain and some types of musculoskeletal pain may be treated with pallidotomy. Spinal cord stimulation of the dorsal column may be an option for radicular/peripheral neuropathic pain.[40]

Postradiation Myelopathy

Radiation myelopathy is an injury to the spinal cord caused by ionizing radiation that is commonly categorized into early and delayed forms. A transient, early delayed myelopathy may occur weeks to a few months after radiation. It is characterized by Lhermitte sign, the brief, electric shock sensation down the spine or extremities caused by flexion of the neck. Treatment is usually not required as the symptoms typically resolve spontaneously over 3-6 months. If the symptoms are severe, carbamazepine or gabapentin may provide some relief. Late delayed myelopathy may be seen 6-12 months after radiation treatment. Unlike early radiation-induced myelopathy, it is usually irreversible. Symptoms may initially be mild such as decreased temperature sensation progressing over several months or may be severe such as acute onset paraplegia occurring in a matter of hours to days. Treatment most commonly begins with glucocorticoids; however, none of the treatments suggested consistently provide effective long-term results. Other therapies used include bevacizumab, a monoclonal antibody against VEGF-A, and hyperbaric oxygen.[41]

Poststroke Pain

Several different types of pain are reported in patients following stroke.[42] Central poststroke pain (CPSP), spasticity pain, shoulder pain, complex regional pain syndrome, and headache are the more common pain disorders.

Central poststroke pain is characterized by a gradual onset of painful sensation just as sensory loss seems to be improving. Three components of pain make up CPSP: constant pain, spontaneous intermittent pain, and hyperalgesia/allodynia. Pharmacologic therapies include TCAs, SSRIs, lamotrigine, and gabapentin/pregabalin. IV lidocaine and ketamine have also been used. Nonpharmacologic therapies include motor cortex stimulation and repetitive transcranial magnetic stimulation. Spasticity pain is typically treated with local neuromuscular blockade or pharmacological treatment as discussed in the multiple sclerosis section.

Glenohumeral subluxation and contractures are common after stroke. Prevention with passive range of motion and stabilization is very important. Subluxation is typically treated with mechanical stabilization. Contractions may be treated with medications such as NSAIDs, acetaminophen, antispasmodics, transcutaneous neuromuscular electrical stimulation, functional electrical stimulation, and botulinum toxin. Surgical procedures for contractures include tendon release, rotator cuff repairs, and scapular mobilization.

Complex regional pain syndrome does not have a definitive treatment. Current treatments focus on reducing pain, maintaining joint mobility, and restoring function. Occupational and physical therapy are an integral part of treating CRPS. Stellate ganglion nerve block may be performed to inhibit sympathetic effects. Other therapies used to treat CRPS include desensitization, motor imagery, and mirror therapy. Treating depression and anxiety is another component of the treatment plan that should not be overlooked. Pharmacologic treatments include memantine, gabapentin, carbamazepine, heterocyclic antidepressants, bisphosphonates, and oral steroids.

Posttraumatic Spinal Cord Injury Pain

Pain is a common finding following spinal cord injury and is categorized as nociceptive or neuropathic. Nociceptive pain includes spasticity and musculoskeletal pain, which has previously been discussed in the multiple sclerosis and Parkinson's sections. First-line treatment for neuropathic pain includes gabapentin or pregabalin and amitriptyline in patients with coexisting depression. Lamotrigine is an alternative medication specifically for incomplete spinal cord injuries. Intravenous lidocaine, ketamine, and morphine provide significant pain relief; however, these medications are not as practical for outpatient use. Duloxetine has shown benefit in patients with central neuropathic pain. Nonpharmacological therapies include cranial stimulation, transcutaneous neuromuscular electrical stimulation, and cognitive-behavioral therapy.[43,44]

Syringomyelia

Syringomyelia is defined as a fluid-filled cyst or cavity within the spinal cord typically found between C2 and T9. While there are several causes of syringomyelia including infection, inflammation, neoplasm, and trauma, it most commonly occurs with Chiari I malformation. It is a chronic, progressive condition that may fluctuate in severity over time. Pain is a common presenting symptom and can be radicular, radiating through the shoulders in a capelike distribution, between the scapula and/or central cord pain. Nearly half of patients will experience a burning, pins and needles, or stretching sensation. Nonsurgical treatment consists of managing pain and maintaining functional capacity and quality of life. Analgesics, antidepressants, antiepileptic drugs, and GABA analogs have been used to treat pain or painful paresthesias. Patients with neurologic deterioration or intractable pain should be referred for surgical decompression and/or shunt placement. The goal of surgical intervention is to restore normal CSF flow.[45,46]

Acute Disseminated Encephalomyelitis

Acute disseminated encephalomyelitis is an inflammatory, immune-mediated demyelinating disorder predominantly affecting the white matter tracts of the central nervous system. It typically affects children and is commonly preceded by a viral infection. It is characterized by acute onset encephalopathy with multifocal neurologic deficits determined by the location of the lesion that progresses rapidly. Common neurologic deficits seen in ADEM include unilateral or bilateral pyramidal signs, cranial nerve palsies, optic neuritis with or without visual loss, speech impairment, hemiplegia, ataxia, seizures, and spinal cord syndrome. Standard of care for ADEM is high-dose corticosteroids. In severe cases or for patients who do not respond to steroids, plasmapheresis with or without corticosteroids and IVIG have shown some benefit. Hypothermia or decompressive craniotomy has been performed for cases of fulminant ADEM and cerebral edema.[47,48]

Acute Pain of the Nervous System

Rheumatic Etiologies of Acute Nervous System Pain

Rheumatic diseases are a common source of pain, and a leading cause of disability. These often present as joint pain in the extremities. Nerve endings are distributed in the interstitial and perivascular tissue of the joint capsule. Joint receptors consist of four types. Type I receptors are corpuscles supplied by a small myelinated fiber that slowly adapt to stretch. Type II receptors are larger myelinated fibers that rapidly adapt to acceleration. Type III receptors are largest with extensive myelin branches into ligaments with slow adaptation at high thresholds. Type IV is fine unmyelinated fibers and acts as nociceptors.[49]

In assessing all patients with rheumatic diseases, understanding a thorough history is helpful to diagnosis and includes the involvement of different systems, the extent of pain, and how the patients' life is affected. Physical examination routinely involves thorough examination of skin and joints for external findings of chronic inflammation. Diagnostic studies can range from standard imaging to blood tests evaluating inflammatory markers, titers of certain antibodies, microscopy of synovial fluid, or potential biopsy samples. However, no one single screening test is ideal for all rheumatologic diseases.

Osteoarthritis is characterized by the progressive loss of articular cartilage leading to joint pain and limited movement, from either primary idiopathic etiology or secondary to trauma or congenital abnormality. As chondrocytes disappear, subchondral bone thickens form osteophytes in joint margins, which can be seen on x-ray films. The inability of chondrocytes to maintain the balance between synthesis and breakdown leads to release of degradative enzymes, triggering synovial macrophages to release metalloproteinases that further inhibit type II collagen. Osteoarthritis commonly affects the first carpometacarpal, hips, knees, and interphalangeal joints.

While the pain from osteoarthritis is largely from mechanical receptors and nociceptors, rheumatoid arthritis is inflammatory with proliferation of synovium and neutrophils accumulation in response to cytokines. Synovial B cells synthesize immunoglobulins, forming complexes in joint capsules, triggering chemotactic phagocytosis by polymorphic leukocytes and release of destructive proteolytic enzyme. Rheumatoid arthritis commonly affects women more than men, with joint erosions causing classic metacarpal-phalangeal ulnar deviation, however, can affect multiple organ systems.[49] Rheumatic vasculitis in small and medium vessels can cause mononeuritis multiplex, intestinal perforation, or cardiac manifestations. Synovial components of the cervical spine can cause atlantoaxial instability—subluxation—that can present as radicular or claudication cervical pain, lead to vascular compromise (vertebral artery) impacting consciousness, and must be evaluated for anesthetic safety prior to surgery. Treatment often begins with anti-inflammatory medications and occupational therapy; however, immunomodulating disease-modifying antirheumatic drugs are being utilized earlier to minimize and prevent erosive joint changes that lead to disability.

Spondyloarthropathies are also inflammatory arthritis types, however, seronegative for RF (rheumatoid factor) immunoglobulin complexes. Ankylosing spondylitis is an enthesitis, causing inflammation at tendon and ligament insertions, ossifying longitudinal ligaments and disc annuli, causing pathognomonic "bamboo spine," and impairing functional movement. This can cause multilevel neuroforaminal stenosis or cauda equina syndrome. Ankylosing spondylitis can propagate to iritis, upper pulmonary fibrosis, and aortic dilation impairing conduction or valvular function as well. Reactive arthritis, or Reiter syndrome, can cause asymmetric arthropathy affecting predominantly lower extremities and activate nociceptors from urinary or ocular inflammation.[50] Psoriatic inflammation can lead to joint abnormalities, dermatologic changes resulting in pruritus, and similarly controlled by quelling inflammation.

Crystal arthropathies also cause acute pain. Deposits of calcium pyrophosphate dihydrate or urate crystals in the articular cartilage and periarticular structures can be extremely painful.[49] Both are consequence of disordered metabolism—pyrophosphate or purines, respectively—leading to accumulation and crystallization at lower temperatures in the extremital joints, causing chronic inflammatory joint changes and tophi formations. Calcium pyrophosphate dihydrate shows short rhomboid crystals with weak birefringence when analyzing synovial fluid. In contrast, urate crystals are long needle-shaped with strongly negative birefringence to polarized light. These can be secondary to overproduction of metabolites or deficiency of enzymatic degradation, poor renal clearance, alcohol or high-purine consumption, and pharmaceutical effects like diuretics.[49]

Further rheumatologic conditions that can result in acute pain include polymyalgia rheumatica, polymyositis, Sjögren syndrome, and lupus. Each leads to inflammation, causing acute and chronic pains, by affecting many organ systems. Often these syndromes can be debilitating to normal life functions. Activation of nociceptors and mechanoreceptors transmit this pain. Controlling the pain is best achieved by targeting underlying inflammatory processes and immunomodulation.

Metabolic Causes of Acute Nervous System Pain

Painful neuropathies from metabolic origins are numerous; however, here, we will discuss more prevalent etiologies: diabetes, uremia, and amyloidosis. Treatment involves addressing underlying metabolic derangements; however, neurologic recovery and symptomatic resolve are variable.

Diabetic neuropathy is often a symmetric distal polyneuropathy affecting neurons in length-dependent fashion, attributing to the classic "stocking-glove" progression of paresthesias. This pain may be due to pathology at multiple sites in the nervous system. Osmotic and glycemic disturbance of myelin may affect sensation and proprioception. There has also been demonstration of altered sodium channel expression in primary afferent neurons, dysregulation of inhibitory interneurons at the spinal cord, and altered descending pain inhibition. Similar mechanisms of pain have been hypothesized in patients with metabolic syndrome, which is characterized by cluster of findings: central obesity, fasting hyperglycemia, hypertension, and dyslipidemias: hypertriglyceridemia or low high-density lipids.

Uremic neuropathy is another peripheral neuropathy, attributed to diminished renal filtration and accumulation of organic waste products. It occurs in patients with reduced glomerular filtration at end-stage renal disease, and is prevalent in 60%-100% of patients on dialysis. Uremic neuropathy is a distal symmetric sensorimotor polyneuropathy, affecting lower extremities typically caused by segmental axonal demyelination. Although the exact mechanism is unknown, multifactorial etiology is likely secondary to electrolyte derangements and toxin accumulation. Hyperkalemia and hyperphosphatemia cause chronic nerve depolarization, disrupting normal ionic gradients, and calcium-mediated processes that cause axonal death. Accumulation of guanidine compounds, parathyroid hormone, and myoinositol are associated with free radical activity that leads to. Symptoms vary but include paresthesias, paradoxical heat sensations, hyperalgesia, and restless leg syndrome that escalate into weakness and muscular atrophy, poor balance, and impaired tendon reflexes. Uremic optic neuropathy causing visual deterioration is documented. Uremic neuropathy is also associated with vitamin deficiencies—such as thiamin, zinc, or biotin—which can independently cause neurologic degradation. Overall, diagnosis is best by nerve conduction, and treatment consists of renal replacement, either through hemodialysis or peritoneal dialysis or transplantation.[51]

Amyloid neuropathy is a common early manifestation of amyloidosis, caused by extracellular deposition of low molecular weight proteinaceous fibrils in antiparallel beta-pleated sheets. While there are many protein precursors, all are lardaceous under gross and microscopic pathology, with characteristic apple-green birefringence under polarized light with Congo red stain. Soluble glycosaminoglycan monomers aggregate into oligomeric structures that become insoluble deposits in a variety of tissues—conjunctiva, pulmonary, skin, cardiac, urinary, or nervous tissue. Amyloidosis causes a peripheral and autonomic neuropathy. Autonomic impact can manifest as abnormal pupillary reflexes, anhidrosis, impotence, or orthostasis. Prognosis can be grim; however, treatment focuses on decreasing transthyretin synthesis or stabilizing tetramers to prevent deposition, and there can be benefit from hepatic transplantation.

REFERENCES

1. Burch RC, Loder S, Loder E, Smitherman TA. The prevalence and burden of migraine and severe headache in the United States: updated statistics from government health surveillance studies. *Headache*. 2015;55(1):21-34.
2. Marmura MJ, Silberstein SD, Schwedt TJ. The acute treatment of migraine in adults: the American headache society evidence assessment of migraine pharmacotherapies. *Headache*. 2015;55(1):3-20.
3. Tepper SJ. Acute treatment of migraine. *Neurol Clin*. 2019;37(4):727-742.
4. Binfalah M, Alghawi E, Shosha E, Alhilly A, Bakhiet M. Sphenopalatine ganglion block for the treatment of acute migraine headache. *Pain Res Treat*. 2018;2018:2516953.

5. Oswald JC, Schuster NM. Lasmiditan for the treatment of acute migraine: a review and potential role in clinical practice. *J Pain Res*. 2018;11:2221-2227.
6. Diener HC, Dodick D, Evers S, et al. Pathophysiology, prevention, and treatment of medication overuse headache. *Lancet Neurol*. 2019;18(9):891-902.
7. Dasgupta B, Borg FA, Hassan N, et al. BSR and BHPR guidelines for the management of giant cell arteritis. *Rheumatology (Oxford)*. 2010;49(8):1594-1597.
8. Loghin M, Levin VA. Headache related to brain tumors. *Curr Treat Options Neurol*. 2006;8(1):21-32.
9. Muehlschlegel S. Subarachnoid hemorrhage. *Continuum (Minneap Minn)*. 2018;24(6):1623-1657.
10. Friedman DI, Rausch EA. Headache diagnoses in patients with treated idiopathic intracranial hypertension. *Neurology*. 2002;58(10):1551-1553.
11. Ferro JM. Prognosis and treatment of cerebral vein and dural sinus thrombosis. *Clin Adv Hematol Oncol*. 2005;3(9):680-681.
12. Ferro JM, Bousser MG, Canhão P, et al. European Stroke Organization guideline for the diagnosis and treatment of cerebral venous thrombosis—Endorsed by the European Academy of Neurology. *Eur Stroke J*. 2017;2(3):195-221.
13. Boulton AJ, Vinik AI, Arezzo JC, et al. Diabetic neuropathies: a statement by the American Diabetes Association. *Diabetes Care*. 2005;28(4):956-962.
14. Schreiber AK, Nones CF, Reis RC, Chichorro JG, Cunha JM. Diabetic neuropathic pain: physiopathology and treatment. *World J Diabetes*. 2015;6(3):432-444.
15. Tesfaye S, Boulton AJ, Dickenson AH. Mechanisms and management of diabetic painful distal symmetrical polyneuropathy. *Diabetes Care*. 2013;36(9):2456-2465.
16. Watson CP, Moulin D, Watt-Watson J, Gordon A, Eisenhoffer J. Controlled-release oxycodone relieves neuropathic pain: a randomized controlled trial in painful diabetic neuropathy. *Pain*. 2003;105(1–2):71-78.
17. Oyibo SO, Prasad YD, Jackson NJ, Jude EB, Boulton AJ. The relationship between blood glucose excursions and painful diabetic peripheral neuropathy: a pilot study. *Diabet Med*. 2002;19(10):870-873.
18. Cohen JI. Herpes zoster. *N Engl J Med*. 2013;369(18):1766-1767.
19. Devor M. Rethinking the causes of pain in herpes zoster and postherpetic neuralgia: the ectopic pacemaker hypothesis. *Pain Rep*. 2018;3(6):e702.
20. Schmader K. Herpes zoster and postherpetic neuralgia in older adults. *Clin Geriatr Med*. 2007;23(3):615-632, vii-viii.
21. Caraceni A, Martini C, Zecca E, et al. Breakthrough pain characteristics and syndromes in patients with cancer pain. An international survey. *Palliat Med*. 2004;18(3):177-183.
22. Rosenblum A, Marsch LA, Joseph H, Portenoy RK. Opioids and the treatment of chronic pain: controversies, current status, and future directions. *Exp Clin Psychopharmacol*. 2008;16(5):405-416.
23. Fokke C, van den Berg B, Drenthen J, Walgaard C, van Doorn PA, Jacobs BC. Diagnosis of Guillain-Barré syndrome and validation of Brighton criteria. *Brain*. 2014;137(Pt 1):33-43.
24. Tosun A, Dursun Ş, Akyildiz UO, Oktay S, Tataroğlu C. Acute motor-sensory axonal neuropathy with hyperreflexia in Guillain-Barré syndrome. *J Child Neurol*. 2015;30(5):637-640.
25. Ruts L, Drenthen J, Jongen JL, et al. Pain in Guillain-Barré syndrome: a long-term follow-up study. *Neurology*. 2010;75(16):1439-1447.
26. Pentland B, Donald SM. Pain in the Guillain-Barré syndrome: a clinical review. *Pain*. 1994;59(2):159-164.
27. Johnson DS, Dunn MJ. Remifentanil for pain due to Guillain-Barré syndrome. *Anaesthesia*. 2008;63(6):676-677.
28. Jennette JC, Falk RJ, Bacon PA, et al. 2012 revised International Chapel Hill Consensus Conference Nomenclature of Vasculitides. *Arthritis Rheum*. 2013;65(1):1-11.
29. van Mook WN, Hulsewé-Evers RP. Critical illness polyneuropathy. *Curr Opin Crit Care*. 2002;8(4):302-310.
30. Shim H, Rose J, Halle S, Shekane P. Complex regional pain syndrome: a narrative review for the practising clinician. *Br J Anaesth*. 2019;123(2):e424-e433.
31. Schütz SG, Robinson-Papp J. HIV-related neuropathy: current perspectives. *HIV AIDS (Auckl)*. 2013;5:243-251.
32. Yoon SY, Oh J. Neuropathic cancer pain: prevalence, pathophysiology, and management. *Korean J Intern Med*. 2018;33(6):1058-1069.
33. Cai Z, Li Y, Hu Z, et al. Radiation-induced brachial plexopathy in patients with nasopharyngeal carcinoma: a retrospective study. *Oncotarget*. 2016;7(14):18887-18895.
34. Ismail A, Pop-Vicas A, Opal S. Spinal epidural abscess. *Med Health R I*. 2012;95(1):21-22.
35. Bilgrami M, O'Keefe P. *Neurologic Diseases in HIV Infected Patients*. 1st ed. Elsevier; 2014.
36. Foley KM. Opioids and chronic neuropathic pain. *N Engl J Med*. 2003;348(13):1279-1281.
37. Foley PL, Vesterinen HM, Laird BJ, et al. Prevalence and natural history of pain in adults with multiple sclerosis: systematic review and meta-analysis. *Pain*. 2013;154(5):632-642.
38. Maarbjerg S, Di Stefano G, Bendtsen L, Cruccu G. Trigeminal neuralgia—diagnosis and treatment. *Cephalalgia*. 2017;37(7):648-657.

39. Truini A, Galeotti F, Cruccu G. Treating pain in multiple sclerosis. *Expert Opin Pharmacother*. 2011;12(15):2355-2368.
40. Geroin C, Gandolfi M, Bruno V, Smania N, Tinazzi M. Integrated approach for pain management in Parkinson disease. *Curr Neurol Neurosci Rep*. 2016;16(4):28.
41. Rampling R, Symonds P. Radiation myelopathy. *Curr Opin Neurol*. 1998;11(6):627-632.
42. Wunsch H, Angus DC, Harrison DA, et al. Variation in critical care services across North America and Western Europe. *Crit Care Med*. 2008;36(10):2787-2793, e1-e9.
43. Widerström-Noga E. Neuropathic pain and spinal cord injury: phenotypes and pharmacological management. *Drugs*. 2017;77(9):967-984.
44. Paolucci S, Martinuzzi A, Scivoletto G, et al. Assessing and treating pain associated with stroke, multiple sclerosis, cerebral palsy, spinal cord injury and spasticity. Evidence and recommendations from the Italian Consensus Conference on Pain in Neurorehabilitation. *Eur J Phys Rehabil Med*. 2016;52(6):827-840.
45. Vandertop WP. Syringomyelia. *Neuropediatrics*. 2014;45(1):3-9.
46. Todor DR, Mu HT, Milhorat TH. Pain and syringomyelia: a review. *Neurosurg Focus*. 2000;8(3):E11.
47. Alper G. Acute disseminated encephalomyelitis. *J Child Neurol*. 2012;27(11):1408-1425.
48. Pohl D, Alper G, Van Haren K, et al. Acute disseminated encephalomyelitis: updates on an inflammatory CNS syndrome. *Neurology*. 2016;87(9 Suppl 2):S38-S45.
49. Gardner G. *Bonica's Management of Pain*. 4th ed. Lippincott Williams & Wilkins; 2010.
50. Jovey RD, Ennis J, Gardner-Nix J, et al. Use of opioid analgesics for the treatment of chronic noncancer pain—a consensus statement and guidelines from the Canadian Pain Society, 2002. *Pain Res Manag*. 2003;8 Suppl A:3A-28A.
51. Walk D, Backonja M. *Bonica's Management of Pain*. 4th ed. Lippincott Williams & Wilkins; 2010.

18

Gastrointestinal System and Acute Visceral Pain

Ken Lee, Alan David Kaye, and Henry Liu

Introduction

The gastrointestinal (GI) system consists of a hollow muscular tubelike organ from the mouth to the anus, measuring about 30 ft long in cadaveric specimens.[1] Its primary functions are ingestion, motility, digestion, absorption, and excretion. Connected to the proximal small bowel are accessory solid organs, namely the liver, gallbladder, and pancreas.[1] In this chapter, the focus is on acute noncancer visceral pain related to the intra-abdominal structures of the GI tract. Data published from the Agency for Healthcare Research and Quality indicate abdominal pain as the most common medical chief complaint in the emergency department, accounting for 4.5 million visits in 2006 and 6 million visits in 2014.[2] This 32% uptrend along with a broader differential diagnosis represents an important challenge for clinicians to understand and treat patients with acute abdominal pain.

Gastrointestinal Neuroanatomy

Innervation of the GI Tract

The viscera, or internal organs, of the GI tract are innervated by the autonomic nervous system, which includes the enteric, sympathetic, and parasympathetic nervous systems.[3] The enteric system is built into the walls of the GI tract, consisting of the myenteric (Auerbach) plexus between smooth muscle layers and the submucosal (Meissner) plexus. They function to regulate motility, secretion, and perfusion and are under modulation by the sympathetic and parasympathetic nervous systems. Sympathetic stimulation predominately inhibits GI function, such as decreased peristalsis, decreased luminal secretions, and vasoconstriction of intestinal vascular beds. The preganglionic sympathetic nerve fibers come from the intermediolateral nuclei of the thoracolumbar spinal cord (T5-L2). Most of these fibers synapse within the sympathetic chain, but a subset bypasses the sympathetic chain forming splanchnic nerves and synapses in groups of ganglia at the anatomical midline, such as the celiac plexus. The respective postganglionic sympathetic nerve fibers ultimately synapse at the target GI viscera, including the enteric plexuses. Conversely, the parasympathetic nervous system predominantly stimulates GI function, such as increased peristalsis and secretions, sphincter relaxation, and vasodilation of intestinal vascular beds. Preganglionic parasympathetic fibers, sometimes referred to as the craniosacral outflow, either travel within the vagus nerve for the proximal GI tract or arise from the lateral gray horn of the sacral cord forming the pelvic splanchnic nerve for the distal GI tract.[1] These fibers then synapse onto ganglia adjacent to the target organ within the myenteric and submucosal plexuses (Fig. 18.1).

Visceral Pain and Pathways

Visceral pain is derived from noxious stimuli within the organs themselves and transmitted by the autonomic nervous system. Pain signals of the GI tract are first sensed by the free nerve endings of afferent A-δ and unmyelinated C fibers within the connective tissue of visceral organs.[4] These afferent fibers travel predominately within sympathetic fibers, splanchnic nerves, and their respective sympathetic plexuses and synapse onto the dorsal horn of the spinal cord. The cell body of such afferent fibers is found within the dorsal root ganglion. The dorsal horn is a critical junction whereby afferent pain signals are constantly modulated by the local and descending interneuron activities. From here, the second-order projections form ascending afferent bundles to the brainstem and diencephalon structures such as the thalamus, hypothalamus, periaqueductal gray, and reticular formation. The spinothalamic tract is one such pain pathway (see Fig. 18.1). Finally, the third-order neurons in the thalamus send projections onto the somatosensory cortex.

As mentioned, visceral pain is primarily mediated by sympathetic nerve pathways. There is some contribution to pain signaling in the distal GI tract, namely the distal colon and rectum, via the parasympathetic pelvic splanchnic nerve.[1] However, the parasympathetic system serves a more physiological role, with afferents signaling fullness, nausea, and distention, and efferents promoting secretions, motility, and sphincter relaxation. This is primarily mediated by the vagus nerve.

Somatic Pain and Referred Pain

Somatic pain is caused by noxious stimuli to superficial structures including the parietal peritoneum, abdominal wall muscles, and skin. Somatic pain is sensitive to crushing and cutting types of injury, whereas visceral pain is primarily induced by inflammation, ischemia, and distention.[5] Somatic pain is also transmitted by free nerve endings of afferent A-δ and C fibers but in a denser distribution and hence better localized than visceral pain. Somatic afferent fibers are carried by the ventral rami of thoracoabdominal nerves rather than with the

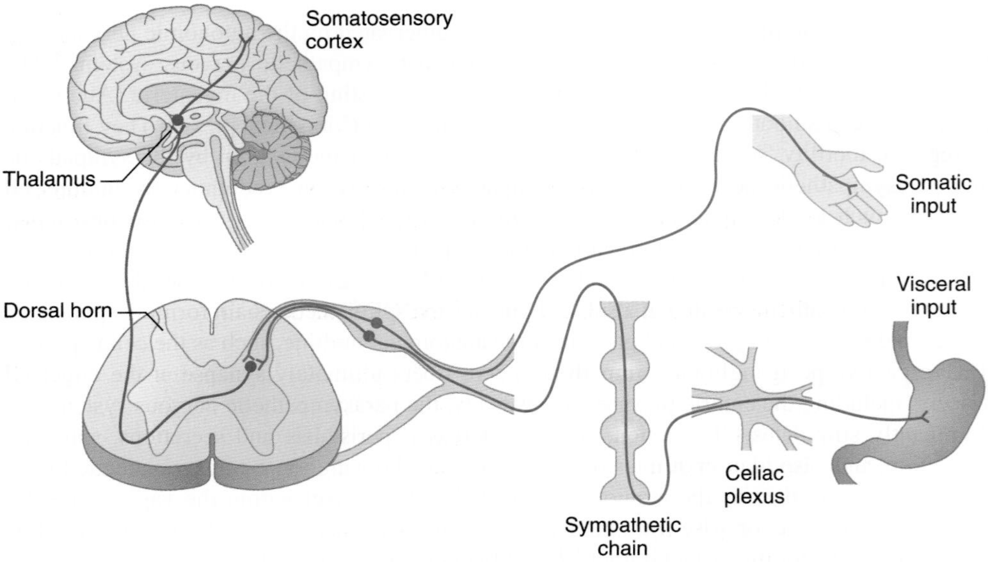

FIGURE 18.1 Visceral and somatic pain pathways. Visceral input (*red*) travels through a prevertebral plexus, in this case the celiac plexus, the sympathetic chain, and synapses to second-order neurons in the dorsal horn. This then ascends to the thalamus to synapse to third-order neurons, which ultimately synapse in the somatosensory cortex. Somatic input (*blue*) may synapse onto the same dorsal horn interneuron, giving rise to referred pain.

sympathetic pathway, demonstrating why visceral pain stimuli are associated with emotional disturbances and autonomic dysregulation such as nausea. From the spinal cord, somatic pain signals share the same ascending tracts as visceral signals.[5]

The convergence of somatic and visceral pain afferents at the level of the spinal cord gives rise to a phenomenon known as referred pain.[5] Defined as pain experienced at a site distant from the noxious stimulus, this process is mediated by somatic and visceral afferents forming synapses onto the same interneuron of the dorsal horn (see Fig. 18.1). A classic example can be illustrated by myocardial ischemia (visceral stimulus) presenting as pain in the left arm (somatic sensation).

Etiologies of Abdominal Pain

The Inflammatory Response

Inflammation is a complex immunological process in response to tissue injury or infection and accounts for a majority of acute abdominal pain syndromes (Table 18.1). The inflammatory process involves an intricate interplay of cells and chemical mediators to protect and repair the damaged site. This process causes several unwanted effects including redness, swelling, heat, and pain. These signs of inflammation are largely a consequence of vasodilation and increased blood flow to the damaged tissue in order to deliver repair factors. Pain, on the other hand, is thought to be an adaptive mechanism to encourage immobility and ultimately facilitate repair.[6] Several inflammatory mediators are responsible for transmission of pain. Initially, local macrophages release acute phase reactants bradykinin and TNF-α upon tissue injury. It is well established that bradykinin, a nine-amino acid peptide, is a primary mediator of inflammatory hyperalgesia via activation of B1 and B2 receptors of sensory afferent nerve endings. Interestingly, B2 receptors are constitutively expressed, whereas B1 receptors are inducible in the presence of cytokines, endotoxins, and injured tissues.[7] TNF-α, on the other hand, initiates a cascade of interleukin synthesis and release including IL-6, IL-1, and IL-8, appropriately creating a milieu of inflammatory mediators. IL-6 and IL-1β upregulate prostaglandins by inducing arachidonic acid availability and cyclooxygenase-2 (COX-2) activity. IL-8 stimulates release of adrenergic amines such as norepinephrine. Both prostaglandins and adrenergic amines are implicated in lowering the threshold for pain transmission at sensory afferents.[6]

Ischemia

Ischemic pain is primarily caused by inadequate oxygen delivery. This is most often encountered in peripheral vascular diseases; however, mesenteric ischemia is a diagnosis associated

TABLE 18.1 COMPARING ETIOLOGIES OF VISCERAL GI PAIN

Etiology	Mechanisms	Receptors and Mediators	Example
Inflammation	Infection Structural damage to mucosa	Cytokines Prostaglandins Adrenergic amines	Peptic ulcer disease Appendicitis
Ischemia	Occlusion of mesenteric vessels	Lactic acidosis and free radicals Acid-sensing ion channel	Acute mesenteric ischemia
Obstruction/ Distention	Intra-abdominal adhesions Neoplasms	Mucosal mechanoreceptors	Small bowel obstruction

with severe GI pain. At the cellular level, a lack of oxygen halts the electron transport chain and oxidative phosphorylation of ATP. Without ATP, the sodium-potassium pump fails to maintain a proper electrochemical gradient leading to membrane damage and reactive oxygen species formation.[8] In addition, hypoxia leads to anaerobic metabolism and lactic acidosis. Sensory A-δ and C fibers are stimulated by acidosis via a H^+-gated cation channel termed ASIC (acid-sensing ion channel).[9] Various metabolites involved in ischemia including lactate, ATP, ADP, and free radicals can further sensitize afferent fibers to noxious stimuli.[10] Finally, ischemic tissue injury elicits a local cytokine response, and inflammatory mechanisms described above likely contribute to ischemic pain.

Obstruction/Distention

The last source of GI pain comes from the distention and stretch of tissue. This is perhaps best demonstrated by an obstructed lumen and subsequent distention of the organ walls proximal to the obstruction, such as a gallstone obstructing the biliary tree or adhesions externally compressing the small bowel. There appears to be subsets of mechanosensitive receptors differentiated in their location and sensitivity. Mechanoreceptors in the mucosa and serosa primarily respond to blunt probing, whereas mechanoreceptors in smooth muscle primarily respond to circumferential stretching.[11] In addition, nerve endings associated with intramural blood vessels are also stimulated by stretch and distention of the hollow viscera.[12] From *in vivo* studies, both low-threshold and high-threshold mechanosensitive afferent fibers have been characterized. Low-threshold afferents account for the majority (75%-80%) of the studied samples and are activated by low distending pressures (<5 mm Hg) but are capable of sensing in the noxious range (25-30 mm Hg). High-threshold afferents account for the minority (20%-25%) and are only activated by pain-eliciting pressures above 25-30 mm Hg. Thus, low-threshold afferents likely encode normal physiological sensations (ie, satiety), whereas high-threshold afferents give rise to acute pathological conditions.

Mechanoreceptors and chemoreceptors likely overlap in the nerve endings of A-δ and C afferent fibers. It has been demonstrated in animal studies that mechanosensitive afferents not only respond to but are sensitized by chemical and thermal insults such as in the setting of inflammation. However, not all afferents are inherently capable of mechanoreception. Termed mechanically insensitive afferents (MIAs), these make up 25% of innervation of the mouse colon.[13] They can, interestingly, acquire temporary mechanosensitivity after exposure to inflammatory mediators. This suggests an integral role of both inherently mechanosensitive afferents and MIAs in propagating and maintaining pain in the inflammatory process.

Differential Diagnosis of Acute Abdominal Pain

History and Physical Examination Findings

The differential diagnosis of acute abdominal pain is broad, and evaluation should begin with the patient's history. The initial location of pain informs on the possible organ involved based simply on anatomy. The onset, duration, severity, quality of pain, as well as exacerbating and remitting factors further narrow the diagnosis. Associated symptoms can give important clues, such as constipation with small bowel obstruction or jaundice with cholestatic conditions. A thorough interrogation of past medical history, for example, heavy alcohol use or previous abdominal surgeries, is also helpful. Symptoms that may signal impending clinical deterioration include high fever, protracted vomiting, syncope, and sudden change in pain severity.

A physical examination should first focus on vital signs and general appearance to quickly determine the acuity of abdominal pain. Tachycardia and hypotension suggest a state of shock; both hypovolemic and distributive shock can be seen in GI emergencies. Determining the presence or absence of classic peritoneal signs (guarding, rigidity, rebound tenderness) is also a priority. Once deemed clinically stable, examine the area of pain with inspection, percussion, palpation, and auscultation.

Laboratory Testing

The need for lab tests should be guided by the history and physical examination. Practically, however, especially for toxic-appearing patients arriving in the emergency department, a broad panel of blood work is typically sent. A basic metabolic panel evaluates electrolyte derangements and renal function in the setting of GI losses and hypovolemia. A complete blood count identifies leukocytosis and bandemia in support for ongoing infection. Liver function tests are important for hepatobiliary etiologies, while amylase and lipase help diagnose pancreatitis. Urinalysis, urine culture, and pregnancy test are typically obtained to rule out genitourinary and gynecological causes.

Imaging Studies

There are multiple imaging modalities available to evaluate acute abdominal pain, and recommendations of which to use largely depend on the location of symptoms. Right upper quadrant pain should be imaged by ultrasonography, despite nuclear cholescintigraphy having slightly superior sensitivity and specificity, given its lower cost and quicker to perform.[14] Left upper quadrant pain has a broad differential and should initially be evaluated by computed tomography (CT), although upper endoscopy is reasonable if gastric or esophageal pathology is suspected from the history and physical examination. Right lower quadrant has a likely diagnosis of appendicitis best evaluated by CT with IV contrast, while left lower quadrant pain has a likely diagnosis of diverticulosis best evaluated by CT with IV and oral contrast. Plain radiographs are useful as a quick tool to detect air under the diaphragm and thus a frank perforation of intraperitoneal viscus or dilated loops of bowel to suggest a bowel obstruction. Finally, obstetrics patients follow a different diagnostic pathway and typically involve abdominal or transvaginal ultrasound to avoid radiation exposure.

Common Organ-Based Differential Diagnoses

Stomach

The stomach is the most proximal organ of the GI tract to be found in the intraperitoneal space. It is perfused by a rich vascular supply with multiple collaterals, making true ischemic pain a rare phenomenon.[15] Thus, gastric pain most commonly arises from inflammation of the mucosa in conditions such as gastritis and peptic ulcers. The gastric body is relatively distensible, and with the oral cavity immediately upstream as a pressure relief valve, emesis is typically an early symptom, rather than pain. Peptic ulcer disease has a prevalence of 1 in 1000 person-years in the U.S. population.[16] Common etiologies include chronic nonsteroidal anti-inflammatory drug (NSAID) use leading to downregulation of acid-protecting prostaglandins, and *Helicobacter pylori* infection resulting in both a blunting of mucosal defense mechanisms and an increase in gastric acid production. Patients with peptic ulcer disease suffer from dull epigastric pain typically associated with ingestion of food, as it stimulates gastric acid production. Diagnosis can be made by history and physical examination alone but often confirmed by upper endoscopy (Table 18.2). Stool antigen or urea breath test can establish *H pylori* status. Significant morbidity and mortality can result from erosion of ulcer into the aforementioned rich vasculature causing hemorrhage or transmural perforation causing frank peritonitis and acute abdomen requiring immediate surgical intervention.

TABLE 18.2 **COMMON ORGAN-BASED DIFFERENTIAL DIAGNOSES OF VISCERAL GI PAIN**

Organ	Diagnosis	Signs/Symptoms	Labs	Imaging/ Diagnostic procedure
Stomach	Peptic ulcer disease	Epigastric pain associated with meals	Stool antigen or urea breath test for *H pylori*	Upper endoscopy
Pancreas	Pancreatitis	Constant epigastric pain radiating to the back	Elevated lipase and amylase	CT or MRI
Hepatobiliary tree	Cholecystitis	Colicky RUQ pain, maybe referred to R scapula	Elevated ESR and CRP	Ultrasound or CT
	Cholangitis	Similar to above, more likely to have fever and chills	Elevated LFTs (alkaline phosphatase)	Ultrasound or CT or MRCP
	Acute hepatitis	As above, with possible encephalopathy, jaundice, ascites	Elevated LFTSs (AST and ALT)	Liver biopsy
Bowels	Small bowel obstruction	Periumbilical colicky pain associated with no stool or flatus	No specific labs	CT with oral and IV contrast
	Mesenteric ischemia	Sudden onset severe pain	Elevated lactic acid	CT or MR angiography
	Diverticulitis	Constant LLQ pain	No specific labs	CT with oral and IV contrast
Appendix	Appendicitis	Poorly localized periumbilical pain progressing to sharp RLQ pain	No specific labs	Ultrasound or CT

Pancreas

The pancreas is a vital organ of the GI tract, producing powerful enzymes found in bile important in the digestion of food. As such, any damage to the structural integrity of the pancreas can lead to significant inflammation. Acute pancreatitis represents a leading cause of hospital admissions in the United States, accounting for over 300 000 per year.[17] The presence of gallstones confers the highest risk of acute pancreatitis likely secondary to obstruction of the biliary tree and reflux of bile into the pancreatic parenchyma. Chronic alcohol use is the other major etiology, with a proposed mechanism of overproduction of enzymes by pancreatic cells. Patients present with a history of epigastric pain associated with nausea and vomiting that persists for hours. The pain is often described as a crescendoing and eventually constant, and about 50% report radiation of pain to the back. Not surprisingly, physical examination would demonstrate epigastric tenderness to palpation. Laboratory findings of elevated serum lipase and amylase are both sensitive and specific to acute pancreatitis especially early in the course of disease. Both CT and MRI are appropriate imaging modalities to evaluate acute pancreatitis with the former being more widely available and expeditious, while the latter utilizes safer IV contrast agents and nonionizing radiation suitable for pregnant patients.[18]

Gallbladder and biliary tree

The gallbladder is nestled behind the liver and is a storage site for bile before release into the duodenum. Precipitation of bile products leads to the formation of gallstones, with a majority of gallstone containing mainly cholesterol and a minority containing mainly bilirubin in patients with chronic hemolysis.[19] Gallstones are very common, found in about 10%-15% of the adult U.S. population, although they typically do not cause significant symptoms.[20] Cholecystitis and cholangitis represent inflammatory processes secondary to obstruction of the gallbladder and/or bile duct system, respectively. This obstruction most commonly results from gallstones but can also arise from malignancies or strictures. Presenting signs and symptoms are similar between these conditions, including right upper quadrant pain, fever, chills, and upregulation of inflammatory markers. The right upper quadrant pain is described as poorly localized and colicky and can be referred to the right lower scapula or posterior ribs. Cholangitis may additionally present with jaundice and corresponding elevations in liver function tests (especially ALT and AST), lipase, and amylase. Imaging is imperative for diagnosis, with abdominal ultrasound and CT being most widely employed. Cholecystitis is characterized by gallbladder enlargement and wall thickening, pericholecystic fluid, and presence of gallstones, while the additional finding of common bile duct dilation suggests cholangitis.[21] More advanced imaging with magnetic resonance cholangiopancreatography utilizes MRI to delineate a higher resolution of the pathology and location of lesion.[22] This modality has allowed clinicians to reserve the invasive endoscopic retrograde cholangiopancreatography to be solely performed as a therapy (ie, extracting an obstructing gallstone) rather than for diagnosis.

The liver is a major organ of the biliary tree and can certainly suffer from hepatitis in the setting of an obstructing gallstone. However, acute hepatitis and liver failure are more commonly induced by acetaminophen overdose and viral infection. These patients present with a constellation of findings, including right upper quadrant pain, but more worrisome are profound encephalopathy, depressed synthetic function, jaundice, abdominal ascites, and intravascular volume depletion.[23] Imaging is often unhelpful, and a liver biopsy is required for definitive diagnosis.

Bowels

The small and large intestine account for the majority of the GI tract, by length and by mass. As a result, there are multiple opportunities for dysfunction leading to acute pain, including small bowel obstruction, mesenteric ischemia, and diverticulitis. Small bowel obstructions are common, responsible for 15 out of 100 admissions for abdominal pain and 350 000 admissions every year.[24] There are a number of extraluminal and intraluminal etiologies for mechanical blockages of the small bowel. However, the majority of small bowel obstruction is from intraperitoneal adhesions, tumors, and hernias, accounting for 80% of all cases. Acute pain from small bowel obstruction is often periumbilical in location, colicky in nature, and peaks every few minutes related to clustered contractions, increase in intraluminal pressure, and circumferential stretch of bowel walls.[25] Associated symptoms include nausea, vomiting, and inability to pass flatus or stool. On physical examination, patients may have high-pitched or hypoactive bowel sounds, hyperresonance on percussion, and hernias or masses on palpation in addition to tenderness. Diagnostic studies include initial imaging with radiograph to rapidly detect dilated loops of bowel or intraperitoneal free air indicating a bowel perforation. An abdominal CT, ideally with oral and intravenous contrast, can provide additional details such as the site of obstruction, the severity (partial vs complete), the etiology (eg, masses or hernias), and inflammatory changes.

Acute mesenteric ischemia is a less common phenomenon encompassing 0.09%-0.2% of surgical admissions; however, it carries a high mortality rate of about 50%.[26] It is characterized by interrupted blood flow to the intestine, namely from arterial and venous embolism or thrombosis, but also from nonocclusive low flow state to the mesenteric vasculature. Patients typically present with sudden onset severe abdominal pain, typically out of proportion of unremarkable physical examination findings. Associated symptoms include nausea, vomiting, and rectal bleeding. If clinical suspicion is high enough and patient is hemodynamically unstable, emergent laparotomy to resect necrosed bowel is indicated. Otherwise, either CT or MRI angiography are appropriate modalities to localize the site of occlusion.

Diverticulitis is a sequela of diverticulosis, where outpouchings of the colonic wall become acutely inflamed. Over half of Americans over the age of 60 have diverticulosis. It is thought to develop at points of weakness in the colonic wall where the vasa recta penetrate the muscular layer, combined with abnormal contractile forces causing the herniation of mucosa and submucosa.[27] Interestingly, by modern estimates, <5% of patients with diverticula develop acute diverticulitis. The pathophysiology of diverticulitis is not entirely understood. The classic theory of a sentinel obstruction of the diverticulum neck causing bacterial overgrowth and ischemia has been challenged, as recent studies point to chronic inflammation and alterations in gut microbiome as important etiologies.[27,28] Abdominal pain is typically described as constant in nature and located in the left lower quadrant given the higher likelihood of diverticulosis in the sigmoid colon.[29] Physical examination would elicit tenderness in the same area, unless frank perforation develops resulting in hemodynamic instability and peritoneal signs of guarding, rigidity, and rebound tenderness. Diagnosis is made by abdominal CT with oral and intravenous contrast, which would reveal presence of diverticula with bowel wall thickening, as well as pericolonic fat stranding.[30]

Appendix

The appendix is a vestigial blind-ended pouch coming off of the cecum. Acute appendicitis is exceedingly common, with a lifetime risk of 1 in 15 in the United States, costing about $3 billion annually to the health care system.[31] One-third of patients present with a perforation requiring emergent surgery. Similar to diverticulitis, pathogenesis is classically believed to arise from appendicolith obstruction, commonly from fecal matter, calculi, infection, or neoplasms. However, most patients with appendicitis do not have appendicolith on imaging, and incidentally found appendicoliths do not develop appendicitis.[32] Onset of abdominal pain is typically periumbilical initially and poorly localized in nature, consistent with visceral pain signaling pathways. As inflammation progresses involving the peritoneal wall, which also suggests impending perforation, pain migrates to the well-known McBurney point in the right lower quadrant. The quality of pain here is described as localized and sharp, consistent with somatic pain pathways. Abdominal pain is associated with anorexia, nausea, and vomiting. Both abdominal CT and abdominal ultrasound can be used for diagnosis.

Treatment of GI Visceral Pain

Ideally, the primary management of the acute GI pain is to address the underlying source. For small bowel obstructions, employ bowel rest, intravenous fluids, and if warranted, surgical approach to relieve the obstruction. For gallstone pancreatitis, proceed with endoscopic retrograde cholangiopancreatography for extraction. However, patients can have excruciating pain, which must be specifically treated before their pathology is resolved. The mainstay therapy continues to be pharmacological, especially intravenous medications, since most GI conditions necessitate strict fast requirement. Peripheral nerve blocks and other interventional pain procedures are rarely offered in the context of acute visceral pain but will be briefly discussed as adjuncts to postoperative pain control after GI surgery and in cases of chronic pain.

Pharmacological

Almost all classes of pain medications have been used in the treatment of acute visceral pain; however, there is a lack of studies that specifically teased out efficacy in treating visceral from somatic and neuropathic pain.[33] Since the transmission of visceral pain relies on multiple neurotransmitters and receptors, no agent alone would likely provide complete analgesia. Acetaminophen, NSAIDs, and opioids are the most commonly utilized, although there exists an exhaustive list of analgesics that are useful in treating visceral pain including gabapentinoids, antispasmodics, antidepressants, *N*-methyl-D-aspartate antagonists, and alpha-2 receptor agonists.

Acetaminophen and NSAIDs are both efficacious in treating visceral GI pain, with a synergistic effect demonstrated in an animal model.[34,35] Acetaminophen is known to potentially cause liver function test increases even at the recommended dose, thus extreme caution must be taken when used in patients with acute liver injury from biliary tree pathology.[36] NSAIDs should not be used in treating gastritis or peptic ulcer, as it may be one of the major culprits of gastric mucosal injury.

Opioids have a role in visceral pain. Opioids have predictably superb efficacy and are usually prescribed in the emergency department or initial inpatient admission for patients experiencing intense acute pain. However, given the context of the U.S. opioid epidemic, practitioners are now increasingly judicious in their prescribing of opioids and they now rely more on opioid-sparing adjuncts for pain control. Opioids impair GI motility as well as central activity in the chemoreceptor trigger zone, promoting nausea and vomiting. As such, opioids can exacerbate patients with small bowel obstruction.[37] Opioids also induce increased phasic pressure at the sphincter of Oddi and may lead to spasmodic biliary pain.[38] It was traditionally believed that morphine had a greater effect on sphincter of Oddi pressure. Increasing sphincter of Oddi tone in conditions such as biliary colic may exacerbate an already high-pressure biliary tree; however, opioids are still commonly used for these conditions in practice.

Nonpharmacological

As mentioned, the use of interventional pain procedures is limited in this patient population due to the relative short time-course of pain and the adequacy of pharmacological agents to bridge them until their underlying condition is resolved. There are instances where nerve blocks are offered. Commonly, acute GI pain requires a surgical intervention such as appendectomy for appendicitis or exploratory laparotomy with bowel resection for small bowel obstruction. Depending on the surgical site, different nerve blocks can be employed—transversus abdominis plane, rectus sheath, quadratus lumborum—all aimed at anesthetizing branches of thoracic and lumbar sensory nerves. Such peripheral nerve blocks of the trunk are very effective in ameliorating postoperative incisional pain as it is transmitted through the somatic afferent pain pathway (see Fig. 18.1).

On the other hand, visceral pain (ie, residual inflammation of the organ itself) is poorly covered by peripheral nerve blocks and requires sympathetic blockade. Again, these are rarely done in the acute setting but are utilized in patients suffering from chronic abdominal pain, for example, GI malignancies and chronic pancreatitis. Sympathetic fibers of most GI structures, including the stomach, pancreas, biliary tree, small intestine, and proximal colon, traverse through the celiac plexus, while sympathetic fibers from descending colon, sigmoid, and proximal rectum traverse through the superior hypogastric plexus.[39] Fluoroscopy- or CT-guided sympathetic blockade of these structures provided effective abdominal pain control of visceral origin. Local anesthetics are used for temporary relief or as a trial before proceeding to neurolysis using alcohol or phenol for more long-lasting results. Spinal cord stimulation has also been shown to have positive outcomes in improving chronic visceral abdominal pain.[40]

Acupuncture is a technique used widely in traditional Chinese medicine and has recently been adapted into some alternative and complementary medicine programs throughout U.S. medical institutions. It involves placing thin needles into various locations in the skin to produce an analgesic effect, which likely occurs through endogenous opioids like enkephalin, beta-endorphin, and dynorphin.[41] There have been multiple randomized controlled trials, especially in the Chinese literature, documenting the efficacy of acupuncture in treating abdominal pain. For example, treatment at two acupuncture points improved pain scores in acute pancreatitis.[42] However, those studies are criticized for being poorly designed and biased.[43] As such, the efficacy of acupuncture remains unclear and has not been introduced into clinical practice. Other acupuncturelike analgesic modalities potentially working in similar mechanism, such as transcutaneous electrical nerve stimulation, are efficacious in alleviating abdominal pain.[44]

REFERENCES

1. Agur A, Dalley A, Moore K. Abdomen. In: Agur A, Dalley A, Moore K, eds. *Moore's Essential Clinical Anatomy*. 6th ed. Wolters Kluwer; 2019:253-317.
2. Moore BJ, Carol S, Owens PL. Trends in Emergency Department Visits, 2006–2014. Healthcare Cost and Utilization Project; Statistical Brief #227. Agency for Healthcare Research and Quality; September 2017.
3. Mark LO, Sabouri AS. Gastrointestinal physiology and pathophysiology. In: Miller RD, Eriksson I, Fleisher LA, Wiener-Kronish JP, Cohen NH, Young WL, eds. *Miller's Anesthesia*. 9th ed. Elsevier; 2014:403-419.
4. Almeida TF, Roizenblatt S, Tufik S. Afferent pain pathways: a neuroanatomical review. *Brain Res*. 2004;1000(1–2):40-56. doi:10.1016/j.brainres.2003.10.073
5. Steeds C. The anatomy and physiology of pain. *Surgery*. 2016;34(2):55-59. doi:10.1016/j.mpsur.2015.11.005
6. Chen L, Deng H, Cui H, et al. Inflammatory responses and inflammation-associated diseases in organs. *Oncotarget*. 2017;9(6):7204-7218. doi:10.18632/oncotarget.23208
7. Golias CH, Charalabopoulos A, Stagikas D, Charalabopoulos K, Batistatou A. The kinin system—bradykinin: biological effects and clinical implications. Multiple roles of the kinin system—bradykinin. *Hippokratia*. 2007;11(3):124-128.
8. Romanelli MR, Thayer JA, Neumeister MW. Ischemic pain. *Clin Plast Surg*. 2020;47(2):261-265. doi:10.1016/j.cps.2019.11.002
9. Waldmann R, Champigny G, Bassilana F, Heurteaux C, Lazdunski M. A proton-gated cation channel involved in acid-sensing. *Nature*. 1997;386(6621):173-177. doi:10.1038/386173a0
10. Queme LF, Ross JL, Jankowski MP. Peripheral mechanisms of ischemic myalgia. *Front Cell Neurosci*. 2017;11:419. doi:10.3389/fncel.2017.00419
11. Bielefeldt K, Gebhar G. Visceral pain: basic mechanisms. In: McMahon S, Koltzenburg M, Tracey I, Turk DC, eds. *Wall & Melzack's Textbook of Pain*. 6th ed. Elsevier; 2013:703-717.
12. Humenick A, Chen BN, Wiklendt L, et al. Activation of intestinal spinal afferent endings by changes in intra-mesenteric arterial pressure. *J Physiol*. 2015;593(16):3693-3709. doi:10.1113/JP270378
13. Prato V, Taberner FJ, Hockley JRF, et al. Functional and molecular characterization of mechanoinsensitive "silent" nociceptors. *Cell Rep*. 2017;21:3102-3115. doi:10.1016/j.celrep.2017.11.066
14. Revzin MV, Scoutt LM, Garner JG, Moore CL. Right upper quadrant pain: ultrasound first! *J Ultrasound Med*. 2017;36:1975-1985. doi:10.1002/jum.14274
15. Tang SJ, Daram SR, Wu R, Bhaijee F. Pathogenesis, diagnosis, and management of gastric ischemia. *Clin Gastroenterol Hepatol*. 2014;12(2):246-252.e1. doi:10.1016/j.cgh.2013.07.025
16. Lin KJ, García Rodríguez LA, Hernández-Díaz S. Systematic review of peptic ulcer disease incidence rates: do studies without validation provide reliable estimates? *Pharmacoepidemiol Drug Saf*. 2011;20(7):718-728. doi:10.1002/pds.2153
17. Krishna SG, Kamboj AK, Hart PA, Hinton A, Conwell DL. The changing epidemiology of acute pancreatitis hospitalizations: a decade of trends and the impact of chronic pancreatitis. *Pancreas*. 2017;46(4):482-488. doi:10.1097/MPA.0000000000000783
18. Sun H, Zuo HD, Lin Q, et al. MR imaging for acute pancreatitis: the current status of clinical applications. *Ann Transl Med*. 2019;7(12):269. doi:10.21037/atm.2019.05.37
19. Lammert F, Gurusamy K, Ko CW, et al. Gallstones. *Nat Rev Dis Primers*. 2016;2:16024. doi:10.1038/nrdp.2016.24
20. Cao AM, Eslick GD. Epidemiology and pathogenesis of gallstones. In: Cox M, Eslick G, Padbury R, eds. *The Management of Gallstone Disease*. Springer, Cham; 2018. https://doi.org/10.1007/978-3-319-63884-3_3
21. Miura F, Okamoto K, Takada T, et al. Tokyo Guidelines 2018: initial management of acute biliary infection and flowchart for acute cholangitis. *J Hepatobiliary Pancreat Sci*. 2018;25(1):31-40. doi:10.1002/jhbp.509
22. Lee SL, Kim HK, Choi HH, et al. Diagnostic value of magnetic resonance cholangiopancreatography to detect bile duct stones in acute biliary pancreatitis. *Pancreatology*. 2018;18(1):22-28. doi:10.1016/j.pan.2017.12.004

23. Stravitz RT, Lee WM. Acute liver failure. *Lancet*. 2019;394(10201):869-881. doi:10.1016/S0140-6736(19)31894-X
24. Rami Reddy SR, Cappell MS. A systematic review of the clinical presentation, diagnosis, and treatment of small bowel obstruction. *Curr Gastroenterol Rep*. 2017;19(6):28. doi:10.1007/s11894-017-0566-9
25. Shi XZ, Lin YM, Hegde S. Novel insights into the mechanisms of abdominal pain in obstructive bowel disorders. *Front Integr Neurosci*. 2018;12:23. doi:10.3389/fnint.2018.00023
26. Bala M, Kashuk J, Moore EE, et al. Acute mesenteric ischemia: guidelines of the World Society of Emergency Surgery. *World J Emerg Surg*. 2017;12:38. doi:10.1186/s13017-017-0150-5
27. Strate LL, Morris AM. Epidemiology, pathophysiology, and treatment of diverticulitis. *Gastroenterology*. 2019;156(5):1282-1298.e1. doi:10.1053/j.gastro.2018.12.033
28. Munie ST, Nalamati SPM. Epidemiology and pathophysiology of diverticular disease. *Clin Colon Rectal Surg*. 2018;31(4):209-213. doi:10.1055/s-0037-1607464
29. Swanson SM, Strate LL. Acute colonic diverticulitis [published correction appears in Ann Intern Med. 2020 May 5;172(9):640]. *Ann Intern Med*. 2018;168(9):ITC65-ITC80. doi:10.7326/AITC201805010
30. Kandagatla PG, Stefanou AJ. Current status of the radiologic assessment of diverticular disease. *Clin Colon Rectal Surg*. 2018;31(4):217-220. doi:10.1055/s-0037-1607466
31. Ferris M, Quan S, Kaplan BS, et al. The global incidence of appendicitis: a systematic review of population-based studies. *Ann Surg*. 2017;266(2):237-241. doi:10.1097/SLA.0000000000002188
32. Khan MS, Chaudhry MBH, Shahzad N, et al. Risk of appendicitis in patients with incidentally discovered appendicoliths. *J Surg Res*. 2018;221:84-87. doi:10.1016/j.jss.2017.08.021
33. Davis MP. Drug management of visceral pain: concepts from basic research. *Pain Res Treat*. 2012;2012:265605. doi:10.1155/2012/265605
34. Tomić MA, Vucković SM, Stepanović-Petrović RM, Ugresić ND, Prostran MS, Bosković B. Synergistic interactions between paracetamol and oxcarbazepine in somatic and visceral pain models in rodents. *Anesth Analg*. 2010;110(4):1198-1205. doi:10.1213/ANE.0b013e3181cbd8da
35. Fraquelli M, Casazza G, Conte D, Colli A. Non-steroid anti-inflammatory drugs for biliary colic. *Cochrane Database Syst Rev*. 2016;9(9):CD006390. doi:10.1002/14651858.CD006390.pub2
36. Hayward KL, Powell EE, Irvine KM, Martin JH. Can paracetamol (acetaminophen) be administered to patients with liver impairment? *Br J Clin Pharmacol*. 2016;81(2):210-222. doi:10.1111/bcp.12802
37. Kassam AF, Kim Y, Cortez AR, Dhar VK, Wima K, Shah SA. The impact of opioid use on human and health care costs in surgical patients. *Surg Open Sci*. 2020;2(2):92-95. doi:10.1016/j.sopen.2019.10.001
38. Camilleri M, Lembo A, Katzka DA. Opioids in gastroenterology: treating adverse effects and creating therapeutic benefits. *Clin Gastroenterol Hepatol*. 2017;15:1338-1349. doi:10.1016/j.cgh.2017.05.014
39. Cornman-Homonoff J, Holzwanger DJ, Lee KS, Madoff DC, Li D. Celiac plexus block and neurolysis in the management of chronic upper abdominal pain. *Semin Intervent Radiol*. 2017;34(4):376-386. doi:10.1055/s-0037-1608861
40. Kapural L, Gupta M, Paicius R, et al. Treatment of chronic abdominal pain with 10-kHz spinal cord stimulation: safety and efficacy results from a 12-month prospective, multicenter, feasibility study. *Clin Transl Gastroenterol*. 2020;11(2):e00133. doi:10.14309/ctg.0000000000000133
41. Han JS. Acupuncture and endorphins. *Neurosci Lett*. 2004;361(1–3):258-261. doi:10.1016/j.neulet.2003.12.019
42. Li J, Zhao Y, Wen Q, Xue Q, Lv J, Li N. Electroacupuncture for severe acute pancreatitis accompanied with paralytic ileus:a randomized controlled trial. *Zhongguo Zhen Jiu*. 2016;36(11):1126-1130. doi:10.1370 3/j.0255-2930.2016.11.002
43. Paley CA, Johnson MI. Acupuncture for the relief of chronic pain: a synthesis of systematic reviews. *Medicina*. 2020;56:6. doi:10.3390/medicina56010006
44. Chen KB, Huang Y, Jin XL, Chen GF. Electroacupuncture or transcutaneous electroacupuncture for postoperative ileus after abdominal surgery: a systematic review and meta-analysis. *Int J Surg*. 2019;70:93-101. doi:10.1016/j.ijsu.2019.08.034

19

Acute Genitourinary System Related Pain

Wesley R. Pate and Natalie P. Tukan

Introduction

There are many causes of acute genitourinary pain, ranging from very common conditions like urinary tract infections to more rare diagnoses like testicular torsion. The etiology of pain can sometimes be clearly delineated based on history and physical exam, while other conditions require more testing to differentiate between diagnostic possibilities. Management can vary widely depending on the diagnosis and can include a variety of treatments including oral and parenteral analgesics, surgical procedures, antibiotics, and local and regional anesthetic techniques. This chapter, while not exhaustive, will focus on the background, diagnosis, and treatment of several of the most important causes of acute genitourinary pain.

Urinary Tract Infections

Background

Urinary tract infections (UTIs) are one of the most common infections in adults. They can involve the lower urinary tract confined to the bladder (cystitis) and/or the upper urinary tract with infection of the renal parenchyma (pyelonephritis).[1] Infections in otherwise healthy individuals with normal urinary tracts are the most common and are referred to as uncomplicated UTIs. Complicated UTIs are associated with factors like structurally or functionally abnormal urinary tracts, immunocompromised hosts, and nosocomial infections. Infection in males is generally considered a complicated UTI.[2]

Women have a tenfold greater incidence of UTI compared to men throughout the reproductive years until declining to a 2:1 difference in older adulthood.[3] The lifetime risk of UTI for women is estimated at 60%.[4] The gender difference in infection rates can be explained by women's short urethras facilitating migration of perineal bacteria into the bladder, whereas men's longer urethras have more ability to clear bacteria through voiding before reaching the bladder.[3] Recent sexual activity is also an important risk factor for infection, as this further facilitates the transit of bacteria through the urethra.[3] Pyelonephritis is usually caused by an ascending infection from the lower urinary tract but can be caused by hematogenous or lymphatic spread, although this is very rare in healthy, nonhospitalized patients.[1] Ultimately, host factors related to genetic variations and anatomic, physiologic, or functional urologic abnormalities (like neurogenic bladder, diabetes, or incomplete voiding) play a large role in whether bacteria entering the bladder are likely to bind to mucosal surfaces and cause infection.[1,3]

More than three-quarters of outpatient UTIs and more than 90% of cases of pyelonephritis in young, healthy women are caused by *Escherichia coli*, with other gram-negative rods comprising normal colonic flora contributing to most of the remaining infections.[3,5] *Staphylococcus saprophyticus* is also a causative bacteria in about 10% of sexually active women.[3]

Symptoms and Diagnosis

Acute bacterial cystitis generally presents with symptoms of dysuria, urinary frequency, and urinary urgency due to bacteria irritating the urethral and bladder mucosa. More rare presenting symptoms include suprapubic tenderness or hematuria.[1] The differential diagnosis for cystitis includes other acute pathologies like pyelonephritis, urethritis, bladder calculi, acute bacterial prostatitis (ABP), or vaginitis. Chronic urinary tract etiologies like interstitial cystitis, chronic pelvic pain syndrome, or overactive bladder are additional diagnostic considerations.[6]

Acute pyelonephritis most commonly presents with flank pain, systemic symptoms like fever and chills, and may also have lower urinary tract symptoms, although presentation can vary widely.[5] In addition to distinguishing pyelonephritis from cystitis, the differential diagnosis includes other urinary tract causes like urolithiasis, gynecologic etiologies like pelvic inflammatory disease, and abdominal pathologies like appendicitis or cholecystitis. Urolithiasis is particularly likely if the flank pain radiates to the groin.[5] Increased vaginal discharge would suggest that a gynecologic etiology is more likely, and imaging is important to elucidate suspected abdominal pathology.

The diagnosis of cystitis is primarily via urinalysis from a clean-voided midstream urine sample with pyuria and/or bacteriuria in combination with bothersome urinary symptoms. If urinary bacteria are identified in the absence of UTI symptoms, this is classified as asymptomatic bacteriuria rather than bacterial cystitis and does not require treatment except in special circumstances like pregnancy or in patients undergoing certain urologic procedures.[7] For cases of suspected pyelonephritis, a urine culture is also obtained to confirm the pathogen and antimicrobial susceptibility.[1] Imaging should be considered in patients more likely to have complicated infections like patients with a history of urolithiasis or known abnormal urinary tract anatomy, or patients with persistent symptoms despite appropriate antibiotic therapy.[6]

Treatment

The cornerstone of management for UTIs is appropriate antimicrobial treatment to eradicate the causative organism(s). Per IDSA guidelines, the first-line recommended antimicrobials in the United States for acute cystitis, depending on factors like availability and local resistance patterns, are nitrofurantoin, trimethoprim-sulfamethoxazole, and fosfomycin. For acute pyelonephritis, treatment should always be based on the antimicrobial susceptibilities from the urine culture, with inpatient parenteral vs outpatient oral treatment depending on the clinical status of the patient and comorbidities.[5,8] With proper antimicrobial treatment, symptoms of cystitis are markedly improved or even completely resolved within 24 hours, and those of pyelonephritis within about 48 hours.[3] Persistent fever or ongoing symptoms after this time raises concern for an alternative diagnosis like obstruction from urolithiasis or the development of a renal or perinephric abscess.[5]

Temporizing options for pain include analgesics like phenazopyridine and nonsteroidal anti-inflammatory drugs (NSAIDs). Phenazopyridine is an azo dye that functions as a urinary analgesic by exerting a local anesthetic action on urinary mucosa.[9] Several studies examining the use of NSAIDs vs antibiotics suggest that although many women may recover with symptom management only, their symptoms resolve more quickly and have less risk of progression to pyelonephritis when treated with antibiotics, pointing toward the utility of NSAIDs as an adjunctive, rather than sole, treatment strategy.[10-12] Patients with debilitating symptoms may also require brief therapy with opioid medications.[3]

In patients with recurrent UTIs, prophylactic measures are also important in managing symptoms, with several options depending on frequency and severity of infections and patient preference. These measures include patient-initiated treatment at the onset of UTI symptoms, daily antibiotic prophylaxis for between 3 and 12 months, or postcoital prophylaxis for women whose UTIs are related to sexual activity.[13] For nonantibiotic options, there is low-grade evidence that cranberry extracts can decrease the rate of recurrent UTI, as they contain proanthocyanidins which prevent the adhesion of bacteria to the urothelium.[3,13] Other tested measures like lactobacillus probiotics or increased water intake have not been shown to have any clinical effect.[13]

Urolithiasis and Renal Colic

Background

Urolithiasis refers to formation of urinary calculi, or stones, anywhere along the entire genitourinary tract. Most commonly, stones form in the collecting system that drain the kidneys, and the presence of these calculi is referred to as nephrolithiasis. Issues with stones occur when they cause obstruction of the kidney or infections within the urinary tract. Pain with stones most commonly involves the passage of a stone through the ureter, and there are patients who consider this the most painful experience of their life.

Risk factors for urolithiasis include obesity, dietary factors, diabetes mellitus, urine characteristics, family history, certain genetic conditions, and arid environments.[14] Gender is also important, as stone disease affects men more than women, though the gender gap has been narrowing over time. Estimates of age distribution of urolithiasis show significant variability between studies, although overall stone disease is rare in the pediatric population.[15]

Recent analysis of the National Health and Nutrition Examination Survey data estimates the prevalence of kidney stones in the United States at 8.8%, with higher rates in men (10.6%) vs women (7.1%).[16] Interestingly, the percentage of patients who form another stone within 5 years after an initial episode has been estimated to be as high as 30%-40%.[17] The prevalence and incidence of kidney stones globally, including in the United States, has been increasing. Various reasons for this increase have been suggested, including changes in diet patterns, increased obesity rates, and increased identification of asymptomatic stones found incidentally on imaging.[15,18] The majority of stones are composed of calcium oxalate, alone or in addition to calcium phosphate, with the remainder composed of uric acid, struvite, and cystine.[14]

Symptoms and Diagnosis

Pain from urinary calculi varies between patients and is often episodic, and the pain is intermittent and described as "colicky" as the stone moves and the ureter spasms. The stones typically cause pain when passing through the ureter, as opposed to when it is in the kidney or immobile in the ureter.[19] It is unknown why the pain arises, although two theories exist: rapid dilation of the collecting system that compresses the renal parenchyma vs urinary extravasation.[19] The pain also differs based on the stone location within the urinary system as a reflection of referred pain from the corresponding dermatomes. For example, in the renal pelvis and proximal ureter, pain presents in the costovertebral angle and flank and can be confused with conditions like pyelonephritis, cholecystitis, or acute pancreatitis depending on the side of the stone. In the distal ureter, pain radiates to the groin as a manifestation of referred pain from the ilioinguinal or genitofemoral nerve and needs to be distinguished from conditions like testicular torsion or epididymitis.[20] A patient with stone colic will often be unable to lie still, which is in contrast to other acute abdominal pathologies, in which the patient does not move in order to prevent pain.[19,20]

Diagnosis of stones is made with imaging, with noncontrast computed tomography considered the gold standard with reported 97% sensitivity and 98% specificity (Fig. 19.1).[15] Imaging with the patient in prone position is most informative because for very distal stones at the ureterovesical junction, prone position can distinguish if the stone is still in the ureter

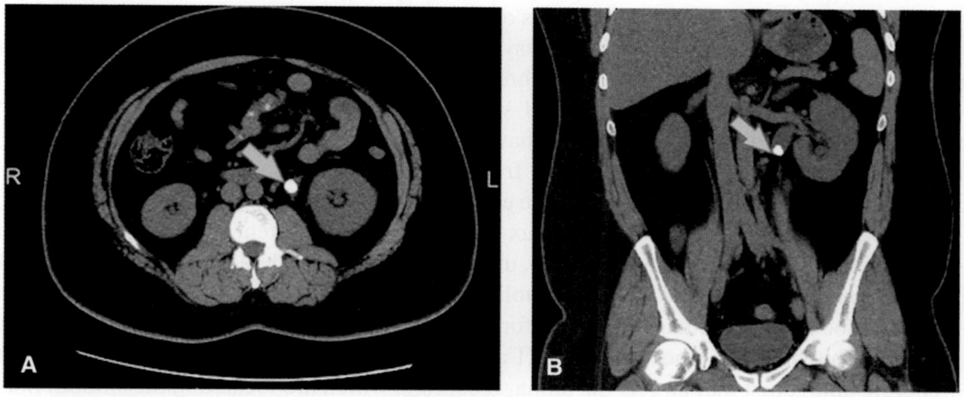

FIGURE 19.1 Images from a noncontrast renal protocol CT scan of a patient with a ureteral stone in the proximal third of the left ureter (*arrows*) in the (**A**) axial and (**B**) coronal views. (Adapted from Pena A, Ferretti JA. Stone disease imaging: there is more to x-rays than what we see! In: Schulsinger D, ed. *Kidney Stone Disease*. Springer; 2015.)

or has passed into the bladder.[21] Ultrasonography has emerged in recent years has a low-cost and radiation-free modality; however, its role in patients with suspected renal colic remains controversial, as sensitivities and specificities that have been reported in the literature vary widely.[22] A review by Ray et al. found a pooled sensitivity and specificity of 45% and 94%, respectively, for ureteric stones and 45% and 88%, respectively, for renal stones.[23] Additionally, scenarios that increase difficulty of identification of stones using ultrasonography include stones <3 mm due to absence of acoustic shadow, ureteral stones that can be obscured by bowel gas, and stones that abut the echogenic renal sinus fat.[22,23] Two groups of patients in which the AUA, EAU, and ACR recommend ultrasound as first-line imaging modality to avoid radiation exposure are pediatric patients (<14 years old) and pregnant patients.[24-26] In addition to imaging, labs should include determination of white blood cell count and serum creatinine to see if leukocytosis or acute kidney injury are present, respectively. Urinalysis and urine culture should also be obtained to evaluate for urinary infection.

Treatment

Treatment of stones in the urinary tract first and foremost involves determination if a stone should be managed medically or surgically in the acute setting. Reasons to intervene earlier include signs of urinary sepsis with obstruction, acute kidney injury that does not respond to fluid resuscitation, obstruction in a solitary kidney, inability to tolerate oral intake, or poor pain control. Urgent intervention in the acute setting involves placement of a ureteral stent or percutaneous nephrostomy tube in order to bypass the stone and decompress the renal collecting system.[27] For patients with uncomplicated ureteral stones <10 mm, American Urologic Association (AUA) guidelines suggest offering observation with pain control and aggressive fluid hydration. If the stone is in the distal ureter, patients can be offered medical expulsive therapy (MET) with the addition of alpha-adrenergic blockers.[27] Management of pain is crucial in this time period, especially if the stone is to be managed medically over the course of several weeks. Options for pain control include a variety of analgesics like acetaminophen, NSAIDs, and opioids. Choice of agents depends greatly on the clinical course of the patient. Intravenous opioids and NSAIDs are often used to quickly and effectively manage severe pain in the acute setting. If a patient is to be managed medically outpatient, oral options are utilized.[19] For patients who fail medical management with either re-presentation with intractable pain or do not spontaneously pass the stone after multiple weeks, surgical intervention is often pursued. Options for eradication of stone are highly dependent on stone characteristics, location, and patient preference. Types of intervention include extracorporeal shock wave lithotripsy, ureteroscopy and laser lithotripsy, percutaneous nephrolithotomy, and rarely laparoscopic and robotic stone removal or nephrectomy.[27]

In patients who have required ureteral stenting, side effects with the stent in place are extremely common with 80% of patients having at least one symptom.[28] These include flank and suprapubic pain, hematuria, dysuria, frequency, urgency, infection, incomplete emptying, incontinence, and encrustation.[28,29] The etiology of these symptoms, while not completely understood, is thought to be related to reflux of urine through the stent during voiding, as well as movement of the stent within the kidney, ureter, and bladder.[30] Medications that target stent-related pain include alpha-blockers, anticholinergics, and pregabalin.

Alpha-blockers are primarily utilized for treatment of hypertension and benign prostatic hyperplasia but have off-label use for MET and ureteral stent pain.[30] Tamsulosin is an alpha-adrenergic antagonist that targets the alpha$_1$ receptors, which are located in the smooth muscle of the prostate, bladder neck, and ureter. Its use in MET and ureteral stent pain is related to the presence of these receptors in the ureter, with the highest density in the distal ureter.[30] Their role in MET is supported by the aforementioned AUA/Endourologic Society guidelines in which their recommendation is specifically for distal ureteral stones <10 mm, as no clear benefit was demonstrated for proximal or mid-ureteral stones in their meta-analysis.[27] With respect to stent discomfort, alpha-blockers help to dilate the ureteral lumen, decrease ureteral spasms and motility, relax trigonal smooth muscle, as well as decrease intravesical pressure and reflux through relaxation of the bladder neck.[30] Patients should be counseled on side effects of orthostatic hypotension, dizziness, headache, fatigue, and retrograde ejaculation.

The role of anticholinergics in urology is predominantly used for overactive bladder, but they are also used in ureteral stent-related pain. Data are controversial about whether they provide a benefit as a monotherapy or in combination with alpha-blockers. Physiologically, anticholinergics are thought to decrease detrusor overactivity that is associated with bothersome voiding symptoms.[30] Whether used alone or in combination with other agents, it is important to consider side effects of anticholinergics that include dementia, blurred vision, headache, dry mouth, orthostatic hypotension, ileus, and urinary retention.

Pregabalin is the last agent that has had recent evidence emerge for its role in ureteral stent pain. A study by Ragab et al. randomized 489 patients who underwent ureteroscopy with stent placement to combination anticholinergic and pregabalin, anticholinergic only, pregabalin only, and placebo. They showed that all groups had lower symptom scores than the placebo group. The hypothesis behind the role of pregabalin in stent pain is by decreasing firing of unmyelinated C fibers with mechanical irritation.[31]

Priapism

Background

Priapism, as defined by the American Urological Association, is a persistent penile erection lasting at least 4 hours that is either unrelated to, or continues hours beyond, sexual stimulation.[32] There are three types of priapism: ischemic, nonischemic, and stuttering. Ischemic priapism is characterized by cavernosal venoocclusion, which is essentially a form of compartment syndrome. Nonischemic priapism has a high cavernous arterial inflow, and stuttering priapism is a form of ischemic priapism with periods of detumescence in between recurrent painful erections.[32] Ischemic priapism lasting over 24 hours can have up to a 90% risk of long-term erectile dysfunction, making prompt diagnosis and management essential.[33] Conversely, nonischemic priapism is not an emergency and usually resolves with conservative management.

Priapism is rare, with epidemiological studies from the past two decades citing incidence between 0.84 and 5.34 cases per 100 000 male person years.[34-36] Over 95% of cases are ischemic in origin.[37] Historically, ischemic priapism has been attributed to sickle cell disease in about two-thirds of pediatric cases and one-quarter of adult cases, with a greater proportion of adult cases due to alternative etiologies such as iatrogenic from intracavernosal injections for erectile dysfunction or from erectogenic medications like trazodone.[33]

Symptoms and Diagnosis

The diagnosis of priapism is considered to be unmistakable, with the primary goal in differentiating between ischemic vs nonischemic priapism. Key features on history, physical examination, and testing can help differentiate between the different types of priapism. Ischemic priapism is painful with a fully rigid penis, patients are more likely to have a history of hematologic abnormalities like sickle cell disease or a history of recent intracavernosal vasoactive drug injections, and cavernosal blood gases will usually be hypoxic, hypercarbic, and acidotic.[32] In contrast, nonischemic priapism is rarely painful, does not cause a fully rigid erection, has normal cavernosal blood gases, and is more likely to be associated with a history of recent perineal trauma.[37] Color duplex ultrasonography is considered an alternative or adjunct to cavernosal blood gas sampling; patients with ischemic priapism have little to no blood flow in the cavernosal arteries as opposed to normal to high flow in nonischemic priapism.[32]

Treatment

The AUA guidelines for treatment of ischemic priapism include therapeutic aspiration, with or without irrigation, followed by intracavernosal injection of sympathomimetics, whose vasoactive properties facilitate detumescence by causing alpha-mediated vasoconstriction within the corpora cavernosa.[32] The most common drug used is the alpha-1 agonist phenylephrine, as it minimizes cardiovascular side effects of systemic absorption as compared to other agents like norepinephrine or epinephrine. Still, monitoring patients during and after intracavernosal injection is critical as patients can develop systemic side effects like hypertension, headache, and reflex bradycardia. If aspiration and sympathomimetic injections fail, surgical shunts can be considered as a rescue option, with several different options for shunting procedures, though they are not a first-line option due to morbidity and success rate.[32] More recently, early implantation of a penile prosthesis is gaining traction as a management strategy for improved long-term outcomes in cases of refractory ischemic priapism, in particular for patients with longer duration of priapism who will almost certainly develop erectile dysfunction.[38,39]

Most cases of nonischemic priapism will resolve with observation alone and there is no role for aspiration—other than to obtain a cavernosal blood gas sample—nor for injection of sympathomimetic agents. Should the priapism not resolve spontaneously or patients request treatment, selective arterial embolization with interventional radiology can be considered, with surgical intervention as a last resort.[32]

Although avoiding long-term complications is the primary goal in ischemic priapism, management of pain is an important adjunct while awaiting detumescence. Providers can consider systemic analgesia with acetaminophen, NSAIDs, or low-dose opioids. For patients with sickle cell disease in whom ischemic priapism may be triggered by a sickle cell crisis, opioid analgesia and hydration are particularly important.[40] Local anesthesia in the form of a ring block or dorsal penile nerve block can be useful in managing the pain associated with priapism as well as providing analgesia for the therapeutic interventions of aspiration and pharmacologic detumescence.[40] A penile ring block is simply circumferential subcutaneous injection of local anesthetic. The technique has been described by several authors, including in a comparative study for anesthesia in adults undergoing circumcision, in which 10 mL of 1:1

mixture of 1% lidocaine and 0.5% bupivacaine was injected subcutaneously in a ring around the base of the penis, with more anesthetic (~⅔) on the dorsal aspect of the penis.[41]

The dorsal penile nerve block, which is more targeted, has also been utilized for multiple other penile conditions including paraphimosis, penile trauma, and circumcision.[42] The dorsal nerves of the penis are formed from branches of the pudendal nerves (S2-4) at the base of the penis and travel deep to Buck fascia, but superficial to the tunica albuginea encasing the corporal bodies, to provide the primary sensory innervation to the penile skin.[42,43] Traditionally, a dorsal penile block has been performed via a landmark-based approach near the origin of the dorsal nerves. The blind technique requires large volumes of local anesthetic to achieve sufficient anesthetic effect and risks inadvertent injection into the corpora cavernosa, failed anesthesia, or local anesthetic toxicity.[42] More recently, an ultrasound-guided technique has been used as an alternative to the landmark-based approach, which more precisely anesthetizes the dorsal nerves and minimizes the risks of the blind technique.

The general steps include placing a high-frequency probe transversely at the dorsal base of the penis with the patient in the supine position and identifying Buck fascia superficial to the corpora cavernosa.[42] The needle tip is visualized penetrating Buck fascia in an in-plane approach, and small-volume local anesthetic—<10 mL—is injected with visualization of spread between the fascia and the corporal bodies (Figs. 19.2 and 19.3).[42,43] Only plain local anesthetic should be used, as the addition of epinephrine increases the risk of penile ischemia and necrosis. Importantly, the deep dorsal vein and paired dorsal arteries lie between Buck fascia and the corpora, and care must be taken to avoid intravascular injection.[43] As with other ultrasound-guided blocks, aspiration and ultrasound visualization are used to confirm proper

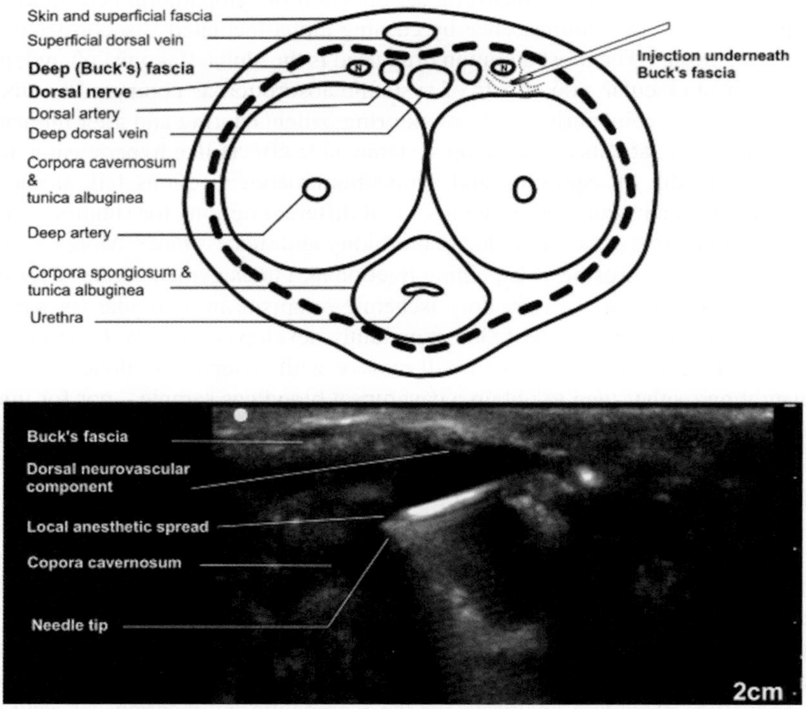

FIGURE 19.2 **Top Panel.** Cross-sectional anatomy at the base of the penis showing the injection site beneath Buck fascia for a dorsal penile nerve block. **Bottom Panel.** Ultrasound image showing needle tip placement underneath Buck fascia with hypoechoic local anesthetic displacing the corpora cavernosum downward. (From Flores S, Herring AA. Ultrasound-guided dorsal penile nerve block for ED paraphimosis reduction. *Am J Emerg Med.* 2015;33:863.e3-865.)

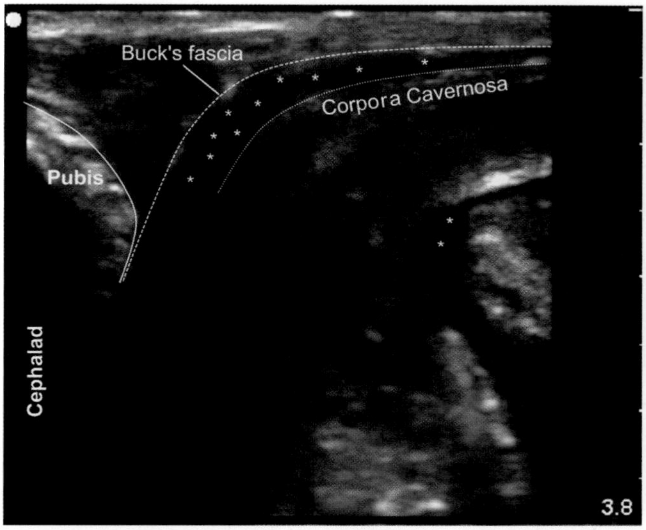

FIGURE 19.3 Ultrasound image of the penis in a sagittal view after injection of local anesthetic for a dorsal penile nerve block. (Adapted from Flores S, Herring AA. Ultrasound-guided dorsal penile nerve block for ED paraphimosis reduction. *Am J Emerg Med.* 2015;33:863.e3-865.)

needle placement. An additional benefit of the dorsal penile nerve block is that since Buck fascia is continuous around the circumference of the penis, a single injection can provide circumferential anesthesia.[42]

Paraphimosis

Background

Paraphimosis is defined as the inability to reduce a retracted prepuce, more commonly referred to as foreskin. This is in contrast to phimosis, in which a foreskin cannot be retracted over the penis. The word comes from Greek origin as "para" means resembling and "phimosis" means muzzling or restriction, though is sometimes spelled "paraphymosis" as "phyma" means swelling.[44] Paraphimosis is a rare condition, with 0.2% incidence in uncircumcised boys 4 months to 12 years old and estimated at ~1% in males over 16 years of age.[45,46]

Paraphimosis results from the inability to reduce the foreskin back over the penile glans. This most commonly occurs when a normal foreskin is retracted and then negligently left in that position for a prolonged time period (Fig. 19.4). Less commonly, an erection in patients with phimosis can allow retraction of the foreskin over the glans. In both scenarios, the circumferentially narrow skin known as the paraphimotic band, or preputial band, is immovable behind the corona of the glans.[44,47] During a paraphimosis, there is a series of physiologic events that lead to swelling of both the glans and inner prepuce. Compression from the paraphimotic band leads to decreased venous return, which causes tumescence of the glans, and an inability of the foreskin to retract spontaneously. Edema occurs in both the inner prepuce and glans from lymphatic and vascular congestion, respectively. This edema worsens the strangulation effect and makes it increasingly difficult to resolve the paraphimosis the longer it is present.[44,47] While it is possible that a prolonged paraphimosis could lead to glans necrosis from compromised arterial supply, this is rare and most commonly erosions and micro-ulcerations occur in the constricting paraphimotic band and edematous inner prepuce and glans.[44]

Symptoms and Diagnosis

Paraphimosis is considered a urologic emergency due to the risk of tissue ischemia and necrosis with prolonged time without reduction. It is diagnosed by clinical history and most

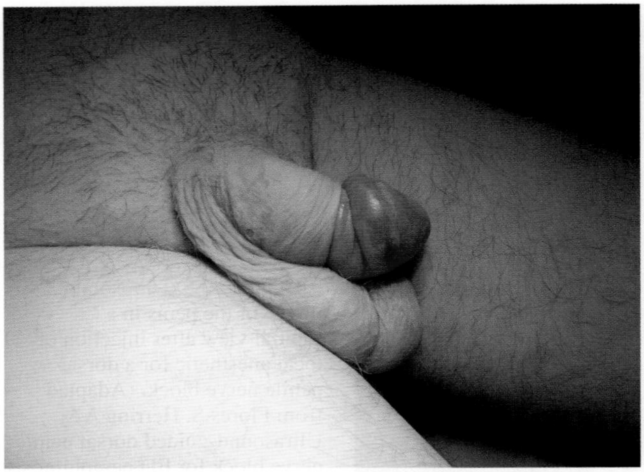

FIGURE 19.4 Paraphimosis of 4 days duration. (From http://commons.wikimedia.org/wiki/File:Paraphimosis.jpg)

importantly, physical exam showing painful, swollen, and edematous glans and foreskin.[47,48] Paraphimosis is often associated with delayed presentation, which occurs due to social embarrassment, lack of caretaker in the elderly, or not recognizing its presence in younger children.[44] One study suggested that only 4% of patients presented within a few hours, 20% within 24 hours, and the majority (68%) between 2 and 4 days.[49] The most common alternative diagnosis is pseudo-paraphimosis, which describes situations that mimic paraphimosis due to swelling of the prepuce. Reported etiologies of this phenomenon include genital piercing, chancroid, syphilitic balanitis, angioedema, insect bite, contact allergy from celandine juice, use of autoerotic metal rings, and coitus-associated penile injuries.[50-55]

Treatment

Treatment of paraphimosis centers around reduction of the swollen foreskin back over the glans. There are numerous methods for manual reduction including simple manual reduction, use of adjuvants to manual reduction, instrument-associated reductions, and surgical reductions.[44,47] Detailed explanation of these different techniques are out of the scope of this chapter, and often urologic consultation is recommended for assistance with reduction. Circumcision in the acute emergent setting is not very common as suturing inflamed and edematous tissue leads to inferior outcomes.[44,47] Interval elective circumcision is important in patients who want to prevent future episodes, in those with phimosis, or in situations in which laceration or ulceration occurred prior to resolution.[44]

Reduction of paraphimosis is often extremely painful, so in addition to use of oral and intravenous pain medications, several anesthetic techniques exist in order to make reduction more tolerable. These techniques include dorsal penile nerve block, penile ring block, topical anesthetics, or conscious sedation. Dorsal penile nerve block and penile ring block were previously described in the section on priapism and involves the same technique for paraphimosis.

As for topical anesthetics and procedural sedation, there was a retrospective cohort study by Burstein and Paquin in 2017 that compared these two techniques for use in reduction of paraphimosis in children <18 years old. Application of topical anesthetic in this study included LET gel (lidocaine 4%, epinephrine 0.1%, tetracaine 0.5%) or lidocaine hydrochloride 2% jelly, followed by wrapping with occlusive dressing for 30 minutes prior to paraphimosis reduction. Procedural sedation was implemented in patients with no contraindications with dosing of ketamine at 1-2 mg/kg initial dose with subsequent doses as needed. They found no difference in reduction success between topical anesthetic vs procedural sedation;

however, topical anesthetic resulted in less adverse events and shorter emergency department length of stay.[56]

Penile Fracture

Background

A penile fracture is a rupture of the tunica albuginea of the penis, which can happen with bending of an erect penis, generally during either sexual intercourse or forceful masturbation.[57] Penile fracture is rare, with the estimated incidence in the United States just over 1 per 100 000 males per year, but is an important diagnosis as delayed management risks long-term morbidity including erectile dysfunction and penile deformity.[58]

Symptoms and Diagnosis

The classic presentation of a penile fracture is the description of an audible crack or snap during intercourse followed by immediate detumescence (loss of erection) and onset of pain, with penile ecchymosis and swelling noted on physical exam.[57] The appearance is often described as an "eggplant deformity" due to the swelling, ecchymosis, and deviation away from the side of the defect in the tunica (Fig. 19.5).[59] History and examination are often sufficient for diagnosis, but ultrasound or MRI can be used as a diagnostic modality to search for defects in the tunica albuginea when the diagnosis is uncertain. Ultrasound is becoming more popular as a low-cost and easily available imaging option (Fig. 19.6), while MRI is highly sensitive and specific but limited by cost and availability.[60,61] Retrograde urethrography is also indicated in cases of suspected urethral injury.[62] The main differential diagnosis for a penile fracture is penile ecchymosis or superficial penile hematoma, which, in contrast to penile fracture, lacks disruption of the tunica albuginea and intracavernous hematoma.[62]

Treatment

For patients in whom penile fracture is suspected, the AUA guidelines recommend urgent surgical exploration and repair, including evaluation for concomitant urethral injury, which can be present in up to a quarter of cases.[57] The primary concern with delayed surgical treatment is a higher risk of complications like impaired erectile function or penile curvature.[63] However, some studies suggest that delayed surgical repair, after edema subsides, facilitates

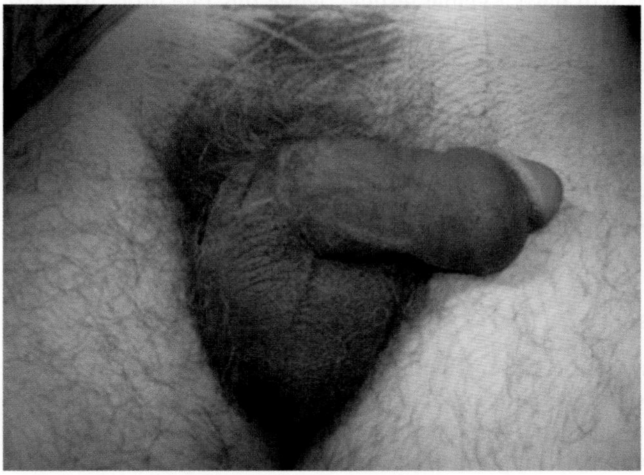

FIGURE 19.5 Classic "eggplant deformity" appearance of a penile fracture with swelling, ecchymosis, and deviation away from the side of the defect. This penile fracture was sustained during intercourse. (From Morey AF, Simhan J. Genital and lower urinary tract trauma. In: Partin AW, Dmochowski RR, Kavoussi LR, Peters CA, eds. *Campbell-Walsh-Wein Urology*. 12th ed. Elsevier; 2020; with permission.)

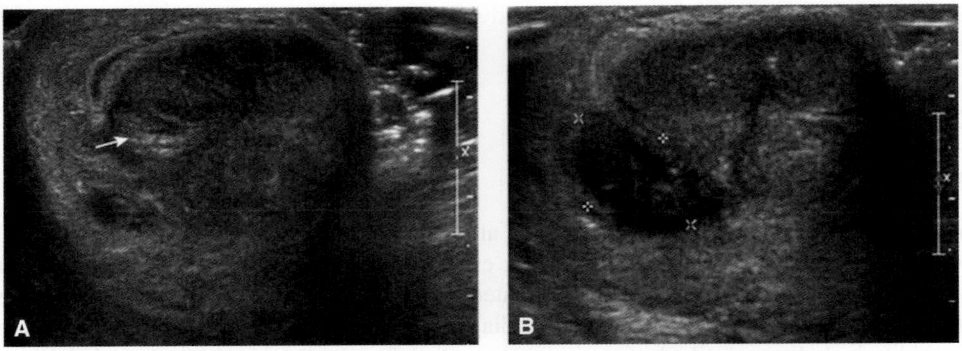

FIGURE 19.6 Ultrasound examination in a patient with a suspected penile fracture. **A.** Evidence of ruptured tunica albuginea (*arrow*). **B.** Hematoma adjacent to the ruptured tunica. (From Morey AF, Simhan J. Genital and lower urinary tract trauma. In: Partin AW, Dmochowski RR, Kavoussi LR, Peters CA, eds. *Campbell-Walsh-Wein Urology*. 12th ed. Elsevier; 2020.)

less-invasive localization and repair of the tear in the tunica albuginea and does not necessarily have worse long-term outcomes.[64-66] Analgesia has a minimal role in treatment for patients undergoing immediate repair other than as a temporizing measure. For patients planned for delayed surgical repair, ice or hot compresses, anti-inflammatory medications, and antibiotics form the mainstay of preoperative therapy.[66] If an alternative diagnosis like penile ecchymosis or superficial penile hematoma is made, conservative management similarly includes ice and NSAIDs, as well as application of a compressive dressing for 1-2 weeks, along with abstinence from sexual activity for a month.[62]

Testicular Torsion

Background

Testicular torsion occurs when the testis twists around the spermatic cord and results in interruption of blood supply to the testis, with the risk of ischemia and infarction if not detorsed. Testicular torsion is most common in children and adolescents, with an annual incidence of 3.8 per 100 000 boys <18 years old, but should be considered in men of any age with acute scrotal pain or swelling.[67] Torsion is a surgical emergency, as salvage of the affected testicle is strongly linked to time to detorsion. Nearly all patients who undergo surgical detorsion within 6 hours of the onset of symptoms will have a viable testicle, while this rate drops to <60% viability after 12 hours and essentially to nonviability by 24 hours.[68]

There are two categories of testicular torsion: intravaginal and extravaginal. Intravaginal torsion involves the testicle rotating around the spermatic cord inside the tunica vaginalis, sometimes related to a deformity in which the testicle does not adhere normally to the posterior scrotal wall, called a bell clapper deformity.[69] Extravaginal torsion, which is much more rare, occurs in neonates either prenatally or postnatally and involves torsion of the entire spermatic cord including the tunica vaginalis.[70] Only intravaginal torsion will be further discussed in this chapter.

Symptoms and Diagnosis

The classic patient with testicular torsion presents with severe, sudden onset, testicular pain, often with associated nausea or vomiting. Differential diagnoses can include a variety of scrotal pathologies, but epididymitis and appendiceal torsion are two of the most likely diagnoses from which testicular torsion should be distinguished.[69] Examination findings consistent with

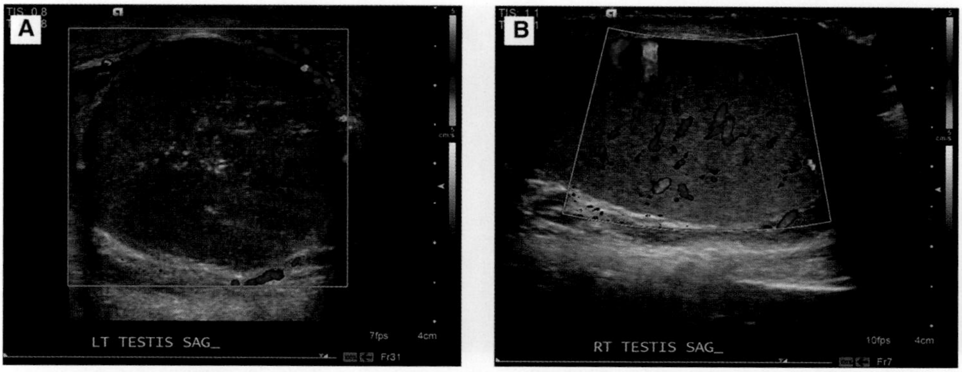

FIGURE 19.7 Color Doppler scrotal ultrasound demonstrating left-sided testicular torsion. **A.** Left testis with no detectable blood flow. **B.** Right testis with normal blood flow. (From Wang J-H. Testicular torsion. *Urol Sci*. 2012;23(3):85.)

torsion include an extremely tender, high-riding testis, absent cremasteric reflex and thick spermatic cord.[71] The absent cremasteric reflex is the most sensitive finding for torsion on physical exam.[72] In epididymitis, discomfort tends to be more gradual and mild than in torsion, and patients are more likely to have dysuria and scrotal erythema or edema.[72]

Appendiceal torsion, in contrast to testicular torsion, involves twisting and spontaneous infarction of the embryological remnants known as the testicular and epididymal appendages. Patients can present with acute scrotal pain and swelling similar to testicular torsion but are less likely to have systemic symptoms like nausea and vomiting.[69] On examination, patients have a normal testicular lie and isolated tenderness to palpation at the superior pole of the testis, with the potential for the "blue dot sign" from the appearance of the infarcted appendage through the skin.[72] Appendiceal torsion is usually managed conservatively with warm baths, anti-inflammatory medications, and temporary activity restrictions.[73]

Patients whose history and examination favor testicular torsion should expeditiously undergo a scrotal Doppler ultrasound to assess for the absence of arterial blood flow to the testis indicative of torsion (Fig. 19.7).[68] Color Doppler ultrasound is very sensitive and specific for confirming suspected testicular torsion, with estimated 100% sensitivity and 97% specificity.[72]

Treatment

Urgent surgical exploration is indicated for any patient with suspected torsion for detorsion of the affected testicle, if viable, as well as orchiopexy of both testicles to minimize the chance of recurrence. Patients with delayed presentations or who are otherwise found to have a nonviable testis on exploration will undergo orchiectomy in lieu of detorsion (Fig. 19.8).[71] Testicular torsion is one of the most acutely painful genitourinary diagnoses, but the role for pain management is somewhat limited, since surgical exploration for definitive management should occur as quickly as possible after the diagnosis. Certainly, analgesic or anxiolytic medications can be part of a preoperative anesthetic plan. Some clinicians will attempt manual detorsion as a temporizing measure to restore blood flow and alleviate pain while awaiting surgery.[74] Performing manual detorsion is painful, so patients can receive analgesic medication, light sedation, or local anesthetic via a spermatic cord block prior to the procedure.[69,75]

Spermatic cord block is more frequently used as a technique to provide anesthesia to the scrotal contents for outpatient urologic procedures like vasovasostomy, hydrocelectomy, or orchiectomy but has also been employed for manual detorsion.[75,76] Like many other regional anesthesia techniques, this block was historically performed as a landmark-based blind

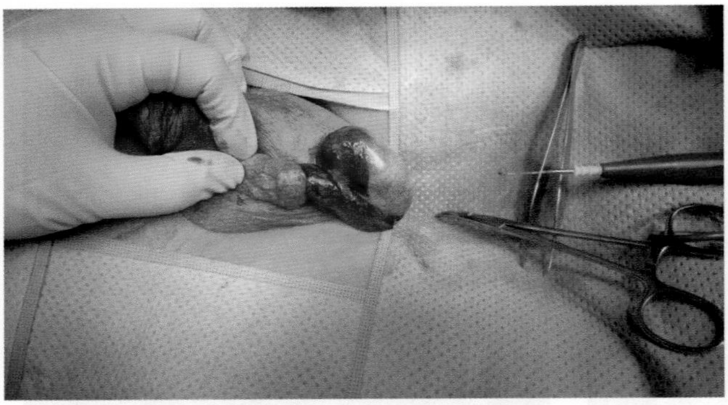

FIGURE 19.8 Intraoperative appearance of infarcted right testis. (From Tang YH, Yeung VH, Chu PS, Man CW. A 55-year-old man with right testicular pain: too old for torsion? *Urol Case Rep.* 2017;11:74-75.)

injection of local anesthetic, with ultrasound guidance now gaining popularity as a way to maximize block efficacy while minimizing the risk of intravascular injection, hematoma, or injury to the contents of the spermatic cord.[77]

The technique as described by Wipfli et al. uses a high-frequency probe in a transverse orientation at the inguinoscrotal junction distal to the superficial inguinal ring, with the best visualization achieved with an assistant gently pinching the spermatic cord and pulling it to the skin surface (Fig. 19.9).[77] The spermatic cord is first identified as a half-rounded structure, and subsequently its contents are identified, with the testicular artery having pulsatile flow on Doppler ultrasound and the vas deferens lacking flow, though both are round and noncompressible (Fig. 19.10). Using an out of plane view with the spermatic cord in short axis, the needle tip is aimed toward the vas deferens before injecting local anesthetic, with the goal to fill the spermatic cord with the local anesthetic around and between the testicular artery and vas deferens (Fig. 19.11).[77] The local anesthetic used will likely depend on institutional preferences but ~10 mL with several additional milliliters for scrotal skin infiltration should be sufficient.[75,77]

Acute Prostate Infections

Background

Prostatitis is common in men with an estimated 35%-50% reporting symptoms in their lifetime.[78] The National Institute of Health classifies prostatitis into four categories. Category I

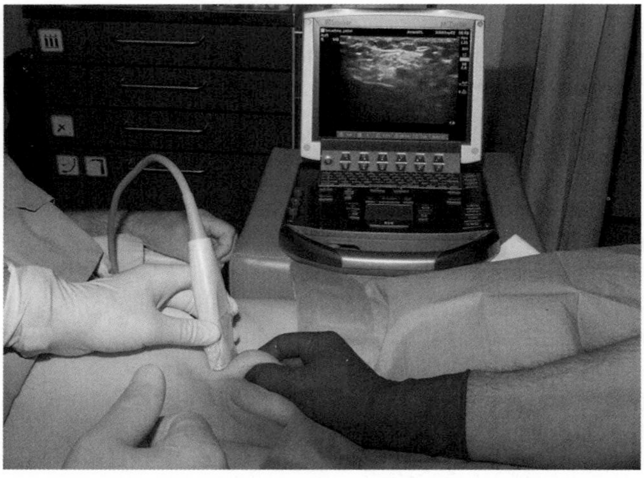

FIGURE 19.9 Proper positioning for ultrasound-guided spermatic cord block with transverse orientation of the ultrasound transducer. Note that the spermatic cord is grasped and lifted to the skin surface for better visualization. (From Wipfli M, Birkhäuser F, Luyet C, Greif R, Thalmann G, Eichenberger U. Ultrasound-guided spermatic cord block for scrotal surgery. *Br J Anaesth.* 2011;106(2):255-259.)

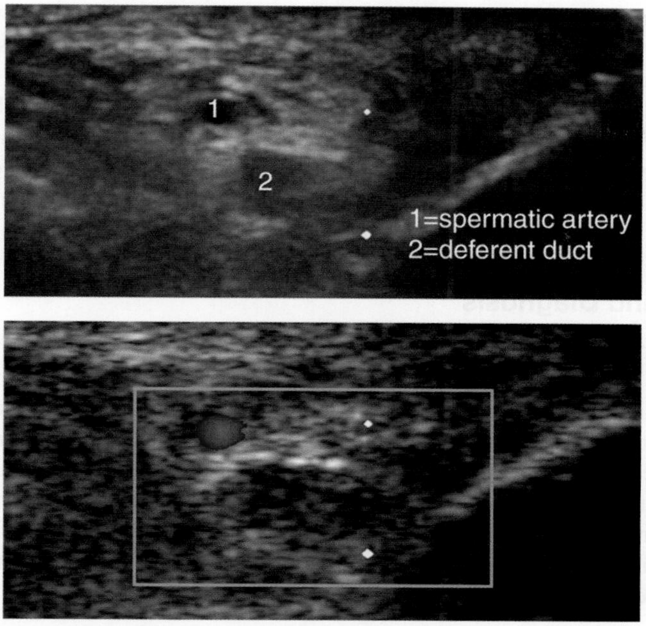

FIGURE 19.10 Ultrasound image of the spermatic cord. **Top Panel.** Compressed spermatic cord with hypoechoic spermatic artery and ductus deferens. Venous plexus compressed and not visible. **Bottom Panel.** Application of color Doppler to differentiate the spermatic artery from the ductus deferens. (From Wipfli M, Birkhäuser F, Luyet C, Greif R, Thalmann G, Eichenberger U. Ultrasound-guided spermatic cord block for scrotal surgery. *Br J Anaesth.* 2011;106(2):255-259.)

is ABP, with the other three categories being either chronic in nature or asymptomatic. Prostatitis most commonly (>90%) of the time is category III, or chronic abacterial prostatitis, also referred to as chronic pain pelvic pain syndrome.[78] This section is devoted to ABP given the importance of its role in acute genitourinary pain. It is bimodal in distribution and most commonly occurs in ages 20-40 years old as well as 70-79 years old.[79] While overall not a common diagnosis, when it occurs, it is often associated with either an immunocompromised state, bladder outlet obstruction, or procedural manipulation of the prostate.[80] The responsible bacterial organism is usually from the Enterobacteriaceae family, with *Escherichia coli* accounting for an estimated 50%-90% of cases. Sexually transmitted organisms have also been implicated including *Neisseria gonorrhoeae*, *Chlamydia trachomatis*, and *Ureaplasma*

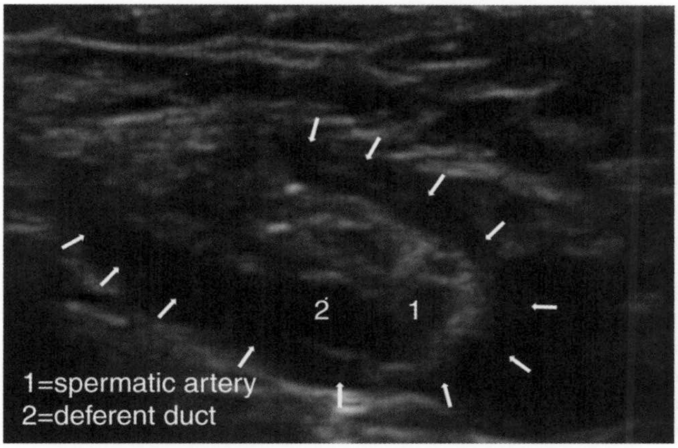

FIGURE 19.11 Ultrasound appearance of spermatic cord after injection of local anesthetic (*arrows*). (From Wipfli M, Birkhäuser F, Luyet C, Greif R, Thalmann G, Eichenberger U. Ultrasound-guided spermatic cord block for scrotal surgery. *Br J Anaesth.* 2011;106(2):255-259.)

urealyticum. Immunocompromised patients are more likely to have atypical species as etiology, specifically, *Salmonella*, *Mycobacterium*, *Staphylococcus,* and fungal species *Candida and Cryptococcus*.[80]

One potential complication of ABP is development of a prostate abscess, though incidence rates have significantly decreased compared to the preantibiotic era.[81] Immunocompromised patients are especially at risk with incidence rates ranging from 3% to 14% compared to the general population at 0.5%.[81,82] It is crucial to identify patients with prostate abscess as estimated mortality ranges from 3% to as high as 30%.[83]

Symptoms and Diagnosis

Presenting symptoms in patients with ABP are bothersome urinary symptoms (dysuria, urinary frequency, and urgency), urinary retention, fever, malaise, myalgia, and pelvic pain.[81] On physical exam, digital rectal exam will often reveal an enlarged and severely tender prostate.[81] The American Academy of Family Physicians recommends against prostatic massage in patients suspected to have ABP. American Academy of Family Physicians also recommends midstream urinalysis and urine culture to be obtained to identify a causative organism.[84] In a patient with immunocompromised state, sepsis, or clinical worsening despite appropriate treatment, imaging with computed tomography with and without contrast or transrectal ultrasound can be useful to identify prostate abscess.[80,82,85]

Treatment

While ABP is extremely painful and initial pain control with NSAIDs and/or opioids is beneficial, definitive treatment centers on appropriate antibiotic therapy based on results of urine culture and antibiotic sensitivities. Fortunately, most antibiotics have good penetration in the acute state of bacterial prostatitis. One antibiotic to avoid usage of is nitrofurantoin as it does not achieve therapeutic levels in the prostate.[86] Selection of an empiric antibiotic is often dictated by whether the patient is clinically stable. Parenteral piperacillin-tazobactam or a third-generation cephalosporin is more appropriate for a more systemically ill patient, while an oral fluoroquinolone can be utilized in a stable patient. Duration of treatment usually is 2 weeks but can be extended to 4 weeks if the patient had bacteremia on presentation.[86]

Acute bacterial prostatitis can also be associated with urinary retention, and the patient should be evaluated for retention with bladder ultrasound after voiding, called a postvoid residual volume. Placement of a urethral or suprapubic catheter and urology consultation is important in instances of urinary retention.[80] While only studied extensively for chronic prostatitis, alpha-adrenergic blockers may be beneficial to allow relaxation of bladder neck that facilitates better emptying of bladder and decreases intraprostatic reflux.[80,82]

REFERENCES

1. American College of Obstetricians and Gynecologists. ACOG Practice Bulletin No. 91: treatment of urinary tract infections in nonpregnant women. *Obstet Gynecol.* 2008;111(3):785-794. doi:10.1097/AOG.0b013e318169f6ef
2. Cooper KL, Badalato GM, Rutman MP. Infections of the urinary tract. In: Partin AW, Dmochowski RR, Kavoussi LR, Peters CA, eds. *Campbell-Walsh-Wein Urology.* 12th ed. Elsevier; 2020.
3. Payne CK, Potts JM. Urinary tract infection: beyond uncomplicated cystitis. In: Potts JM, ed. *Essential Urology: A Guide to Clinical Practice.* 2nd ed. Springer; 2012.
4. Foxman B, Barlow R, D'Arcy H, Gillespie B, Sobel JD. Urinary tract infection: self-reported incidence and associated costs. *Ann Epidemiol.* 2000;10(8):509-515. doi:10.1097/01.ju.0000155596.98780.82
5. Johnson JR, Russo TA. Acute pyelonephritis in adults [published correction appears in N Engl J Med. 2018 Mar 15;378(11):1069]. *N Engl J Med.* 2018;378(1):48-59. doi:10.1056/nejmcp1702758
6. Hanno PM. Lower urinary tract infections in women and pyelonephritis. In: Hanno PM, Guzzo TJ, Malkowicz SB, Wein AJ, eds. *Penn Clinical Manual of Urology.* 2nd ed. Saunders; 2014.

7. Nicolle LE, Gupta K, Bradley SF, et al. Clinical practice guideline for the management of asymptomatic bacteriuria: 2019 update by the Infectious Diseases Society of America. *Clin Infect Dis.* 2019;68(10):e83-e110. doi:10.1093/cid/ciy1121
8. Gupta K, Hooton TM, Naber KG. International clinical practice guidelines for the treatment of acute uncomplicated cystitis and pyelonephritis in women: a 2010 Update by the Infectious Diseases Society of America and the European Society for Microbiology and Infectious Diseases. *Clin Infect Dis.* 2011;52(5):e103-e120. doi:10.1093/cid/ciq257
9. Huang Y, Li JM, Lai ZH, Wu J, Lu TB, Chen KM. Phenazopyridine-phthalimide nano-cocrystal: release rate and oral bioavailability enhancement. *Eur J Pharm Sci.* 2017;109:581-586. doi:10.1016/j.ejps.2017.09.020
10. Gágyor I, Bleidorn J, Kochen MM, Schmiemann G, Wegscheider K, Hummers-Pradier E. Ibuprofen versus fosfomycin for uncomplicated urinary tract infection in women: randomised controlled trial. *BMJ.* 2015;351:h6544. doi:10.1136/bmj.h6544
11. Kronenberg A, Butikofer L, Odutayo A, et al. Symptomatic treatment of uncomplicated lower urinary tract infections in the ambulatory setting: randomised, double blind trial. *BMJ.* 2017;359:j4784. doi:10.1136/bmj.j4784
12. Vik I, Bollestad M, Grude N, et al. Ibuprofen versus pivmecillinam for uncomplicated urinary tract infection in women-A double-blind, randomized non-inferiority trial. *PLoS Med.* 2018;15(5):e1002569. doi:10.1371/journal.pmed.1002569
13. Anger J, Lee U, Ackerman AL, et al. Recurrent uncomplicated urinary tract infections in women: AUA/CUA/SUFU guideline. *J Urol.* 2019;202(2)282-289. doi:10.1097/JU.0000000000002963
14. Humphreys MR, Lieske JC. Evaluation and medical management of kidney stones. In: Potts JM, ed. *Genitourinary Pain and Inflammation: Diagnosis and Management.* Humana Press; 2016.
15. Miller NL, Borofsky MS. Evaluation and medical management of urinary lithiasis. In: Partin AW, Dmochowski RR, Kavoussi LR, Peters CA, eds. *Campbell-Walsh-Wein Urology.* 12th ed. Elsevier; 2020.
16. Scales CD Jr, Smith AC, Hanley JM, Saigal CS; Urologic Diseases in America Project. Prevalence of kidney stones in the United States. *Eur Urol.* 2012;62(1):160-165. doi:10.1016/j.eururo.2012.03.052
17. Johnson CM, Wilson DM, O'Fallon WM, Malek RS, Kurland LT. Renal stone epidemiology: a 25-year study in Rochester, Minnesota . *Kidney Int.* 1979;16(5):624-631. doi:10.1038/ki.1979.173
18. Romero V, Akpinar H, Assimos DG. Kidney stones: a global picture of prevalence, incidence, and associated risk factors. *Rev Urol.* 2010;12(2–3):e86-e96.
19. Palmieri M, Dave SK. Managing your pre-operative and post-operative pain. In: Schulsinger DA, ed. *Kidney Stone Disease: Say NO to Stones!* Springer International Publishing; 2016.
20. Stoller ML. Urinary stone disease. In: McAninch JW, Lue TF, eds. *Smith & Tanagho's General Urology.* 19th ed. McGraw-Hill; 2020. Accessed September 07, 2020. https://accessmedicine-mhmedical-com.ezp-prod1.hul.harvard.edu/content.aspx?bookid=2840&sectionid=241660803
21. Meissnitzer M, Meissnitzer T, Hruby S, et al. Comparison of prone vs. supine unenhanced CT imaging in patients with clinically suspected ureterolithiasis. *Abdom Radiol (NY).* 2017;42(2):569-576. doi:10.1007/s00261-016-0918-1
22. Brisbane W, Bailey MR, Sorensen MD. An overview of kidney stone imaging techniques. *Nat Rev Urol.* 2016;13(11):654-662. doi:10.1038/nrurol.2016.154
23. Ray AA, Ghiculete D, Pace KT, Honey RJ. Limitations to ultrasound in the detection and measurement of urinary tract calculi. *Urology.* 2010;76(2):295-300. doi:10.1016/j.urology.2009.12.015
24. Coursey CA, Casalino DD, Remer EM, et al. ACR Appropriateness Criteria® acute onset flank pain—suspicion of stone disease. *Ultrasound Q.* 2012;28(3):227-233. doi:10.1097/RUQ.0b013e3182625974
25. Fulgham PF, Assimos DG, Pearle MS, Preminger GM. Clinical effectiveness protocols for imaging in the management of ureteral calculous disease: AUA technology assessment. *J Urol.* 2013;189(4):1203-1213. doi:10.1016/j.juro.2012.10.031
26. Türk C, Petřík A, Sarica K, et al. EAU guidelines on interventional treatment for urolithiasis. *Eur Urol.* 2015;69:475-482.
27. Assimos D, Krambeck A, Miller NL, et al. Surgical management of stones: American Urological Association/Endourological Society Guideline, PART II. *J Urol.* 2016;196(4):1161-1169. doi:10.1016/j.juro.2016.05.091
28. Joshi HB, Okeke A, Newns N, Keeley FX Jr, Timoney AG. Characterization of urinary symptoms in patients with ureteral stents. *Urology.* 2002;59(4):511-516. doi:10.1016/s0090-4295(01)01644-2
29. Fischer KM, Louie M, Mucksavage P. Ureteral stent discomfort and its management. *Curr Urol Rep.* 2018;19(8):64. doi:10.1007/s11934-018-0818-8
30. Koprowski C, Kim C, Modi PK, Elsamra SE. Ureteral stent-associated pain: a review. *J Endourol.* 2016;30(7):744-753. doi:10.1089/end.2016.0129
31. Ragab M, Soliman MG, Tawfik A, et al. The role of pregabalin in relieving ureteral stent-related symptoms: a randomized controlled clinical trial. *Int Urol Nephrol.* 2017;49(6):961-966. doi:10.1007/s11255-017-1561-7
32. Montague DK, Jarow J, Broderick GA, et al. American Urological Association guideline on the management of priapism. *J Urol.* 2003 (reviewed 2010);170(4):1318-1324. doi:10.1097/01.ju.0000087608.07371.ca

33. Levey HR, Segal RL, Bivalacqua TJ. Management of priapism: an update for clinicians. *Ther Adv Urol.* 2014;6(6):230-244. doi:10.1177/1756287214542096
34. Eland IA, van der Lei J, Stricker BH, Sturkenboom MJ. Incidence of priapism in the general population. *Urology.* 2001;57(5):970-972. doi:10.1016/s0090-4295(01)00941-4
35. Roghmann F, Becker A, Sammon JD, et al. Incidence of priapism in emergency departments in the United States. *J Urol.* 2013;190(4):1275-1280. doi:10.1016/j.juro.2013.03.118
36. Earle CM, Stuckey BG, Ching HL, Wisniewski ZS. The incidence and management of priapism in Western Australia: a 16 year audit. *Int J Impot Res.* 2003;15(4):272-276. doi:10.1038/sj.ijir.3901018
37. Broderick GA, Kadioglu A, Bivalacqua TJ, Ghanem H, Nehra A, Shamloul R. Priapism: pathogenesis, epidemiology, and management. *J Sex Med.* 2010;7(1 Pt 2):476-500. doi:10.1111/j.1743-6109.2009.01625.x
38. Zacharakis E, Garaffa G, Raheem AA, Christopher AN, Muneer A, Ralph DJ. Penile prosthesis insertion in patients with refractory ischaemic priapism: early vs delayed implantation [published correction appears in BJU Int. 2016 Apr;117(4):E7]. *BJU Int.* 2014;114(4):576-581. doi:10.1111/bju.12686
39. Ralph DJ, Garaffa G, Muneer A, et al. The immediate insertion of a penile prosthesis for acute ischaemic priapism. *Eur Urol.* 2009;56(6):1033-1038. doi:10.1016/j.eururo.2008.09.044
40. Berger R, Billups K, Brock G, et al. Report of the American Foundation for Urologic Disease (AFUD) thought leader panel for evaluation and treatment of priapism. *Int J Impot Res.* 2001;13(suppl 5):S39-S43. doi:10.1038/sj.ijir.3900777
41. Szmuk P, Ezri T, Ben Hur H, Caspi B, Priscu L, Priscu V. Regional anaesthesia for circumcision in adults: a comparative study. *Can J Anaesth.* 1994;41(12):1181-1184. doi:10.1007/BF03020658
42. Flores S, Herring AA. Ultrasound-guided dorsal penile nerve block for ED paraphimosis reduction. *Am J Emerg Med.* 2015;33:863.e3-863.e865. doi:10.1016/j.ajem.2014.12.041
43. Rose G, Costa V, Drake A, Siadecki SD, Saul T. Ultrasound-guided dorsal penile nerve block performed in a case of zipper entrapment injury. *J Clin Ultrasound.* 2017;45(9):589-591. doi:10.1002/jcu.22459
44. Fahmy MA. Paraphimosis. In: Fahmy MA, ed. *Normal and Abnormal Prepuce.* Springer International Publishing; 2020.
45. Herzog LW, Alvarez SR. The frequency of foreskin problems in uncircumcised children. *Am J Dis Child.* 1986;140(3):254-256.
46. Bragg BN, Leslie SW. Paraphimosis. In: *StatPearls.* StatPearls Publishing; 2020.
47. Simonis K, Rink M. Paraphimosis. In: Merseburger A, Kuczyk M, Moul J, eds. *Urology at a Glance.* Springer; 2014.
48. Manjunath AS, Hofer MD. Urologic emergencies. *Med Clin North Am.* 2018;102(2):373-385. doi:10.1016/j.mcna.2017.10.013
49. Jadhav SE, Jadhav SS. Clinical study of proportion of predisposing events and causes of paraphimosis. *Indian J Appl Res.* 2013;3:373-374.
50. Jones SA, Flynn RJ. An unusual (and somewhat piercing) cause of paraphimosis. *Br J Urol.* 1996;78(5):803-804. doi:10.1046/j.1464-410x.1996.25435.x
51. Harvey K, Bishop L, Silver D, Jones T. A case of chancroid. *Med J Aust.* 1977;1(26):956-957.
52. Nadimi AE, Carver CM. Syphilis presenting with paraphimosis: painless no longer. *J Am Acad Dermatol.* 2016;74(5):AB154.
53. Mainetti C, Scolari F, Lautenschlager S. The clinical spectrum of syphilitic balanitis of Follmann: report of five cases and a review of the literature. *J Eur Acad Dermatol Venereol.* 2016;30(10):1810-1813. doi:10.1111/jdv.13802
54. Fariña LA, Alonso MV, Horjales M, Zungri ER. Balanopostitis alérgica de contacto y parafimosis por aplicación tópica de jugo de celidonia [Contact-derived allergic balanoposthitis and paraphimosis through topical application of celandine juice]. *Actas Urol Esp.* 1999;23(6):554-555.
55. Verma S. Coital penile trauma with severe paraphimosis. *J Eur Acad Dermatol Venereol.* 2005;19(1):134-135. doi:10.1111/j.1468-3083.2004.00955.x
56. Burstein B, Paquin R. Comparison of outcomes for pediatric paraphimosis reduction using topical anesthetic versus intravenous procedural sedation. *Am J Emerg Med.* 2017;35(10):1391-1395. doi:10.1016/j.ajem.2017.04.015
57. Morey AF, Brandes S, Dugi DD III, et al. Urotrauma: AUA guideline. *J Urol.* 2014 (amended 2017);192(2):327-335. doi:10.1016/j.juro.2014.05.004
58. Rodriguez D, Li K, Apoj M, Munarriz R. Epidemiology of penile fractures in United States Emergency Departments: access to care disparities may lead to suboptimal outcomes. *J Sex Med.* 2019;16(2):248-256. doi:10.1016/j.jsxm.2018.12.009
59. Morey AF, Simhan J. Genital and lower urinary tract trauma. In: Partin AW, Dmochowski RR, Kavoussi LR, Peters CA, eds. *Campbell-Walsh-Wein Urology.* 12th ed. Elsevier; 2020.
60. Zare Mehrjardi M, Darabi M, Bagheri SM, Kamali K, Bijan B. The role of ultrasound (US) and magnetic resonance imaging (MRI) in penile fracture mapping for modified surgical repair. *Int Urol Nephrol.* 2017;49(6):937-945. doi:10.1007/s11255-017-1550-x

61. Saglam E, Tarhan F, Hamarat MB, et al. Efficacy of magnetic resonance imaging for diagnosis of penile fracture: a controlled study. *Investig Clin Urol.* 2017;58(4):255-260. doi:10.4111/icu.2017.58.4.255
62. Metzler IS, Reed-Maldonado AB, Lue TF. Suspected penile fracture: to operate or not to operate? *Transl Androl Urol.* 2017;6(5):981-986. doi:10.21037/tau.2017.07.25
63. Bozzini G, Albersen M, Otero JR, et al. Delaying surgical treatment of penile fracture results in poor functional outcomes: results from a large retrospective multicenter European study. *Eur Urol Focus.* 2018;4(1):106-110. doi:10.1016/j.euf.2016.02.012
64. Naraynsingh V, Hariharan S, Goetz L, Dan D. Late delayed repair of fractured penis. *J Androl.* 2010;31(2):231-233. doi:10.2164/jandrol.109.008268
65. el-Assmy A, el-Tholoth HS, Mohsen T, Ibrahiem el-HI. Does timing of presentation of penile fracture affect outcome of surgical intervention? *Urology.* 2011;77(6):1388-1391. doi:10.1016/j.urology.2010.12.070
66. Nasser TA, Mostafa T. Delayed surgical repair of penile fracture under local anesthesia. *J Sex Med.* 2008;5(10):2464-2469. doi:10.1111/j.1743-6109.2008.00851.x
67. Zhao LC, Lautz TB, Meeks JJ, Maizels M. Pediatric testicular torsion epidemiology using a national database: incidence, risk of orchiectomy and possible measures toward improving the quality of care. *J Urol.* 2011;186(5):2009-2013. doi:10.1016/j.juro.2011.07.024
68. Ludvigson AE, Beaule LT. Urologic emergencies. *Surg Clin North Am.* 2016;96(3):407-424. doi:10.1016/j.suc.2016.02.001
69. Bourke MM, Silverberg JZ. Acute scrotal emergencies. *Emerg Med Clin North Am.* 2019;37:593-610.
70. Callewaert PR, Van Kerrebroeck P. New insights into perinatal testicular torsion. *Eur J Pediatr.* 2010;169(6):705-712. doi:10.1007/s00431-009-1096-8
71. Ross JH. Pediatric potpourri. In: Potts JM, ed. *Essential Urology: A Guide to Clinical Practice.* 2nd ed. Springer; 2012.
72. Kadish HA, Bolte RG. A retrospective review of pediatric patients with epididymitis, testicular torsion, and torsion of testicular appendages. *Pediatrics.* 1998;102(1 Pt 1):73-76. doi:10.1542/peds.102.1.73
73. Hills-Dunlap JL, Rangel SJ. Pediatric surgery. In: Doherty GM, ed. *Current Diagnosis & Treatment: Surgery.* 15th ed. McGraw-Hill; 2020. Accessed July 19, 2020.
74. Demirbas A, Demir DO, Ersoy E, et al. Should manual detorsion be a routine part of treatment in testicular torsion? *BMC Urol.* 2017;17(1):84. doi:10.1186/s12894-017-0276-5
75. Kiesling VJ, Schroeder DE, Pauljev P, et al. Spermatic cord block and manual reduction: primary treatment for spermatic cord torsion. *J Urol.* 1984;132(5):921-923. doi:10.1016/s0022-5347(17)49947-2
76. Kaye KW, Lange PH, Fraley EE. Spermatic cord block in urologic surgery. *J Urol.* 1982;128(4):720-721. doi:10.1016/s0022-5347(17)53154-7
77. Wipfli M, Birkhäuser F, Luyet C, Greif R, Thalmann G, Eichenberger U. Ultrasound-guided spermatic cord block for scrotal surgery. *Br J Anaesth.* 2011;106(2):255-259. doi:10.1093/bja/aeq301
78. Potts JM. Prostatitis and chronic pelvic pain syndrome. In: Potts JM, ed. *Essential Urology.* Springer; 2012.
79. Roberts RO, Lieber MM, Rhodes T, Girman CJ, Bostwick DG, Jacobsen SJ. Prevalence of a physician-assigned diagnosis of prostatitis: the Olmsted County Study of Urinary Symptoms and Health Status Among Men. *Urology.* 1998;51(4):578-584. doi:10.1016/s0090-4295(98)00034-x
80. Khan FU, Ihsan AU, Khan HU, et al. Comprehensive overview of prostatitis. *Biomed Pharmacother.* 2017;94:1064-1076. doi:10.1016/j.biopha.2017.08.016
81. Ackerman AL, Parameshwar PS, Anger JT. Diagnosis and treatment of patients with prostatic abscess in the post-antibiotic era. *Int J Urol.* 2018;25(2):103-110. doi:10.1111/iju.13451
82. Reddivari AKR, Mehta P. Prostate abscess. In: *StatPearls.* November 2019. Accessed September 1, 2020. https://www.statpearls.com/kb/viewarticle/27832
83. Ludwig M, Schroeder-Printzen I, Schiefer HG, Weidner W. Diagnosis and therapeutic management of 18 patients with prostatic abscess. *Urology.* 1999;53(2):340-345. doi:10.1016/s0090-4295(98)00503-2
84. Coker TJ, Dierfeldt DM. Acute bacterial prostatitis: diagnosis and management. *Am Fam Physician.* 2016;93(2):114-120.
85. Chou YH, Tiu CM, Liu JY, et al. Prostatic abscess: transrectal color Doppler ultrasonic diagnosis and minimally invasive therapeutic management. *Ultrasound Med Biol.* 2004;30(6):719-724. doi:10.1016/j.ultrasmedbio.2004.03.014
86. Lipsky BA, Byren I, Hoey CT. Treatment of bacterial prostatitis. *Clin Infect Dis.* 2010;50(12):1641-1652. doi:10.1086/652861

20

Acute Endocrine System–Related Pain

Erica Seligson, Matthew B. Allen, and Richard D. Urman

Introduction

Pain related to diseases of the endocrine system is diverse in its clinical manifestations, pathophysiology, and management. The following chapter describes evaluation and treatment of pain related to diabetes, hypoadrenalism, thyroiditis, and parathyroid dysfunction.

Pain Related to Diabetes

Diabetes affects 425 million people worldwide, a number expected to exceed 600 million by 2045.[1] Up to one-third of patients with diabetes will develop painful diabetic peripheral neuropathy (pDPN), making it the most common complication related to diabetes and the most common form of neuropathy.

Clinical Features

Painful diabetic neuropathy (pDPN) was initially described in 1885 as a "burning and unremitting quality, often with a nocturnal exacerbation."[2] Risk factors for neuropathy among diabetics include age, duration of disease, and poor glycemic control.[1] Patients typically describe a constellation of positive and negative sensory symptoms, including dysesthesias (ie, burning, shooting, or electric shock–like pain), paresthesias, and numbness. The symptoms typically present in a symmetric, "stocking and glove" distribution but can extend proximally with disease progression.[3] Common features on physical examination include impaired proprioception and sensation of light touch, temperature, vibration, and pinprick.[1] Ankle deep tendon reflexes are typically diminished or absent.[1]

The differential diagnosis for peripheral neuropathy includes a variety of systemic illnesses (eg, chronic kidney or liver disease, monoclonal gammopathies, inflammatory polyneuropathies, vasculitides), medication side effects, toxic exposures, hereditary disorders, and nutritional deficiencies. Clinical features suggesting a nondiabetic cause of neuropathy include focal or asymmetric symptoms, rapid onset, nonlength dependence, and predominance of motor weakness. Relevant laboratory studies include fasting blood glucose, complete blood count, comprehensive metabolic profile, erythrocyte sedimentation rate, vitamin B_{12}, and thyroid-stimulating hormone. Further diagnostic testing may include screening for markers of rheumatologic disease or paraneoplastic syndromes and electrodiagnostic testing.

Pathophysiology

The pathology of pDPN is characterized by a number of pathogenetic mechanisms, many of which are attributed to the harmful effects of hyperglycemia and resulting metabolic changes.

Yagihashi et al. described that long-term hyperglycemia causes a downstream metabolic cascade, consisting of polyol pathway hyperactivity, advanced glycation end products, and increased reactive oxygen species.[4] These products activate protein kinases, which compromise both endoneurial microvessels and neural tissues, ultimately resulting in functional and structural changes of peripheral neuropathy. Additionally, there are metabolic aberrations at the level of the nerve, which elicit inflammatory reactions via cytokine release and macrophage migration to support the development of neuropathy. Finally, the inflammation mediates both ischemia and reperfusion and accelerates the underlying nerve injury.[4]

The development of pDPN also appears to involve central sensitization and altered central pain processing. As the thalamus is integrally involved in the nociceptive pathway, it is plausible to suggest that alterations in this area may contribute to the pathogenesis of pDPN. Some evidence suggests an imbalance between excitatory and inhibitory neurotransmitters in the CNS of patients with pDPN; specifically, a higher glutamate/GABA ratio within the thalamus of these patients has been described.[5]

Management

While glycemic control is a cornerstone of diabetes management, its impact on the development of neuropathic pain is variable. The Diabetes Control and Complications Trial found tight glycemic control resulted in a 60% reduction in the rate of neuropathic pain in type 1 diabetics, but the same does not appear to be true for patients with type 2 diabetes.[6] There are currently no drugs recommended for prevention or reversal of pDPN. Management therefore centers on treatment of symptoms with the aim of improving functional status and quality of life.

Treatment guidelines recommend the following as first- or second-line agents: pregabalin, gabapentin, duloxetine, venlafaxine, and amitriptyline.[7] Only pregabalin, duloxetine, fluoxetine, and tapentadol are FDA approved for pDPN (Table 20.1). Choice of agent is driven

TABLE 20.1 FDA-APPROVED DRUGS FOR TREATMENT OF DIABETIC NEUROPATHY

Drug	Starting Dose	Maximum Dose	Common Side Effects	Favorable Comorbidities (Based on Side Effect Profile/ Mechanism of Action)	Unfavorable Comorbidities (Based on Side Effect Profile/ Mechanism of Action)
Gabapentin	100-300 mg tid	1200 mg tid	Dizziness, fatigue, drowsiness, and ataxia	Insomnia, essential tremor, restless legs syndrome	Substance use disorder
Pregabalin	75 mg bid	150 mg bid			
Duloxetine	20-30 mg bid	120 mg qd	Nausea, dry mouth, somnolence, fatigue	Depression, anxiety	Patients at risk of serotonin syndrome (eg, those on other serotonergic drugs)
Amitriptyline	25 mg qhs	150 mg qd (either 150 mg qd or 75 mg qhs)	Drowsiness, dry mouth, constipation, difficulty urinating, dizziness, sexual dysfunction, and headache		Prolonged QT interval, cardiac arrhythmia

by patient-specific consideration of side effect profile and comorbid conditions. For further information on use of antidepressants and gabapentinoids for pain, see Chapter 36.

Gabapentin and pregabalin are γ-aminobutyric (GABA) mimetics that cause analgesia via high affinity binding and modulation of calcium channel α2-δ proteins in the dorsal root ganglion.[8] Modulation of these channels reduces the number of synaptic vesicles that fuse within the presynaptic membrane, thus limiting the release of neurotransmitters (GABA, glutamate, noradrenaline, substance P, and calcitonin gene–related peptide) into the synapse. Gabapentin has also been shown to inhibit ectopic discharge activity from injured peripheral nerves. Finally, there is some evidence to support its antiallodynic effects due to either enhanced inhibitory input of GABA-mediated pathways and antagonism of both NMDA receptors and calcium channels in the CNS.[9]

A systematic review and meta-analysis of trials of gabapentin for pDPN demonstrated an NNT for benefit (NNTB) of 5.9 to reduce pain intensity by at least 50% at gabapentin doses of 1200 mg or more.[1] Furthermore, a double-blind, placebo-controlled multicentre study of 165 patients with pDPN reported a statistically significant reduction in mean daily pain score in the gabapentin group, with an NNT being 3.8.[9] Because of nonlinear pharmacokinetics, gabapentin is typically started at lower doses (eg, 100-300 mg three times daily) and gradually up-titrated to effect.[10] Maximum dose is 1200 mg three times daily.

The evidence for pregabalin is equally strong. A systematic review and meta-analysis demonstrated an NNT of 7.8 to reduce pain by at least 50% using a pregabalin dose of 600 mg daily.[11] Pregabalin is more potent than gabapentin, is typically started at a dose of 75 mg twice daily, and increased as necessary to a maximum daily dose of 300 mg (although the maximum dose is 600 mg in Europe and pregabalin doses up to 600 mg per day are approved for other indications). Both gabapentin and pregabalin are renally excreted and require dose adjustment in patients with impaired renal function.

Nearly two-thirds of patients taking gabapentinoids for neuropathic pain report a side effect, the most common being dizziness, fatigue, drowsiness, and ataxia.[11] Although drug interactions are thought to be uncommon due to lack of protein binding and metabolism, coadministration of gabapentin and pregabalin with opioids and benzodiazepines does increase the risk of overdose and death. Concerns about recreational use of gabapentinoids has led to prescribing restrictions and further underlines the need for caution when prescribing these drugs in patients with substance use disorders.[1] Gabapentin and pregabalin's side effect profile makes them rational options for patients with insomnia, essential tremor, or restless legs syndrome. Acute discontinuation of gabapentinoids can result in withdrawal symptoms including anxiety, insomnia, and headaches, so tapering prior to discontinuation is recommended.[1]

Mirogabalin is an emerging α2-δ subunit ligand for the treatment of neuropathic pain, which has shown excellent analgesic effects and safety profiling in recent randomized controlled trials. Unlike gabapentin and pregabalin, which are nonselective ligands for the α2-δ-1 and α2-δ-2, mirogabalin is more selective for the α2-δ-1 subunit and may be a promising option for neuropathic pain in the future.[1]

Serotonin and norepinephrine reuptake inhibitors

Duloxetine inhibits serotonin and norepinephrine reuptake, which enhances the descending inhibition of pain associated with pDPN. Several placebo-controlled randomized controlled trials have found duloxetine to be superior to placebo for pDPN at doses of 60 and 120 mg.[12] The data comparing duloxetine to other agents are mixed. Two RCTs and a pooled analysis showed it to be superior to pregabalin 300 mg,[13-15] while others found it to have similar or inferior efficacy to the gabapentinoids. The NNTB of duloxetine 60 mg daily for 50% reduction in pain is 5.0.

Venlafaxine is another SNRI commonly used in the treatment of pDPN and has shown to be superior to placebo at doses of 150/225 mg; however, the studies are small and limited, with some reported cases of atrial fibrillation, nausea, headache, and insomnia.[16] Overall,

SNRIs are well-tolerated. Their mechanism of action and clinical effect make them rational choices for patients with comorbid depression and/or anxiety. Importantly, coadministration of SNRIs with serotonergic drugs, particularly tramadol or monoamine oxidase inhibitors, increases the risk of serotonin syndrome and should be avoided.[17] Unlike duloxetine, venlafaxine does not have FDA approval for treating pDPN.

Amitriptyline

Among the tricyclic antidepressants (TCAs), amitriptyline is most commonly used for the treatment of neuropathic pain and pDPN. The exact analgesic mechanism of these agents is poorly understood but involves inhibition of noradrenaline and serotonin reuptake from the synaptic cleft, anticholinergic inhibition, indirect dopaminergic action, and sodium channel blockade.[18-20]

Although amitriptyline has been used as a first-line agent for neuropathic pain for decades, reliable data to support its use are limited. One systematic review found amitriptyline to be more effective than placebo in pDPN, though other network meta-analyses have found amitriptyline to have the second lowest efficacy (above placebo only) with the lowest safety profile and lowest benefit-risk balance.[21] The Cochrane Collaboration review concluded that there is a lack of supportive unbiased evidence for a beneficial effect.[11]

The dose for neuropathic pain is 10-25 mg, with up-titration over a period of weeks to a maximum dose of 75 mg daily. TCAs are well-absorbed orally, and their lipophilicity allows them to be widely distributed and penetrable into the central nervous system.[7] However, given their first-pass metabolism in the liver, they have inconsistent bioavailability and require 6-8 weeks of up-titration to achieve effective analgesia. Side effects largely stem from anticholinergic action and include drowsiness, dry mouth, constipation, difficulty urinating, dizziness, sexual dysfunction, and headache. Amitriptyline is arrhythmogenic and should be avoided in patients with prolonged QT interval and other cardiac comorbidities.

Opioids

Tapentadol ER, which is a relatively new, centrally acting μ-opioid receptor agonist, is the fourth and final drug approved by the FDA for use in neuropathic pain at a range of 50-700 mg daily. This drug inhibits norepinephrine and serotonin reuptake and has a strong affinity at the μ receptor, the latter of which interrupts synaptic transmission of ascending pain signals at the level of the spinal cord and activates descending inhibition. Three large RCTs have demonstrated effective analgesia in patients with pDPN taking tapentadol compared with placebo.[22-24] Tapentadol's lower potential for misuse compared to traditional opioids makes this drug a favorable choice in adult patients with pDPN.

Tramadol is another centrally acting synthetic opioid but has weaker affinity at the μ-opioid receptor when compared with tapentadol. Overall, evidence to support tramadol's efficacy in relieving pDPN is limited. Early studies of the drug were promising; however, a Cochrane Collaboration review found the evidence of quality to be low for its analgesic benefit in these patients; furthermore, the incidence of adverse events including serotonin syndrome, confusion, dizziness, and seizures is not insignificant. Despite these shortcomings, tramadol at doses of 200-400 mg daily is often used as a second- or third-line therapy or for breakthrough pain, in those patients who did not respond to or experienced symptoms from first-line therapies.

The use of traditional opioid agonists is discouraged as first-line treatment for diabetic neuropathic pain. Despite these recommendations, use of opioids in pDPN management often precedes that of other drugs. Oxycodone, morphine, and methadone are the strongest opioids used in the treatment of diabetic neuropathic pain,[25] with some studies demonstrating significant analgesia compared with placebo.[26] However, the aforementioned studies were of short duration and did not evaluate the risk of opioid use disorder in patients with DPN. One Cochrane Collaboration review looked at the use of ten different opioids in patients with neuropathic pain and determined an improvement in mean pain scores of 1.5 points (out of 10) compared with placebo.[27] As is widely recognized, these agents carry an increased risk of overdose events, development of opioid use disorder, and drug diversion. Their long-term use is associated with systemic complications including fractures, myocardial infarctions, and endocrinological dysfunction.[28]

A number of additional therapies have been trialed in patients with neuropathic pain, though there is limited evidence to support their use. Sodium valproate, carbamazepine, oxcarbazepine, topiramate, lacosamide, phenytoin, levetiracetam, and zonisamide have all been examined in these patients without meaningful, reproducible success. A Cochrane overview of antiepileptic drugs for neuropathic pain reported no or insufficient evidence of efficacy. More recently, there is emerging evidence that some neurosurgical treatments, for example, invasive neuromodulation, may be effective for patients with medication refractory PDN. One systematic review and meta-analysis of the existing evidence provided by two RCTs supports the use of tonic spinal cord stimulation (t-SCS) in the treatment of medication refractory severe PDN. This therapy involves regular electrical pulses (~50 Hz) delivered to the dorsal columns, evoking paresthesias in the area of pain and operating through a gate control mechanism to compete out other pain signals.

Overall, pDPN continues to represent a therapeutic challenge, as its pathogenesis is incompletely understood. The pharmacological treatments are largely symptomatic[5]; all current guidelines support a personalized approach with a minimum start, which is tailored to the maximum response with the least side effects.

Pain Related to Disorders of the Thyroid

There is a small population of patients who suffer from painful thyroid diseases. Among them, subacute thyroiditis (SAT) and painful Hashimoto thyroiditis (pHT) are the two most common.

Clinical Features of Subacute Thyroiditis

Subacute thyroiditis (SAT; also called de Quervain thyroiditis) is a self-limited viral inflammatory disorder, most commonly seen in females between the ages of 40-50 years, with an incidence of 12.1 cases per 100 000/year.[29] SAT follows an unpredictable clinical course; however, the natural history usually involves three-to-four phases over the course of several months. In the acute phase, patients present with acute onset of unilateral or bilateral thyroid pain, radiating to the jaw or ears and exacerbated by coughing or head movements. Physical examination reveals an enlarged and exquisitely tender thyroid gland. Fever and symptoms associated with thyrotoxicosis including palpitations, sweating, and weight loss are common, as is a preceding upper respiratory tract infection. Thyroid hormones spill into the circulation due to acute inflammation and are responsible for a transient hyperthyroidism (high serum free T4 and T3, low serum TSH). Transient asymptomatic euthyroidism follows, and a short phase of subclinical hypothyroidism evolves in most patients (normal free T4 and T3, high TSH).[30] Approximately 15% of patients develop permanent hypothyroidism requiring thyroid replacement therapy.[29] While the clinical features of SAT are sufficient to establish the diagnosis, additional laboratory findings include an elevation of nonspecific inflammatory markers (ESR and CRP), elevated transaminases and leukocytosis.

Management of Subacute Thyroiditis

Treatment recommendations focus on relieving both thyroid pain and symptoms of hyperthyroidism if present. Symptomatic relief for mild-moderate pain is typically achieved with a short course of NSAIDs or aspirin. However, for patients with severe neck pain or systemic symptoms, glucocorticoids are recommended, which may also shorten disease duration.[30] Typically, a 2- to 8-week course of oral prednisone provides adequate relief, with the goal being to find the lowest possible dose that provides relief and reducing the dose by 5 to 10 mg every week.

Clinical Features of Painful Hashimoto Thyroiditis

Classically, SAT arises in the absence of a previously known underlying thyroid disease.[31] This is a distinct entity from pHT, which is a rare variant and acute exacerbation of Hashimoto thyroiditis. In fact, a literature review of all case reports of pHT from 1957 to 2019 identified only 70 patients, predominantly young adult women, the majority of whom have a known history of thyroid disease as evidenced by the presence of antithyroid antibodies. The presentation is usually fever with insidious, progressive pain, or acute intolerable thyroid pain in the absence of a preceding viral illness. Many of these patients are initially misdiagnosed with SAT but are re-evaluated given poor response to medical treatment with NSAIDs, glucocorticoids, or levothyroxine.[32]

Management of Painful Hashimoto Thyroiditis

Total thyroidectomy is the gold standard for the treatment of pHT and is the only intervention demonstrative of long-term relief based on case reports and case series.[31]

Pathophysiology

In SAT, neck pain is thought to be a result of thyroid inflammation, either from a viral infection or a post viral inflammatory process, ultimately damaging thyroid follicles and activating proteolysis of thyroglobulin stored within the follicles. This process also accounts for the transient biochemical hyperthyroidism. The pathophysiology of thyroid-related pain in pHT, however, remains unknown. One popular hypothesis attributes the pain to capsular stretching due to rapid thyroid enlargement; however, many patients experience pain even if the size of the thyroid gland remains the same or becomes atrophic.[31]

Finally, there are other more causes of neck pain, both of thyroidal and nonthyroidal origin that must be excluded. A differential diagnosis of thyroid-related neck pain includes acute infectious (suppurative) thyroiditis, Riedel thyroiditis, primary thyroid lymphoma, and hemorrhage into a thyroid nodule. Nonthyroidal causes of painful neck include gastroesophageal reflux or spasm, neck muscle contractures, dental pain, and referred pain from angina.

Pain Related to Disorders of the Parathyroid

The classical signs and symptoms of primary hyperparathyroidism (PHPT) reflect the combined effects of increased PTH secretion and hypercalcemia, known as "bones, stones, abdominal groans, and psychiatric overtones."

Clinical Features

In the United States, PHPT has a prevalence of 0.86%, with the majority of cases affecting women ages 50-60 years old.[33] Most cases of PHPT (90%) occur from a sporadic and benign adenoma that produces PTH, while 10% are familial forms (multiple adenoma or hyperplasia) and 1% from parathyroid carcinoma.[33]

The most common presenting symptom is isolated bony pain, though PHPT can also cause pain related to pathological fractures, skeletal deformities, and generalized muscle weakness. This symptomatology is due to the catabolic action of PTH resulting in reduced bone mineral density, typically in the distal radius and hip, and in more severe cases, the lumbar spine.[33] Painful rheumatologic manifestations are also described in patients with PHPT; the presence of arthralgias and myalgias predominantly affecting the proximal shoulder and pelvic muscles often mimics polymyalgia rheumatica, whereas widespread pain and fatigue can lead to a misdiagnosis of fibromyalgia.[34] In addition to musculoskeletal complaints, patients may suffer severe abdominal pain, pancreatitis, and peptic ulcer disease, as elevated serum calcium levels can lead to a reduction in neuromuscular excitability and hypergastrinemia.[33] Finally, painful nephrolithiasis is a well-described manifestation of the hypercalciuria of PTPH, with ~2%-8% of patients with kidney stones carrying an underlying diagnosis of PHPT.

While elevated levels of calcium and parathyroid hormone typically confirm the diagnosis, additional laboratory testing with focus on intact PTH, 24-hour urinary calcium, and serum 25-hydroxyvitamin D should be undertaken to distinguish PHPT from other disease processes that may present with bodily pain in conjunction with hypercalcemia. A differential diagnosis includes occult malignancy, both humoral hypercalcemia of malignancy via PTH-related protein, as well as malignancy via direct bone destruction, familial hypocalciuric hypercalcemia, secondary hyperparathyroidism, and granulomatous diseases.

Pathophysiology

Plasma total calcium levels are finely regulated by PTH, with strict control being necessary to ensure proper functioning of cellular signaling, muscle contraction, and bone remodeling. The parathyroid glands respond to calcium variations through calcium-sensitive receptors on the main cells; in PHPT, there is abnormal parathyroid activity with its cells losing sensitivity to calcium concentration, overproducing PTH, ultimately resulting in hypercalcemia.[33] While in 80%-90% of cases the diagnosis is made in the context of *asymptomatic* hypercalcemia, the remainder of patients experience a constellation of painful symptoms related to the effects of hypercalcemia.

Management

Parathyroid surgery is recommended to all patients with classical symptoms or complications of PHPT. In these patients, surgical intervention is curative, improving bone mineral density, thereby decreasing fracture risk, reducing the risk of nephrolithiasis, and improving important quality of life measurements including bodily pain.[35]

Pain Related to Disorders of the Adrenal Gland

The painful manifestations of adrenal insufficiency are less well described in the literature compared with those of diabetes mellitus and thyroid disease. As the clinical features of hypoadrenalism can be quite subtle, there is often a delay in arriving at the correct diagnosis. Furthermore, the lack of research-based classification of its painful features makes studying this syndrome at an epidemiologic level rather challenging.

Clinical Features

Pain has been described in cases of both adrenal crisis (also called acute adrenal insufficiency or addisonian crisis) and in milder, chronic hypoadrenal states. Adrenal crisis is a life-threatening condition, defined as an acute deterioration in health status associated with hypotension and features that resolve within 1-2 hours after glucocorticoid administration.[36] The disease carries a mortality rate of 0.5/100 patients per year and arises from an absolute or relative deficiency of cortisol, ultimately leading to insufficient tissue glucocorticoid activity to maintain homeostasis.[36] In addition to shock, approximately one-third patients experience gastrointestinal distress, including abdominal tenderness and guarding, nausea, and vomiting. Diffuse myalgias, musculoskeletal, and lower back pain have also been described. In cases of adrenal necrosis (caused by hemorrhage, emboli, or sepsis), abdominal, flank, and back pain occur in up to 85% of patients.[37]

While an adrenal crisis is the most severe manifestation of adrenal insufficiency, chronic hypoadrenalism can also be painful. Although not often recognized, up to 13% of patients with chronic adrenal insufficiency report musculoskeletal symptoms including myalgias, arthralgias, stiffness, muscle cramps, and lower back pain.[38] A number of review articles have described cases of hypoadrenalism in which musculoskeletal symptoms were the prominent clinical feature. In 2008, Sathi et al. outlined three cases of adrenal insufficiency, the first in a patient with chronic knee arthralgias; further investigation of malaise, weight loss, and chronic hypotension ultimately led to the correct diagnosis of adrenal insufficiency, and symptoms resolved with hydrocortisone.[39] Others had a constellation of chronic, diffuse total-body myalgias, often associated with physical examination deformities such as flexion contractures. Similarly, once the diagnosis of hypoadrenalism was made, cortisol replacement therapy with either hydrocortisone or fludrocortisone led to symptom resolution. Importantly, in these cases, delay in arriving at the correct diagnosis was spent ruling out other causes such as systemic lupus erythematosus, rheumatoid arthritis, polymyalgia rheumatica, and fibromyalgia.[39] Finally, one study identified 10 patients with idiopathic primary hypoadrenalism who experienced chest and abdominal pain as their presenting symptom, ultimately found to be related to hypoadrenal serositis.[40]

As acute adrenal insufficiency is rarely an independent process, the differential diagnosis can be quite broad depending on the underlying etiology. In patients with altered mental status, gastrointestinal distress, pyrexia, and hypotension, adrenal crisis should be considered. Notably, abdominal distress can be such a predominating symptom of an adrenal crisis that it leads to an erroneous diagnosis of gastroenteritis. Features supporting chronic hypoadrenalism include chronic fatigue, muscle weakness, abdominal pain, hypotension, weight loss, headache, and skin changes. As described, it is often difficult to make a definitive diagnosis of chronic hypoadrenalism given the subtlety of symptoms; a broader differential includes amyotrophic lateral sclerosis, myasthenia gravis, polymyositis, sarcoid myopathy, temporal arteritis, and osteomalacia. Concomitant features to aid in the diagnosis include characteristic electrolyte perturbations such as hyponatremia, hyperkalemia, and hypoglycemia. Additional laboratory abnormalities include eosinophilia, normochromic normocytic anemia, hypercalcemia, and low or normal aldosterone.[39] Investigation to determine the precipitating cause of an adrenal crisis is important, whether that is sepsis, infection, trauma, physical or emotional stress, myocardial infarction, or nonadherence to glucocorticoid replacement therapy. In a patient with no known adrenal pathology who presents with hypotension refractory to fluids, vasopressors, and appropriate management otherwise, adrenal crisis should be at the top of the differential.

Pathophysiology

The pathophysiology of hypoadrenal pain itself is poorly understood but ultimately depends on the underlying etiology. Generally speaking, cortisol deficiency results in a loss of the normal suppressive action of endogenous glucocorticoids on inflammatory cytokines. The subsequent rapid increase in cytokine levels can precipitate malaise and diffuse pain.[36] Others have posited that the painful musculoskeletal manifestations may be due to a corticosteroid deficiency–induced skeletal muscle wasting, as some patients treated with corticosteroids demonstrate increased muscle fiber proportion and diameter.[38] Finally, cortisol may influence pain processing through corticosteroid receptors in the spinal cord dorsal horn, which plays a critical role in the mediation of nociceptive pain transmission.[41]

Management

Once a diagnosis of adrenal crisis is made, intravenous hydrocortisone 100 mg should be administered, followed by 200 mg every 24 hours as a continuous infusion or in 50 mg boluses every 6 hours, with subsequent doses tailored to the clinical response.[36] Hydrocortisone is preferred given its physiological glucocorticoid pharmacokinetics, plasma protein binding, tissue distribution ,and balanced glucocorticoid-mineralocorticoid effects. During an adrenal crisis, crystalloid fluid should be given according to standard resuscitation protocols with adjustment for the patient's relevant comorbidities. Concomitant diagnosis and management of the precipitating illness is required. After management of adrenal crisis, hydrocortisone doses should be tapered over a period of 3 days to the patient's maintenance dose, while assessment of preventable precipitating events and prevention strategies are undertaken.

Conclusion

Endocrine disorders can be manifested by various painful symptoms. Early diagnosis and treatment of hormonal imbalance is critical to relieve painful symptoms.

REFERENCES

1. Alam U, Sloan G, Tesfaye S. Treating pain in diabetic neuropathy: current and developmental drugs. *Drugs*. 2020;80(4):363-384.
2. Pavy FW. Introductory address to the discussion on the clinical aspect of glycosuria. *Lancet*. 1885;126(3250):1085-1087.
3. Raghu ALB, Parker T, Aziz TZ, et al. invasive electrical neuromodulation for the treatment of painful diabetic neuropathy: systematic review and meta-analysis. *Neuromodulation*. 2021;24(1):13-21. 10.1111/ner.13216.
4. Yagihashi S, Mizukami H, Sugimoto K. Mechanism of diabetic neuropathy: where are we now and where to go? *J Diabetes Investig*. 2011;2:18-32.
5. Schreiber AK, Nones CFM, Reis RC, Chichorro JG, Cunha JM. Diabetic neuropathic pain: physiopathology and treatment. *World J Diabetes*. 2015;6(3):432-444.
6. Albers JW, Herman WH, Pop-Busui R, et al. Effect of prior intensive insulin treatment during the Diabetes Control and Complications Trial (DCCT) on peripheral neuropathy in type 1 diabetes during the Epidemiology of Diabetes Interventions and Complications (EDIC) Study. *Diabetes Care*. 2010;33(5):1090-1096.
7. Khdour MR. Treatment of diabetic peripheral neuropathy: a review. *J Pharm Pharmacol*. 2020;72(7):863-872.
8. Taylor CP. Mechanisms of analgesia by gabapentin and pregabalin–calcium channel alpha2-delta [Cavalpha2-delta] ligands. *Pain*. 2009;142(1-2):13-16.
9. Rose MA, Kam PC. Gabapentin: pharmacology and its use in pain management. *Anaesthesia*. 2002;57: 451-462.
10. Bockbrader HN, Wesche D, Miller R, Chapel S, Janiczek N, Burger P. A comparison of the pharmacokinetics and pharmacodynamics of pregabalin and gabapentin. *Clin Pharmacokinet*. 2010;49(10):661-669.
11. Derry S, Bell RF, Straube S, Wiffen PJ, Aldington D, Moore RA. Pregabalin for neuropathic pain in adults. *Cochrane Database Syst Rev*. 2019;(1):CD007076.
12. Raskin J, Pritchett YL, Wang F, et al. A double-blind, randomized multicenter trial comparing duloxetine with placebo in the management of diabetic peripheral neuropathic pain. *Pain Med*. 2005;6(5):346-356.
13. Tesfaye S, Wilhelm S, Lledo A, et al. Duloxetine and pregabalin: high-dose monotherapy or their combination? The "COMBO-DN study"—a multinational, randomized, double-blind, parallel-group study in patients with diabetic peripheral neuropathic pain. *Pain*. 2013;154(12):2616-2625.
14. Tanenberg RJ, Clemow DB, Giaconia JM, Risser RC. Duloxetine compared with pregabalin for diabetic peripheral neuropathic pain management in patients with suboptimal pain response to gabapentin and treated with or without antidepressants: a post hoc analysis. *Pain Pract*. 2014;14(7):640-648.
15. Griebeler ML, Morey-Vargas OL, Brito JP, et al. Pharmacologic interventions for painful diabetic neuropathy: an umbrella systematic review and comparative effectiveness network meta-analysis. *Ann Intern Med*. 2014;161(9):639-649.
16. NICE. *Neuropathic pain in adults: pharmacological management in non-specialist settings* [CG173]. 2013. https://www.nice.org.uk/guidance/cg173.
17. Knadler MP, Lobo E, Chappell J, Bergstrom R. Duloxetine: clinical pharmacokinetics and drug interactions. *Clin Pharmacokinet*. 2011;50(5):281-294.

18. Lawson K. A brief review of the pharmacology of amitriptyline and clinical outcomes in treating fibromyalgia. *Biomedicines*. 2017;5(2):24.
19. Chong MS, Hester J. Diabetic painful neuropathy: current and future treatment options. *Drugs*. 2007;67(4):569-585.
20. Sindrup SH, Otto M, Finnerup NB, Jensen TS. Antidepressants in the treatment of neuropathic pain. *Basic Clin Pharmacol Toxicol*. 2005;96(6):399-409.
21. Rudroju N, Bansal D, Talakokkula ST, et al. Comparative efficacy and safety of six antidepressants and anticonvulsants in painful diabetic neuropathy: a network meta-analysis. *Pain Phys*. 2013;16(6):E705-E714.
22. Vinik AI, Shapiro DY, Rauschkolb C, et al. A randomized withdrawal, placebo-controlled study evaluating the efficacy and tolerability of tapentadol extended release in patients with chronic painful diabetic peripheral neuropathy. *Diabetes Care*. 2014;37(8):2302-2309.
23. Niesters M, Proto PL, Aarts L, Sarton EY, Drewes AM, Dahan A. Tapentadol potentiates descending pain inhibition in chronic pain patients with diabetic polyneuropathy. *Br J Anaesth*. 2014;113(1):148-156.
24. Vadivelu N, Kai A, Maslin B, Kodumudi G, Legler A, Berger JM. Tapentadol extended release in the management of peripheral diabetic neuropathic pain. *Ther Clin Risk Manag*. 2015;11:95-105.
25. Chou R, Fanciullo GJ, Fine PG, et al.; American Pain Society–American Academy of Pain Medicine Opioids Guidelines Panel. Clinical guidelines for the use of chronic opioid therapy in chronic noncancer pain. *J Pain*. 2009;10(2):113-130.
26. Finnerup NB, Attal N, Haroutounian S, et al. Pharmacotherapy for neuropathic pain in adults: a systematic review and meta-analysis. *Lancet Neurol*. 2015;14(2):162-173.
27. McNicol ED, Midbari A, Eisenberg E. Opioids for neuropathic pain. Cochrane *Database Syst Rev*. 2013;(8):CD006146.
28. Paone D, Dowell D, Heller D. Preventing misuse of prescription opioid drugs. *City Health Information*. 2011;30:23-30.
29. Fatourechi V, Aniszewski JP, Fatourechi GZ, Atkinson EJ, Jacobsen SJ. Clinical features and outcome of subacute thyroiditis in an incidence cohort: Olmsted County, Minnesota, study. *J Clin Endocrinol Metab*. 2003;88:2100-2105.
30. Benbassat CA, Olchovsky D, Tsvetov G, Shimon I. Subacute thyroiditis: clinical characteristics and treatment outcome in fifty-six consecutive patients diagnosed between 1999 and 2005. *J Endocrinol Invest*. 2007;30:631-635.
31. Rotondi M, Capelli V, Locantore P, Pontecorvi A, Chiovato L. Painful Hashimoto's thyroiditis: myth or reality? *J Endocrinol Invest*. 2017;40(8):815-818.
32. Peng CC, Huai-En Chang R, Pennant M, Huang HK, Munir KM. A literature review of painful Hashimoto thyroiditis: 70 published cases in the past 70 years. *J Endocr Soc*. 2019;4(2):bvz008.
33. Oberger Marques JV, Moreira CA. Primary hyperparathyroidism. *Best Pract Res Clin Rheumatol*. 2020;34(3):101514. https://doi.org/10.1016/j.berh.2020.101514
34. Borgia AR, et al. Hiperparatiroidismo, una causa olvidada de dolor músculo-esquelético difuso. *Reumatol Clin*. 2012. http://dx.doi.org/10.1016/j.reuma.2012.02.008
35. Ambrogini E, Cetani F, Cianferotti L, et al. Surgery or surveillance for mild asymptomatic primary hyperparathyroidism: a prospective, randomized clinical trial. *J Clin Endocrinol Metab*. 2007;92(8):3114e21.
36. Rushworth RL, Torpy DJ, Falhammar H. Adrenal crisis. *N Engl J Med*. 2019;381(9):852-861.
37. Rao RH, Vagnucci AH, Amico JA. Bilateral massive adrenal hemorrhage: early recognition and treatment. *Ann Intern Med* 1989;110:227.
38. Hoshino C, Satoh N, Narita M, Kikuchi A, Inoue M. Painful hypoadrenalism. *BMJ Case Rep*. 2011;2011: bcr0120113735.
39. Sathi N, Makkuni D, Mitchell WS, Swinson D, Chattopadhyay C. Musculoskeletal aspects of hypoadrenalism: just a load of aches and pains?. *Clin Rheumatol*. 2009;28(6):631-638.
40. Tucker WS Jr, Niblack GD, McLean RH, et al. Serositis with autoimmune endocrinopathy: clinical and immunogenetic features. *Medicine (Baltimore)*. 1987;66:138.
41. Pinto-Ribeiro F, Moreira V, Pêgo JM, et al. Antinociception induced by chronic glucocorticoid treatment is correlated to local modulation of spinal neurotransmitter content. *Mol Pain*. 2009;5:41.

21

Acute Ear, Nose, and Throat Pain

Lauren K. Eng, Matthew R. Eng, Sahar Shekoohi, Elyse M. Cornett, and Alan David Kaye

Ear Pain

Ear Anatomy

Inflammation or irritation of the cranial nerves V (trigeminal nerve), VII (facial nerve), IX (glossopharyngeal nerve), X (vagus nerve), or cervical nerves C1 through C3 may result in ear pain, otherwise known as otalgia.[1] Otalgia can be classified as either primary otalgia or secondary otalgia. Primary otalgia is ear pain that results from the ear itself, and secondary otalgia is ear pain that results from another primary source[2] (Table 21.1). The ear anatomy includes the auricle, the external auditory meatus and canal, the tympanic membrane, and the middle ear.

Primary Otalgia

In children, primary otalgia is typically the presenting symptom for otitis media or otitis externa.[2-4] Not often present in adults, this diagnosis is found in higher prevalence among children. Otitis media and otitis externa are inflammatory conditions and can be acute or chronic. Acute otitis media presents with a recent history of upper respiratory illness and an inflamed tympanic membrane. Acute otitis media is the most common cause of primary otalgia in children. Otitis externa usually presents with a recent history of water exposure (ie, swimming) with drainage or discharge present from the auditory canal. Primary otalgia can also result following surgery, from trauma, skin pathology or irritation, viral infection, or sunburn.

Secondary Otalgia

Secondary otalgia is more common in adults and is referred ear pain as a result of another underlying pathology.[5] Secondary otalgia may result from temporomandibular jaw (TMJ) syndrome, pharyngitis, tonsillitis, dental causes, cervical spine arthritis, or malignancy involving the head, neck, or chest. TMJ syndrome causes otalgia during chewing or talking and is accompanied by crepitus or tenderness at the joint of the TMJ. Infections to the sinuses, pharynx, and tonsils may also result in secondary otalgia. Similarly, dental infections may also cause secondary otalgia, especially when molars are involved. Investigation of secondary otalgia should include a thorough history as well as examination of the face, mouth, dentition, neck, and pharynx. Special consideration should be taken to rule out malignancy in high-risk patients. For example, malignancy of the chest can cause referred otalgia via the vagus nerve (CN X). Other sources such as gastroesophageal reflux, myofascial pain, salivary gland disorders, sinusitis, myocardial infarction, temporal arteritis, or thoracic aneurysms are atypical possible causes of otalgia.

TABLE 21.1 CLASSIFICATIONS OF OTALGIA

Primary otalgia	Otitis media
	Otitis externa
Secondary otalgia	TMJ syndrome
	Pharyngitis
	Tonsillitis
	Dental etiologies
	Cervical spine arthritis
	Head/neck/chest malignancies
Neuralgias	Trigeminal
	Sphenopalatine
Postsurgical otalgia	Myringotomy
	Mastoidectomy
	Tympanoplasty

Neuralgia

Inflammation of cranial nerves V, VII, and IX is commonly implicated in otalgia.[5] Most common neuralgias are trigeminal and sphenopalatine. Pain can be elicited by palpation of the middle ear and mastoid with an otherwise normal ear examination.

Postsurgical Otalgia

Otalgia can occur after surgical procedures involving the ear and mastoid. Surgical procedures such as myringotomy/tube insertion, middle ear, or mastoid procedures may result in postsurgical otalgia.[6-9] Pain is commonly seen after mastoidectomy and is characterized by tenderness to the mastoid cavity. In addition to postsurgical pain, these procedures are often accompanied by postoperative nausea and vomiting. Postoperative pain for patients who have undergone a mastoidectomy or tympanoplasty typically have pain for up to 2 weeks. This pain is managed by oral pain medication such as ibuprofen or acetaminophen.[8] Perioperative pain control for children who are undergoing myringotomy procedures may be treated with either intranasal or intravenous fentanyl.[7] In addition, local anesthetic or steroidal injections may be used to treat acute postoperative pain.[6]

Acute Pain Management in Primary Otalgia

In the case of primary otalgia arising from acute processes like otitis media or externa, management includes the use of topical antimicrobials combined with oral nonsteroidal anti-inflammatory agents or acetaminophen. Pain resolved in fewer days in the pediatric population when treated with antibiotics.[10] Other options for acute pain associated with otitis media are topical procaine or lidocaine preparations, in the absence of tympanic membrane (TM) perforation. In AOM with persistent pain, if a topical antimicrobial has not been given, one should be started.

In treatment of acute otitis externa, providers should recommend analgesics based on severity of pain. Patients with persistent pain should be reevaluated for other causes of otalgia or different antimicrobial therapy should be recommended.

Acute Pain Management in Secondary Otalgia and Referred Pain

In referred pain or secondary otalgia, therapy should focus on treating the primary source.[2,3,5] Correct diagnosis of the causative source of pain is, therefore, most important. Initial treatment of secondary otalgia may be addressed with oral NSAIDs. Since opioids mask signs and symptoms necessary for diagnosis, they should be avoided. The patient should be reexamined if persistent pain is experienced for 2-3 weeks despite treatment. For short-term relief or breakthrough pain relief is desired, local anesthesia should be considered. For involvement of the nasopharynx, spray or specific nerve blocks may be considered. For involvement of the larynx, the patient may gargle or transtracheal 4% lidocaine may be considered. For involvement of the ear canal, application of topical local anesthetic or injection of the chorda tympani has been effective. While unusual, a multitude of primary sources can present as ear pain, so a thorough history and physical examination of the patient with proper diagnosis is the most effective start to treating secondary otalgia.

Nose Pain

Nose Anatomy

The external nose is pyramidal shape and composed of skin, dorsal nasal bone, and upper and lower cartilages. The medial and lateral crura and columella contribute to the tip of nose. Internal nose includes septum, which divides the nose into two nostrils. The lateral wall includes superior, middle, and inferior turbinates.

Etiology

Chronic nasal pain can be caused by various inflammatory and infectious etiologies. Nose picking can lead to nasal mucosal infection with *Staphylococcus aureus* that can develop ulceration, pain, and bleeding. HSV-1 infection can also involve nasal mucosa. *Mycobacterium*, syphilis and rhinoscleroma, and fungal infection can cause nasal sore less commonly. Intranasal drugs such as cocaine can also cause chronic nasal sore. Immunocompromised patients can develop *Pseudomonas aeruginosa* infection that can affect nasal mucosa.[11] Benign and malignant tumors in the sinonasal area and acute and chronic rhinitis mostly present with nasal congestion and discharge and less commonly nasal pain. Trauma is one of the most common noninfectious causes of nose pain. Sarcoidosis is a rare medical condition that can cause inflammation and formation of granuloma and cause nose pain. Septal perforation is another uncommon cause of nose pain, which can be caused by cancer or cocaine abuse or rhinoplasty side effect.

Acute Throat Pain

Introduction

Acute sore throat is one of the most common complaints among patients that refer to clinics. Most of acute pharyngitis caused by viral infection are self-limited, while symptoms usually overlap between viral and other types of acute pharyngitis. To avoid inappropriate antibiotic treatment and to determine which patients have serious conditions, for example, airway obstruction, a comprehensive systematic approach is needed.

Throat Anatomy

The esophagus, windpipe (trachea), voice box (larynx), tonsils, and epiglottis are all located in the throat. The pharynx is a muscular tube that extends downward from the back of the nose to the neck. It is divided into three sections: the nasopharynx, the oropharynx, and the laryngopharynx, sometimes known as the hypopharynx. The epiglottis is a flap of tissue located at the back of the neck beneath the tongue. Its primary purpose is to cover the windpipe (trachea) during eating, preventing food from entering the airway.[12]

Etiology

Causes of sore throat are categorized as noninfectious and infectious. Respiratory viruses and group A *Streptococcus* (GAS) are the most common infectious causes.

Infectious Causes

Respiratory viruses, including SARS-CoV-2

A total of 25-45% of acute pharyngitis cases are related to viral infections. Adenovirus, coronaviruses, and rhinovirus are the most common causes of viral pharyngitis. Other types of viruses such as influenza virus, parainfluenza virus, RSV, and enterovirus are less common causes of acute viral pharyngitis. Respiratory virus can cause other symptoms, including nasal congestion, cough, sneezing, and conjunctivitis with sore throat. Fever is usually low grade in this group, except with COVID-19.[13,14]

Group A Streptococcus

Approximately 5-15% of acute pharyngitis is caused by GAS, and this microbe is the most common cause of bacterial pharyngitis. Signs and symptoms in this group include sore throat, pharyngeal edema, fever, tonsillar exudates, and cervical lymphadenopathy. GAS can invade beyond the pharynx and cause cellulitis and abscess and also it can be related to immune-mediated complications, for example, rheumatic fever.[15-18]

Other bacteria

Group C and G *Streptococcus*

Roughly 5-10% of acute pharyngitis cases are caused by these types of bacteria, and the prevalence is less common than GAS pharyngitis. Signs and symptoms are similar to GAS infection; however, they are not associated with immune-mediated complications, for example, glomerulonephritis or rheumatic fever.

Mycoplasma and *Chlamydia* species

These bacteria cause acute pharyngitis mostly in children and young adults, and they usually involve lower respiratory tract as well.[19,20]

Corynebacterium diphtheriae

This type of infection is rare but should be considered specially in patients who traveled to areas with unknown vaccination history. Signs and symptoms include gradually onset sore throat, low-grade fever, cervical lymphadenopathy, and gray membrane that bleeds if dislodged.

HIV and sexually transmitted infections

Acute HIV infection

A total of 40% of patients with acute HIV infection develops acute pharyngitis. Pharyngeal exudates are rare, and these patients usually have painful mucocutaneous lesions. Fever and cervical lymphadenopathy are also seen in these patients.

Neisseria gonorrhoeae

This type of pharyngitis is mostly common in homosexual men. Signs and symptoms include sore throat, pharyngeal exudates, and cervical lymphadenopathy.

Treponema pallidum

A total of 50% of patients with secondary syphilis present with pharyngitis. Mucous patches on oral mucosa and tongue covered by pink/gray membrane are usually seen on examination. Rash on palms and soles with generalized lymphadenopathy are other common symptoms in this condition. Symptoms usually occur months after primary exposure.

Epstein-Barr virus and other herpes viruses

Approximately 85% of patients with infectious mononucleosis present with acute pharyngitis. Signs and symptoms include high fever, tender posterior cervical lymphadenopathy, and patchy pharyngeal exudates with palatal petechiae. Symptoms are usually prolonged in this group and often last 2-3 weeks. CMV can also cause acute pharyngitis; however, symptoms are usually milder than EBV infection. Herpes simplex virus infection can also present with acute pharyngitis. Most common signs and symptoms in patients with HSV-1 infection are pharyngeal erythema and exudates with cervical lymphadenopathy. HSV-2 can also present with pharyngitis following orogenital contacts with similar symptoms.[20,21]

Noninfectious Causes

Medications including ACE inhibitors and some chemotherapeutics can cause acute sore throat. Allergic rhinitis and sinusitis are among other most common causes. Patients with gastroesophageal reflux disease can also present with acute sore throat. Smoking or exposure to secondhand smoke or dry air can also cause pharyngitis symptoms. Autoimmune disorders, including Behçet syndrome, Kawasaki disease, and periodic fever with aphthous stomatitis, pharyngitis, and adenitis (PFAPA) are the other important causes of pharyngitis.[22]

REFERENCES

1. Önerci M, Önerci TM. Ear anatomy. In: *Diagnosis in Otorhinolaryngology*. Springer; 2009.
2. Neilan RE, Roland PS. Otalgia. *Med Clin North Am*. 2010;94(5):961-971.
3. Ely JW, Hansen MR, Clark EC. Diagnosis of ear pain. *Am Fam Physician*. 2008;77:621-628.
4. Earwood JS, Rogers TS, Rathjen NA. Ear pain: diagnosing common and uncommon causes. *Am Fam Physician*. 2018;97(1):20-27.
5. Charlett SD, Coatesworth AP. Referred otalgia: a structured approach to diagnosis and treatment. *Int J Clin Pract*. 2007;61(6):1015-1021.
6. Lawhorn CD, Bower CM, Brown RE, et al. Topical lidocaine for postoperative analgesia following myringotomy and tube placement. *Int J Pediatr Otorhinolaryngol*. 1996;35(1):19-24.
7. Dewhirst E, Fedel G, Raman V, et al. Pain management following myringotomy and tube placement: intranasal dexmedetomidine versus intranasal fentanyl. *Int J Pediatr Otorhinolaryngol*. 2014;78(7):1090-1094.
8. Watcha MF, Ramirez-Ruiz M, White PF, Jones MB, Lagueruela RG, Terkonda RP. Perioperative effects of oral ketorolac and acetaminophen in children undergoing bilateral myringotomy. *Can J Anaesth*. 1992;39(7):649-654.
9. Güven M, Kara A, Yilmaz MS, Demir D, Güven EM. Comparison of incidence and severity of chronic postsurgical pain following ear surgery. *J Craniofac Surg*. 2018;29(6):e552-e555.
10. Venekamp RP, Sanders SL, Glasziou PP, Del Mar CB, Rovers MM. Antibiotics for acute otitis media in children. *Cochrane Database Syst Rev*. 2015;(6):CD000219.
11. Gaafar HA, Gaafar AH, Nour YA. Rhinoscleroma: an updated experience through the last 10 years. *Acta Otolaryngol*. 2011;131(4):440-446.
12. Albahout KS, Lopez RA. Anatomy, head and neck, pharynx. In: *StatPearls [Internet]*. StatPearls Publishing; 2021. [cited 2021 Aug 17]. http://www.ncbi.nlm.nih.gov/books/NBK544271/
13. Huovinen P, Lahtonen R, Ziegler T, et al. Pharyngitis in adults: the presence and coexistence of viruses and bacterial organisms. *Ann Intern Med*. 1989;110(8):612–616.
14. Bisno AL. Acute pharyngitis. *N Engl J Med*. 2001;344(3):205-211.

15. Snow V, Mottur-Pilson C, Cooper RJ, Hoffman JR; American Academy of Family Physicians, American College of Physicians-American Society of Internal Medicine, et al. Principles of appropriate antibiotic use for acute pharyngitis in adults. *Ann Intern Med.* 2001;134(6):506-508.
16. Centor RM, Atkinson TP, Ratliff AE, et al. The clinical presentation of Fusobacterium-positive and streptococcal-positive pharyngitis in a university health clinic: a cross-sectional study. *Ann Intern Med.* 2015;162(4):241-247.
17. Shulman ST, Bisno AL, Clegg HW, et al. Clinical practice guideline for the diagnosis and management of group A Streptococcal pharyngitis: 2012 update by the Infectious Diseases Society of America. *Clin Infect Dis.* 2012;55(10):1279-1282. Oxford Academic [Internet]. [cited 2021 Aug 17]. https://academic.oup.com/cid/article/55/10/e86/321183
18. Llor C, Madurell J, Balagué-Corbella M, Gómez M, Cots JM. Impact on antibiotic prescription of rapid antigen detection testing in acute pharyngitis in adults: a randomised clinical trial. *Br J Gen Pract.* 2011;61(586):e244-e251.
19. Waites KB, Atkinson TP. The role of Mycoplasma in upper respiratory infections. *Curr Infect Dis Rep.* 2009;11(3):198-206.
20. Glezen WP, Clyde WA Jr, Senior RJ, Sheaffer CI, Denny FW. Group A Streptococci, mycoplasmas, and viruses associated with acute pharyngitis. *JAMA.* 1967 Nov 6;202(6):455-460.
21. Luzuriaga K, Sullivan JL. Infectious mononucleosis. *N Engl J Med.* 2010;362(21):1993-2000. [cited 2021 Aug 17]. https://www.nejm.org/doi/full/10.1056/nejmcp1001116
22. Renner B, Mueller CA, Shephard A. Environmental and non-infectious factors in the aetiology of pharyngitis (sore throat) [Internet]. *Inflamm Res.* 2012;61(10):1041-1052. [cited 2021 Aug 17]. https://www.ncbi.nlm.nih.gov/pmc/articles/PMC3439613/

22

Acute Dermatologic Disorders

Jennifer S. Xiong

Introduction

There are various acute dermatologic conditions that can present with symptoms of moderate to severe cutaneous pain. Examples of such painful dermatologic disorders include, but are not limited to, the continuum of Stevens-Johnson syndrome and toxic epidermal necrolysis, pyoderma gangrenosum (PG), hidradenitis suppurativa, and calciphylaxis. Involvement of dermatology consultants early on in presentation is recommended for diagnostic and therapeutic guidance for all acute dermatologic disorders. Pain management is an important aspect of therapeutic management in acute dermatologic disorders, and it is frequently guided by the World Health Organization's proposed analgesic ladder for stepwise approach to pain management.[1]

Stevens-Johnson Syndrome and Toxic Epidermal Necrolysis

Stevens-Johnson syndrome and toxic epidermal necrolysis (SJS/TEN) make up a continuum of severe cutaneous adverse reactions that are characterized by fever, systemic disturbance, and significant epidermal sloughing that is associated with high morbidity and mortality. SJS/TEN are commonly triggered by various medications (eg, sulfa drugs, antiseizure drugs, and antibiotics), and as such, rapid recognition of SJS/TEN and withdrawal of culprit medications are critical for adequate control and reduction in mortality of this severe reaction. The mainstay of treatment for SJS/TEN is supportive care.

Stevens-Johnson syndrome and toxic epidermal necrolysis are characterized by painful mucocutaneous necrosis and epidermal detachment (Fig. 22.1) and, together, are part of a disease continuum classified based on pattern of lesions and on extent of epidermal detachment. SJS is classified by widespread erythematous macules with detachment of epidermis, affecting <10% of body surface area, whereas TEN involves detachment of epidermis above 30% of body surface area. SJS/TEN overlap is a third classification, which describes patients with epidermal detachment between 10% and 30% of body surface area[2] (Fig. 22.2). Differential diagnosis for presentation includes viral exanthems, other drug rashes, and erythema multiform; however, SJS/TEN may be differentiated by its characteristic severe cutaneous pain.

Cutaneous pain is a prominent feature in SJS/TEN, with skin pain often out of proportion to cutaneous findings. The presence of severe dermatologic pain should alert evaluating physicians to consider SJS/TEN on the differential, for early recognition is imperative for reduction in mortality. Dermatology consultation should be made as soon as possible to further guide diagnosis and management. Diagnostic workup may involve skin biopsy for histopathologic examination; however, histologic findings are neither specific nor diagnostic. Diagnosis relies heavily on the presence of clinical features, which include history of drug exposure, prodrome

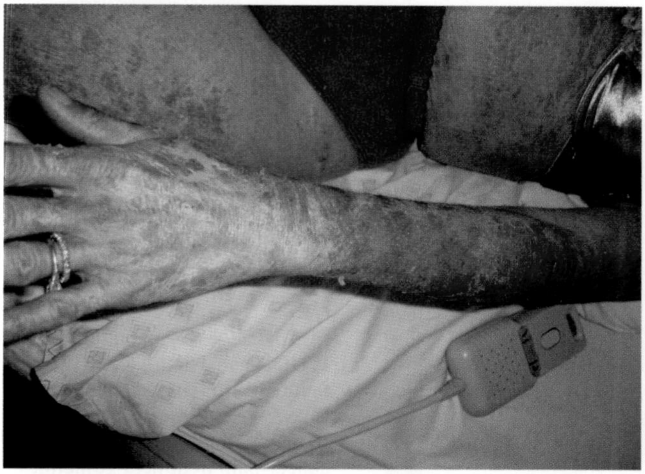

FIGURE 22.1 Epidermal sloughing and detachment associated with SJS/TEN. (From Ofoma UR, Chapnick EK. Fluconazole induced toxic epidermal necrolysis: a case report. *Cases J*. 2009;2:9071. doi:10.1186/1757-1626-2-9071)

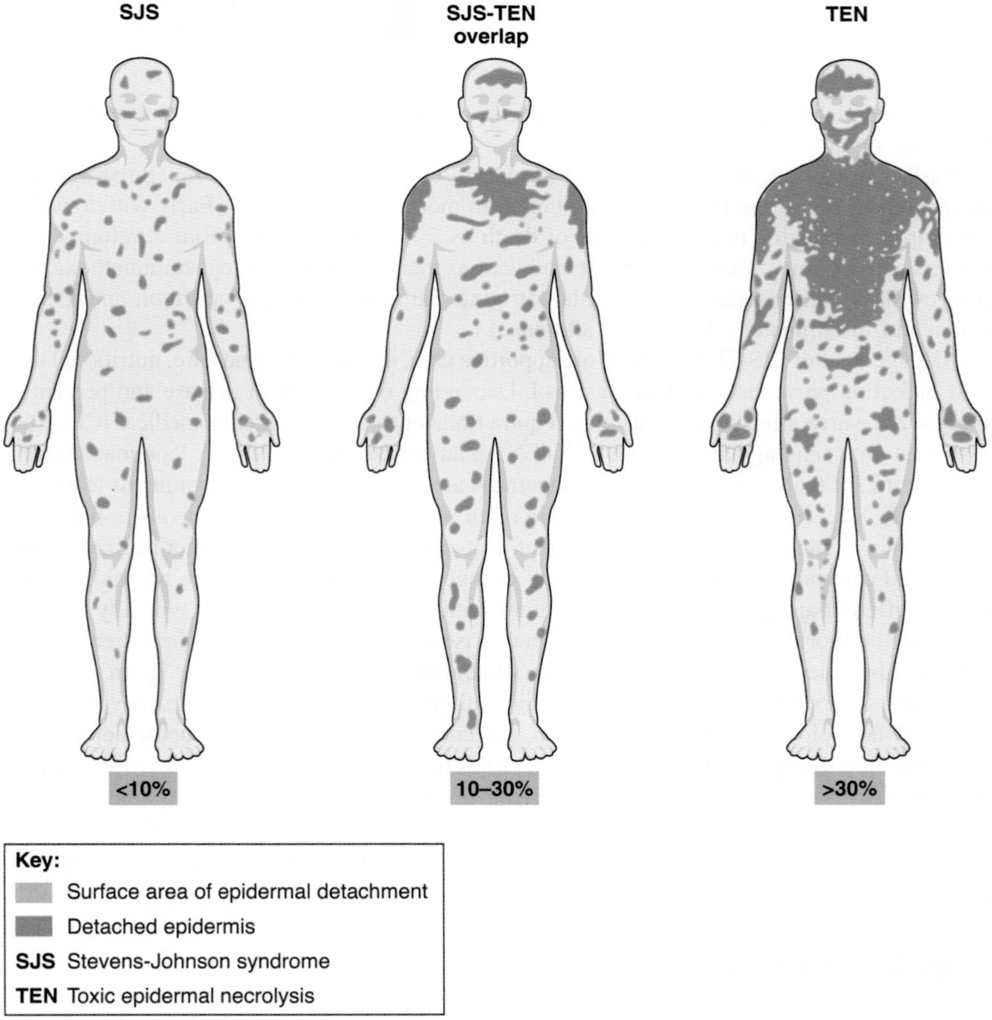

FIGURE 22.2 Representation of SJS, SJS-TEN overlap, and TEN, illustrating percent body surface area affected by epidermal detachment. (From Harr T, French LE. Toxic epidermal necrolysis and Stevens-Johnson syndrome. *Orphanet J Rare Dis*. 2010;5:39.)

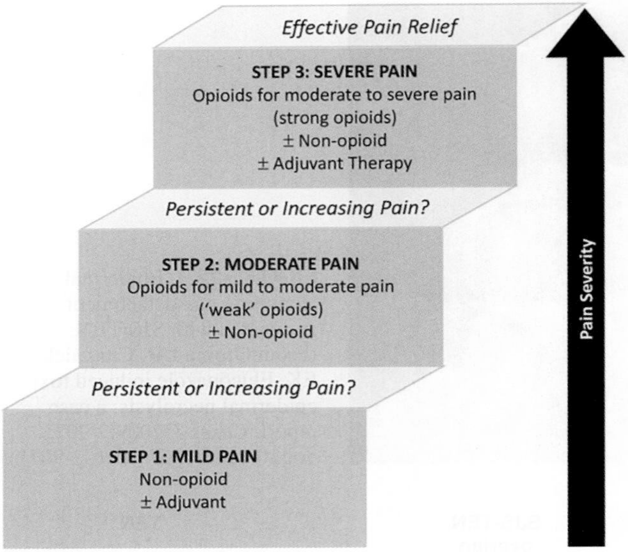

FIGURE 22.3 Adaptation of the WHO Analgesic Ladder. (From Samuelly-Leichtag G, Adler T, Eisenberg E. Something must be wrong with the implementation of cancer-pain treatment guidelines. A lesson from referrals to a pain clinic. *Rambam Maimonides Med J*. 2019;10(3):e0016.)

of fever and malaise, painful progressive rash, severely painful mucosal erosions, and positive Nikolsky sign.[3]

Early recognition and withdrawal of suspected culprit medication is imperative for adequate control of the reaction and for reduction in mortality of SJS/TEN. Early withdrawal of the culprit medication may reduce risk of death by 30% for each day before development of blisters and erosions.[4] Common culprit medications include antibiotics (eg, sulfamethoxazole, doxycycline), antiepileptic drugs (eg, lamotrigine, carbamazepine), allopurinol, and nonsteroidal anti-inflammatory drugs (eg, diclofenac).

Management of SJS/TEN consists of supportive care, including wound care, nutritional support, infection prevention, and pain control. Depending on severity of disease and percent of body surface area affected, patients may require transfer to a burn center or medical ICU experienced with managing patients with SJS/TEN for advanced supportive care. Pain management is a significant feature of SJS/TEN management as cutaneous pain is a prominent feature of the SJS/TEN reaction, with severe skin pain often out of proportion to cutaneous findings and most severe at sites of epidermal detachment. Cutaneous pain will also further be exacerbated by wound care procedures such as dressing changes. While there have been no studies comparing different analgesic regimens in patients with SJS/TEN, treatment is typically initiated based on the World Health Organization's step-wise analgesic ladder.[5] Therefore, treatment of SJS/TEN pain depends on intensity of pain, which can be described numerically on a scale of increasing severity from 0 to 10. For mild pain with intensity rating <4, patients may be treated with oral nonopioid analgesics (eg, aspirin, acetaminophen) that may be supplemented with mild oral opioids (eg, codeine) or synthetic opioids (eg, tramadol). For moderate to severe pain with intensity >4, patients should receive regularly scheduled opioids (eg, morphine, fentanyl) delivered enterally, by PCA, or by infusion, with regular around-the-clock re-evaluation of pain score (Fig. 22.3). For severe pain uncontrolled by standard adjuncts and parenteral opioids, patients may require ketamine-based sedation or general anesthesia.[6]

Pyoderma Gangrenosum

Pyoderma gangrenosum is a rare inflammatory and ulcerative neutrophilic dermatosis that ranks among the most painful of skin disorders.[1]

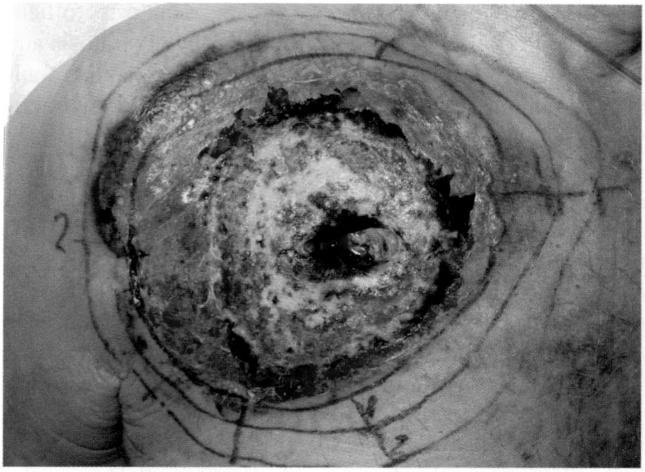

FIGURE 22.4 Large ulcer of pyoderma gangrenosum with violaceous borders and necrotic center. (From Inan I, Myers PO, Braun R, et al. Pyoderma gangrenosum after totally implanted central venous access device insertion. *World J Surg Onc*. 2008;6:31.)

Pyoderma gangrenosum presentation classically begins with small tender papules or pustules on the lower extremities that gradually evolve into large painful ulcers with distinctly violaceous undermined borders[7] (Fig. 22.4). Typical findings of PG ulcers include central site of necrosis with surrounding ulceration of the epidermis and dermis with an inflammatory cell infiltrate. PG most commonly occurs in adults aged 50s to 60s, with more than 50% of patients affected by PG also suffering from an underlying systemic disease (eg, chronic inflammatory bowel disease, inflammatory arthritis, hematologic malignancy).[7] Associated symptoms of PG may often include fevers, myalgias, and arthralgias.

Differential diagnosis for PG includes similar-appearing cutaneous ulcerations resulting from infection, malignancy, vasculitis, and diabetes. Diagnostic testing may include biopsy of the lesion for determination of the presence of neutrophilic infiltrate; however, histopathological findings are often variable and nonspecific.[7] As such, diagnosis of PG is ultimately one of exclusion after all other etiologies of leg ulceration have been ruled out[1]; there or no pathognomonic clinical or histologic features of PG.

There presently is no published gold standard targeted therapy or algorithm for treatment of PG, and current practice has been largely empirical and based on limited data from case studies and randomized control trials. In general, patients may be treated with a combination of topical or systemic therapies that suppress the inflammatory process associated with PG (eg, corticosteroids, topical tacrolimus, cyclosporine, infliximab).[8] Careful wound care measures are also implemented for optimization of wound healing. Treatment of associated systemic disorder may also help to reduce severity of PG.

An important consideration of PG treatment includes pain management. The deep and severe inflammatory process and ulceration associated with PG can result in debilitating pain, with patients often describing the pain as "stabbing" in quality. Wound manipulation from required repeated dressing changes will further exacerbate such pain. Sufficient pain management should be implemented with enteral and/or parenteral analgesic medications by following the World Health Organization analgesic ladder guidelines.[5] Hyperbaric oxygen therapy has been showing in several case studies to significantly reduce pain associated with PG while aiding in wound healing by elevating oxygen tension in ulcers; however, the application of hyperbaric oxygen therapy is limited as it is both expensive and not widely available.[9]

Hidradenitis Suppurativa

Hidradenitis suppurativa (HS) is a painful inflammatory disease that is characterized by painful relapse-remitting boil-like lesions located commonly in the intertriginous skin areas like the axilla and groin. Pathogenesis of HS has been hypothesized to be related to follicular occlusion from ductal keratinocyte proliferation, leading to follicular hyperkeratosis and plugging.[10] Diagnosis is based on classic clinical features, and treatment may require analgesics ranging from nonsteroidal anti-inflammatory drugs to oral opiates to addition of anticonvulsants and selective serotonin reuptake inhibitors/serotonin-norepinephrine reuptake inhibitors.

Presentation of HS varies in severity, with severity of pain strongly correlating with quality of life. The disease consists of painful, deep-seated inflammatory nodules, predominantly occurring in intertriginous areas (eg, axillae, inguinal area, inframammary regions, scrotum, etc.) with associated sinus tract formation, comedones, odorous abscesses, and scarring (Fig. 22.5). Differential diagnosis for HS includes acne vulgaris, Crohn disease abscess manifestations, granuloma inguinale, and follicular pyodermas. The diagnosis of HS relies on a thorough history and physical examination and is supported by three main clinical features: typical lesions (multiple deep-seated inflamed nodules, tombstone comedones, sinus tracts, abscesses, and/or fibrotic scars), typical locations (axillae, groin, inframammary areas; often bilateral distribution), and relapses and chronicity.[11] Due to the painful and acute or chronic nature of the disease, patients with HS are at high risk for depression and anxiety.[12]

Management of HS includes wound and skin care, reducing burden of disease, and pain management. Proper wound care involves wound dressing with simple petrolatum for minimization of skin trauma. Common medications used for reducing burden of disease include topical clindamycin, oral tetracycline, metformin, antiandrogenic agents (eg, spironolactone, oral contraceptives), clindamycin-rifampin combination therapy, acitretin, and oral dapsone. Acute inflammatory nodules may benefit from intralesional corticosteroid injections or punch debridement.

Adequate pain management for patients with HS is imperative, as inadequate treatment of pain may increase risk of anxiety and depression.[12] While anti-inflammatory drugs can decrease pain associated with HS, adjunctive pain medications like topical analgesics and oral acetaminophen are typically necessary to manage pain in HS patients. If pain management is inadequate with those agents, oral opiates can be considered by following the World Health Organization's step-wise analgesic ladder. Additionally, anticonvulsants, tricyclics, selective serotonin reuptake inhibitors, and serotonin-norepinephrine reuptake inhibitors possess neuropathic pain-relieving properties that not only offer long-term pain control in patients with HS but may also address any co-occurring depression.[13]

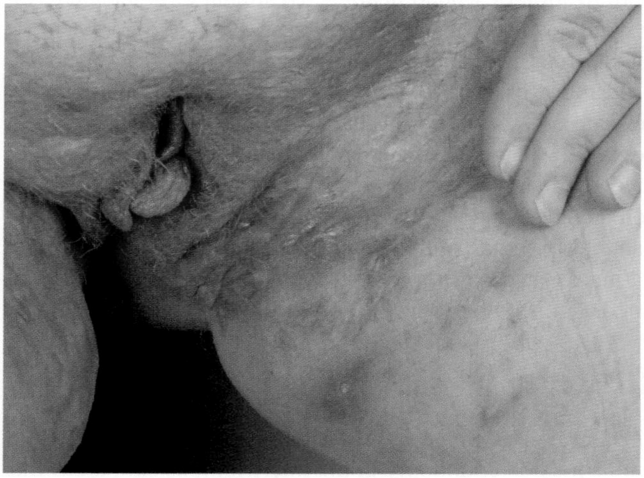

FIGURE 22.5 Hidradenitis suppurativa in the perineal area. (From Alharbi Z, Kauczok J, Pallua N. A review of wide surgical excision of hidradenitis suppurativa. *BMC Dermatol.* 2012;12:9.)

Calciphylaxis

Calciphylaxis, also known as calcific uremic arteriolopathy, is a rare and serious complication seen in patients with end-stage renal disease. It presents with excruciatingly painful skin ischemia and necrosis secondary to small vessel vasculopathy within the dermis and subcutaneous adipose tissue.[14] Management of calciphylaxis is supportive, with emphasis on pain management and palliative care as the prognosis for calciphylaxis is poor, with mortality rates of up to 80%.[15]

Calciphylaxis presents as lesions of painful ischemic necrosis. Common sites of calciphylaxis formation include areas with greatest adiposity, including distal and proximal lower extremities, trunk, and proximal upper extremities.[14] Characteristic lesions of calciphylaxis include violaceous, indurated, plaquelike nodules that eventually progress into necrotic ulcers with eschars (Fig. 22.6). Differential diagnosis for calciphylaxis includes warfarin necrosis, vasculitis, atherosclerosis, cholesterol embolization, and cellulitis. Diagnosis of calciphylaxis is based on examination findings of the typical painful ulcerated lesion with a black eschar. Skin biopsy may also prove helpful to confirm the diagnosis when uncertain, and as such, involvement of dermatology consultants is advantageous during initial evaluation.

Pathogenesis of calciphylaxis is poorly understood, with progression to subcutaneous and vascular calcification and injury. Management typically consists of supportive care involving wound care, infection treatment, management of electrolyte abnormalities, optimizing dialysate in dialysis patients, and pain management per the World Health Organization's analgesic pain ladder guidelines. Sodium thiosulfate, which has calcium-chelating and antioxidant properties, has also become an emerging pharmacologic option acting to increase clearance of calcium from the body and to reduce vascular calcification.[16] Ultimately, presentation of calciphylaxis is a sign of poor prognosis, as development of calciphylaxis ulcers are associated

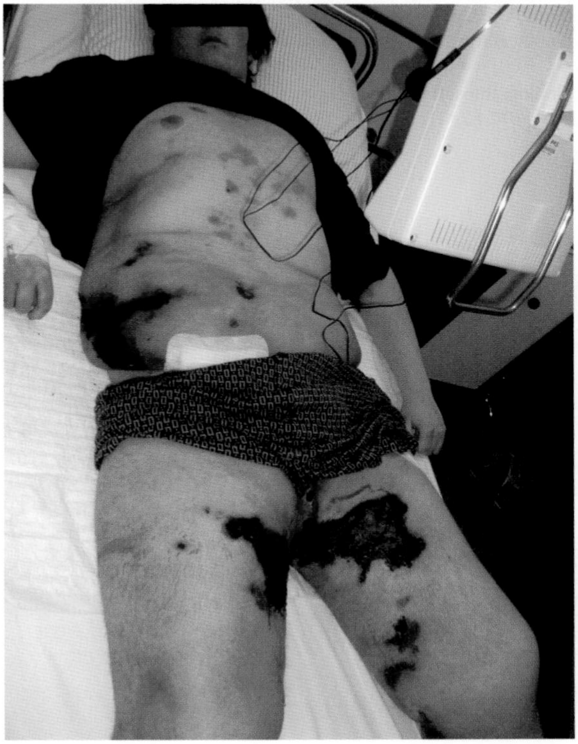

FIGURE 22.6 Calciphylaxis in bilateral lower extremities and abdominal wall. (From Tsolakidis S, Grieb G, Piatkowski A, et al. Calciphylaxis—a challenging & solvable task for plastic surgery? A case report. *BMC Dermatol.* 2013;13:1.)

with a mortality rate as high as 80%.[15] Early involvement of palliative care specialists may be beneficial for assistance with worsening prognosis, escalating analgesic regimens, and for assistance with bridge to terminal care.[14]

REFERENCES

1. Beiteke U, Bigge S, Reichenberger C, Gralow I. Pain and pain management in dermatology. *J Dtsch Dermatol Ges*. 2015;13(10):967-987.
2. Bastuji-Garin S. Clinical classification of cases of toxic epidermal necrolysis, Stevens-Johnson syndrome, and erythema multiforme. *Arch Dermatol*. 1993;129(1):92-96.
3. Schwartz R, McDonough P, Lee B. Toxic epidermal necrolysis. *J Am Acad Dermatol*. 2013;69(2):187.e1-187.e16.
4. Garcia-Doval I, LeCleach L, Bocquet H, Otero X, Roujeau J. Toxic epidermal necrolysis and Stevens-Johnson syndrome: does early withdrawal of causative drugs decrease the risk of death? *Arch Dermatol*. 2000;136(3):323-327.
5. WHO. WHO's cancer pain ladder for adults. Published 2020. https://www.who.int/cancer/palliative/painladder
6. Valeyrie-Allanore L, Ingen-Housz-Oro S, Colin A, Thuillot D, Sigal M, Binhas M. Prise en charge de la douleur dans le syndrome de Stevens-Johnson/Lyell et les autres dermatoses bulleuses étendues. *Ann Dermatol Venereol*. 2011;138(10):694-697.
7. Burns T, Breathnach S, Cox N, Griffiths C. *Rook's Textbook of Dermatology*. 8th ed. Wiley-Blackwell;2010.
8. Brooklyn T, Dunnill G, Probert C. Diagnosis and treatment of pyoderma gangrenosum. *BMJ*. 2006;333(7560):181-184.
9. Tutrone W, Green K, Weinberg J, Caglar S, Clarke D. Pyoderma gangrenosum: dermatologic application of hyperbaric oxygen therapy. *J Drugs Dermatol*. 2007;6(12):1214-1219.
10. von Laffert M, Stadie V, Wohlrab J, Marsch W. Hidradenitis suppurativa/acne inversa: bilocated epithelial hyperplasia with very different sequelae. *Br J Dermatol*. 2010;164(2):367-371.
11. Jemec G. Hidradenitis suppurativa. *N Engl J Med*. 2012;366(2):158-164.
12. Brennan F, Carr D, Cousins M. Pain management: a fundamental human right. *Anesth Analg*. 2007;105(1):205-221.
13. Horváth B, Janse I, Sibbald G. Pain management in patients with hidradenitis suppurativa. *J Am Acad Dermatol*. 2015;73(5):S47-S51.
14. Polizzotto M, Bryan T, Ashby M, Martin P. Symptomatic management of calciphylaxis: a case series and review of the literature. *J Pain Symptom Manage*. 2006;32(2):186-190.
15. Fine A, Zacharias J. Calciphylaxis is usually non-ulcerating: risk factors, outcome and therapy. *Kidney Int*. 2002;61(6):2210-2217.
16. Yu Z, Gu L, Pang H, Fang Y, Yan H, Fang W. Sodium thiosulfate: an emerging treatment for calciphylaxis in dialysis patients. *Case Rep Nephrol Dial*. 2015;5(1):77-82.

23

Acute/Chronic Infection Diseases and Postherpetic Neuralgia Considerations in Pain Management

Karla Samaniego, Varsha D. Allampalli, Alexandra R. Cloutet, Stephen P. Patin, Vijayakumar Javalkar, Elyse M. Cornett, and Alan David Kaye

Introduction

Pain is defined as an unpleasant sensory and emotional experience associated with or resembling that associated with actual or potential tissue damage.[1] Chronic pain is commonly defined as any pain that lasts more than 12 weeks. Typically, pain is a feature of many infectious processes such as abscess, urinary tract infection, or any bacterial infection that causes an inflammatory process. The main scope of this chapter is focused on neuralgia, such as postherpetic neuralgia (PHN), where the pain is a result of the involvement of the neurological pathways resulting in neuropathic pain. Neuropathic pain is different from nociceptive pain. Nociceptive pain is a result of tissue damage that results in secondary activation of the neural pathways. Neuropathic pain or neuralgia is related to nervous system lesions or dysfunction and could be due to different mechanisms such as peripheral nervous system sensitization, deafferentation, or neurogenic inflammation.[2,3]

Postherpetic neuralgia is one of the commonly encountered neuralgia related to infections in clinical practice. The incidence of herpes zoster (HZ) is ~4 cases per 1000 population, with a total burden of about 1 million cases annually in the United States. About 15% of adults with HZ develops PHN, and there are ~150 000 new cases in the United States annually.[4] After the initial varicella infection, the virus persists in the dorsal root ganglia and cranial ganglia, such as geniculate ganglion. Reactivation of the virus can occur through reduced cell-mediated immunity due to stress, illness, medication, aging, or idiopathic cause's results in shingles.[5]

The clinical hallmark of PHN includes a rash consisting of erythematous papules in a dermatomal distribution followed by lancinating or burning pain in the dermatomal distribution. Thoracic and lumbar dermatomes are commonly affected. Usually, the pain persists for 3 months or more following HZ.[6] In immunocompromised patients, multidermatomal involvement is seen.[7] Reactivation of the varicella-zoster virus (VZV) at geniculate ganglion presents with a vesicular rash on the ear accompanied by facial nerve paralysis,[8] which is referred to as Ramsay Hunt syndrome. Reactivation of the latent virus in the trigeminal ganglion with involvement of the ophthalmic division of the trigeminal nerve leads to ocular zoster, which may causes keratitis, scleritis, uveitis, retinitis, and choroiditis.[9] Rarely involvement of the other cranial nerves such as the abducens and vagus nerve without typical skin rash has been described.[10] Other neurological complication of HZ infection includes encephalitis, motor neuropathy,[11] myelitis,[12] stroke,[13] and Guillain-Barré syndrome.[14] This chapter focuses on chronic and acute infection diseases, their evaluation, diagnosis, and differential diagnosis.

Pathophysiology

Varicella-zoster virus is a type of human herpes virus that causes two distinct diseases, varicella (chickenpox) and HZ (shingles). This DNA virus remains latent within the sensory ganglia following the resolution of chickenpox. Conditions leading to decreased cellular immunity cause reactivation of the virus. Transportation of the VZV along peripheral nerves is associated with acute neuritis.[15] Damaged peripheral and central nerve fibers may develop a lower threshold for action potentials and discharge spontaneously, resulting in peripheral sensitization.[16] Multiple peripheral and central mechanisms contribute to PHN. Qualitatively different types of pain that characterize PHN probably have different underlying mechanisms.[17]

Acute HZ is characterized by hemorrhagic inflammation of the peripheral nerve, dorsal root, and dorsal root ganglion. Inflammation can extend centrally into the spinal cord and leptomeninges.[18] There is a paucity of autopsy data related to PHN cases. One study reported five cases, three with severe PHN and two with no persistent pain.[19] Patients with persistent pain had associated dorsal horn atrophy and cellular, axonal, and myelin loss with fibrosis in the sensory ganglion. It was interesting to note that axonal and myelin loss in the nerve and/or sensory root was not specific to patients with pain.

Neurotransmitters implicated in causing PHN are unknown. Postmortem study of the affected dorsal horn from one patient with PHN failed to demonstrate differences in the levels of these neurotransmitters when compared with the unaffected side.[20] The same study was unable to demonstrate a deficiency of opiate receptors in the affected dorsal horn. Evaluation of cytokine profiles extracted from skin punch biopsies of dermatomes affected by PHN found no significant differences when compared with skin biopsies from the normal contralateral side,[21] but intraepidermal nerve fiber density was found to be lower in affected skin as compared to unaffected skin.

Epidemiology and Risk Factors

One in every three persons develops HZ during their lifetime.[22] It is estimated that 5%-20% of those with HZ can develop PHN.[23] The frequency and severity of PHN increase with advancing age, occurring in 20% of people aged 60-65 years who have had acute HZ and in more than 30% of people aged >80 years.[24] In addition to age, risk factors for developing PHN after HZ include the presence of a prodrome (defined as pain and/or abnormal sensations before rash onset), severe rash (defined as >50 lesions: papules, vesicles, or crusted vesicles), and severe pain during the acute phase.[25] A recent meta-analysis also identified ophthalmic involvement as a risk factor. Additional possible risk factors included systemic lupus erythematosus, diabetes, and recent trauma.[26] Immunocompromised patients are at increased risk of VZV reactivation as well as neurological complications.[12]

Lai and Yew[27] identified five studies ($N = 4169$) for meta-analysis and demonstrated that family history is a significant risk factor for HZ infection (OR = 3.03; 95% CI, 1.86-4.94). One proposed genetic mechanism involves human leukocyte antigens (HLAs), specifically HLA-A, which are responsible for presenting peptides to $CD8^+$ receptors to elicit an immune response. IE6862 is a VZV transcription factor protein and is responsible for eliciting $CD8^+$ response. A study conducted by Meysman et al.[28] found that patients who had lower HLA-A presentation ability of IE62 protein had a 60% greater risk of HZ.

Being of the Black race appears to be protective against HZ in comparison to Caucasians. Black individuals may have elevated exposure to varicella leading to cell-mediated immunity.[29] Genetic variations, racial differences in reporting and seeking medical care, could be other possible explanations.[30]

Evaluation and Diagnosis

Postherpetic neuralgia is generally underdiagnosed in the context of primary care due to the chronic nature of the pain that this disease is characterized by. It is most often a clinical diagnosis and requires a good history and physical examination. The index of suspicion for this disease should also increase in older patients. The risk of developing PHN increases with age, and the Olmsted County Study found that 73% of its participants with PHN were above the age of 60.[31] The criteria for diagnosis include a prior HZ infection with a unilateral rash in a dermatomal distribution; (the most frequently affected nerves being thoracic, cervical, and trigeminal) and persistent (eg, greater than or equal to 3 months) burning or lancinating pain, allodynia, paresthesia, or hyperalgesia in or around the same dermatomal distribution on the body as the zoster rash.[32] Approximately 90% of people with PHN report allodynia. Another common manifestation of the disease is anesthesia in the affected dermatomes. People tend to report deficits in vibratory, tactile, thermal, and pinprick sensation.[33] Checking for the presence of a cutaneous scar may also be useful for people who cannot recall the presence or distribution of the zoster infection.[34] Additionally, some people report autonomic changes on the skin affected, such as increased sweating.[34]

When diagnosing PHN, it is important to be aware that there are variants that do not conform to the widely accepted diagnostic criteria for this disease. One of those is referred to as zoster sine herpete (ZSH), where those inflicted with prolonged burning pain and allodynia did not report a preceding zoster rash, though this is considered atypical.[35] Diagnosing ZSH may require more than a history and physical.

Diagnosing PHN is generally done without the use of laboratory testing. However, serological testing for VZV IgG and IgM titers is available.[32] These tests are generally unwarranted for typical cases of PHN as they are neither sensitive nor specific. However, they may be useful in atypical presentations of disease such as ZSH.[32] Additionally, it can be difficult to distinguish a vesicular lesion caused by VZV from one caused by the herpes simplex virus. Immunofluorescent staining of skin scrapings can be used to characterize the virus present.[32]

There are some new and promising biomarkers. A new biomarker called galectin-3 is being studied for its role in the pathogenesis of PHN. Galectin-3 is part of the galectin-binding lectin family and has many proinflammatory effects on the body. Levels of this biomarker have been found to be higher in patients with a history of VZV who developed PHN when compared with patients with a history of VZV who did not develop PHN. In the future, this may be a valuable diagnostic tool in atypical PHN.[36] There is also preliminary evidence that MRI may hold utility in diagnosing atypical PHN as well as help in differentiating HZ from PHN as we continue to identify differences in regional brain activity between these two diseases.[37] See Table 23.1.

Differential Diagnosis and Treatment/Management

In the setting of acute pain potentially associated with an infectious etiology, a host of differential diagnoses should be considered. The differential diagnoses should be guided by clinical information, namely the demographic data, history of present illness, and physical examination. This information can help the clinician classify the type of pain and, subsequently, the possible causative infection responsible for the pain.[38]

With an increased prevalence of diabetes, and because of the overlap in clinical symptoms with other causes of neuropathic pain, diabetic neuropathy should be considered high in the differential list of patients with neuropathic pain.[39] Chronic CNS conditions, such as multiple sclerosis, Parkinson disease, syringomyelia, and others, should be considered; testing should

TABLE 23.1 DIAGNOSING POSTHERPETIC NEURALGIA

History
Advanced age
The patient reports a history of unilateral dermatomal rash
Pain is chronic in nature (greater than or equal to 3 months)
Pain interferes with activities of daily living
Physical examination
Presence of cutaneous scarring in dermatomal distribution
Allodynia, hyperalgesia, hypoalgesia present
Sensory deficits with tactile, thermal, vibratory stimuli
Autonomic changes on skin
Laboratory testing
PHN diagnosis does not require laboratory testing
VZV IgG and IgM titers can aid in diagnosis of subclinical disease
Immunofluorescence staining can distinguish between VZV and herpes simplex virus infection

From Nalamachu S, Morley-Forster P. Diagnosing and managing postherpetic neuralgia. *Drugs Aging*. 2012;29(11):863-869.

be expanded on further clinical evaluation. General radiculopathies (eg, cervical, thoracic, lumbosacral) should be considered as the nerve entrapments involved with these conditions can mimic neuropathic pain of other conditions. Toxin-related neuropathies (ie, alcohol, chemotherapy, etc.) can be identified through a thorough history.[40] Infectious etiologies of neuropathic pain include both human immunodeficiency virus and HZ from reactivated VZV.[41] To a lesser extent, cytomegalovirus can cause similar symptoms and should be considered.

Postherpetic neuralgia is both the most common complication of HZ and one of the more difficult complications to treat. The best way to treat is by prevention, particularly with the HZ vaccine.[42] The vaccine, whether the live attenuated mechanism or the glycoprotein E mechanism, aims to increase VZV-specific cell-mediated immunity in hopes of preventing both the reactivation of the virus and the risk of PHN for those that do experience reactivation.[43,44] Broadly, this vaccination is recommended for those 50 years of age or older; however, providers should consider special cases.

For those in which HZ (and therefore postherpetic neuralgia) prevention was not achieved, treatment begins with oral and topical medications. First-line therapy includes oral tricyclic antidepressants (TCAs), which have mechanisms to relieve psychological symptoms (inhibition of noradrenaline and serotonin uptake) and provide analgesic effects (alpha-2-adrenergic receptor blockade).[45] However, clinicians must consider the large side effect profile of TCAs with the patient's state of health. For this reason, additional first-line therapies include gabapentinoid agents such as oral pregabalin or gabapentin and lidocaine 5% patches. Many clinicians choose to initially prescribe a gabapentinoid medication first to avoid these anticholinergic, alpha-blockade-associated, and antihistaminergic effects.[46] Extended-release formulations such as gralise, an extended-release gastroretentive gabapentin medication, provides efficacy and reduced side effects related to slow release allowing for higher blood levels and once a day dosing. Other medical treatments include capsaicin creams, many of which are sold at common drug stores; however, there are limited data related to effectiveness. SNRIs/SSRIs (serotonin-norepinephrine reuptake inhibitors and selective serotonin reuptake inhibitors) have also been used, albeit with similar outcomes as TCAs. Ketamine infusions (NMDA antagonists) have recently become popular, but data are mostly anecdotal at this time.[47]

Invasive options to treat postherpetic neuralgia include Botox injections, local anesthetic injections for their sympathetic blockade effects, spinal cord stimulation, or even epidural/intrathecal injections. Data are limited in the effectiveness of most invasive treatments, though.

Likewise, with the exception of Botox injections, the side effect profile of these treatments is often considerable and undesirable.[48]

Conclusion

Neuralgia resulting from infectious disease affects a large number of people, and it is most unfortunate with regard to PHN that more people do not receive the highly effective shingles vaccine. PHN is a neuropathic pain syndrome that can last for months or even years after resolution of shingles, typically waxes and wanes, and is more prevalent in females and in the elderly. The HZ rash results from reactivation of the VZV. It is estimated that ~1 in 3 adults will develop HZ in their lifetime, which amounts to ~1 million new cases in the United States annually. Of those who develop HZ, about 15% or 150 000 will experience PHN as a complication. The pain associated with PHN can be debilitating and have a severe impact on activities of daily living and overall quality of life.

The precise mechanism for the development of PHN is not fully understood. Damage to central and peripheral nerves may be a result of inflammation associated with VZV reactivation and can lead to peripheral sensitization; however, the neurotransmitters involved in this process is unknown. As a result of this peripheral sensitization, patients with PHN experience allodynia, hyperalgesia, and pain that is either constant or intermittent. Risk factors for development of PHN include advanced age, immunocompromised state, prodrome, severe rash, and severe pain during the acute phase of HZ. Diagnosis of PHN is based on history and physical examination. The relevant history for diagnosis includes prior history of rash with HZ virus in a dermatomal distribution and pain that persists in the same dermatomal area for at least 3 months. Physical examination may reveal scarring from a prior rash as well as sensory deficits or autonomic changes to the skin. Lab testing is available but unnecessary unless the patient has an atypical presentation of PHN (eg, with no prior history of rash). For atypical presentations, use of a biomarker galectin-3 and MRI show promise for diagnosing atypical PHN.

First-line management of PHN involves oral and topical medications. TCAs are considered first-line, but because of their considerable side effect profile, other first-line options include gabapentinoids and lidocaine 5% patches. For those experiencing pain that is refractory to treatment with oral or topical medications, invasive treatment options are available as well. These include Botox injections, spinal cord stimulation, injection of local anesthetics, and epidural/intrathecal injections; however, data on the effectiveness of invasive treatments are limited.

In summary, since PHN is both debilitating and oftentimes refractory to treatment, prevention of HZ is the most important form of management. The best form of prevention is the HZ vaccine, which is recommended for individuals over the age of 50 to prevent reactivation of VZV or development of PHN.

REFERENCES

1. Raja SN, Carr DB, Cohen M, et al. The revised International Association for the Study of Pain definition of pain: concepts, challenges, and compromises. *Pain*. 2020;161(9):1976-1982.
2. Kerstman E, Ahn S, Battu S, Tariq S, Grabois M. Neuropathic pain. In: *Handbook of Clinical Neurology [Internet]*. Elsevier; 2013:175-187. https://linkinghub.elsevier.com/retrieve/pii/B9780444529015000150
3. Nicholson B. Differential diagnosis: nociceptive and neuropathic pain. *Am J Manag Care*. 2006;12(9 Suppl):S256-S262.
4. https://www.cdc.gov/shingles/hcp/clinical-overview.html#:~:text=Postherpetic%20neuralgia%20(PHN)%20is%20the,herpes%20zoster%20increases%20with%20age
5. Hadley GR, Gayle JA, Ripoll J, et al. Post-herpetic neuralgia: a review. *Curr Pain Headache Rep*. 2016;20(3):17.

6. Hadley GR, Gayle JA, Ripoll J, et al. Erratum to: post-herpetic neuralgia: a review. *Curr Pain Headache Rep.* 2016;20(4):28.
7. Lewis DJ, Schlichte MJ, Dao H. Atypical disseminated herpes zoster: management guidelines in immunocompromised patients. *Cutis.* 2017;100(5):321;324:330.
8. Jeon Y, Lee H. Ramsay Hunt syndrome. *J Dent Anesth Pain Med.* 2018;18(6):333-337.
9. Gnann JW. Varicella-zoster virus: atypical presentations and unusual complications. *J Infect Dis.* 2002;186(Suppl 1):S91-S98.
10. Joo T, Lee YC, Kim TG. Herpes zoster involving the abducens and vagus nerves without typical skin rash: a case report and literature review. *Medicine (Baltimore).* 2019;98(19):e15619.
11. Gopal KVT, Sarvani D, Krishnam Raju PV, Rao GR, Venkateswarlu K. Herpes zoster motor neuropathy: a clinical and electrophysiological study. *Indian J Dermatol Venereol Leprol.* 2010;76(5):569-571.
12. Nagel MA, Gilden D. Neurological complications of varicella zoster virus reactivation. *Curr Opin Neurol.* 2014;27(3):356-360.
13. Amlie-Lefond C, Gilden D. Varicella zoster virus: a common cause of stroke in children and adults. *J Stroke Cerebrovasc Dis.* 2016;25(7):1561-1569.
14. Kang J, Sheu J, Lin H. Increased risk of Guillain-Barré syndrome following recent herpes zoster: a population-based study across Taiwan. *Clin Infect Dis.* 2010;51(5):525-530.
15. Burke BL, Steele RW, Beard OW, Wood JS, Cain TD, Marmer DJ. Immune responses to varicella-zoster in the aged. *Arch Intern Med.* 1982;142(2):291-293.
16. Gharibo C, Kim C. Postherpetic neuralgia: an overview of the pathophysiology, presentation, and management. *Pain Medicine News.* 2011;8.
17. Fields HL, Rowbotham M, Baron R. Postherpetic neuralgia: irritable nociceptors and deafferentation. *Neurobiol Dis.* 1998;5(4):209-227.
18. Denny-Brown D. Pathologic features of herpes zoster: a note on "geniculate herpes." *Arch Neur Psych.* 1944;51(3):216.
19. Watson CPN, Deck JH, Morshead C, Van der Kooy D, Evans RJ. Post-herpetic neuralgia: further post-mortem studies of cases with and without pain. *Pain.* 1991;44(2):105-117.
20. Watson CPN, Morshead C, Van der Kooy D, Deck J, Evans RJ. Post-herpetic neuralgia: post-mortem analysis of a case. *Pain.* 1988;34(2):129-138.
21. Üçeyler N, Valet M, Kafke W, Tölle TR, Sommer C. Local and systemic cytokine expression in patients with postherpetic neuralgia. *PLoS One.* 2014;9(8):e105269.
22. Harpaz R, Ortega-Sanchez I, Seward J. Prevention of herpes zoster recommendations of the Advisory Committee on Immunization Practices (ACIP). *MMWR Recomm Rep.* 2008;6(57):1-30.
23. Klompas M, Kulldorff M, Vilk Y, Bialek SR, Harpaz R. Herpes zoster and postherpetic neuralgia surveillance using structured electronic data. *Mayo Clin Proc.* 2011;86(12):1146-1153.
24. Fashner J, Bell AL. Herpes zoster and postherpetic neuralgia: prevention and management. *Am Fam Physician.* 2011;83(12):1432-1437.
25. Nagasako EM, Johnson RW, Griffin DRJ, Dworkin RH. Rash severity in herpes zoster: correlates and relationship to postherpetic neuralgia. *J Am Acad Dermatol.* 2002;46(6):834-839.
26. Forbes HJ, Thomas SL, Smeeth L, et al. A systematic review and meta-analysis of risk factors for postherpetic neuralgia. *Pain.* 2016;157(1):30-54.
27. Lai YC, Yew YW. Risk of herpes zoster and family history: a meta-analysis of case-control studies. *Indian J Dermatol.* 2016;61(2):157-162.
28. Meysman P, De Neuter N, Bartholomeus E, et al. Increased herpes zoster risk associated with poor HLA-A immediate early 62 protein (IE62) affinity. *Immunogenetics.* 2018;70(6):363-372.
29. Schmader K, George LK, Burchett BM, Hamilton JD, Pieper CF. Race and stress in the incidence of herpes zoster in older adults. *J Am Geriatr Soc.* 1998;46(8):973-977.
30. Joon Lee T, Hayes S, Cummings DM, et al. Herpes zoster knowledge, prevalence, and vaccination rate by race. *J Am Board Fam Med.* 2013;26(1):45-51.
31. Yawn BP, Saddier P, Wollan PC, St Sauver JL, Kurland MJ, Sy LS. A population-based study of the incidence and complication rates of herpes zoster before zoster vaccine introduction. *Mayo Clin Proc.* 2007;82(11):1341-1349.
32. Gruver C, Guthmiller KB. Postherpetic neuralgia. In: *StatPearls* [Internet]. StatPearls Publishing; 2021 [cited 2021 May 1]. http://www.ncbi.nlm.nih.gov/books/NBK493198/
33. Bowsher D. Pathophysiology of postherpetic neuralgia: towards a rational treatment. *Neurology.* 1995;45(12 Suppl 8):S56-S57.
34. Nalamachu S, Morley-Forster P. Diagnosing and managing postherpetic neuralgia. *Drugs Aging.* 2012;29(11):863-869.
35. Gilden DH, Wright RR, Schneck SA, Gwaltney JM Jr, Mahalingam R. Zoster sine herpete, a clinical variant. *Ann Neurol.* 1994;35(5):530-533.
36. Wang T, Fei Y, Yao M, Tao J, Deng J, Huang B. Correlation between galectin-3 and early herpes zoster neuralgia and postherpetic neuralgia: a retrospective clinical observation. *Pain Res Manag.* 2020;2020.

37. Cao S, Li Y, Deng W, et al. Local brain activity differences between herpes zoster and postherpetic neuralgia patients: a resting-state functional MRI study. *Pain Physician*. 2017;20(5):E687-E699.
38. Alpay Kanitez N, Celik S, Bes C. Polyarthritis and its differential diagnosis. *Eur J Rheumatol*. 2019;6(4):167-173.
39. Forouhi NG, Wareham NJ. Epidemiology of diabetes. *Medicine*. 2014;42(12):698-702.
40. Nicholson B. Differential diagnosis: nociceptive and neuropathic pain. *Am J Manag Care*. 2006;12(9):7.
41. Gershon AA, Breuer J, Cohen JI, et al. Varicella zoster virus infection. *Nat Rev Dis Primers*. 2015;1(1):15016.
42. Lang P-O, Ferahta N. Recommandations pour le traitement et la prévention du zona et des douleurs associées chez la personne âgée. *Rev Med Interne*. 2016;37(1):35-42.
43. Weinberg A, Zhang JH, Oxman MN, et al. Varicella-Zoster virus–specific immune responses to herpes zoster in elderly participants in a trial of a clinically effective zoster vaccine. *J Infect Dis*. 2009;200(7):1068-1077.
44. Weinberg A, Lazar AA, Zerbe GO, et al. Influence of age and nature of primary infection on varicella-zoster virus–specific cell-mediated immune responses. *J Infect Dis*. 2010;201(7):1024-1030.
45. Obata H. Analgesic mechanisms of antidepressants for neuropathic pain. *Int J Mol Sci*. 2017;18(11):2483.
46. Argoff CE. Review of current guidelines on the care of postherpetic neuralgia. *Postgrad Med*. 2011;123(5):134-142.
47. Kim YH, Lee PB, Oh TK. Is magnesium sulfate effective for pain in chronic postherpetic neuralgia patients comparing with ketamine infusion therapy? *J Clin Anesth*. 2015;27(4):296-300.
48. Johnson RW, Rice ASC. Postherpetic neuralgia. *N Engl J Med*. 2014;371(16):1526-1533.

SECTION III

Special Populations

24

Pediatric Patient

Lindsey K. Xiong, Cassandra M. Armstead-Williams, and Sonja A. Gennuso

Introduction

Regional anesthesia in pediatric patients has recently gained popularity. It has a documented protective effect in reducing noxious surgical stress, provides superior analgesia, and reduces the minimum alveolar concentration of volatile anesthetic agents. Well-established evidence proves that inadequate analgesia in the neonate results in biobehavioral changes and modulates future pain responses in childhood. For example, former neonatal intensive care patients exposed to noxious stimuli demonstrate an exaggerated response to pain in the primary somatosensory cortex, and anterior cingulate cortex, and insult on functional magnetic resonance imaging studies. Regional anesthesia also facilities minimal airway instrumentation thus allowing a spontaneously breathing patient for some surgical procedures.[1] Table 24.1 outlines the advantages of regional anesthesia in children.

In addition to providing pain coverage with minimal to no opioid use, regional anesthesia is generally safe. These techniques should only be performed by specialized pediatric anesthesiologists. Mild sedation to general anesthesia is employed in pediatric regional anesthesia because children tend to be less cooperative than their adult counterparts.[2]

Advances in ultrasound technology have allowed practitioners to provide adequate postoperative pain relief, therefore reducing opioid consumption, the incidence of postoperative nausea and vomiting, and respiratory complications (Table 24.2). The French-Language Society of Pediatric Anesthesiologists (ADARPEF) published large prospective studies demonstrating the safety of regional anesthesia performed under general anesthesia in children. Complications are reported at a rate of 0.12% with a 95% confidence interval. In that percentage, complications were four times greater in children <6 months old receiving a caudal block (1.9% of 18 650 caudal blocks).[3,4]

Additional data from the Pediatric Regional Anesthesia Network registry and the UK National Pediatric Epidural Audit support a low incidence of complications of regional anesthesia in children. Common complications were related to catheter malfunctions such as disconnection, displacement, and disconnection. Other complications related to neuraxial anesthetic techniques were transient neurological defect (2.4 in 10 000) without permanent sequelae, two cases of epidural abscesses, one case of postdural puncture headache, and five cases of severe neuropathy/radiculopathy with resolution over a 10-month period.[5]

Technical Considerations of Ultrasound Use in Children

Safe performance of increased use of regional anesthesia in the pediatric population requires adequate integrated training in needling techniques and ultrasound imaging.[6]

TABLE 24.1 **ADVANTAGES OF REGIONAL ANESTHESIA IN CHILDREN**

Patient benefits	Decreased risk of postoperative apnea in premature infants
	Reduced MAC • Potentially decreased neurotoxicity • Reduced risk of general anesthesia • Smoother emergence
	Decreased stress hormonal response
	Reduced requirement for postoperative ventilator support
	Better postoperative pain management
	Decreased intraoperative blood loss
	Improved GI function and postoperative appetite
	Maintained hemodynamic stability: Up to 8 years of age
Hospital benefits	Reduced length of stay
	Faster discharge from first-stage recovery
	Reduced need for postoperative ventilatory support

Advantages are as compared to patients receiving generalized anesthesia.
Note: Adapted from NYSORA.com/foundations-of-regional-anesthesia/sub-specialities/pediatric-anestheisa.

High-frequency ultrasound probes of 10-15 MHz are recommended in children. The active transducer surface length should be between 25 and 30 mm. Nerve appearance can be variable; the nerve diameter and frequency and angle of the ultrasound beam can determine whether the nerve appears as a hypo- or hyperechoic structure. Generally, neural structures like plexuses that are more central and compact structures tend to generate more hypoechoic images. On the contrary, peripheral terminal nerves have a more hyperechoic appearance. The in-plane (IP) technique is preferred in pediatric regional anesthesia. This IP technique facilitates visualization of the entire length of the needle during block placement.[7]

Anatomical and Physiological Differences Between Pediatric and Adult Patients

Anatomical, physiological, and pharmacokinetic differences exist in neonates, infants, older children, and adults. Increased systemic absorption and accumulation of local anesthetics are more likely to occur in infants secondary to their increased cardiac output and immature hepatic function (Table 24.3).

TABLE 24.2 **ADVANTAGES OF ULTRASOUND USE IN PEDIATRIC REGIONAL ANESTHESIA**

More precise needle placement/reduced tissue damage
Decreased volume of local anesthetic
Visualization of anatomical variations and structures
Decreased need for a peripheral nerve stimulator
Allows for facial plane blocks
Higher block success rate
Faster block onset
No ionizing radiation

TABLE 24.3 **KEY DIFFERENCE BETWEEN PEDIATRIC AND ADULT ANATOMY AND PHYSIOLOGY**

Anatomical	Characteristics	Clinical Concerns
	Neonates: Spinal cord ends at L3 (adults at L1) Intercristal line is at L5-S1 (adults at L4-L5) Dural sac terminates at S3-S4 (adults at S2)	Increased risk of dural puncture when performing caudal anesthesia Perform spinal anesthesia below L4
	Shorter neural diameter Incomplete myelin sheath Less connective tissue around the endoneurium	Increased risk of prolonged motor block and early onset of both sensory and motor blocks
	Smaller, more superficial tendons, vessels, and nerves	Increased risk of injury to neural and surrounding structures
Physiological	**Characteristics**	**Clinical Concerns**
	Poor lumbar orthosympathetic component in children	Less risk of developing hypotension following neuraxial anesthesia
	Lower concentration of alpha-1-acid glycoprotein in babies <1 year Hepatic biotransformation of LA is decreased in babies <9 months	Increased risk of free concentration of local anesthetic in the serum following repeated doses and/or continuous infusions
	Higher cardiac output: • Higher amount of cardiac sodium-gated channels open • Higher systemic absorption	Higher risk of cardiac toxicity

Note: Adapted from BJA Education: General Principles of Regional Anesthesia in Children. Management of local anesthetic toxicity in children.

Local Anesthetics

Local anesthetics are lipid-soluble weak bases that work by binding the voltage-dependent sodium channel. This binding prevents effective depolarizing of the cell membrane and blocks conduction of afferent pain signals and efferent motor transmission. Local anesthetics also block potassium and calcium channels at higher concentrations.

Local anesthetics are classified as esters or amides. Ester local anesthetics are rapidly metabolized by plasma pseudocholinesterases, whereas amides require cytochrome P-450 enzymes from the liver for metabolism. The hepatic biotransformation necessary for amide local anesthetics is immature at birth. In contrast, plasma pseudocholinesterases are present in neonates.

Human serum albumin and alpha-1-acid glycoprotein (AGP) are two proteins in the blood to which local anesthetics bind. Although concentrations of AGP are low in the serum, it is the primary protein that binds local anesthetics. At birth, the concentration of AGP is low. Infants and neonates have a higher free fraction of local anesthetics than adults. This possibly increases their risk of systemic local anesthetic toxicity.

A rare and catastrophic life-threatening complication of local anesthetics is local anesthetic systemic toxicity (LAST). The majority of cases occur in infants with an incidence of 0.76-1.6:10 000. Early recognition of LAST is challenging because most often children receiving regional anesthesia are sedated or under general anesthesia. According to the ADARPEF study, one case of LAST resulted in convulsions. Similarly, the UK epidural audit reported two respiratory failures and one seizure.[8]

Rapid identification of LAST is necessary to avoid circulatory collapse and death. LAST causes acute neurological and cardiovascular manifestations (Table 24.4). Airway management,

TABLE 24.4 SYSTEMIC SIGNS OF LAST

Cardiovascular signs
Vasoconstriction at low concentrations
Vasodilation at high concentrations
Negative inotropic effect
Decreased myocardial contractility
Depressed rapid phase of depolarization of Purkinje fibers
Depressed spontaneous firing of sinoatrial node
Central nervous system signs
Auditory and visual disturbances
Light-headedness and dizziness
Tremors and muscle twitching
Seizures

oxygenation, ventilation, and life support are the initial steps of LAST treatment. Further treatment requires lipid resuscitation with the lipid emulsion Intralipid. Recent guidelines from The Society of Pediatric Anesthesia and the ESRA/ASRA joint committee limit the maximum cumulative amount of lipid resuscitation therapy to 10 mL/kg. Table 24.5 outlines the treatment of LAST in pediatric patients according to Society of Pediatric Anesthesia guidelines.

The local anesthetics of choice in pediatric regional anesthesia are levobupivacaine and ropivacaine. Amide local anesthetics tend to have greater lipid solubility, greater stability to hydrolysis, a longer duration of action, and a lower incidence of allergic reactions. ESRA/ASRA joint committee suggests the use of preservative-free intrathecal morphine or clonidine to improve both the duration of blocks and the quality of analgesia. For peripheral nerve blocks, alpha-2-agonists, clonidine and dexmedetomidine, improve postoperative analgesia compared with plain local anesthetic.[9]

Neuraxial Anesthesia in Children

Caudal and Epidural Anesthesia

Epidural analgesia can be achieved at the thoracic, lumbar, or caudal level. In addition to superior postoperative pain management, epidural analgesia is beneficial in lowering the amount

TABLE 24.5 SPA GUIDELINES: MANAGEMENT OF LAST IN PEDIATRIC PATIENTS

Cease injection of local anesthetic
Call for assistance
Give 100% oxygen, maintain airway, consider intubation
Give a benzodiazepine if seizures occur
Max of 1 µg/kg epinephrine to treat hypotension
Avoid beta-blockers, calcium channel blockers, propofol, and vasopressin
Administer 20% IV lipid emulsion 1.5 mg/kg over 1 minute
Begin IV infusion of 20% lipid emulsion at 0.25 mL/kg/min
Titrate the infusion to 0.5 mL/kg/min if cardiovascular stability is compromised
Repeat boluses of 20% lipid emulsion up to 4.5 mL/kg every 3-5 minutes until hemodynamic stability is achieved
Max dose should not exceed 10 mL/kg
Adhere to CPR/PALS/APLS guidelines
Maintain adequate sometimes prolonged chest compressions
Consider cardiopulmonary bypass/ECMO if spontaneous circulation does not occur after 6 minutes
Monitor/correct hypercarbia, hyperkalemia, acidosis

Note: Adapted from BJA Education: General Principles of Regional Anesthesia in Children. Management of local anesthetic toxicity in children: SPA guidelines.

of circulating stress hormones, facilitating weaning from mechanical ventilation, and enabling earlier ambulation. General considerations must be taken into account such as room temperature, minimizing heat loss, and monitoring of vital signs.

There are various anatomical differences that should be noted in children compared with adults. The conus medullaris is at L3 in neonates and infants. This is true until about 1 year old when the conus medullaris is at L1 as in adults. Children also have a more narrow and flat sacrum. The sacral plate does not ossify until around 8 years old. Younger children tend to have a more cephalic sacral hiatus, and the dural sac may end more caudally around S4 in children <1 year old. Neonates and infants have a proportionally smaller pelvis compared to adults. Therefore, Tuffier line, the imaginary line that stretches across the top of the iliac crests, corresponds to the L4-L5 or L5-S1 interspace in children as opposed to L3-L4 in adults. This makes this landmark appropriate for all pediatric patients.

Infants and neonates have double the amount of cerebrospinal fluid (CSF) at about 4 mL/kg compared to 2 mL/kg of the adult. The majority of CSF in a child is in the spinal canal. The nonmyelinated spinal cord of neonates allows a lower concentration of local anesthetic to be used to achieve analgesia.

Various formulas can be used to determine the depth of the epidural space from the skin in children. A rough estimate of the length from the skin to the epidural spaces is 1 mm/kg body weight. 0.05 multiplied by the weight in kilograms plus 0.8 will give an estimation of the depth in centimeters (cm). The depth in centimeters can also be estimated by the child's age in years. For example, depth (cm) is equal to 0.15 multiplied by age in years plus 1.

Analgesia can be obtained with a single injection of medications or a continuous infusion. Body weight is used to predict the spread of local anesthetic. A volume per weight dosage is therefore used (Table 24.6). For example, a dilute solution of local anesthetic can be used at a

TABLE 24.6 ASRA/ESRA RECOMMENDATIONS FOR A SINGLE INJECTION LA DOSE FOR NEURAXIAL ANESTHESIA AND PNB IN CHILDREN

Nerve Block	Drug and Contraction	Dose (mL/kg)
Upper limb	Ropivacaine 0.2%, bupivacaine, levobupivacaine 0.25%	0.5-1.5
Lower limb	Ropivacaine 0.2%, bupivacaine, levobupivacaine 0.25%	0.5-1.5
Facial plane blocks	Ropivacaine 0.2%, bupivacaine 0.25%	0.2-0.75
Caudal	Ropivacaine 0.2%, levobupivacaine 0.25%	0.5-1.2
Spinal	Weight <5 kg hyperisobaric bupivacaine 0.5% Weight 5-15 kg hyperisobaric bupivacaine 0.5% Weight > 15 kg hyperisobaric bupivacaine 0.5% Tetracaine 0.5%	1 0.4 0.3 0.5-1
Intrathecal adjuncts		
	Epinephrine 1:200 000	
	Fentanyl	2 μg/kg
	Preservative-free morphine	10-20 μg/kg
	Clonidine	1-2 μg/kg
PNB adjuncts		
	Clonidine	Minimally effective dose
	Dexmedetomidine	Minimally effective dose

dose of 1.0 mL/kg to a maximum volume of 20 mL at the caudal level. For children <20 kg, 0.5 mL/kg will achieve a sacral surgical level, 1.0 mL/kg will achieve a high lumbar surgical level, 1.25 mL/kg will achieve a low thoracic surgical level (NYSORA). 0.1% ropivacaine or 0.125% bupivacaine at a rate of 0.2 mg/kg/h for neonates and 0.4 mg/kg/h for older children for 48 hours has been proved as safe and effective analgesia and avoids cumulative toxicity.

Epinephrine, opioids, clonidine, and ketamine are well-studied adjuvants for epidural anesthesia in the pediatric population. 1:200 000 epinephrine is useful to decrease the systemic absorption rate of local anesthetic. It also possibly reveals inadvertent intravascular injection. Epidural opioids such as fentanyl and morphine prolong the duration of analgesia; however, they can result in nausea and vomiting, respiratory depression, itching, and urinary retention (Table 24.7). Therefore, opioid adjuvants appear to be more beneficial for monitored inpatients. For single injection caudal anesthesia, 2 μg/kg of fentanyl along with the local anesthetic solution is recommended. For continuous epidural infusions, 1-2 μg/mL of fentanyl along with 0.1% bupivacaine has shown success in children. Fentanyl should be avoided in neonatal epidural infusions. Pulse oximetry monitoring is recommended for opioid use in children secondary to the possibility of respiratory depression. 30-90 μg/kg of caudal morphine has been suggested and enhances the level of blockade because morphine is a hydrophilic molecule and spreads rostrally. An acceptable alternative to epidural opioids to prolong the duration of action of local anesthetics without unwanted side effects is clonidine. Clonidine stimulates the descending noradrenergic medullospinal pathways and inhibits the release of nociceptive neurotransmitters in the dorsal horn of the spinal cord. For a single-injection epidural, 1-5 μg/kg of clonidine has been effective. 0.1 μg/kg/h clonidine in epidural infusions is beneficial without causing hypotension and bradycardia. Finally, low doses of preservative-free ketamine enhance the analgesic effects of local anesthetics. 1 mg/kg of ketamine has been used as a sole epidural anesthetic. 0.23-0.5 mg/kg of ketamine have been added to single-injection epidural anesthetics without psychotomimetic effects. However, controversy exists surrounding the use of ketamine in neonates. It is unclear whether ketamine produces apoptotic neurodegeneration or is actually neuroprotective in the developing brain.

Spinal Anesthesia

Spinal anesthesia is most often used in preterm infants undergoing surgery for an inguinal hernia repair. However, it has been successfully used for a variety of procedures such as abdominal, urological, and orthopedic procedures in children. When considering spinal anesthesia for a child, important factors to take into consideration are the child's airway, length of the procedure, surgical site, and surgical position. A major contraindication for spinal anesthesia in a nonsedated child is a surgery what will be longer than 60 minutes. Other contraindications include children with ventricular shunts, poorly controlled seizures, severe anatomical deformities, systemic infection or infection at the puncture site, underlying coagulopathy, hemodynamic instability, and neuromuscular diseases.

TABLE 24.7 COMPLICATIONS OF EPIDURAL ANESTHESIA

Neurologic Injury	Epidural Hematoma	Infection
PDPH	Total spinal anesthesia	LAST
Pruritus	Nausea and vomiting	Urinary retention
Sedation	Respiratory depression	Hyperventilation

PDPH, postdural postural headache; LAST, local anesthetic systemic toxicity.

TABLE 24.8 SPINAL DOSING OF 0.5% BUPIVACAINE IN CHILDREN <10 KG

Dose (mg/kg)	Age (months)	Weight (kg)
1	1	3
0.8	2	4
0.6	3	5
0.4	>4	6

For children that weigh <10 kg, 0.5-1 mg/kg of 0.5% bupivacaine is used for spinal anesthesia. Possible additives are an epinephrine wash, 1 μg/kg clonidine, or 10 μg/kg morphine (for cardiac surgery). Typical doses for 0.5% bupivacaine are listed in Table 24.8.

Prior to spinal placement, general considerations should be taken into account based on the patient's age and if sedation/general anesthesia will be used in conjunction with a spinal anesthetic. For example, the OR should be warmed and heating lamps and/or warming blankets may be used to preserve the infant's temperature. Prior to block placement, standard monitoring devices such as the blood pressure cuff, electrocardiogram, and pulse oximeter should be placed. If a eutectic mixture of local anesthetic cream is used, the risk of methemoglobinemia must be considered for very small preterm neonates.

Spinal placement can be accomplished in the sitting or lateral position. An assistant is necessary to hold the child in place. If the sitting position is the position of choice, care must be taken to avoid neck flexion, which could cause an airway obstruction in infants. Neck flexion does not assist the placement of the spinal block in infants. Tuffier line, the imaginary line that stretches across the top of the iliac crests, corresponds to the L4-L5 or L5-S1 interspace in infants. However, in older children, this area corresponds to L3-L4 interspace as in adults. The midline approach is generally recommended; a short 22- or 25-gauge spinal needle is often used. The correct dose of spinal local anesthetic should be calculated and prepared in an insulin syringe because the total dose of local anesthetic must be taken into account. This volume includes the volume corresponding to the hub of the needle. Children have a soft ligament flavor. The dura may not have the characteristic feel as the adult dura has once it is penetrated. Local anesthetic drugs may be administered slowly once clear CSF is exiting the needle. Once the medication is injected, avoid lifting the infant's lower limbs and the Trendelenburg position as this can result in total spinal anesthesia. In children over 2 years old, the Bromage scale can be used to assess the block. For example, if the patient has free movement of the knees and feet, no block is present. A partial block will result in free movement of the feet with isolated knee flexion. If the patient is unable to flex the knees but can flex the feet, this is an almost complete block. A complete block results in the inability to move the feet or legs. The pinprick or response to cold stimuli can be used to assess the block in infants. The anesthetist should observe changes in ventilation rate and pattern to determine the level of blockade. Table 24.9 covers adverse effects of spinal anesthesia in children.

Peripheral Nerve Blocks in Children

Head and Neck Blocks

Head and neck blocks are sensory nerve blocks that are increasing in popularity because of their safety profile, postoperative analgesic effects, and ease to place.

Supraorbital and supratrochlear nerves (V1 division of the trigeminal nerve)

V1 of the trigeminal nerve (5th cranial nerve) gives rise to the supraorbital, supratrochlear, and ophthalmic nerves. V1 passes through the cranium at the superior orbital fissure before dividing into the frontal, lacrimal, and nasociliary nerves. The supraorbital and supratrochlear nerves are both frontal nerve branches that pass through the supraorbital and supratrochlear notches. These nerves are responsible for the innervation of the frontal scalp, forehead, medial upper eye, and the nasal bridge. Supraorbital and supratrochlear nerve blocks are indicated for procedures at or cephalic to the eyebrow and upper eyelid region. These procedures include ventriculoperitoneal shunt placement, Ommaya reservoir placement in neonates, skin lesions of the scalp, and midline skin procedures.

Following induction, the supraorbital foramen is located by palpating the midline of the orbital rim. This location correlates to the midpoint of the pupil. The distance of the infraorbital foramen from the midline is about 21 mm plus 0.5 multiplied by the age in years. Cleanse the skin. Advance the needle through the skin until bone is contacted. Withdraw the needle about 1 mm, and check for a negative aspiration. Then inject 0.5-2 mL of local anesthetic (0.25% bupivacaine with 1:200 000 epinephrine). Apply pressure to the area to spread local anesthetic and prevent formation of a hematoma. Although rare, complications of this block are intravascular injection, hematoma, and trauma to the eye globe.

Infraorbital nerve (V2 division of the trigeminal nerve)

The infraorbital nerve is a branch of the maxillary nerve. It passes through the infraorbital foramen before dividing into the inferior palpebral, external nasal, and superior labial nerves. V2 supplies sensation to the lower eyelid and orbital floor, the upper lip, tip of the nose, and a portion of the nasal septum. The infraorbital block is useful for patients undergoing cleft lip repair, nasal septum repair, and endoscopic sinus surgery.[10]

Two different techniques can be used to block the infraorbital nerve. The first is the extraoral approach. The infraorbital foramen is palpated on the floor of the orbital rim. A 27-gauge needle is advanced through this foramen. After negative aspiration, up to 1 mL of local anesthetic is placed into the area. Following removal of the needle, apply pressure for 1 minute.

The second technique is the intramural approach. At the first premolar tooth, a needle is advanced through the buccal mucosa in the direction of the infraorbital foramen. A 70° bend in the needle facilitates passing the needle on the maxillary process. Aspirate before injecting up to 1 mL of local anesthetic to the area. Place a finger externally at the infraorbital foramen to prevent penetration of the globe. Sensation to this area will be numb for several hours. Therefore, prevention should be in place to reduce biting the upper lip.

Greater palatine nerve (V2)

The mucous membrane of the hard palate and gums are innervated by the greater palatine nerve. This is a common block for cleft palate repair. The greater palatine nerve arises from the pterygopalatine ganglion, passes through the greater palatine foramen, and lies in a groove of the hard palate. Following induction, the patient is positioned supine with the need in a neutral midline position. A bite block keeps the mouth open. The palatine foramen is medial and anterior to the first molar. Aspiration and injection of 1 mL of local anesthetic in the mucosa are performed using a 27-gauge needle.

V3 mandibular division of the trigeminal nerve

V3 supplies sensation to portions of the temporoparietal scalp, lower lip, and lower jaw. The mental nerve exits the mental foramen at the level of the midline in line with the supraorbital and infraorbital foramina. It is the most targeted nerve in children. Following induction of general anesthesia, a 27-gauge needle is directed at the level of the lower incisor toward the infraorbital foramen. After negative aspiration, 1.7 mL is injected. In order to block the lateral scalp, 1-2 mL of local anesthetic is deposited at the midpoint between the pinna and the angle of the eye to block the auriculotemporal nerve.

Greater occipital nerve

Cervical root C2 generates the greater occipital nerve. This nerve innervates the posterior portions of the scalp. This block is useful for analgesia of the scalp for posterior fossa surgery and chronic occipital neuralgia. Following induction, this nerve block is performed by palpating the occipital protuberance. The occipital artery runs inferior and lateral to the occipital protuberance. Once the artery is identified via palpation, a 27-gauge needle is advanced lateral to the artery. Following negative aspiration, 1.5-2 mL of 0.25% bupivacaine with 1:200 000 epinephrine is injected.

The ultrasound can also be used to perform a greater occipital nerve block. The C1 vertebra spinous process is identified. Move caudal to identify the bifid C2 vertebra. Rotate a linear probe by 90°, and scan laterally to identify the greater occipital nerve running along the obliques wapitis muscle. Using a 27-gauge needle, aspirate and inject 2 mL of local anesthetic solution using an in plane approach.

Greater auricular nerve (superficial cervical plexus)

The superficial cervical plexus innervates the posterior auricular area, lateral scalp, anterior-lateral skin of the neck, and the parotid gland. It is derived from C2-C4 nerve roots. At the level of the cricoid, it wraps around the sternocleidomastoid (SCM) and divides into four branches: great auricular, lesser occipital, supraclavicular, and transverse cervical nerves. Blockade of the superficial cervical plexus provides analgesia for otoplasty, thyroid surgery, tympanomastoid surgery, and procedures for the anterior neck. Following induction, a line is drawn from Chassaignac tubercle at C6 to the posterior border of the clavicular head of the SCM. A 27-gauge needle with a 60° bend is advanced along the posterior border of the SCM. Following negative aspiration, up to 3 mL of local anesthetic (1-3 mL of 0.25% bupivacaine with epinephrine 1:200 000) is deposited. This block may be accompanied by Horner syndrome, which is unequal pupil size, eyelid drooping, raising of the lower eyelid, and light-colored iris. Additional complications that may arise are intravascular injection, blockage of the deep cervical plexus, recurrent laryngeal nerve paralysis, unilateral phrenic nerve paralysis, and hematoma.[11]

Nerve of Arnold

The auricular branch of the vagus nerve is the nerve of Arnold. It supplies sensory innervation to the lower half of the tympanic membrane and the auditory canal. This block provides analgesia for myringotomy. Following induction, 0.5-1 mL of local anesthetic is injected into the cartilage of the posterior tragus.

Upper Extremity Pediatric Blocks

The brachial plexus supplies nerves of the upper extremity. The plexus is derived from ventral rami of C5-C8 and part of the ventral ramus of T1. Ultrasound guidance should be employed for these blocks. 0.5-1 mL/kg of bupivacaine or ropivacaine can be used safely as well as dexmedetomidine to prolong the nerve blocks. The most common approaches to the brachial plexus in children are the interscalene, supraclavicular, infraclavicular, and axillary blocks. The interscalene block is rarely used in younger children because of limited indications and increased incidence of complications. Complications of upper extremity blocks include hematoma, intramural injection, intravascular injection, and pneumothorax (with the exception of the axillary block).[12]

TABLE 24.9 COMPLICATIONS OF SPINAL ANESTHESIA IN CHILDREN

Hypotension[a]	Bradycardia
PDPH[b]	Transient radicular symptoms
Total spinal anesthesia	

[a]Hypotension is uncommon in children. However, if a fluid bolus is needed, 10 mL/kg can be given.
[b]0.3 mL/kg of blood is used for an epidural blood patch for persistent PDPH in children.

Interscalene block

This block provides excellent analgesia for older children and teenagers undergoing shoulder surgery and surgery of the proximal humerus and lateral two-thirds of the clavicle. The ultrasound probe is oriented at in the transverse plane at the level of the cricoid cartilage on the lateral border of the SCM muscle. Alternatively, the nerve bundle can be located at the supraclavicular view and then traced cranially to where C5, C6, and C7 nerve roots align like a "stop light." Complications of this block are potentially fatal. These complications include pneumothorax, vertebral artery injection, and intrathecal injection. Although ultrasound guidance reduces complications, a successful interscalene block is associated with Horner syndrome, recurrent laryngeal nerve block, and hemidiaphragmatic paralysis.

Supraclavicular block

The trunks and divisions of the brachial plexus are covered by the supraclavicular nerve block. The supraclavicular nerve block is indicated for surgical procedures of the upper arm. This portion of the brachial plexus is located in the supraclavicular fossa lateral and superficial to the subclavian artery. Note that the first rip will be inferior and medial to the brachial plexus, and the lung pleura is usually within 2 cm of the plexus. Complications of this block include pneumothorax, intraneural, and intravascular injection.[11]

Infraclavicular block

The infraclavicular nerve block blocks the brachial plexus at the level of the cords. It is useful for surgical procedures below the elbow. The pectoralis major and pectoralis minor muscles are located superficial to the cords, and they will run medial and inferior to the coracoid process of the scapula. The axillary vessels are deep to the cords. The medial cord is between the axillary artery and vein, and the posterior cord runs deep to the artery. Complications of this nerve block are pneumothorax and puncture of vascular structures.[12]

Lower Extremity Blocks

Femoral block

The femoral nerve is formed by the dorsal rami of L2-L4. After leaving the lumbar plexus, it runs inferior to the inguinal ligament and superficial to the iliopsoas muscle. It is lateral to the femoral artery and vein. It provides sensation to the anterior and medial thigh, and parts of the femur, hip, and knee joint. The femoral nerve block is therefore useful to provide analgesia for hip and femur fractures, patellar injuries, and anterior thigh injuries. Complications of the femoral nerve block include hematoma formation, intravascular and intraneural injection, and infection.[13]

Saphenous block

The saphenous nerve is a cutaneous branch of the femoral nerve. It supplies sensation to the knee and medial lower leg. If blocked proximally at the adductor canal, it provides analgesia to the knee joint. If the saphenous is blocked distally, analgesia is provided to the medial lower leg.

Sciatic block

The sciatic nerve arises in the sacral plexus and is composed of nerve fibers from L4-S3. A sciatic nerve block provides analgesia to the posterior thigh, lower leg, and foot. The sciatic nerve can be blocked in the subgluteal region and in the popliteal fossa.

Complications of the sciatic nerve block are the same for the femoral nerve block.

Trunk Blocks

Transversus abdominal plane (TAP) block

The TAP block provides analgesia to the anterior abdominal wall. The transversus abdominis plane contains thoracolumbar nerve roots and is located between the internal oblique and transversus abdominis muscle layers. The TAP block is indicated for postoperative pain control of abdominal incisions. Complications of the TAP block are infection, LAST, bowel puncture, and intravascular injection.

Ilioinguinal/iliohypogastric nerve block

This block provides postoperative analgesia of the inguinal region and scrotum. It provides superior pain relief following hydrocelectomy, inguinal hernia repair, and orchiopexy. Complications of this nerve block include infection, LAST, bowel puncture, intravascular injection, and femoral nerve palsy.

Rectus sheath block

The rectus sheath is formed by the aponeuroses of the external oblique, internal oblique, and transversus abdominis muscles and encases the rectus abdominis muscle with anterior and posterior sheaths. This block is useful for midline abdominal incisions such as in umbilical hernia repair and laparoscopic procedures. Complications include infection, LAST, bowel puncture, and intravascular injection.[14]

REFERENCES

1. Suresh S, Schaldenbrand K, Wallis B, De Oliveira GS. Regional anaesthesia to improve pain outcomes in paediatric surgical patients: a qualitative systematic review of randomized controlled trials. *Br J Anaesth.* 2014;113(3):375-390.
2. Liu Y, Seipel C, Lopez ME, et al. A retrospective study of multimodal analgesic treatment after laparoscopic appendectomy in children. *Paediatr Anaesth.* 2013;23(12):1187-1192.
3. Ecoffey C, Lacroix F, Giaufré E, Orliaguet G, Courrèges P; Association des Anesthésistes Réanimateurs Pédiatriques d'Expression Française (ADARPEF). Epidemiology and morbidity of regional anesthesia in children: a follow-up one-year prospective survey of the French-Language Society of Paediatric Anaesthesiologists (ADARPEF). *Paediatr Anaesth.* 2010;20(12):1061-1069.
4. Giaufré E, Dalens B, Gombert A. Epidemiology and morbidity of regional anesthesia in children: a one-year prospective survey of the French-Language Society of Pediatric Anesthesiologists. *Anesth Analg.* 1996;83(5):904-912.
5. Suresh S, Long J, Birmingham PK, De Oliveira GS. Are caudal blocks for pain control safe in children? An analysis of 18,650 caudal blocks from the Pediatric Regional Anesthesia Network (PRAN) database. *Anesth Analg.* 2015;120(1):151-156.
6. Bosenberg A. Regional anaesthesia in children: an update. *South Afr J Anaesth Analg.* 2013;19(6):282-288.
7. Boretsky KR. Regional anesthesia in pediatrics: marching forward. *Curr Opin Anaesthesiol.* 2014;27(5):556-560.
8. Llewellyn N, Moriarty A. The national pediatric epidural audit. *Paediatr Anaesth.* 2007;17(6):520-533.
9. Richman JM, Liu SS, Courpas G, et al. Does continuous peripheral nerve block provide superior pain control to opioids? A meta-analysis. *Anesth Analg.* 2006;102(1):248-257.
10. Chiono J, Raux O, Bringuier S, et al. Bilateral suprazygomatic maxillary nerve block for cleft palate repair in children: a prospective, randomized, double-blind study versus placebo. *Anesthesiology.* 2014;120(6):1362-1369.
11. Kapral S, Krafft P, Eibenberger K, Fitzgerald R, Gosch M, Weinstabl C. Ultrasound-guided supraclavicular approach for regional anesthesia of the brachial plexus. *Anesth Analg.* 1994;78(3):507-513.
12. Marhofer P, Sitzwohl C, Greher M, Kapral S. Ultrasound guidance for infraclavicular brachial plexus anaesthesia in children. *Anaesthesia.* 2004;59(7):642-646.
13. Marhofer P, Harrop-Griffiths W, Willschke H, Kirchmair L. Fifteen years of ultrasound guidance in regional anaesthesia: part 2—Recent developments in block techniques. *Br J Anaesth.* 2010;104(6):673-683.
14. Kaye AD, Green JB, Davidson KS, et al. Newer nerve blocks in pediatric surgery. *Best Pract Res Clin Anaesthesiol.* 2019;33(4):447-463.

25

Acute Pain Management Considerations in the Older Adult

Sarahbeth R. Howes, Tyson Hamilton, Elyse M. Cornett, and Alan David Kaye

Introduction

Many treatments for chronic pain in the older adult are not well studied related to limitations of the patient population. Limitations include society's stigma in assuming pain is a part of aging, frail patient population with presumably multiple comorbidities, and polypharmacy associated with treating comorbidities.[1,2] Nevertheless, pain is reported in 60% independent and 80% dependent long-term geriatric patients.[3] Despite a high incidence in the elderly, pain is most likely underreported between the assumption that pain is related to aging, communication barriers in patient-physician exams or provider-staff assessments, poorly identified pain attributing it to another preexisting comorbidity, cognitive impairment, patient anxiety to report pain as it may reflect the progression of current, preexisting disease or fear of addiction to prescribed medications, and physician fear of prescribing due to polypharmacy.[1-4]

The World Health Organization (WHO) current guidelines for treating pain includes a stepwise approach, beginning with nonopioids for mild pain, adding a weak opioid for moderate to severe pain, or replacing it with a strong opioid if pain relief is not achieved, classifying the pain as severe.[3,5] Pain in the geriatric population can be thought of in two ways: cancer-related vs non–cancer-related.[3] Opioid use is efficacious for cancer-related pain; however, pain management options for non–cancer-related pain are small.[3] Geriatric non–cancer-related pain is most identified as arthritic pain, such as osteoarthritis and rheumatoid arthritis.[3] In addition, postherpetic neuralgia (PHN) and chronic systemic disease-induced pain are also common causes.[1,3] The pathophysiology behind the pain produced by each of these conditions is different, yet the options for treating pain remain nonetheless the same.

In addition to the different modalities of pain, there are several limitations of elderly patients. The pharmacodynamics and pharmacokinetics in the older adult are heavily researched, all of which show how aging impacts the ability to metabolize common analgesic medications.[1] Given the prevalence of diabetes and heart conditions, it is difficult to combat pain management with current medications, like nonsteroidal anti-inflammatory drugs (NSAIDs), which are associated with cardiovascular and renal complications.[1] Not to mention the overall increase in depression and dementia within this age group, whose neuronal pathways are newly identified as overlapping with pain neuronal pathways.[6]

Evidence shows a relationship between chronic pain and a patient's outlook in management, especially if that outlook is bleak.[1] For example, a study showed patients receiving a total knee arthroscopy (TKA) who underwent a one-time perioperative Acceptance and Commitment Therapy (ACT) workshop decreased opioid use and achieved pain relief faster than the control group who did traditional standard of care treatment.[7] Group-based education and exercise are not inferior to individualized cognitive functional therapy in pain reduction.[8] Current international guidelines for chronic low back pain (CLBP) suggest psychological therapy

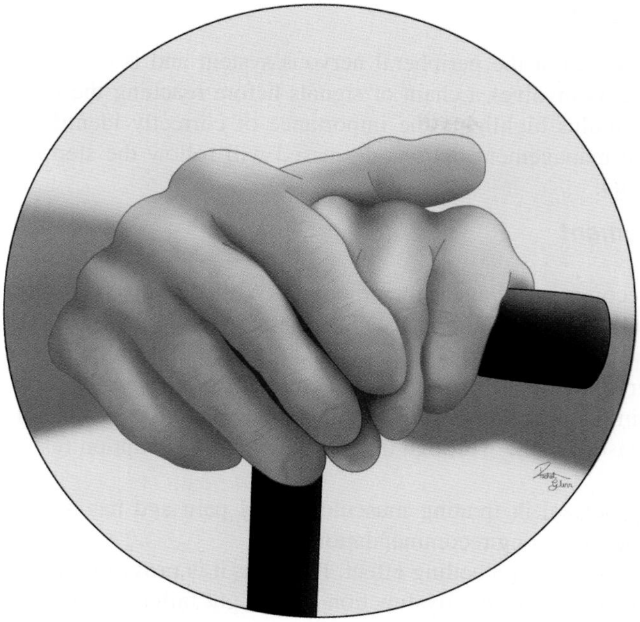

FIGURE 25.1 Elderly patient using the physical support of a walking cane due to uncontrolled pain. (Drawing by Rachel Glenn, medical illustrator.)

in addition to exercise.[9] With this evidence, geriatric pain is best relieved when using a multimodal, biopsychosocial approach[1,8,10] (Fig. 25.1).

Treatment/Management

Importance of the Basics: Proper History and Physical

Treatment management must first begin with a proper history and physical to best identify and characterize the type of pain ailing the patient. Lack of knowledge on how to evaluate pain in older adults, especially those who are dependent on staff-provider communications because of assisted living or long-term care facilities, can be a major hindrance in correctly assessing the type of pain.[4] The likelihood of this pain resulting from current comorbid conditions or previous surgeries is high.[1] Authentic patient history is important when considering pharmacological treatment options, which will be limited by other medical conditions and possible drug interactions. A good quality physical provides background when considering roles of other treatment teams, such as physical therapy, occupational therapy, psychological intervention, or interventional therapies. From there, the physician can identify the patient's attitude regarding pain and align treatment options with goals of care.

Nonpharmacological Management

When considering rehabilitation, it is important to understand rehabilitation programs are utilized with the goal to restore function; however, if restoration is unlikely, the treatment can be focused on improving patient disability.[1] For instance, it is well known from studies dating back to the 1990s that strength-training exercises can improve pain and mobility in patients with osteoarthritis.[1] Properly educated and supervised patients are more likely to adhere to recommended training, with encouragement and group exercises increasing positive social interactions and overall hopefulness toward possible pain resolution.[1] Physical therapy has proven to block the transduction of pain signals from the peripheral nervous system to the central nervous system (CNS).[1] Providers must contemplate these nonpharmacological, lower-risk treatment modalities and consider their ability to compliment pain regression through a biopsychosocial approach, perhaps even before considering more risky pharmacological options.

Pharmacological Management

Physiologically, pain begins as a signal at the peripheral nervous system and is eventually transduced to the CNS.[1] This process involves a chain of signals before reaching the CNS. Their individualized activation stimulus highlights the importance of correctly identifying the type of pain. Pharmacological management options discussed will follow the stepwise approach currently advised by WHO.

Mild pain: nonopioid management

Acetaminophen

Acetaminophen is the first-line recommended agent for mild pain. While the mechanism of action of acetaminophen is not fully understood, it is accepted that acetaminophen works at both the central and peripheral levels.[5] Centrally it is thought that acetaminophen inhibits pain by stimulating the descending serotoninergic pathways.[5] Molecularly it is thought that acetaminophen acts specifically within the peroxidase site of bifunctional enzyme prostaglandin H synthase (PGSH), cyclooxygenase (COX).[5] Through this, the enzymatic disruption results in peripheral inhibition of COX.[5]

Acetaminophen is particularly helpful in treating musculoskeletal pain and has a good safety profile (high quality of evidence, strong recommendation).[10]

In contrast to opioids, acetaminophen has a ceiling effect; however, it is proven up to 4 g of the drug does not result in evidence of hepatic dysfunction or outright failure.[3] Important considerations for use include recognizing acetaminophen, like most drugs, is metabolized by the liver. It is recognized that an aged liver may delay the clearance of drugs.[10] Of note, acetaminophen use is an absolute contraindication in patients with liver failure.[10]

In contrast to NSAIDs, acetaminophen does not have any anti-inflammatory properties, strictly acting as an analgesic and antipyretic.[3,5] This disadvantage is detrimental given that the top geriatric non–cancer-causing pain conditions in the elderly are arthritic inflammatory diseases like osteoarthritis and rheumatoid arthritis.[11] Further research also suggests that uncontrolled inflammatory pain can result in a cycle of pain due to the induced neurogenic inflammation. Direct tissue injury, as seen with "wear and tear" diseases like osteoarthritis, results in inflammation mediators through the conversion of arachidonic acid into prostaglandins and stimulation of nociceptors that transmit the brain to the CNS.[3,12]

NSAIDs

Nonsteroidal anti-inflammatory drugs (NSAIDs) can be used in addition or independent from acetaminophen. NSAIDs inhibit the conversion of arachidonic acid to prostaglandin H_2 (PGH2), by inhibiting PGHS (COX). Thus, it prevents the development of COX and subsequent prostaglandins (D series), prostacyclin, and thromboxanes from synthesizing.[5] This mechanism of action is the reason NSAIDs are characterized as analgesic, antipyretic, and anti-inflammatory drugs.[5]

NSAID use in the elderly is limited related to their unwanted side effects. Side effects vary based on the specificity of NSAIDs. Since COX has two isoenzymes, COX-1 (PGHS-1) and COX-2 (PGHS-2), NSAIDs can be classified as nonselective or selective.[1,5] Nonselective NSAIDs inhibit both COX-1 and COX-2, while selective NSAIDs inhibit COX-2. Both are associated with cardiovascular risks, renal toxicity, and GI side effects ranging from mild dyspepsia, nausea, diarrhea, to severe mucosal damage in the GI tract associated with increased morbidity and mortality.[1] Selective COX-2 NSAIDs can decrease the incidence of unwanted GI side effects.[1]

Moderate pain: nonopioid management + weak opioid

There is a lack of clinical evidence regarding which opioid would be most safe, efficacious, and tolerable in addition to acetaminophen use in compliance with WHO's stepwise approach because of lack of RCT with elderly patients.[2] This lack of evidence further supports the importance of physician-based clinical judgment.[2] Opioid use in the elderly is sometimes avoided by clinicians due to misbelief in propagating delirium.[3] Multiple studies have countered that misbelief proving that, in fact, undertreated pain worsens delirium in the elderly or actually propagates cognitive decline.[3,6,13] Research also argues that chronic pain can be an attributable risk factor for early death.[13] Thus, opioid is recommended for moderate to severe pain or pain that reduces quality of life.[10]

The following are considered weak opioids: codeine, dihydrocodeine, tramadol, and tapentadol.[1,2,14] Weak opioids used in combination with acetaminophen include hydrocodone, propoxyphene, and oxycodone.[10] International guidelines recognize low-dose morphine or oxycodone for WHO's step II ladder.[15]

Codeine

Codeine is a weak acting opioid and is less associated with hip fractures when compared to tramadol.[16]

Dihydrocodeine

Dihydrocodeine is derivative of codeine, with analgesic effects similar to codeine if not twice as potent to codeine and tramadol, although research data are limited.[17,18]

Tramadol

Tramadol is a weak opioid, and there is a paucity of studies conducted among elderly patients. It is advantageous over NSAIDs since its perceived risk of cardiovascular and GI side effects were less.[16] It also has advantages over stronger opioids since it has a lower risk of respiratory depression.[16] The known side effects involve reducing the seizure threshold with patients using other serotonergic drugs and/or a history of seizures.[1] Studies also suggest a correlation between tramadol and an increased risk in falls. However, research is limited.[16]

Tapentadol

Tapentadol is a newer weak opioid, whose advantages show negligible analgesic active metabolites and lesser GI side effects. However, current released research reveals poorly conducted trials without significant evidence to support its use over other well-studied opioids.[2]

Hydrocodone

Hydrocodone is metabolized into two metabolites: hydromorphone and dihydrocodeine.[19] Hydrocodone's use is limited given its combination with acetaminophen, and the maximum recommended acetaminophen dose is 4 g/day.[20] However, as of 2014, the FDA restricted each dose of hydrocodone maximum dose of 325 mg of acetaminophen per dose.[21]

Propoxyphene (Dextropropoxyphene)

Significant side effects in the elderly led to its market withdrawal did not change the chronic pain management in the geriatric population.[2]

Oxycodone

Oral oxycodone was titrated to assess the safety of utilizing smaller doses when smaller doses (acting as a weaker opioid) were preferred and deemed successful in patients with swallowing difficulties or whose overall risk of accidental overdose was increased.[1]

Morphine

Low-dose morphine is recognized as a possible implication to pain management for moderate pain.[15] Liquid morphine was observed to reduce non–cancer-related pain in patients with an average age of 75.[2] Morphine is metabolized to an active product, morphine 6-glucuronide, and therefore, reduced renal function in an elderly patient must be evaluated. Further research is needed.

Severe pain: nonopioid management + strong opioid

The preferred evidence-based add-ons for step III opioid therapy include morphine, fentanyl, oxycodone, and buprenorphine.[2] A study evaluating long-term opioid use showed improvement in social engagement and functional status in nursing home residents.[1] Pain, specifically chronic pain greatly limiting the quality of life, is associated with an increased risk of depression.[13] Improvement in pain treatment is proven to improve sleep, implying that pain, sleep, and depression in nursing home patients can be resolved with proper pain management.[6]

Fentanyl

This is a short-acting synthetic opioid that is effective in both cancer-related pain and chronic pain. As of 2011, intranasal fentanyl was approved for acute breakthrough pain in cancer patients.[22] In a study comparing oral transmucosal fentanyl with intranasal fentanyl among cancer patients, intranasal fentanyl was superior.[2] In an open-label study comparing intranasal fentanyl to IV hydromorphone, intranasal fentanyl was very likely noninferior to IV hydromorphone.[22] Intranasal fentanyl is fast acting and thus results in faster pain relief to cancer patients presenting to the emergency department with acute pain. [22] This patient population also was randomized and included older adults, >65 year old.[22]

Buprenorphine

Transdermal buprenorphine was recently explored and found to have better benefit older patients >65 year old vs younger patients.[1] Buprenorphine is a partial agonist with kappa antagonist action. Additionally, buprenorphine was explored in patients with chronic comorbidities and transdermal patches were deemed satisfactory and effective in alleviating their pain.[2] The ease in use of this medication proved increase in patient compliance and was associated with decrease in risk of toxicities with conventional application.[2] Another added benefit of buprenorphine transdermal system (TDS) is not requiring adjustment for renal insufficiency due to its hepatic clearance. A noted side effect among patients with depression using TDS exhibited worsening depressive symptoms resulting in 52% of patients withdrawing from the study compared to acetaminophen.[23] In a randomized, placebo-controlled trial, nursing home patients with advance dementia using TDS withdrew related to increased psychiatric and neurologic adverse events.[23] The same study also showed decrease in day time activities within the first week of TDS use in patients with advanced dementia.[23] Buprenorphine is the only opioid demonstrating a ceiling effect for respiratory depression.

The use of opioids in cancer pain

The criteria for selecting analgesics for pain treatment in the elderly include, but are not limited to, overall efficacy, overall side-effect profile, onset of action, drug interactions, abuse potential, and practical issues, such as cost and availability of the drug, and the severity and type of pain (nociceptive, acute/chronic, etc.). At any given time, the order of choice in the decision-making process can change. This consensus is based on evidence-based literature (extended data are not included and chronic, extended-release opioids are not covered). There are various driving factors relating to prescribing medication, including availability of the compound and cost, which may, at times, be the main driving factor. The transdermal formulation of buprenorphine is available in most European countries, particularly those with high opioid usage, except for France; however, the availability of the sublingual formulation of buprenorphine in Europe is limited, as it is marketed in only a few countries, including Germany and Belgium. The opioid patch is experimental at present in the United States and the sublingual formulation has dispensing restrictions, and therefore, its use is limited. It is evident that the population pyramid is upturned. Globally, there is going to be an older population that needs to be cared for in the future. This older population has expectations in life, in that a retiree is no longer an individual who decreases their lifestyle activities. The "baby boomers" in their 60s and 70s are "baby zoomers"; they want to have a functional active lifestyle. They are willing to make trade-offs regarding treatment choices and understand that they may experience pain, providing that can have increased quality of life and functionality. Therefore, comorbidities—including cancer and noncancer pain, osteoarthritis, rheumatoid arthritis, and PHN—and patient functional status need to be taken carefully into account when addressing pain in the elderly. WHO step III opioids are the mainstay of pain treatment for cancer patients, and morphine has been the most used for decades. In general, high level evidence data (Ib or IIb) exist, although many studies have included only few patients. Based on these studies, all opioids are considered effective in cancer pain management (although parts of cancer pain are not or only partially opioid sensitive), but no well-designed specific studies in the elderly cancer patient are available. Of the two opioids that are available in transdermal formulation, for example, fentanyl and buprenorphine, fentanyl is the most investigated, but based on published data, both seem to be effective, with low toxicity and good tolerability profiles, especially at low doses. The use of opioids in non-cancer–related pain: Evidence is growing that opioids are efficacious in noncancer pain (treatment data mostly level Ib or IIb), but need individual dose titration and consideration of the respective tolerability profiles. Again, no specific studies in the elderly have been performed, but it can be concluded that opioids have shown efficacy in noncancer pain, which is often due to diseases typical for an elderly population. When it is not clear which drugs and which regimes are superior in terms of maintaining analgesic efficacy, the appropriate drug should be chosen based on safety and tolerability considerations. Evidence-based medicine, which has been incorporated into best clinical practice guidelines, should serve as a foundation for the decision-making processes in patient care; however, in practice, the art of medicine is realized when we individualize care to the patient. This strikes a balance between the evidence-based medicine and anecdotal experience. Factual recommendations and expert opinion both have a value when applying guidelines in clinical practice. The use of opioids in neuropathic pain: The role of opioids in neuropathic pain has been under debate in the past but is nowadays more and more accepted; however, higher opioid doses are often needed for neuropathic pain than for nociceptive pain. Most of the treatment data are level II or III and suggest that incorporation of opioids earlier on might be beneficial. Buprenorphine shows a distinct benefit in improving neuropathic pain symptoms, which is considered a result of its specific pharmacological profile. The use of opioids in elderly patients with impaired hepatic and renal function: Functional impairment of excretory organs is common in the elderly, especially with respect to renal function. For all opioids except buprenorphine, half-life of the active drug and metabolites is increased in the elderly and in patients with renal dysfunction. It is, therefore, recommended that, except for buprenorphine, doses be reduced, a longer time interval be used between doses, and creatinine clearance be monitored. Thus, buprenorphine appears to be the top-line choice for opioid treatment in the elderly. Opioids and respiratory depression: Respiratory depression is a significant threat for opioid-treated patients with underlying pulmonary condition or receiving concomitant CNS drugs associated with hypoventilation. Not all opioids show equal effects on respiratory depression: buprenorphine is the only opioid demonstrating a ceiling for respiratory depression when used without other CNS depressants. The different features of opioids regarding respiratory effects should be considered when treating patients at risk for respiratory problems, therefore careful dosing must be maintained. Opioids and immunosuppression: Age is related to a gradual decline in the immune system: immunosenescence, which is associated with increased morbidity and mortality from infectious diseases, autoimmune diseases, and progression of cancer, and decreased efficacy of immunotherapy, such as vaccination. The clinical relevance of the immunosuppressant effects of opioids in the elderly is not fully understood; however, there are significant data that opioids suppress natural killer cells and pain itself may also cause immunosuppression. Providing adequate analgesia can be achieved without significant adverse events, opioids with minimal immunosuppressive characteristics should be used in the elderly. The immunosuppressive effects of most opioids are poorly described, and this is one of the problems in assessing true effect of the opioid spectrum, but there is some indication that higher doses of opioids correlate with increased immunosuppressant effects. Taking into consideration all the very limited available evidence from preclinical and clinical work, buprenorphine can be recommended, while morphine and fentanyl cannot. Safety and tolerability profile of opioids: The adverse event profile varies greatly between opioids. As the consequences of adverse events in the elderly can be serious, agents should be used that have a good tolerability profile (especially regarding CNS and gastrointestinal effects) and that are as safe as possible in overdose especially regarding effects on respiration. Slow dose titration helps to reduce the incidence of typical initial adverse events such as nausea and vomiting. Sustained release preparations, including transdermal formulations, increase patient compliance.

Adjuvant therapy

The three-step pain management ladder recommended by WHO encourages utilization of adjuvant therapy throughout all three tiers. This is important to recognize, as it further reiterates the importance of a multimodal, biosocial approach to pain management. Multiple studies mentioned provided evidence in a relationship between pain, depression, dementia, and sleep. Thus, highlighting the importance of a proper history and physical to identify all comorbid conditions that could be worsening pain conditions.[1,4,6,13,23] Effective advent therapy proven to improve pain in the older adult consists of TCAs, SSRIs, SNRIs, gabapentin, muscle relaxants, memantine, and low-dose naltrexone.[1,2,10] All these adjuvants are advised to be used with caution, each with its own unique side effects among the geriatric population. The goal of this section is to further emphasize the multimodal, biopsychosocial approach for pain management in the elderly, recognizing that all drugs are unique to the individual.[3,6,8,10]

Conclusion

Pain in the elderly is a complicated subject but has profound implications on the quality of life and functionality of these individuals. Without proper pain management, patients often report a variety of different comorbidities in addition to limited independence. Acute pain management in elderly patients requires that practitioners keep in mind the unique barriers and challenges that may present. Elderly patients often have CNS, liver, kidney, and other physical barriers to effective assessment and management but may also often have other challenges such as polypharmacy, changes in pain perception, and other pharmacokinetic changes. Therefore, in these patients, the pain assessment technique may require modification, and/or, alternative agents may be required in their treatment. With a proper understanding of these challenges, practitioners can help to achieve improved main control with appropriate use of treatment modalities and using a careful, multidisciplinary approach to management.

REFERENCES

1. Schwan J, Sclafani J, Tawfik VL. Chronic pain management in the elderly. *Anesthesiol Clin.* 2019;37(3):547-560.
2. Prostran M, Vujović KS, Vučković S, et al. Pharmacotherapy of pain in the older population: the place of opioids. *Front Aging Neurosci* [Internet]. 2016[cited 2021 Apr 29];8:144. https://www.ncbi.nlm.nih.gov/pmc/articles/PMC4909762/
3. Borsheski R, Johnson QL. Pain management in the geriatric population. *Mo Med.* 2014;111(6):508-511.
4. Resnick B, Boltz M, Galik E, et al. Pain assessment, management and impact among older adults in assisted living. *Pain Manag Nurs Off J Am Soc Pain Manag Nurses.* 2019;20(3):192-197.
5. Jóźwiak-Bebenista M, Nowak JZ. Paracetamol: mechanism of action, applications and safety concern. *Acta Pol Pharm.* 2014;71(1):11-23.
6. Blytt KM, Bjorvatn B, Husebo B, Flo E. Effects of pain treatment on sleep in nursing home patients with dementia and depression: a multicenter placebo-controlled randomized clinical trial. *Int J Geriatr Psychiatry.* 2018;33(4):663-670.

7. Dindo L, Zimmerman MB, Hadlandsmyth K, et al. Acceptance and commitment therapy for prevention of chronic post-surgical pain and opioid use in at-risk veterans: a pilot randomized controlled study. *J Pain Off J Am Pain Soc*. 2018;19(10):1211-1221.
8. O'Keeffe M, O'Sullivan P, Purtill H, Bargary N, O'Sullivan K. Cognitive functional therapy compared with a group-based exercise and education intervention for chronic low back pain: a multicentre randomised controlled trial (RCT). *Br J Sports Med*. 2020;54(13):782-789.
9. Recommendations | Low back pain and sciatica in over 16s: assessment and management | Guidance | NICE [Internet]. NICE; [cited 2021 May 3]. https://www.nice.org.uk/guidance/ng59/chapter/Recommendations#non-invasive-treatments-for-low-back-pain-and-sciatica
10. Kaye AD, Baluch A, Scott JT. Pain management in the elderly population: a review. *Ochsner J*. 2010;10(3):9.
11. Berenbaum F. Osteoarthritis as an inflammatory disease (osteoarthritis is not osteoarthrosis!). *Osteoarthritis Cartilage*. 2013;21(1):16-21.
12. Matsuda M, Huh Y, Ji R-R. Roles of inflammation, neurogenic inflammation, and neuroinflammation in pain. *J Anesth*. 2019;33(1):131-139.
13. Domenichiello AF, Ramsden CE. The silent epidemic of chronic pain in older adults. *Prog Neuropsychopharmacol Biol Psychiatry*. 2019;93:284-290.
14. Pharmacological management of chronic pain—BPJ 16 September 2008 [Internet]. [cited 2021 May 3]. https://bpac.org.nz/BPJ/2008/September/chronic.aspx
15. Luppi M. Randomized trial of low-dose morphine versus weak opioids in moderate cancer pain. [cited 2021 May 3]. https://core.ac.uk/reader/54012989?utm_source=linkout
16. Wei J, Lane NE, Bolster MB, et al. Association of tramadol use with risk of hip fracture. *J Bone Miner Res*. 2020;35(4):631-640.
17. Leppert W, Woroń J. Dihydrocodeine: safety concerns. *Expert Rev Clin Pharmacol*. 2016;9(1):9-12.
18. Leppert W. Dihydrocodeine as an opioid analgesic for the treatment of moderate to severe chronic pain. *Curr Drug Metab*. 2010;11(6):494-506.
19. Cone EJ, Heltsley R, Black DL, Mitchell JM, Lodico CP, Flegel RR. Prescription opioids. II. Metabolism and excretion patterns of hydrocodone in urine following controlled single-dose administration. *J Anal Toxicol*. 2013;37(8):486-494.
20. American Geriatrics Society Panel on the Pharmacological Management of Persistent Pain in Older Persons. Pharmacological management of persistent pain in older persons: pharmacological management of persistent pain in older persons. *J Am Geriatr Soc*. 2009;57(8):1331-1346.
21. Manchikanti L, Atluri S, Kaye AM, Kaye AD. Hydrocodone bitartrate for chronic pain. *Drugs Today Barc Spain 1998*. 2015;51(7):415-427.
22. Banala SR, Khattab OK, Page VD, Warneke CL, Todd KH, Yeung S-CJ. Intranasal fentanyl spray versus intravenous opioids for the treatment of severe pain in patients with cancer in the emergency department setting: a randomized controlled trial. *PLoS ONE [Internet]*. 2020 Jul 10 [cited 2021 May 3];15(7). https://www.ncbi.nlm.nih.gov/pmc/articles/PMC7351205/
23. Erdal A, Flo E, Aarsland D, et al. Tolerability of buprenorphine transdermal system in nursing home patients with advanced dementia: a randomized, placebo-controlled trial (DEP.PAIN.DEM). *Clin Interv Aging*. 2018;13:935-946.

26

Pregnant Patient

Kelly S. Davidson and Carmen Labrie-Brown

Introduction

Pregnant patients are a unique population requiring special consideration in regards to pain management for a number of reasons. When approaching management of pain in the parturient, one must consider the effect that a medication will have on the mother, the fetus and the pregnancy. The physiologic changes that occur during pregnancy can cause the patient pain prior to the onset of labor. The pain is usually musculoskeletal in nature and secondary to the body stretching and growing to accommodate the developing fetus.[1]

Labor itself is known to be a painful experience, however each woman experiences labor differently due to a multitude of factors including, cultural, social, psychological and physiologic factors.[2] Therefore, the approach to pain management during labor must be individualized for each patient based on their desires and expectations for their labor experience. For many women, labor and childbirth is the most intense pain they will experience in their entire life.[3] In this chapter, we will discuss the safety and efficacy of a variety of pain management techniques available for pregnant patients ranging from nonpharmacologic therapies to neuraxial anesthesia and how to individualize the pain management plan for each patient.

Common Causes of Pain in Pregnant Patients

Ligamentous and Abdominal Wall Pain

Abdominal pain can be a worrisome symptom heralding a miscarriage, especially if it is accompanied by vaginal bleeding and thus should result in prompt evaluation by an obstetrician. Other causes of abdominal pain result from rapid stretching and hematoma formation of the round ligament resulting in pain and tenderness that radiates to the pubic tubercle. Rapid stretching of the rectus abdominal muscle can result in a hematoma within the rectus sheath that produces abdominal wall pain that is exacerbated with flexion of the abdominal muscles. Both conditions are treated with localized heat and, if severe, oral analgesics which we will discuss the safety of later in the chapter.[1]

Low Back Pain and Pelvic Girdle Pain

Low back pain is one of the most common complaints from pregnant women and is caused by a combination of weight gain, predominantly in the abdominal region, and an increase in pregnancy hormones such as relaxin, progesterone, and estrogen, which contribute to joint laxity. The increased weight causes increased axial loading, pelvic tilt with resultant hyperlordosis, and stretching and weakening of abdominal muscles, which can all culminate to cause back and pelvic girdle pain. The incidence increases with increasing gestational age and by 35 weeks, the prevalence of low back pain and pelvic girdle pain reach up to 71.3% and 64.7%, respectively.[4] See Table 26.1 for a summary of the different characteristics of low back pain vs pelvic girdle pain.

TABLE 26.1 **CHARACTERISTICS OF LOW BACK PAIN VS PELVIC GIRDLE PAIN IN PREGNANCY**

Low Back Pain	Pelvic Girdle Pain
May be present prior to pregnancy	Typically not present prior to pregnancy
Pain located in lumbar region	Pain predominantly over sacroiliac joint between the posterior superior iliac crest and gluteal fold
Decreased range of motion in the lumbar region	Pain is intermittent
Tenderness to palpation over paraspinous muscles	Pain frequently associated with walking or standing
Pain is constant	Normal range of motion of lumbar region
Frequently no issues with walking or standing	

While back and pelvic girdle pain are common during pregnancy, it is important to first rule out any red flag symptoms such as bowel or bladder incontinence, radiculopathy, or weakness prior to forming a treatment plan. If the patient has red flag symptoms such as neurologic deficits, then imaging with magnetic resonance imaging (MRI) is warranted. Assuming none of these symptoms are present, it is reasonable to start with conservative therapy such as yoga, water exercises, acupuncture, or physical therapy. Oral analgesics can be used and are discussed in more detail below. Transcutaneous electrical nerve stimulation (TENS) was found to be equivalent to oral acetaminophen or exercise at treating back pain in pregnancy in one randomized controlled trial.[5]

Medications Used to Treat Pain During Pregnancy

When managing acute pain in a pregnant patient, one must consider the effect of each medication on the developing fetus prior to prescribing. Recent changes have been made by the Food and Drug Administration (FDA) who no longer supports the use of the pregnancy category (A, B, C, D, and X) classification system for risk stratification of medications used during pregnancy. This system, initially developed in the 1970s, was designed to help clinicians recognize the type and amount of data available but was instead used as a grading system leading to misinterpretation of recommendations. The implementation of the Pregnancy Lactation and Labeling Rule (PLLR) in 2015 requires each medication label to include data summaries as well the strength of the data to aid clinicians in understanding what data exist prior to prescribing.[6] Here, we discuss medications commonly prescribed for pregnancy and their effects on the developing fetus.

Acetaminophen

Acetaminophen is an antipyretic analgesic that does not share the anti-inflammatory properties of nonsteroidal anti-inflammatory drug (NSAID) and does not affect prostaglandin synthesis. For persistent pain during pregnancy that cannot be controlled with conservative measures such as yoga, acupuncture, or physical therapy, acetaminophen is an acceptable first-line oral analgesic agent in pregnancy as it has no known teratogenic effects and does not cause fetal ductus arteriosis closure in the third trimester.[1]

Opioids

Opioids can be used for short-term relief of acute pain especially following nonobstetric surgery in pregnant women. Morphine, fentanyl, and hydromorphone are all acceptable options for acute pain control when potent parenteral analgesia is necessary for surgical procedures. Post-operatively, a short course of oral analgesics such as oxycodone or hydrocodone combined with acetaminophen are reasonable options to treat pain associated with surgical procedures.[1] Neonatal abstinence syndrome, characterized by difficulty feeding, regulating temperature, as well as respiratory distress and seizures, is a feared complication of chronic opioid use in pregnancy. For this reason, opioids should not be used for prolonged periods during pregnancy if it can be avoided.[7] Patients who have a chronic pain syndrome requiring chronic opioids or have a substance abuse disorder and take methadone fall under the category of chronic pain and will not be discussed in this chapter. Neuraxial administration of hydrophilic opioids such as morphine greatly reduces postoperative opioid consumption when given for cesarean section.[1]

Nonsteroidal Anti-inflammatory Drugs

Nonsteroidal anti-inflammatory drugs (NSAIDs) are a class of medications that cause anti-inflammatory and analgesic properties and are commonly prescribed for musculoskeletal pain; however, caution must be exercised when considering this medication in the parturient. Examples include ibuprofen, naproxen, indomethacin, and ketorolac, the former two of which are available over the counter (OTC).[1] This class of medications poses different risks to the unborn fetus at different gestational ages. The risk of use for short durations in the first trimester appears low but cannot be excluded. The FDA recommends against use of NSAIDs after 20 weeks of gestational age owing to a small but serious risk of renal insufficiency of the fetus and subsequent oligohydramnios. This condition is usually reversed with discontinuation of the medication. It is also recommended to avoid NSAIDs (excluding 81 mg aspirin) after 30 weeks of gestation due to the increased risk of premature closure of the fetal ductus arteriosis.[8]

Ergot Alkaloids

Ergotamine is an effective treatment for migraine headaches but is contraindicated in pregnancy due to its teratogenicity and ability to cause uterine contractions and spontaneous abortion in high doses. Methylergonovine is an ergot alkaloid given to the parturient for treatment of uterine atony.[1]

Pathophysiology of Labor Pain

First Stage of Labor

The first stage of labor is visceral in nature and starts at the onset of labor and extends to full cervical dilation which is considered to be 10 cm. Uterine contraction and resultant myometrial ischemia causes release of leukotrienes, histamine, serotonin, substance P, and bradykinins which stimulate chemoreceptors. This visceral type of pain is transmitted pain via small unmyelinated "C" fibers, which travel with sympathetic fibers and pass through the uterine, cervical, and hypogastric nerve plexuses into the lumbar sympathetic chain. The pain fibers from the sympathetic chain enter the white rami communicantes at the T10-L1 spinal nerves and pass through the posterior nerve roots and synapse in the dorsal horn of the spinal cord.[9]

Second Stage of Labor

The second stage of labor begins with complete cervical dilation and ends with delivery of the fetus. Somatic nerve fibers are responsible for carrying pain signals during the second stage of labor. The transition from the first to second stage of labor involving both somatic and visceral components is reported to cause an increase in pain intensity. Distention of vaginal and perineal tissues causes pain signals to be transmitted to the spinal cord at the level of S2, S3, and S4, primarily via the pudendal nerve. Other nerves involved in signaling pain from the perineum include the ilioinguinal nerve and the genital branch of the genitofemoral nerve. As the fetus descends through the pelvic outlet, rectal pressure gives the parturient the urge to valsalva and push to expel the fetus.[10]

Affects of Uncontrolled Labor Pain on the Fetus

While many young healthy women can tolerate the pain associated with labor and may choose to forgo any pain intervention, pain itself is not necessarily benign. Severe pain such as that present during labor causes neurohumoral, respiratory, and psychological consequences. Intermittent hyperventilation associated with labor can cause hypocarbia, which inhibits ventilatory drive causing maternal and fetal hypoxemia. Hyperventilation can also result in a respiratory alkalosis, which causes a left shift of the oxyhemoglobin curve, and increases the affinity for oxygen of maternal hemoglobin, while decreasing oxygen delivery to the fetus. Epidural analgesia reduces pain and allows the patient to maintain regular respirations resulting in increased oxygen tension for mother and fetus.[11] Elevated plasma catecholamines can decrease uteroplacental perfusion by increasing maternal peripheral vascular resistance. Small primate studies reflected that stress and pain cause fetal acidosis by lowering fetal oxygenation and can also slow fetal heart rate.[12] The psychological consequences of enduring such a traumatic and painful event can contribute to the development of postpartum depression and even posttraumatic stress disorder. One study involving 1288 women having either vaginal or cesarean delivery reported that persistent pain and postpartum depression was related to the severity of acute pain after childbirth and was not related to the type (vaginal vs cesarean) of delivery.[13]

Nonpharmacologic Management of Labor Pain

Women have been bearing children for centuries, long before the modern pain management developments. Many women choose to forgo pharmacologic or regional anesthesia interventions in favor of a more "natural" delivery. A painless delivery does not necessarily correlate with a satisfaction of the birth experience. Nonpharmacologic methods of pain relief such as relaxation techniques, hypnotherapy, and aromatherapy focus on coping with pain rather than eliminating it.

Psychoprophylaxis

Preparation for the childbirth can significantly modify the pain experience and help laboring mothers cope with the pain. The Lamaze method after Dr. Ferdinand Lamaze focuses on breathing techniques and conscious relaxation to decrease pain perception.[14] Preparation reduces the fear and anxiety, which can exacerbate pain. The continuous presence of a support person, such as a doula or midwife, has been shown to reduce pain severity.[1]

Aromatherapy

Aromatherapy has shown to reduce stress levels, which can also help patient's cope with pain, but have not been shown to reduce pain.[1]

Hypnotherapy

Hypnotherapy is a similar concept to psychoprophylaxis and controlled breathing, except it takes a lot more preparation. It takes 4-5 weeks to develop the skills necessary to effectively achieve the hypnotic state that is effective for pain control.[1]

TABLE 26.2 REGIONAL TECHNIQUES FOR LABOR ANALGESIA

Visceral pain (T10-L1) (stage 1 of labor) • Bilateral paracervical blocks (associated with fetal bradycardia, therefore, rarely used) • Intrathecal opioids
Somatic pain (transition and stages 2 and 3 of labor) • Bilateral pudendal nerve blocks • Saddle block (spinal anesthesia) • Low caudal epidural block (S2-S4)
All pain (T10-S4) (stages 1, 2, 3) • Epidural (lumbar or caudal) • Combined spinal epidural (CSE) • Continuous spinal

Transcutaneous Electrical Stimulation

Transcutaneous electrical stimulation (TENS) can be applied to the suprapubic area or lower back depending on where the patient is experiencing pain. TENS units are thought to function by interrupting pain impulse transmission to the brain and may increase endorphin production.[1]

Pharmacologic Options for Labor Pain (Table 26.2)

Intermittent Bolus Opioids

Systemic opioids can be administered via subcutaneous, intramuscular, or intravenous routes to manage labor pain. Subcutaneous and intramuscular routes are painful as they require an injection with each administration but can be useful in facilities where there is a lack of skilled personnel to administer medications intravenously or provide neuraxial analgesia. Intravenous administration of opioids is easier to titrate due to the faster onset and a more predictable effect. Opioids are very lipid soluble (with the exception of morphine), and readily cross the placenta by passive diffusion. Because of this, this class of medication has been observed to compromise fetal well-being during labor to include changes in fetal heart tracing, decreased alertness, and poor feeding. In order to mitigate these adverse fetal effects, use of parenteral opioids should be discontinued in the late second stage of labor, which, as mentioned above, is the most painful for most patients.[15] See Table 26.3 to see a summary of dosing of the following parenteral medications for labor.

The choice of parenteral opioid differs between each facility based on availability and preference of the institution. Nalbuphine is a mixed agonist-antagonist with favorable safety

TABLE 26.3 DOSING REGIMENS FOR PARENTERAL ANALGESIC MEDICATIONS FOR LABOR

Drug	Dose/Interval	Route
Nalbuphine	2.5-10 mg q2-4 hours	IV
Morphine	1-4 mg q1-4 hours	IV
Meperidine	25-50 mg q2-3 hours	IV
Remifentanil	10-30 μg with 2-minute lockout interval and no background infusion	IV via PCA
Fentanyl	10-25 μg with 5- to 10-minute lockout period with 50-100 μg loading dose and no loading dose	IV via PCA

profile due to dose ceiling effect on respiratory depression. It can be dosed 2.5-10 mg IV every 2-4 hours.[16] Morphine is ineffective at providing analgesia at doses required to minimize apnea and is infrequently used intravenously in facilities where neuraxial analgesia is available.[17] Meperidine, known as pethidine in the European literature, is commonly administered for labor analgesia in the United Kingdom and is the most common opioid used for labor in the world. Its use is avoided in the United States, however due to the adverse effects related to the long acting active metabolite, normeperidine. It can take up to 3 to 6 days for the neonate to clear meperidine and its active metabolite normeperidine from its system.[15] Additionally, the accumulation of normeperidine can cause seizures, serotonergic crisis in patients taking monoamine oxidase inhibitors (MAOIs), and is not reversible by naloxone.[18]

Remifentanil

Remifentanil has a rapid onset and short duration of action due to its metabolism by nonspecific tissues and plasma esterases. While the medication rapidly crosses the placenta, it is also rapidly cleared by the fetus and does not carry the same risk of reduced APGAR scores observed with longer acting opioids. It still carries a significant risk of respiratory depression and patients should be monitored closely.[19]

The European RemiPCA SAFE Network hospitals from Germany and Switzerland developed a protocol in 2009 based on current literature for remifentanil PCA that consists of bolus doses of 10-30 μg IV remifentanil, with a lockout interval of 2 minutes, and no background infusion. A loading dose is unnecessary for remifentanil PCA for labor. It is also recommended that in addition to pulse oximetry, end tidal carbon dioxide monitoring should be employed, as it is more sensitive at detecting apnea than pulse oximetry alone. Supplemental oxygen should be avoided unless the patient's oxygen saturation drops below 94% as it can mask signs of apnea. For these reasons, continuous one on one nursing is recommended to monitor for apneic events.[20]

Remifentanil is inferior to epidural anesthesia; however, it could be a viable option in patients where neuraxial anesthesia is contraindicated, for example, in patients receiving prophylactic anticoagulants, or with pathology of the spine that would preclude epidural placement.[9]

Fentanyl

Fentanyl can be administered via PCA in place of remifentanil. It has a favorable side effect profile and provides adequate pain relief based on data from a few small studies. Fentanyl has a longer duration of action than remifentanil but is still relatively short and, like remifentanil, it has no active metabolites. A loading dose of 50-100 μg can be given with a bolus dose of 10-25 μg and a lockout period of 5-10 minutes. It is recommended to avoid a background infusion.[21] As with any opioid PCA, patients receiving fentanyl PCA for labor analgesia require constant nurse monitoring for sedation and respiratory depression.

Nitrous Oxide

Nitrous oxide is an inhaled anesthetic used uncommonly in the United States but is used widely in Canada, Australia, Great Britain, New Zealand, and Finland (to name a few) for labor pain.[22] The US Food and Drug Administration (FDA) has approved new nitrous oxide administrations systems for use in the delivery room in the United States; however, it is by no means widely available. Nitrous oxide is self-administered by the parturient via a face mask over the nose and mouth or with a mouthpiece. A portable tank is equipped with a demand valve that opens with each inhalation and closes with exhalation. The most commonly used mixture is a 50/50 mixture of nitrous oxide and air.[23] The effects of nitrous oxide take up to

50 seconds from administration to produce analgesia, which makes timing challenging. If the parturient waits until the beginning of a contraction to administer the nitrous, the peak analgesic effect will occur after the contraction is ended. In addition, the second stage of labor requires the mother to be alert in order to push and the effects of this medication can cause drowsiness and make this difficult.[22]

Nitrous oxide has a few advantages to other types of pain interventions such as opioids and neuraxial anesthesia that may explain why, while the analgesia is inferior to epidural anesthesia, patient satisfaction is similar to those who choose epidural analgesia. It allows the mother freedom of movement and does not require the frequent monitoring required after epidural placement.[24] It does not cause respiratory depression and, since it is self administered, if the patient is too drowsy, she will be unable to administer more agent while the drug is eliminated via the lungs.[22] There is a long standing concern about the occupational risk of nitrous oxide in causing spontaneous abortion; however, in 2015, the European Society of Anesthesiology Taskforce in 2015 released a statement that there is lack of evidence for a teratogenic effect or increased risk for abortion in women with occupation exposure provided nitrous oxide scavenging equipment is used.[24]

Inhaled anesthetic administration causes environmental pollution, which is why the FDA requires the use of a blender device with a scavenger, which is superior to European nitrous oxide delivery systems with regard to environmental harm. The main side effects reported in patients who chose nitrous oxide for analgesia during labor are nausea, vomiting, and dizziness.[25]

Regional Analgesia Techniques

Paracervical Block

The paracervical block can be performed by infiltration of the bilateral paracervical ganglion located at the posterolateral aspect of the vaginal fornix. It is only useful in treating pain associated with the first stage of labor. Paracervical blocks are not used in the United States for labor due to the tendency to cause fetal bradycardia, and superior analgesic options without such risk.[1]

Pudendal Nerve Block

The pudendal nerve is responsible for sensation of the lower vagina, perineum, and vulva. Bilateral pudendal nerve blocks are useful for providing analgesia during the second stage of labor. In addition, they can supplement an epidural that spares the sacral nerves or if a lumbar sympathetic block was used for the first stage of labor. If forceps delivery is anticipated in a patient without an epidural, bilateral pudendal nerve blocks can be considered. It is performed by injecting the pudendal nerve where it traverses lateral and inferior to the sacrospinal ligament with 10 mL of 0.5% bupivacaine, 3% 2-chloroprocaine, or 1% lidocaine.[1]

Neuraxial Anesthesia

Neuraxial anesthesia for labor and delivery was initially introduced in the 1940s but did not gain popularity until the 1980s largely due to an effort to reduce maternal mortality related to general anesthesia for cesarean delivery. Specifically, term pregnant patients are at an increased risk of airway related to airway complications such as failed endotracheal intubations.[26] Epidural anesthesia is now the primary form of pain control during labor in the United States with 70% of women receiving an epidural for labor analgesia per the 2016 obstetric anesthesia work force survey.[27]

Epidural Anesthesia

The epidural technique involves palpation of the spinous processes of the lumbar vertebrae and introducing a needle using either a paramedian or midline approach between the L3-L4 and L4-L5 vertebrae most commonly. A glass syringe is attached to the needle filled with either air or saline and increased resistance is encountered when the ligamentum flavum is engaged. Once the needle traverses the ligamentum flavum, a "loss of resistance" is felt and a catheter is threaded through the needle leaving 2-5 cm of catheter in the epidural space (Fig. 26.1). The catheter is then secured to the patient's back and attached to an infusion of local anesthetic that is capable of delivering a dilute concentration of anesthetic until the mother delivers the fetus.[1]

There are a few different options when considering epidural infusions, and it varies based on the capability of the epidural pump at each facility. A typical epidural infusion consists of a dilute concentration of local anesthetic (0.0625%-0.125% bupivacaine) that is infused continuously at a rate of 8-12 mL/h. The anesthesiologist can give an additional bolus dose of local anesthetic to achieve the desired dermatomal level and adjust the infusion rate to maintain the desired level of analgesia. Opioids such as fentanyl 2 μg/mL can be added to the infusion for additional analgesia. Patient controlled epidural analgesia (PCEA) pumps allow the patient to administer an additional bolus of the epidural infusion if the baseline infusion is insufficient. An example of settings for a PCEA pump would be 5-8 mL/h with 5-10 mL bolus and a 10-20 minute lockout interval. The most recent development in epidural infusions is referred to as "programmed intermittent bolus." Instead of delivering the local anesthetic mixture as a continuous infusion, it delivers a bolus of medication at scheduled intervals, with or without a PCEA function. It is thought to provide superior analgesia because the medication is able to spread over a larger area and cover both the sacral and mid-lumbar dermatomes, whereas a continuous infusion is likely to cover only the dermatomes closest to the epidural catheter. A typical programmed intermittent bolus regimen would be 6 mL 0.0625% bupivacaine with 2 μg/mL fentanyl every 30 minutes with a patient bolus of 5 mL and a lockout interval of 10 minutes. Studies have shown a low incidence of instrumental delivery and decreased motor

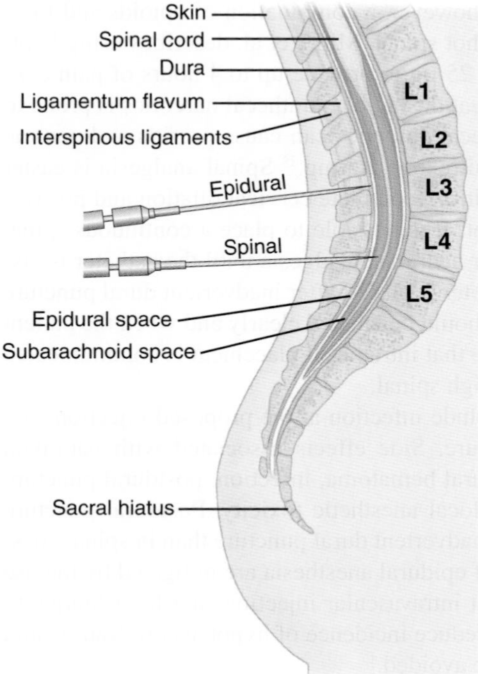

FIGURE 26.1 Epidural placement. The needle travels in between the spinous processes through first the skin, subcutaneous tissue, supraspinous ligament, interspinous ligament, and finally ligamentum flavum to reach the epidural space.

blockade with the programmed intermittent bolus technique without any reduction in patient satisfaction with pain control.[26]

Combined Spinal Epidural Anesthesia

A combined spinal and epidural (CSE) technique can be considered when the patient is in an advanced stage of labor, and it is critical to achieve analgesia quickly. The technique is similar to an epidural. Once the epidural space is identified using the loss of resistance technique, a smaller gauge spinal needle is inserted through the larger needle and punctures the dura. Once clear cerebrospinal fluid returns through the spinal needle, a small dose of local anesthetic is administered into the intrathecal space providing the patient with relief within 2-4 minutes. An epidural can take 15-20 minutes to achieve peak analgesia depending on the type and amount of local anesthetic used for the initial bolus. There are arguments for and against the use of the CSE technique for labor analgesia, and the approach to each patient's analgesia should be individualized. In addition to the rapid onset, there is a more uniform and complete distribution of sensory blockade and greater sacral coverage with a CSE than epidural alone. One argument against CSE is that placement of a spinal will delay discovery of a nonfunctioning epidural until the spinal wears off. The counter argument is that the placement of a spinal through the epidural needle is actually another method of confirming the correct identification of the epidural space and actually increases the likelihood of a functioning epidural. There is also evidence that performing a dural puncture with a 25-g needle without administering a spinal dose can achieve the same effect in regard to sacral dermatomal coverage without the unwanted effects of performing a true CSE.[26] When performing a CSE, adding fentanyl to the spinal mixture should be considered. There is level I evidence that intrathecal fentanyl causes more rapid cervical dilation and can shorten the first stage of labor by up to 100 minutes.[28]

Spinal

Spinal anesthesia is a single injection block that can be utilized if delivery is imminent and analgesia is needed quickly. The duration of spinal anesthesia, lasting only 60-90 minutes, limits its use for labor to the late second stage; however, a combination of opioids and local anesthetic can prolong the duration of a single shot spinal. Minty et al. describes using bupivacaine 2.5 mg, morphine 250 μg, and fentanyl 25 μg to provide up to 4 hours of pain control while allowing the patient to ambulate. Repeat dosing of intrathecal narcotics is prone to tachyphylaxis and is not recommended. Intrathecal narcotics can cause pruritis and nausea, which can be treated with a low dose of oral naltrexone 2.5 mg.[28] Spinal analgesia is easier to perform in the lateral position if the fetal position (complete cervical dilation and positive station) does not permit the patient to sit upright. It is possible to place a continuous spinal catheter, which allows the provider to administer neuraxial analgesia until the catheter is discontinued.[1] Most often, a continuous spinal catheter is placed after inadvertent dural puncture when placing an epidural. Intrathecal catheters should be labeled clearly and when the patient is handed off to another provider, it is imperative that intrathecal placement is communicated to avoid overdosing the catheter and causing a high spinal.

Contraindications to neuraxial anesthesia include infection at the proposed injection site, coagulopathy, and increased intracranial pressure. Side effects associated with neuraxial anesthesia include bleeding in the form of epidural hematoma, infection, postdural puncture headache, hypotension, nausea, vomiting, and local anesthetic toxicity. Postdural puncture headaches are more common in epidurals with inadvertent dural puncture than in spinal anesthetic due to size of the epidural needle. Risks of epidural anesthesia are mitigated by the use of a test dose to reduce incidence of inadvertent intravascular injection, sterile technique to reduce infection, and preemptive fluid bolus to reduce incidence of hypotension. Nausea and vomiting is less common if opioid analgesics are avoided.[1]

Effects of Epidural Analgesia on Labor Progression and Delivery Method

The goal of pain management in labor is to make the patient comfortable without causing any harm to the patient or the unborn fetus. One concern is that epidural analgesia will prolong labor and may increase rate of instrumental or operative delivery. Based on meta-analyses of randomized trials comparing systemic opioids and neuraxial analgesia, it was determined that the first stage of labor is prolonged by 30 minutes and the second stage of labor is prolonged by 15 minutes in the neuraxial group. In the same study, it was observed that instrumental delivery was increased in the neuraxial analgesia group; however, the concentration of bupivacaine used was high at 0.25%, which could be confounding. A more recent study from the Netherlands observed over 600 000 deliveries and while the rate of neuraxial analgesia for labor tripled over a 10-year period, there was no increase in instrumental deliveries. The myth that choosing an epidural for analgesia will increase the chance of cesarean section has been unfounded after a systematic review in 2011 including 38 randomized trials that failed to identify a link between labor epidural analgesia and increased risk for cesarean delivery.[26]

Conclusions

The pregnant patient is complex and each intervention should be considered carefully as it is not only the patient who is affected but also the unborn fetus. Many factors determine how each patient will tolerate the inevitable pain associated with labor, and each patient will need an individualized plan to treat pain based on their physiology, psychology, beliefs, and expectations for labor. Luckily, there are many options discussed above for labor analgesia, and good communication is key to patient safety and satisfaction.

REFERENCES

1. Benzon HT. Chapter 35 managing pain during pregnancy and lactation. In: *Practical Management of Pain*. 5th ed. Philadelphia, PA: Elsevier/Saunders; 2014:474–491.
2. Yadollahi P, Khalaginia Z, Vedadhir A, Ariashekouh A, Taghizadeh Z, Khormaei F. The study of predicting role of personality traits in the perception of labor pain. *Iran J Nurs Midwifery Res*. 2014;19(7 Suppl 1):S97-S102. http://www.ncbi.nlm.nih.gov/pubmed/25949260
3. Thomson G, Feeley C, Moran VH, Downe S, Oladapo OT. Women's experiences of pharmacological and non-pharmacological pain relief methods for labour and childbirth: a qualitative systematic review. *Reprod Health*. 2019;16(1):71. https://doi.org/10.1186/s12978-019-0735-4
4. Casagrande D, Gugala Z, Clark SM, Lindsey RW. Low back pain and pelvic girdle pain in pregnancy. *J Am Acad Orthop Surg*. 2015;23(9):539-549. https://doi.org/10.5435/JAAOS-D-14-00248
5. Sehmbi H, D'Souza R, Bhatia A. Low back pain in pregnancy: investigations, management, and role of neuraxial analgesia and anaesthesia: a systematic review. *Gynecol Obstet Invest*. 2017;82(5):417-436. https://doi.org/10.1159/000471764
6. Byrne JJ, Saucedo AM, Spong CY. Evaluation of drug labels following the 2015 pregnancy and lactation labeling rule. *JAMA Netw Open*. 2020;3(8):e2015094. https://doi.org/10.1001/jamanetworkopen.2020.15094
7. Desai RJ, Huybrechts KF, Hernandez-Diaz S, et al. Exposure to prescription opioid analgesics in utero and risk of neonatal abstinence syndrome: population based cohort study. *BMJ*. 2015;350:h2102. https://doi.org/10.1136/bmj.h2102
8. Nonsteroidal Anti-Inflammatory Drugs (NSAIDs): Drug Safety Communication—Avoid Use of NSAIDs in Pregnancy at 20 Weeks or Later | FDA. n.d. Accessed February 2, 2021. https://www.fda.gov/safety/medical-product-safety-information/nonsteroidal-anti-inflammatory-drugs-nsaids-drug-safety-communication-avoid-use-nsaids-pregnancy-20
9. Labor S, Maguire S. The pain of labour. *Rev Pain*. 2008;2(2):15-19. https://doi.org/10.1177/204946370800200205
10. Braverman F. Labor pain management. In: *Essentials of Pain Management*. Springer New York; 2011. https://doi.org/10.1007/978-0-387-87579-8_22

11. Reynolds F, Sharma SK, Seed PT. Analgesia in labour and fetal acid–base balance: a meta-analysis comparing epidural with systemic opioid analgesia. *BJOG.* 2002;109(12):1344-1353. https://doi.org/10.1046/j.1471-0528.2002.01461.x
12. Morishima HO, Yeh MN, James LS. Reduced uterine blood flow and fetal hypoxemia with acute maternal stress: experimental observation in the pregnant baboon. *Am J Obstet Gynecol.* 1979;134(3):270-275. https://doi.org/10.1016/s0002-9378(16)33032-0
13. Eisenach JC, Pan PH, Smiley R, Lavand'homme P, Landau R, Houle TT. Severity of acute pain after childbirth, but not type of delivery, predicts persistent pain and postpartum depression. *Pain.* 2008;140(1):87-94. https://doi.org/10.1016/j.pain.2008.07.011
14. Lothian JA. Lamaze breathing: what every pregnant woman needs to know. *J Perinat Educ.* 2011;20(2):118-120. https://doi.org/10.1891/1058-1243.20.2.118
15. Smith LA, Burns E, Cuthbert A. Parenteral opioids for maternal pain management in labour. *The Cochrane Database Syst Rev.* 2018;6(6):CD007396. https://doi.org/10.1002/14651858.CD007396.pub3
16. Zeng Z, Lu J, Shu C, et al. A comparison of nalbuphine with morphine for analgesic effects and safety: meta-analysis of randomized controlled trials. *Sci Rep.* 2015;5:10927. https://doi.org/10.1038/srep10927
17. Olofsson C, Ekblom A, Ekman-Ordeberg G, Hjelm A, Irestedt L. Lack of analgesic effect of systemically administered morphine or pethidine on labour pain. *Br J Obstet Gynaecol.* 1996;103(10):968-972. https://doi.org/10.1111/j.1471-0528.1996.tb09545.x
18. Fleet J, Belan I, Jones MJ, Ullah S, Cyna AM. A comparison of fentanyl with pethidine for pain relief during childbirth: a randomised controlled trial. *BJOG.* 2015;122(7):983-992. https://doi.org/10.1111/1471-0528.13249
19. Weibel S, Jelting Y, Afshari A, et al. Patient-controlled analgesia with remifentanil versus alternative parenteral methods for pain management in labour. *Cochrane Database Syst Rev.* 2017;4(4):CD011989. https://doi.org/10.1002/14651858.CD011989.pub2
20. Melber AA, Jelting Y, Huber M, et al. Remifentanil patient-controlled analgesia in labour: six-year audit of outcome data of the RemiPCA SAFE Network (2010-2015). *Int J Obstet Anesth.* 2019;39:12-21. https://doi.org/10.1016/j.ijoa.2018.12.004
21. Miyakoshi K, Tanaka M, Morisaki H, et al. Perinatal outcomes: Intravenous patient-controlled fentanyl versus no analgesia in labor. *J Obstet Gynaecol Res.* 2013;39(4):783-789. https://doi.org/10.1111/j.1447-0756.2012.02044.x
22. Rooks JP. Nitrous oxide for pain in labor—why not in the United States? *Birth.* 2007;34(1):3-5. https://doi.org/10.1111/j.1523-536X.2006.00150.x
23. Likis FE, Andrews JC, Collins MR, et al. Nitrous oxide for the management of labor pain: a systematic review. *Anesth Analg.* 2014;118(1):153-167. https://doi.org/10.1213/ANE.0b013e3182a7f73c
24. Vallejo MC, Zakowski MI. Pro-con debate: nitrous oxide for labor analgesia. *BioMed Res Int.* 2019;2019:4618798. https://doi.org/10.1155/2019/4618798
25. Collins MR, Starr SA, Bishop JT, Baysinger CL. Nitrous oxide for labor analgesia: expanding analgesic options for women in the United States. *Rev Obstetr Gynecol.* 2012;5(3-4):e126-e131. http://www.ncbi.nlm.nih.gov/pubmed/23483795
26. Lim G, Facco FL, Nathan N, Waters JH, Wong CA, Eltzschig HK. A review of the impact of obstetric anesthesia on maternal and neonatal outcomes. *Anesthesiology.* 2018;129(1):192-215. https://doi.org/10.1097/ALN.0000000000002182
27. Traynor AJ, Aragon M, Ghosh D, et al. Obstetric anesthesia workforce survey: a 30-year update. *Anesth Analg.* 2016;122(6):1939-1946. https://doi.org/10.1213/ANE.0000000000001204
28. Minty RG, Kelly L, Minty A, Hammett DC. Single-dose intrathecal analgesia to control labour pain: is it a useful alternative to epidural analgesia? *Can Fam Physician.* 2007;53(3):437-442. http://www.ncbi.nlm.nih.gov/pubmed/17872679

27

Acute Pain Management in the ICU

Farees Hyatali, Franciscka Macieiski, Harish Bangalore Siddaiah, and Alan David Kaye

Introduction

Pain in the critically ill patient is often underreported and misdiagnosed. Such factors that contribute are that these patients may not be able to express themselves due to invasive respiratory support or altered mental function. Pain management in the intensive care unit (ICU) can be challenging due to the severity of illness of critically ill patients. The benefits and risks of pain management techniques and medications should be weighed in lieu of the severity of the patient's illness and their comorbidities as well as the side effects of each technique and medication.[1]

Regional Anesthesia

Peripheral Nerve Blocks

Regional anesthesia in the form of peripheral nerve blocks has been used to decrease postoperative pain in the ICU. Peripheral nerve blocks have the benefit of having less strict anticoagulant guidelines prior to performing the block and less side effects and provide safe effective analgesia. These blocks can be performed via a single injection or via a continuous catheter-based technique.[2]

Fascial plane blocks such as the pectoral 1 and 2 blocks, the erector spinae plane block, as well as the serratus anterior plane blocks have been used for rescue analgesia for cardiac surgical patients who have had severe postsurgical pain and can also improve lung function by reducing splinting from severe thoracic pain.

Patients who have had sternal fractures, sternotomies, and rib fractures have also benefited from ultrasound-guided transversus thoracis plane blocks, which can also decrease pain scores and ultimately improve lung function by reducing splinting secondary to severe pain.

Neuraxial Analgesia

Patients who have suffered rib fractures, as well as those undergoing thoracic and upper and mid abdominal surgeries, can benefit from neuraxial analgesia, in particular, thoracic epidural analgesia.[3,4]

Benefits include reduced pain scores, improved pulmonary function, increased gastric motility, decreased risk of deep vein thrombosis that may assist in early extubation in patients who are intubated, reduced time to initial bowel movement, and reduced morbidity and mortality.

Side effects of neuraxial anesthesia include but not limited to nausea, vomiting, urinary retention, and lower extremity weakness (especially in the case of lumbar epidural). If opiates are added to the local anesthesia administered via these routes, opioid-induced pruritis can also occur. In addition, the choice of using these techniques must be weighed against their possible side effects.

Contraindications to neuraxial interventional techniques include patient refusal, hemodynamic instability, true allergy to local anesthetic drugs, and active anticoagulation (guided by the anticoagulation guidelines from the American Society of Regional Anesthesia).

Analgesics

Opiates

Opiates used for acute perioperative pain management include morphine, hydromorphone, fentanyl, buprenorphine, methadone, remifentanil, sufentanil, alfentanil, and ketamine. These medications can be administered via oral, intravenous, sublingual, intramuscular, and rectal administration. All of these medications provide excellent analgesia, however, they have numerous unwanted side effects and significant abuse potential. Adverse side effects include nausea, vomiting, sedation, opioid-induced respiratory depression, opioid-induced constipation, opioid-induced pruritis, and urinary retention. In addition, they can result in hypoventilation and hypercarbia and can lead to cardiopulmonary compromise in critically ill patients. This may result in these patients requiring respiratory support or may result in prolonged intubation.[5]

Methadone is generally administered to patients who have a history of opiate abuse and are attempting to overcome their addiction. In addition, it can also be used as part of an anesthetic plan to reduce perioperative pain. This drug is generally administered orally or intravenously. Administration of methadone in particular can prolong the QTc interval and can lead to torsade de pointes, which may result in ventricular tachycardia and fibrillation in patients with a history of prolonged QT. A careful review of medications must be performed prior to reduce the risk of increasing the QTc.

Remifentanil may be used as a continuous intravenous infusion at a low rate with a patient controlled bolus as part of patient-controlled analgesia for acute pain management. Remifentanil is unique of all the opiates in that it has a very short half-life and context sensitive half time of ~10 minutes resulting in complete clearance of the opiate from the blood. This is due to the fact that it is metabolized by red blood cell esterases, which rapidly break down the drug in the blood stream.[6]

Sufentanil may be administered by neuraxial or via an intravenous route (as a bolus or continuous infusion) for acute pain management. It is an excellent adjuvant in local anesthetic solutions for neuraxial analgesia and has also been used as an adjuvant to prolong the duration of a spinal anesthetic when used for surgical anesthesia; however, it is associated with opioid-induced pruritis, nausea, and vomiting when used as an intrathecal adjuvant. Sufentanil when used as an infusion has a longer context sensitive half time when compared to remifentanil, and care must be taken with regard to administration of large doses of this medication.

Buprenorphine is another medication used in the perioperative period in patients with a history of opiate abuse. It is generally combined with naloxone to produce buprenorphine/naloxone (naloxone added to reduce the abuse potential of this drug). Buprenorphine is a partial opioid mu agonist and kappa antagonist with a half-life of ~37 hours. When buprenorphine is administered, the drug provides a ceiling effect with regard to analgesia and does not produce as much respiratory depression compared to more potent opiates. This drug is commonly used for withdrawal of opiates in those who have a history of opiate abuse and is generally administered as an oral formulation and in some instances a transdermal patch for this purpose. It has also been approved for pain management. In addition, it can be combined within local anesthetic solutions as an adjuvant related to the fact that it possesses some local anesthetic properties by blocking voltage-gated sodium channels and can thus be administered via epidural or intrathecal routes. In this regard, buprenorphine can be effective in treating drug cravings in opioid-dependent patients in the ICU.

Meperidine is an opioid with local anesthetic properties and an atropine-like structure. Meperidine has been used intrathecally to prolong the duration of spinal anesthesia; however, it has unpleasant side effects of opioid-induced pruritis, constipation, sedation, nausea, and vomiting. When compared to other commercially available opioids used as adjuvants in intrathecal local anesthetic solutions, meperidine has a greater rate of side effects. Currently, meperidine is most commonly used in the ICU for the treatment of postoperative shivering as well as shivering in patients undergoing hypothermia after sudden cardiac arrest. It can also be used to provide analgesia; however, other agents such as fentanyl can provide superior analgesia in comparison.

Tramadol is an opiate with both serotonin and norepinephrine reuptake inhibitor properties that can be administered via oral, intravenous, intramuscular, and intrathecal administration. Side effects include an increased risk of seizures in patients with a history of seizures and an increased chance of serotonin syndrome especially in patients who are taking medications that increase serotonin. It can be considered as an analgesic agent in the ICU; however, there are other agents that can provide a greater quality of analgesia.[7]

Nonsteroidal Anti-inflammatory Agents

These medications inhibit the cyclooxygenase (COX) enzymes of which there are two main types related to pain, COX-1 and -2. COX-2–mediated effects include, pain, inflammation, and fever. These medications work by reducing inflammatory mediators, which provide nociceptive pain. They provide excellent analgesia, especially when incorporated within a multimodal analgesia regimen. It must be noted that these particular agents have a ceiling effect with regard to analgesia. Side effects include nausea, vomiting, gastrointestinal bleeding, increased risk of cardiovascular disease (especially in COX-2–selective nonsteroidal anti-inflammatory drugs of which celecoxib is the only one still available), platelet dysfunction, increased risk of bleeding, and renal dysfunction and these must be considered prior to administration in critically ill patients.[8]

Adjuvants

Dexmedetomidine

Dexmedetomidine, a selective alpha 2 agonist, has been used for sedation but related to local anesthetic properties, it has been used as an adjuvant to pain management. It is given as an infusion (0.2-2 µg/kg/h) and has been used in order to decrease opioid requirements in patients. Dexmedetomidine can be used as a sole analgesia agent or as an adjuvant in order to decrease opioid requirements. It can also be added to peripheral nerve blocks and neuraxial anesthetics to prolong their duration and reduce the opiate consumption of critically ill patients.[9]

Lidocaine

Lidocaine infusions have been used as an adjuvant to pain management as it decreases the opioid requirements for these patients. Lidocaine has antinociceptive and anti-inflammatory properties. It acts on the sodium channels and reduces neuronal transmission. It is especially useful in patients who have contraindications.[10,11]

The infusion is generally administered between 0.5 and 3 mg/kg/h, and care must be taken to avoid systemic toxicity, especially in patients who suffer from cardiac and renal failure (the metabolites of lidocaine may accumulate in these patients and can cause systemic toxicity).

The acid-base status, rate as well as dose of lidocaine, factors that influence the plasma concentration of free lidocaine, altered plasma protein levels, and hepatic or renal function are major factors in determining the patient's risk of toxicity. In patients who are critically ill, their metabolism may be altered leading to an accumulation of lidocaine and its metabolites resulting in an increased risk of systemic toxicity.

Careful monitoring must be used using standard ASA monitors while the infusion is being administered in order to monitor for signs and symptoms of local anesthetic toxicity such as seizures or cardiac arrhythmias. If local anesthetic toxicity is suspected, a serum lidocaine level should be obtained, and equipment and medications needed to treat local anesthetic toxicity should be available including lipid emulsion.

Ketamine

Ketamine infusions have been used as an adjuvant for pain management in the ICU, and numerous studies have demonstrated efficacy with limited side effects. It is an NMDA receptor antagonist and results in a dissociative state when given at anesthetic doses (generally 0.35 mg/kg as a single bolus, followed by an infusion of 0.1-1 mg/kg/h). Subanesthetic doses of ketamine have been used to decrease intraoperative and postoperative pain requirements and has recently been a popular adjuvant in the ICU in order to decrease opioid requirements.[12]

REFERENCES

1. Kaushal B, Chauhan S, Saini K, et al. Comparison of the efficacy of ultrasound-guided serratus anterior plane block, pectoral nerves ii block, and intercostal nerve block for the management of postoperative thoracotomy pain after pediatric cardiac surgery. *J Cardiothorac Vasc Anesth*. 2019;33(2):418-425. doi:10.1053/j.jvca.2018.08.209
2. Yalamuri S, Klinger RY, Bullock WM, Glower DD, Bottiger BA, Gadsden JC. Pectoral fascial (PECS) I and II blocks as rescue analgesia in a patient undergoing minimally invasive cardiac surgery. *Reg Anesth Pain Med*. 2017;42(6):764-766. doi:10.1097/AAP.0000000000000661
3. Fujii S, Roche M, Jones PM, Vissa D, Bainbridge D, Zhou JR. Transversus thoracis muscle plane block in cardiac surgery: a pilot feasibility study. *Reg Anesth Pain Med*. 2019;44(5):556-560. doi:10.1136/rapm-2018-100178
4. Krishna SN, Chauhan S, Bhoi D, et al. Bilateral erector spinae plane block for acute post-surgical pain in adult cardiac surgical patients: a randomized controlled trial. *J Cardiothorac Vasc Anesth*. 2018;33(2):368-375. doi:10.1053/j.jvca.2018.05.050
5. Alford DP, Compton P, Samet JH. Acute pain management for patients receiving maintenance methadone or buprenorphine therapy [published correction appears in Ann Intern Med. 2006 Mar 21;144(6):460]. *Ann Intern Med*. 2006;144(2):127-134. doi:10.7326/0003-4819-144-2-200601170-00010
6. Weibel S, Jelting Y, Afshari A, et al. Patient-controlled analgesia with remifentanil versus alternative parenteral methods for pain management in labour. *Cochrane Database Syst Rev*. 2017;4(4):CD011989. doi:10.1002/14651858.CD011989.pub2
7. Budd K. The role of tramadol in acute pain management. *Acute Pain*. 1999;2(4):189-196. doi:10.1016/S1366-0071(99)80019-9
8. Ho KY, Gwee KA, Cheng YK, Yoon KH, Hee HT, Omar AR. Nonsteroidal anti-inflammatory drugs in chronic pain: implications of new data for clinical practice. *J Pain Res*. 2018;11:1937-1948. doi:10.2147/JPR.S168188
9. Habibi V, Kiabi FH, Sharifi H. The effect of dexmedetomidine on the acute pain after cardiothoracic surgeries: a systematic review. *Braz J Cardiovasc Surg*. 2018;33(4):404-417. doi:10.21470/1678-9741-2017-0253
10. Dunn LK, Durieux ME. Perioperative use of intravenous lidocaine. *Anesthesiology*. 2017;126(4):729-737. doi:10.1097/ALN.0000000000001527
11. Jung S, Ottestad E, Aggarwal A, Flood P, Nikitenko V. 982: Intravenous lidocaine infusion for management of pain in the intensive care unit. *Crit Care Med*. 2020;48(1):470. https://journals.lww.com/ccmjournal/Fulltext/2020/01001/982__INTRAVENOUS_LIDOCAINE_INFUSION_FOR_MANAGEMENT.943.aspx
12. Schwenk ES, Viscusi ER, Buvanendran A, et al. Consensus guidelines on the use of intravenous ketamine infusions for acute pain management from the American Society of Regional Anesthesia and Pain Medicine, the American Academy of Pain Medicine, and the American Society of Anesthesiologists. *Reg Anesth Pain Med*. 2018;43(5):456-466. doi:10.1097/AAP.0000000000000806

28

Acute Pain Management for Orthotopic Liver Transplant Surgery

Islam Mohammad Shehata, Antolin S. Flores, Leonid Gorelik, and Alan David Kaye

Introduction

Liver transplant (LTx) is the most effective treatment for patients with end-stage liver disease.[1] Recovery from such a major procedure is multifaceted; however, meeting postoperative pain control milestones contributes to a shorter hospital stay and accelerates recipient physical and psychological recovery.[2] Conversely, poorly managed acute pain is a strong predictor of long-term disability and poor quality of life.[3,4] Although it is well documented[5,6] that LTx recipients have a decreased analgesic requirement, postoperative pain control is still important. The surgical incision for LTx surgery, specifically the subcostal component and the use of surgical retractors for a prolonged period of time, contributes to the severity of postoperative pain.[7] Pain is further exacerbated related to location of the incision, which gets aggravated with normal activities of recovery, tidal breathing, and even minimal movement, usually necessitating a high analgesia requirement.[8]

Multimodal analgesia is a concept involving regional and systemic analgesia, in the form of opioid and non-opioid medication.[9] It expands the prospects of analgesia to manage pain, decrease neuro-hormonal stress response to surgery, decrease metabolic demand on the newly transplanted liver and facilitate early mobilization and early weaning from mechanical ventilation.[5] Fast tracking anesthesia for early extubation of LTx patients is an emerging concept which mandates optimal perioperative pain management.[10,11] Spontaneously breathing patients have reduced pleural pressure during inspiration, improving venous return and graft perfusion.[12] Thus, to meet the goal of earlier extubation, postoperative pain must be adequately controlled while preserving respiratory drive. As such, the significant role of multimodal analgesia is emphasized in all Enhanced Recovery After Surgery (ERAS) guidelines, especially the intra-abdominal surgeries.[13] However, there are limited data regarding ERAS or other pain management protocols in LTx recipients.[14] Therefore, we aim to provide an overview of the novel nonopioid per oral regimens and regional analgesia modalities for post-LTx analgesia.

Pathophysiology of Post-transplant Analgesia

It is imperative to understand that the pharmacokinetic characteristics of any drug may be altered by the distorted concentrations of plasma proteins, hepatic blood flow, and biliary flow after LTx. Moreover, graft size, graft regeneration, and elevated levels of pro-inflammatory cytokine may be other important factors that alter the metabolic capacity of the transplanted liver.[15] Postoperatively, LTx patients may also have reduced renal function due to intraoperative fluid shifts, suboptimal renal perfusion during the anhepatic phase, or nephrotoxic calcineurin inhibitor immunosuppression therapy.[16]

Systemic Analgesia

Systemic analgesic therapy involves the combination of different analgesic agents that target various pain nociceptive pathways, such as non–steroidal anti-inflammatory drugs (NSAIDs), acetaminophen, gabapentinoids, and opioids.

Opioids have long been the mainstay of intraoperative analgesia in LTx. Postoperative pain has been attributed to many factors including the large surgical incision, extended pressure on the lower ribs from the surgical retractors, intraoperative hemorrhage, higher distribution clearance due to the hyperdynamic circulation of end-stage liver disease, and the enhanced metabolism of the new functioning graft.[7] One of the most commonly used opioids is fentanyl whose metabolism may not be impaired in the presence of poor graft recovery.[17] However, significant reduction in the graft blood flow can interfere with its metabolism that may necessitate dosing adjustment to avoid prolonged sedation, especially if infused throughout the lengthy surgery.[2] Another important element to consider is many patients' history of alcohol or IV drug abuse, which precipitated their presentation for transplantation.[5] Patients with substance abuse disorders may require additional monitoring and regimented control over opioid dispensing.[18]

Due to the growing aversion from administering opioids, clinicians have increasingly looked to employ alternative pain medications.[9] Although acetaminophen is metabolized by the liver, producing a hepatotoxic metabolite, its clinical use up to 3 g/day for 7 days in patients with chronic liver disease was found to be safe and showed no evidence of toxicity in recent studies.[19] However, regular monitoring of liver function tests for early diagnosis of graft worsening is highly recommended due to the high variability of the toxic dose and possibility of smaller doses having an increased risk of causing toxicity as well.[20] Gabapentinoids, such as pregabalin and gabapentin, are becoming increasingly popular components of ERAS protocols.[9] Three recent retrospective studies concluded that a regimen of acetaminophen and gabapentin was associated with decreased opioid consumption, providing evidence for a non–opioid-centered strategy for post-LTx analgesia.[14,21,22] Although no official recommendations include gabapentinoids in LTx pain regimens, recent evidence is supportive.[14,21,22]

NSAIDs provide reliable postoperative pain control in many surgical populations but may not be the safest analgesic modality in LTx patients. NSAIDs have been implicated in hepatocellular damage in addition to other unfavorable effects such as temporary antiplatelet activity and inhibition of prostaglandin synthesis in the gastric mucosa.[23] Moreover, LTx patients have increased risk of renal dysfunction as a result of hemodynamic impairment, dehydration, immunosuppression, and NSAIDs administration.[23]

Fast tracking anesthesia for early extubation of LTx patients is an emerging concept, which mandates optimal perioperative pain management to carefully balance analgesia and respiratory function. This concept was first introduced to LTx in 2002 by Findlay et al. at the Mayo Clinic in a consecutive series of 80 patients where they demonstrated a 60% reduction in intraoperative analgesia with fentanyl (decreased to 23 μg/kg from 50 μg/kg, $P < .001$) and in total mechanical ventilation time (553 minutes vs 1081 minutes, $P < .001$).[10] A more recent review by Aniskevich and Pai in 2015 reported that 60% of their LTx recipients were extubated in the operating room and able to bypass the ICU completely.[11]

Regional Analgesia

Regional analgesia encompasses various techniques including neuraxial analgesia, paraspinal and abdominal wall blocks, and incisional field local anesthetic infiltration. These procedures involve the administration of local anesthetics and/or lower concentration opioids, compared to systemic administration, near the site of nerves carrying afferent pain signals.

There is a growing body of literature demonstrating the safe use of regional analgesia in improving perioperative pain and decreasing the use of systemic analgesia in postsurgical patients.[24]

Pharmacokinetic Properties of Local Anesthetics

The metabolic pathways of local anesthetics in the anhepatic phase and in patients with deranged liver function were not well understood until recently. One of the most commonly used local anesthetics, lidocaine, is metabolized by CYP1A2 and CYP3A4, and its hepatic extraction ratio is 65%, which is much higher than that of ropivacaine (40%), a longer-acting local anesthetic.[25] As a result of the low hepatic extraction ratio of ropivacaine, its total clearance is less related to changes in the hepatic blood flow and depends mostly on hepatic enzyme activity and plasma protein binding.[25] Although the available data on the metabolism of bupivacaine is scant, it is structurally related to ropivacaine with a hepatic extraction ratio of 38%.[25] The current data show that end-stage liver disease has a roughly similar impact on both bupivacaine and ropivacaine clearance.[25]

An increase of bupivacaine plasma concentration was reported in eleven patients who received bilateral intercostal nerve blocks 2 days post liver transplantation with accumulation after repeated doses. However, the results should be interpreted with caution as intercostal blocks are known to have the highest systemic absorption of any neural blockade technique, which is attributed to the high vascularity of the area.[26] A study examining the pharmacokinetics of levobupivacaine used for epidural anesthesia in patients with liver dysfunction showed slower metabolism and an increase of its plasma concentration, which was attributed to levobupivacaine being metabolized by the cytochrome P-450 enzyme.[27]

A double-blinded, randomized, placebo-controlled study comprised of 39 patients undergoing liver resection surgery assigned to receive ropivacaine for transversus abdominis plane (TAP) nerve block demonstrated that the ropivacaine pharmacokinetic profile remained within the safe range.[28]

Hepatic dysfunction itself may not mandate dose adjustment for single-shot regional anesthetic techniques despite the reduction of hepatic clearance, which is offset by the unchanged absorption and the larger volume of distribution and maintenance of α1-acid glycoprotein synthesis. However, the risk of local anesthetic systemic toxicity (LAST) is increased for repeat boluses and continuous infusions, and therefore a dose reduction is recommended.[29]

Abdominal Wall Block

The abdominal wall is supplied by the lower six thoracic and upper two lumbar sensory nerves through a number of plexuses invading the musculature of the abdominal wall. Real-time ultrasonography facilitates the identification of the musculofascial planes and viewing the spread of local anesthetics within.[30]

Ultrasound-guided TAP block is an established analgesic technique for upper abdominal surgery with a notable opioid sparing effect.[31] TAP provides analgesia for the skin, subcutaneous tissue, and peritoneum.[5] Altered hepatic blood flow, hepatic enzyme activity, and plasma protein binding seen in LTx extends the half-life of local anesthetics resulting in possibly increased but safe plasma concentrations.[26,28] Seemingly, TAP is an attractive regional analgesia option in LTx patients.

A pilot study on 17 LTx patients receiving bilateral TAP block found a significant reduction in pain scores and morphine consumption in the first 24 hours postoperatively, facilitating early extubation in comparison to the intravenous morphine comparison group.[32] When pooled with three other trials employing TAP for living donor liver surgery, TAP block group had nearly 30 mg lower morphine requirements at 24 hours for pain mitigation than the conventional intravenous analgesic group.[33] Another recent publication from the Mayo Clinic liver transplant group, Amundson et al., of a nonrandomized, retrospective study of 77 living liver donor patients (29 block vs 48 standard care) demonstrated significantly better analgesia with liposomal bupivacaine TAP block on postoperative day 0 as compared with their standard multimodal analgesia (which included intrathecal hydromorphone). They also noted a reduced time to return of bowel activity and resumption of full diet in the TAP block patients.[34]

Complications after TAP block are rare when the ultrasound-guided technique is used. However, cases of iatrogenic liver trauma have been reported after TAP block.[35,36] Ultrasound-guided placement by a skilled practitioner is essential to reduce incidences of TAP-related trauma.

Another possible regional block for LTx patients is an ultrasound-guided quadratus lumborum block (QLB). The QLB is a fascial plane block with local anesthetic introduced to the thoracic paravertebral space, deep to the transversus abdominis aponeurosis.[37] The QLB can provide a long-lasting analgesic effect and has the advantage of covering all the dermatome segments from L2 caudally to the T7 segment cranially.[35] This block has been used successfully with an opioid-sparing effect in various abdominal surgeries.[38] In contrast, the TAP block is superficial to the transversus abdominis aponeurosis. However, the TAP block may still be preferable to QLB because it is relatively easier to place.[39]

Neuraxial Analgesia

Thoracic epidural analgesia (TEA) has been reported to provide better analgesic effects than intravenous opioids after major abdominal surgery with reduction of the potential hepatotoxicity of parenteral analgesics due to the altered drug metabolism.[40,41] Moreover, it has shown to decrease liver hepatic congestion and surgical blood loss by increasing splanchnic vasodilatation and decreasing the portal vein pressure.[42] There is also evidence suggesting that local anesthetics used in epidural anesthesia exhibit extended action in patients with liver dysfunction due to slower cytochrome P-450 enzyme metabolism, subsequently increasing their plasma concentration.[27]

Thoracic epidural analgesia (TEA) has successfully been deployed in the LTx population.[43] In a 3-year period at the Medical University of Warsaw, 67 patients underwent LTx, of which 47 met criteria for TEA. Fifteen of the 16 excluded patients were due to hepatic encephalopathy. Twenty-two patients received TEA and general anesthesia (GA), while the remaining 25 received GA alone (control). The patients who received TEA and GA were significantly more often extubated in the operating room (70% vs 48%) and had significantly lower visual analog pain scores at rest ($P < .01$ at 18 hours) and with coughing ($P < .003$ at 18 hours).[44]

Not every LTx patient is a candidate for TEA. An epidural hematoma is a rare but devastating complication when the epidural catheter is placed.[45] The risk of incidence is increased in patients with abnormal coagulation profile, like those with impaired hepatic function.[46] Criteria used for TEA is an international normalized ratio (INR) <1.5, activated partial thromboplastin time (aPTT) <45 seconds, and platelet count >70 g/L.[43] TEA's adoption in the LTx patient population has been limited historically due to the underlying coagulation problems and profound blood loss seen in a typical LTx; however, the aforementioned TEA in LTx patients study reported none of the complications in patients receiving TEA.[43] It is, nevertheless, important to attain normal coagulation profile and standard platelet count and correlating the result with the thromboelastometry before placement and removal of epidural catheters. Epidural abscess is another uncommon catastrophic complication (1.1:100 000 blocks) with increased incidence in immunocompromised patients.[47] Therefore, it is crucial to maintain sterility during catheter insertion and vigilant postoperative monitoring for a masked inflammatory response.[47] Clinicians must acknowledge these considerations when weighing the risk-benefit ratio of epidural analgesia in end-stage liver disease patients. The risk of complications in the unique LTx populations compared to the benefits of improving the pain management has made many institutions understandably hesitant to adopt TEA's widespread use.[48]

Paraspinal Block

The erector spinae plane (ESP) block has emerged as an effective novel interfascial plane block, which was recently described by Forero et al. in 2016 to provide thoracic analgesia in both chronic neuropathic pain and acute postsurgical or posttraumatic pain.[49] The ESP block is easy to perform and requires only a single injection in the lower thoracic and upper abdominal areas. Although the location is close in proximity to the neuraxiom, it is superficial to the erector spinae muscle. ESP is therefore regarded as a "low risk" block because the anatomical region is devoid of major blood vessels and away from the pleura.[50]

There are no published reports of ESP in adult LTx recipients. However, there has been proof-of-principal of ESP in LTx recipients via one case report in which two pediatric patients undergoing LTx received ESP blocks with satisfactory analgesic control. When compared with historical opioid consumption rates for this population, these two patients consumed markedly fewer opioid medications, both intraoperative and postoperatively.[51] Ultrasound-guided bilateral ESP block was performed in three adult patients undergoing living donor liver transplantation to provide adequate analgesia (visual analog pain scale <4 during first 24 hours) without complications.[52] Further studies are required to compare ESP block with conventional analgesic techniques for technical simplicity, patient safety, and analgesic efficacy.

Incisional Field Infiltration

Local anesthetic wound infiltration is a simple and safe analgesic modality. Local infiltration has the least risk for systemic absorption of local anesthetic and also carries a lower relative risk related to neuraxial and peripheral nerve blocks in patients with coagulation abnormalities.[53] A randomized controlled trial assessing the analgesic efficacy of continuous wound instillation of ropivacaine in patients undergoing elective open liver resection surgery found a reduction in both morphine consumption and postoperative pain score while better preserving respiratory function.[54]

A meta-analysis comparing the efficacy of the TAP block in abdominal surgery patients showed that wound infiltration was not inferior in reducing opioid consumption during the first 24 hours postoperatively.[55] However, the TAP block had a longer lasting analgesic effect.[55]

Similarly, another meta-analysis showed that incisional field infiltration had comparable analgesic effect to epidural techniques after the first postoperative day in open liver resection patients.[56]

Limitations of Regional Analgesia

The major limitations of regional analgesia in LTx patients are the potential risk of infection and bleeding from the associated coagulopathy.

Only about 10% of LTx patients presented with normal preoperative clotting panel results. Normal hemostasis encompasses three phases: primary, which depends on platelets; secondary, which involves the coagulation pathway; and the last phase, fibrinolysis, which prevents clot over-propagation. End-stage liver disease can cause disruption of all phases by the quantitative and qualitative deficits in circulating platelet counts, synthetic dysfunction of procoagulant factors, antithrombotic, and antifibrinolytic protein.[57]

In case of LTx surgery, a *de novo* coagulopathy presents at the different stages of surgery. During the dissection phase, dilutional coagulopathy develops due to the blood loss and fluid therapy. Coagulopathy during the anhepatic phase is attributed to absence of the synthetic function of the liver-based clotting factors. Moreover, the ischemic reperfusion injury at the neohepatic phase with the released metabolites and the blood loss presents another additive factor for coagulopathy.[58]

Infection represents the leading cause of acute decompensation of chronic liver disease patients with mortality risk ranging from 12% to 52%. Cirrhosis-associated immune dysfunction of chronic liver disease possesses an increased risk for viral, bacterial, fungal, and protozoan infections. Moreover, the risk is aggravated during the perioperative period because of immunosuppressive therapy.[59]

Conclusion

An increasing number of LTxs are performed each year, and the wait list continues to outpace this growth. As such, successful perioperative management is meeting the challenge of postoperative pain control by devising new analgesic regimens that both decrease pain and improve short-term patient outcomes, particularity reducing opioid consumption, while minimizing complications. This review outlines reported pain protocols, with a special emphasis on the emerging regional anesthesia practices. Many of these currently have limited evidence supporting their success, however. Additional clinical studies need to be performed to further compare efficacy and safety, but one can expect regional anesthetic techniques to have a growing and prominent role in postoperative care of LTx patients in the future.

REFERENCES

1. Farkas S, Hackl C, Schlitt HJ. Overview of the indications and contraindications for liver transplantation. *Cold Spring Harb Perspect Med*. 2014;4(5):a015602.
2. Feltracco P, Carollo C, Barbieri S, et al. *Pain Control after Liver Transplantation Surgery*. Elsevier; 2014:2300-2307.
3. Mandell MS, Smith AR, Dew MA, et al. Early postoperative pain and its predictors in the adult to adult living donor liver transplantation cohort study (A2ALL). *Transplantation*. 2016;100(11):2362.
4. Forsberg A, Lorenzon U, Nilsson F, Bäckmana L. Pain and health related quality of life after heart, kidney, and liver transplantation. *Clin Transplant*. 1999;13(6):453-460.
5. Weyker P, Webb C, Mathew L. Pain management in liver transplantation. *Liver Anesthesiology and Critical Care Medicine*. Springer; 2018:507-523.
6. Moretti EW, Robertson KM, Tuttle-Newhall J, Clavien P-A, Gan T-J. Orthotopic liver transplant patients require less postoperative morphine than do patients undergoing hepatic resection. *J Clin Anesth*. 2002;14(6):416-420.
7. Milan Z. Analgesia after liver transplantation. *World J Hepatol*. 2015;7(21):2331.
8. Eghtesad B, Kadry Z, Fung J. Technical considerations in liver transplantation: what a hepatologist needs to know (and every surgeon should practice). *Liver Transpl*. 2005;11(8):861-871.
9. Chadha R, Pai S-l, Aniskevich S, et al. Nonopioid modalities for acute postoperative pain in abdominal transplant recipients. *Transplantation*. 2020;104(4):694-699.
10. Findlay JY, Jankowski CJ, Vasdev GM, et al. Fast track anesthesia for liver transplantation reduces postoperative ventilation time but not intensive care unit stay. *Liver Transpl*. 2002;8(8):670-675.
11. Aniskevich S, Pai S-L. Fast track anesthesia for liver transplantation: review of the current practice. *World J Hepatol*. 2015;7(20):2303.
12. Magder S. Heart-Lung interaction in spontaneous breathing subjects: the basics. *Ann Transl Med*. 2018;6(18):348.
13. Beverly A, Kaye AD, Ljungqvist O, Urman RD. Essential elements of multimodal analgesia in enhanced recovery after surgery (ERAS) guidelines. *Anesthesiol Clin*. 2017;35(2):e115-e143.
14. Lee TC, Bittel L, Kaiser TE, Quillin RC III, Jones C, Shah SA. Opioid minimization after liver transplantation: results of a novel pilot study. *Liver Transpl*. 2020;26(9):1188-1192.
15. Ganesh S, Almazroo OA, Tevar A, Humar A, Venkataramanan R. Drug metabolism, drug interactions, and drug-induced liver injury in living donor liver transplant patients. *Clin Liver Dis*. 2017;21(1):181-196.
16. Pai S-L, Aniskevich S, Rodrigues ES, Shine TS. Analgesic considerations for liver transplantation patients. *Curr Clin Pharmacol*. 2015;10(1):54-65.

17. Smith HS. *Opioid Metabolism*. Elsevier; 2009:613-624.
18. Krahn LE, DiMartini A. Psychiatric and psychosocial aspects of liver transplantation. *Liver Transpl*. 2005;11(10):1157-1168.
19. Benson GD, Koff RS, Tolman KG. The therapeutic use of acetaminophen in patients with liver disease. *Am J Ther*. 2005;12(2):133-141.
20. Larson AM, Polson J, Fontana RJ, et al. Acetaminophen-induced acute liver failure: results of a United States multicenter, prospective study. *Hepatology*. 2005;42(6):1364-1372.
21. Tong K, Nolan W, O'Sullivan DM, Sheiner P, Kutzler HL. Implementation of a multimodal pain management order set reduces perioperative opioid use after liver transplantation. *Pharmacotherapy*. 2019;39(10):975-982.
22. Kutzler HL, Gannon R, Nolan W, et al. Opioid avoidance in liver transplant recipients: reduction in postoperative opioid use through a multidisciplinary multimodal approach. *Liver Transpl*. 2020;26(10):1254-1262.
23. Rubenstein J, Laine L. The hepatotoxicity of non-steroidal anti-inflammatory drugs. *Aliment Pharmacol Ther*. 2004;20(4):373-380.
24. Kumar K, Kirksey MA, Duong S, Wu CL. A review of opioid-sparing modalities in perioperative pain management: methods to decrease opioid use postoperatively. *Anesth Analg*. 2017;125(5):1749-1760.
25. Jokinen MJ, Neuvonen PJ, Lindgren L, et al. Pharmacokinetics of ropivacaine in patients with chronic end-stage liver disease. *Anesthesiology*. 2007;106(1):43-55.
26. Bodenham A, Park G. Plasma concentrations of bupivacaine after intercostal nerve block in patients after orthotopic liver transplantation. *Br J Anaesth*. 1990;64(4):436-441.
27. Ran J, Wang Y, Li F, Zhang W, Ma M. Pharmacodynamics and pharmacokinetics of levobupivacaine used for epidural anesthesia in patients with liver dysfunction. *Cell Biochem Biophys*. 2015;73(3):717-721.
28. Ollier E, Heritier F, Bonnet C, et al. Population pharmacokinetic model of free and total ropivacaine after transversus abdominis plane nerve block in patients undergoing liver resection. *Br J Clin Pharmacol*. 2015;80(1):67-74.
29. Christie LE, Picard J, Weinberg GL. Local anaesthetic systemic toxicity. *BJA Educ*. 2015;15(3):136-142.
30. Finnerty O, Carney J, McDonnell J. Trunk blocks for abdominal surgery. *Anaesthesia*. 2010;65:76-83.
31. Abdelsalam K, Mohamdin O. Ultrasound-guided rectus sheath and transversus abdominis plane blocks for perioperative analgesia in upper abdominal surgery: a randomized controlled study. *Saudi J Anaesth*. 2016;10(1):25.
32. Milan Z, Duncan B, Rewari V, Kocarev M, Collin R. *Subcostal Transversus Abdominis Plane Block for Postoperative Analgesia in Liver Transplant Recipients*. Elsevier; 2011:2687-2690.
33. Sharma A, Goel AD, Sharma PP, Vyas V, Agrawal SP. The effect of transversus abdominis plane block for analgesia in patients undergoing liver transplantation: a systematic review and meta-analysis. *Turk J Anaesthesiol Reanim*. 2019;47(5):359.
34. Amundson AW, Olsen DA, Smith HM, et al. Acute benefits after liposomal bupivacaine abdominal wall blockade for living liver donation: a retrospective review. *Mayo Clinic Proc Innov Qual Outcomes*. 2018;2(2):186-193.
35. Lancaster P, Chadwick M. Liver trauma secondary to ultrasound-guided transversus abdominis plane block. *Br J Anaesth*. 2010;104(4):509-510.
36. Farooq M, Carey M. A case of liver trauma with a blunt regional anesthesia needle while performing transversus abdominis plane block. *Reg Anesth Pain Medicine*. 2008;33(3):274-275.
37. Akerman M, Pejčić N, Veličković I. A review of the quadratus lumborum block and ERAS. *Front Med*. 2018;5:44.
38. Elsharkawy H, El-Boghdadly K, Barrington M. Quadratus lumborum blockanatomical concepts, mechanisms, and techniques. *Anesthesiology*. 2019;130(2):322-335.
39. Baytar Ç, Yılmaz C, Karasu D, Topal S. Comparison of ultrasound-guided subcostal transversus abdominis plane block and quadratus lumborum block in laparoscopic cholecystectomy: a prospective, randomized, controlled clinical study. *Pain Res Manag*. 2019;2019.
40. Garimella V, Cellini C. Postoperative pain control. *Clin Colon Rectal Surg*. 2013;26(3):191.
41. Moraca RJ, Sheldon DG, Thirlby RC. The role of epidural anesthesia and analgesia in surgical practice. *Ann Surg*. 2003;238(5):663.
42. Jacquenod P, Wallon G, Gazon M, et al. Incidence and risk factors of coagulation profile derangement after liver surgery: implications for the use of epidural analgesia—a retrospective cohort study. *Anesth Analg*. 2018;126(4):1142-1147.
43. Trzebicki J, Nicinska B, Blaszczyk B, et al. Thoracic epidural analgesia in anaesthesia for liver transplantation: the 10-year experience of a single centre. *Ann Transplant*. 2010;15(2):35-39.
44. Trzebicki J. Assessment of the value of thoracic segment epidural anesthesia as an element of anesthesia and postoperative management in orthotopic liver transplantation. Dissertation for doctor of medical sciences degree (in Polish). Medical University of Warsaw; 2004.
45. Gulur P, Tsui B, Pathak R, Koury K, Lee H. Retrospective analysis of the incidence of epidural haematoma in patients with epidural catheters and abnormal coagulation parameters. *Br J Anaesth*. 2015;114(5):808-811.

46. Fazakas J, Tóth S, Füle B, et al. *Epidural Anesthesia? No of Course*. Elsevier; 2008:1216-1217.
47. Horlocker TT, Wedel DJ. Regional anesthesia in the immunocompromised patient. *Reg Anesth Pain Med.* 2006;31(4):334-345.
48. Hwang G-S, McCluskey SA. Anesthesia and outcome after partial hepatectomy for adult-to-adult donor transplantation. *Curr Opin Organ Transplant.* 2010;15(3):377-382.
49. Forero M, Adhikary SD, Lopez H, Tsui C, Chin KJ. The erector spinae plane block: a novel analgesic technique in thoracic neuropathic pain. *Reg Anesth Pain Med.* 2016;41(5):621-627.
50. Tsui BC, Kirkham K, Kwofie MK, et al. Practice Advisory on the bleeding risks for peripheral nerve and interfascial plane blockade: evidence review and expert consensus. *Can J Anesth.* 2019;66(11):1356-1384.
51. Moore RP, Liu C-JJ, George P, et al. Early experiences with the use of continuous erector spinae plane blockade for the provision of perioperative analgesia for pediatric liver transplant recipients. *Reg Anesth Pain Med.* 2019;44(6):679-682.
52. Hacibeyoglu G, Topal A, Arican S, Kilicaslan A, Tekin A, Uzun ST. USG guided bilateral erector spinae plane block is an effective and safe postoperative analgesia method for living donor liver transplantation. *J Clin Anesth.* 2018;49:36-37.
53. Collyer T. Regional anaesthesia and patients with abnormalities of coagulation. *Anaesthesia.* 2013;68(12):1286-1287.
54. Chan S, Lai P, Li P, et al. The analgesic efficacy of continuous wound instillation with ropivacaine after open hepatic surgery. *Anaesthesia.* 2010;65(12):1180-1186.
55. Yu N, Long X, Lujan-Hernandez JR, Succar J, Xin X, Wang X. Transversus abdominis-plane block versus local anesthetic wound infiltration in lower abdominal surgery: a systematic review and meta-analysis of randomized controlled trials. *BMC Anesthesiol.* 2014;14(1):121.
56. Bell R, Pandanaboyana S, Prasad KR. Epidural versus local anaesthetic infiltration via wound catheters in open liver resection: a meta-analysis. *ANZ J Surg.* 2015;85(1-2):16-21.
57. Northup P, Reutemann B. Management of coagulation and anticoagulation in liver transplantation candidates. *Liver Transpl.* 2018;24(8):1119-1132.
58. Forkin KT, Colquhoun DA, Nemergut EC, Huffmyer JL. The coagulation profile of end-stage liver disease and considerations for intraoperative management. *Anesth Analg.* 2018;126(1):46-61.
59. Bartoletti M, Giannella M, Tedeschi S, Viale P. Opportunistic infections in end stage liver disease. *Infect Dis Rep.* 2018;10(1):7621.

29

Chronic Pain and the Opioid Tolerant Patient

Chikezie N. Okeagu, Gopal Kodumudi, Boris C. Anyama, and Alan David Kaye

Introduction

Investigation into the experience of pain has captivated medical research for decades. Despite intense focus and several significant advances, many aspects of the etiologies, assessment, and treatments of pain remain shrouded in mystery. This is partially because the perception of pain is diverse and transcends mere sensation, also involving complex emotional, psychological, and social elements.[1-3] The general approach to addressing pain involves first classifying it as either acute or chronic. Relative to chronic pain, acute pain is short lasting and occurs in close temporal proximity to an identifiable cause such as an injury or surgery. This pain usually resolves as the injured tissue heals. When pain lingers longer than the expected time for healing, it is regarded as chronic pain. Chronic pain is typically defined as pain that persists longer than 3-6 months.[4,5] Chronic pain can be the result of a discrete injury, in other words a progression of acute pain, or it can be of insidious onset with difficulty associating it to a distinct event.[3] All pain, but especially chronic pain, can be extremely distressing with debilitating impacts on individuals, families, and society.

Chronic pain inflicts a considerable burden both on a personal and a societal level. It is estimated that chronic pain affects 11%-40% of U.S. adults and ~20% of people worldwide.[6,7] Furthermore, 15%-20% of physician visits are related to chronic pain complaints amounting to a cost of roughly €200 billion yearly in Europe and $150 billion yearly in the United States. Even as staggering as these statistics are, many believe that these estimates are too low and that chronic pain is much more pervasive. Given the enormous diversity of chronic pain syndromes, the exact prevalence of chronic pain is difficult to measure. Moreover, many chronic pain patients suffer in solitude and do not seek medical attention. Chronic pain is also often a comorbidity of other illnesses, which may cause the chronic pain component to be overlooked. For example, according to the World Health Organization, unipolar depression, coronary heart disease, cerebrovascular disease, and traffic accidents will be the leading contributors to the global burden of disease by 2030. Chronic pain is often a component of all of these.[7,8]

In most of the developed world, opioid medications have become a mainstay in the treatment of chronic pain. This is especially pronounced in the United States, where sales of prescription opioids have quadrupled over the last 15-20 years. As a result, 20% of patients with chronic nonmalignant pain are under treatment with opioids.[9] This extensive use has brought with it a multitude of issues, including tolerance, physical dependence, and abuse among users. While these issues are challenges, they also present obstacles to treating acute pain in patients with chronic pain who are managed on opioid medications. In addition to the significant percentage of patients who are opioid-tolerant because of treatment of chronic pain, there are other populations of patients whose tolerance to opioids may present challenges in treating acute pain. These include patients who abuse opioid drugs recreationally (ie, heroin) and former addicts who are enrolled in opioid replacement programs. This chapter, therefore, presents an overview of the management of acute pain in patients with baseline chronic pain and opioid tolerance.

Physiologic Adaptations to Opioid Use

Regular use of opioids can lead to the pharmacologic phenomena of tolerance and dependence. Following continued exposure, a rightward shift in the dose-response curve can occur, leading to increased medication requirements to achieve the same effect. This is known as tolerance and develops to a variety of the drugs' effects, including analgesia, euphoria, sedation, respiratory depression, and nausea. Interestingly, tolerance to miosis and inhibition of bowel motility does not occur. Dependence refers to a state of neuroadaptation such that removal of an agonist, in this case, opioids, results in the onset of withdrawal symptoms. Endogenous opioids are made constantly within the body, for example, enkephalins, dynorphins, and endorphins, and with the delivery of exogenous opioids, there will be a shutdown of endogenous opioid production, resulting in central nervous system hyperarousal. Symptoms of opioid withdrawal include restlessness, anxiety, tachycardia, diaphoresis, abdominal pain, nausea, vomiting, and diarrhea.[10] While unpleasant, opioid withdrawal is not life-threatening. The molecular mechanisms underlying these phenomena are not fully understood but are thought to involve complex neurobiological elements leading to receptor alteration, desensitization, and internalization.[11] Oftentimes, these physiological changes are accompanied by a psychological compulsion to obtain and consume opioid medication. This phenomenon is known as addiction. Addiction is primarily psychological and is characterized by repeated use despite harmful consequences. While it is like and frequently occurs with physical dependence, it is its own distinct entity. Similar to tolerance and dependence, addiction is thought to be multifactorial with complex underlying mechanisms.[9]

Opioid-induced hyperalgesia (OIH) is another adaptation to opioid use that can have detrimental effects. OIH is characterized by a paradoxical increase in pain observed with opioid administration. Before the description of OIH, increasing dosage requirements in patients being treated for pain were attributed to increasing tolerance to the medication and/or progression or exacerbation of the condition responsible for the pain. While these phenomena likely contribute, there is some evidence that OIH also plays a role. Though limited, studies have shown that patients on long-term opioid replacement therapy have a lower tolerance for painful stimuli. Furthermore, some evidence suggests that the onset of OIH may be very rapid as patients who received higher doses of intraoperative opioids reported higher pain scores and consumed more opioids postoperatively. OIH is thought to be the result of a cascade of pronociceptive mediators caused by the docking of opioids onto glial cells in the brain and spinal cord via toll-like receptor-4 (TLR4). Further elucidation of this mechanism may present new targets for treatment.[11]

Assessment and Patient Education

A thorough history and physical is an essential component of the evaluation of any acute pain complaint (Fig. 29.1). The aim should be to collect details regarding the patient's symptoms to help guide treatment decisions. When assessing acute pain in patients with baseline chronic pain and/or opioid tolerance, it is necessary to be aware of some special considerations. First, it is important to review the patient's maintenance chronic pain medications, including usual drugs, doses, and prescribers. Setting aside prejudices and employing a nonjudgmental approach is essential to make the patient comfortable being forthcoming with information regarding both prescribed and illicit substances used for pain control. It is helpful to explain to

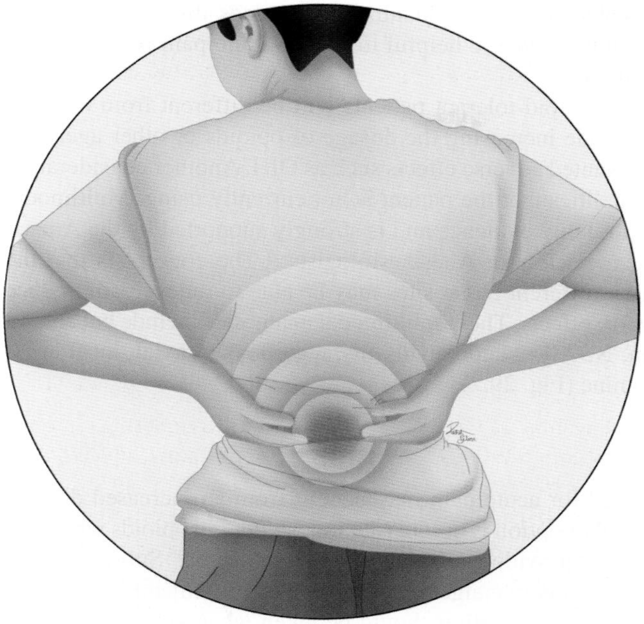

FIGURE 29.1 A patient with low back pain.

the patient that this knowledge is necessary to provide the best possible treatment. Even when dealing with the most trustworthy patients, verification of this information should be sought by checking the labels on the prescription bottles, contacting the prescribing physician or dispensing pharmacy, and/or checking with the appropriate regulatory program(s) (ie, prescription monitoring database). In emergency settings, dose verification may not be possible. In these instances, patients who report opioid use for the management of chronic pain should be assumed to have some level of tolerance and physiologic dependence. As such, the reported daily opioid amount can be given in two to four divided doses to avoid the risk of opioid withdrawal. Patients' response, level of sedation, and respiratory status should be monitored closely until verification can be obtained.[11]

Discussing patient preferences, past experiences, and long-term pain management plans can aid in developing a plan for treatment. Reassurance that treatment of their new acute pain complaints will be prioritized is often helpful. Patients should be made aware that past bad experiences with pain management or opioid addiction will not preclude them from receiving any available treatment options.[11] Notwithstanding, acute pain management in patients who have chronic pain and/or opioid tolerance is uniquely challenging as typical initial treatment measures may be less effective, and as such, it is important to manage patient expectations. Making the patient aware that it may be impossible to safely relieve all of their pain will help them to set realistic expectations for the outcome of treatment.

Treatment

Treating acute pain often involves nonopioid analgesics such as acetaminophen and nonsteroidal anti-inflammatory drugs (NSAIDs). Opioids are usually introduced when the acute pain is moderate to severe.[12] However, acute pain in opioid-tolerated patient can be quite challenging. Health care professionals tend to under treat acute pain in this patient population due to fear of the opioid's pharmacological side effects, iatrogenic drug addiction, and prescription drug diversion. This leads to patients being undertreated, resulting in continuous pain, withdrawal, and a negative experience with health care providers.[13] To avoid stigmatizing this population, alternative measures should be implemented. Individualized care plans that include multimodal analgesic and regional techniques may be helpful to reduce acute pain in this patient population and provide positive outcomes.

Treatment plans for acute pain in opioid-tolerant patients will be different from those of opioid naive patients. This may include increasing the dosage of opioids or other agents to provided pain relief and prevent unwanted adverse effects such as OIH. Another consideration is the exploration of treatment modalities that the patient is not currently using. Multimodal analgesia for pain control has high-quality evidence and is strongly supported by the American Pain Society and the American Society of Anesthesiologists.[14] The concept is that the combination of analgesics acting on different target sites may be able to relieve pain, reduce opioid requirements and their adverse effects. These multimodal analgesics include but are not limited to opiates, acetaminophen, NSAIDs, anticonvulsants, regional/neuraxial, local anesthetics, alpha-2 agonists, and ketamine (Fig. 29.2).

Opioids

Opioid-tolerant patients being treated for acute pain may benefit from an increased dose of their current opioid medication. Another option is opioid rotation; switching opioids when one opioid at a max or near-max dose is not providing adequate analgesic effects.[15] Substituting an opioid with one-half to two-thirds of an equianalgesic opioid is the recommended approach to ensure safety and efficacy. Careful consideration should be taken when switching from a long-acting opioid to a short-acting opioid—related to the risk of withdrawal in these patients. Methadone and buprenorphine can also be beneficial in the acute pain setting. Methadone, an opioid agonist, and *N*-methyl D-aspartate (NMDA), receptor antagonist, given once a day at the baseline dose, can prevent withdrawal symptoms and provide short-term analgesia.[13] An addiction specialist will be needed if a long-acting analgesic is required. Buprenorphine is a partial mu agonist and kappa antagonist. It is also used for withdrawal and has a short analgesic effect. In fact, a small randomized trial suggested that buprenorphine is as effective as morphine for postoperative pain control in children undergoing lateral thoracotomy. Contrarily, buprenorphine use may dampen the efficacy of a full-opioid agonist and lessen their utility in

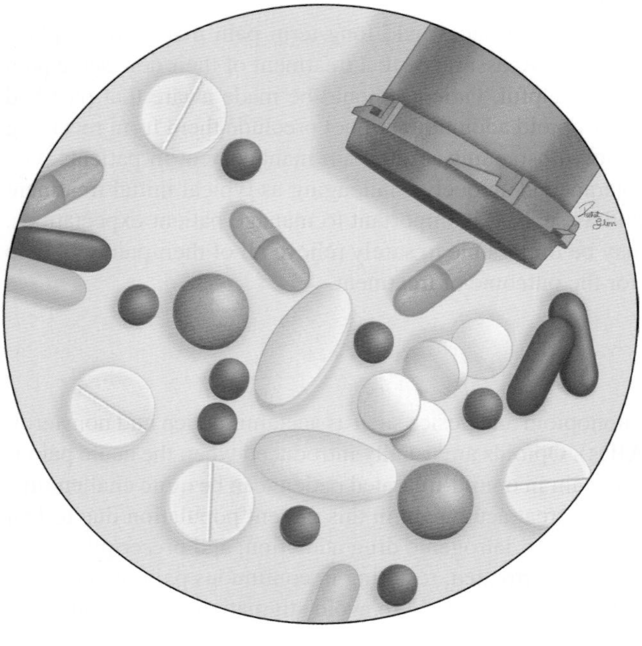

FIGURE 29.2 Pain medication.

the treatment of acute pain.[9] When acute pain is expected in patients who take buprenorphine chronically (eg, postoperative pain from an elective procedure), discontinuing buprenorphine 72 hours prior to surgery will allow a full agonist to provide effective analgesia preoperatively. If the acute pain is unexpected (eg, trauma) and buprenorphine is unable to be discontinued, then intravenous opioid agonists such as fentanyl and sufentanil will be useful to overcome the Mu opioid receptors and provide more effective pain control.

Acetaminophen and NSAIDs

Acetaminophen (or paracetamol) is a commonly used drug for pain. Although there is limited research involving acetaminophen with opioid-tolerant patients in the acute setting, a systemic review concluded that acetaminophen combined with an NSAID provided superior analgesia compared to either drug alone.[13] NSAIDs, nonselective cyclooxygenase (COX) inhibitors (eg, naproxen, ketorolac), and selective COX-2 inhibitors (eg, celecoxib) have been shown to be an effective opioid-sparing choice in opioid-tolerant patients.[13] They also decrease the need for a rescue drug and increase the time needed before a rescue drug is required.

Anticonvulsants

Gabapentin, commonly used to treat chronic neuropathic pain, may also have a role in acute pain management. Some evidence exists to support its use in the perioperative setting.[13] A meta-analysis showed gabapentin reduced pain intensity, decreased opioid consumption, and reduced opioid-related side effects while having a sedative effect in the postoperative period.[11] Despite no improvement in pain relief, pregabalin has also shown to be as effective as gabapentin in reducing opioid consumption and opioid-related side effects in the perioperative setting. Limited studies have shown the effectiveness of gabapentin and pregabalin in the opioid-tolerant patient population, but both drugs should be considered solely as adjuvant therapy and be used concomitantly with other agents.[13]

Regional Anesthesia

Regional anesthesia can be beneficial in providing pain relief in opioid-tolerant patients. Some operations can be performed exclusively with regional anesthesia to prevent the use of opioids.[13] Furthermore, the addition of regional anesthesia to general anesthesia and other traditional protocols provides longer-lasting analgesia. Although typical regional anesthetic techniques provide pain relief for around 1 postoperative day, continuous infusion can extend this period. Lidocaine has both analgesic and anti-inflammatory effects in the acute setting.[14] In fact, intravenous lidocaine has been effective in decreasing opioid requirements, nausea, and vomiting during abdominal surgery.

Alpha-2 Agonists

Alpha-2 agonist (eg, clonidine, dexmedetomidine) can be useful in the withdrawal symptoms in opioid-tolerant patients by suppressing the sympatho-adrenergic response.[13] Clonidine has opioid-sparing analgesia and antihyperalgesic effects that can be helpful in the perioperative setting in providing systemic analgesic.

Ketamine

Ketamine, an NMDA antagonist, has been useful in treating acute pain in opioid-tolerant patients.[11] Ketamine has been shown to reverse morphine tolerance and restore the effectiveness of the opioids in the acute postoperative pain.[13] One study showed that a ketamine infusion in combination with a PCA in the opioid-tolerant patients not only provides postoperative analgesia but may have a role in the prevention of persistent postsurgical pain.[13,14]

Perioperative Management of Patients on Chronic Opiate Therapy

Perioperative pain management of chronic opiate users in the presence of opioid tolerance can be challenging.[11] Goals of perioperative pain management include attaining adequate analgesia and preventing withdrawal. In addition, long-term care must encompass behavioral, psychiatric, and social aspects. These patients require higher opiate doses and are in danger of severe postoperative pain. Furthermore, clinicians and other health care providers often have prejudices and misconceptions of opiate users and abusers that can prevent these patients from attaining proper analgesia.[9] Some of these misconceptions include the beliefs that patients on maintenance therapy with Suboxone or methadone will not require further analgesia or that additional opioids will cause addiction relapse or toxicity (CNS/respiratory depression). However, it has been shown that these patients do not have a higher risk of these side effects.[9]

Prior to the induction of anesthesia and the start of surgery, patients on chronic opiate therapy should take their usual baseline dose of opiates.[9] If the patient is unable to take oral medications, an equianalgesic IV dose of morphine can be given. Equianalgesic tables should be utilized to determine the oral morphine equivalent dose; next, the IV dose can be calculated by using the oral:IV morphine ratio of 3:1.

Intraoperatively, dosages and requirements should be increased based on vital signs of the patient (eg, preventing tachycardia, hypertension). The goal is to decrease the sympathetic mediated pain response. Low-dose ketamine has been shown to decrease opiate requirements and improve pain scores.[10] The Analgesia Nociception Index (measure of heart rate variability) has also been used to direct intraoperative opiate dosing and provide adequate analgesia.[16] Regional anesthesia can result in decreased intraoperative requirements; however, it does not alleviate opiate withdrawal.

In the postoperative period, these opiate-dependent patients require four times the amount of typical postoperative opiate requirements. When compared to opiate naive patients, patients dependent on chronic opiate therapy for malignant pain have been shown to require triple the typical duration of postoperative treatment when compared to opiate naive patients.[17] Multimodal anesthesia, regional anesthesia, and PCAs have been helpful in controlling postoperative pain. Opiate antagonists and mixed agonist-antagonists should be avoided as these can lead to withdrawal symptoms.

Perioperative Management of Opiate Abusers

Patients who have a history of opiate addiction should be differentiated on the time frame of the opiate abuse (former vs current or current and undergoing maintenance opiate therapy). To determine the adequate perioperative opiate dose, it is critical to determine the precise street dose that the patient is using. Next, the street dose should be converted to a daily maintenance morphine or methadone dose for the duration of the perioperative period.[9]

Treatment of Patients Undergoing Methadone or Buprenorphine Maintenance Treatment

Methadone is a long-acting opiate with a half-life of ~23 hours and is taken once a day to decrease opiate abuse; initial maintenance dose is 15-30 mg once a day and is titrated up to an effective dose of 80-120 mg. The maintenance methadone dose should still be taken on the morning of surgery. Methadone can be administered intramuscularly or subcutaneously if the patient is unable to take the oral form. If methadone is not available, an equianalgesic dose of morphine should be administered on the day of surgery.[9]

Buprenorphine is a mixed opiate agonist-antagonist that is also used for maintenance therapy. It is effective from 24 to more than 36 hours, and so it is typically taken once a day sublingually or transdermally; the initial dose is 2-8 mg, titrated up weekly by 4 mg to max dose of 32 mg. The daily buprenorphine maintenance dose should be continued on the day of surgery, with different opiates being used for analgesia. If the daily dose of buprenorphine is low, ¼ of the dose can be given every 6-8 hours.[9]

Conclusion

Providing analgesia to opioid-dependent patients is challenging. The number of opiate-tolerant patients has increased, comprising chronic noncancer pain patients, opiate abusers, and patients on chronic maintenance therapy. Providers must be adept providing adequate perioperative analgesia to these population. This patient population often faces prejudices and misunderstandings from health care providers that can preclude them from achieving adequate analgesia. Physicians should be aware of pharmacologic phenomena such as tolerance, withdrawal, and hyperalgesia; perioperatively, for the chronic opiate user, baseline levels of opioids should be provided on the day of surgery to prevent withdrawal. Short-term use of opioids higher than average opioid dose may be needed. Multimodal analgesia with the addition of adjuvant and nonopioid pharmacological treatment decrease tolerance and OIH.

REFERENCES

1. Hylands-White N, Duarte RV, Raphael JH. An overview of treatment approaches for chronic pain management. *Rheumatol Int*. 2017;37:29-42.
2. Hansen GR, Streltzer J. The psychology of pain. *Emerg Med Clin North Am*. 2005;23:339-348.
3. Mills SEE, Nicolson KP, Smith BH. Chronic pain: a review of its epidemiology and associated factors in population-based studies. *Br J Anaesth*. 2019;123(2):e273-e283.
4. Wijma AJ, van Wilgen CP, Meeus M, Nijs J. Clinical biopsychosocial physiotherapy assessment of patients with chronic pain: the first step in pain neuroscience education. *Physiother Theory Pract*. 2016;32(5):368-384.
5. Derry S, Wiffen PJ, Kalso EA, et al. Topical analgesics for acute and chronic pain in adults—an overview of Cochrane Reviews. *Cochrane Database Syst Rev*. 2017;(5):CD008609.
6. Dahlhamer J, Lucas J, Zelaya C, et al. Prevalence of chronic pain and high-impact chronic pain among adults—United States, 2016. *MMWR Morb Mortal Wkly Rep*. 2018;67(36):1001-1006.
7. Treede RD, Rief W, Barke A, et al. A classification of chronic pain for ICD-11. *Pain*. 2015;156:1003-1007.
8. Van Hecke O, Torrance N, Smith BH. Chronic pain epidemiology and its clinical relevance. *Br J Anaesth*. 2013;111(1):13-18.
9. Coluzzi F, Bifulco F, Cuomo A, et al. The challenge of perioperative pain management in opioid-tolerant patients. *Ther Clin Risk Manag*. 2017;13:1163-1173.
10. Mitra S, Sinatra RS. Perioperative management of acute pain in the opioid-dependent patient. *Anesthesiology*. 2004;101(1):212-227.
11. Huxtable CA, Roberts LJ, Somogyi AA, Macintyre PE. Acute pain management in opioid-tolerant patients: a growing challenge. *Anaesth Intensive Care*. 2011;39(5):804-823.
12. Alford DP, Compton P, Samet JH. Acute pain management for patients receiving maintenance methadone or buprenorphine therapy. *Ann Intern Med*. 2006;144(2):127-134.
13. Shah S, Kapoor S, Durkin B. Analgesic management of acute pain in the opioid-tolerant patient. *Curr Opin Anaesthesiol*. 2015;28(4):398-402.
14. Cooney MF, Broglio K. Acute pain management in opioid-tolerant individuals. *J Nurse Pract*. 2017;13(6):394-399. doi:10.1016/j.nurpra.2017.04.016
15. Adebola A, Duncan N. Acute pain management in patients with opioid tolerance. *US Pharm*. 2017;42(3):28-32. https://www.uspharmacist.com/article/acute-pain-management-in-patients-with-opioid-tolerance
16. Daccache G, Jeanne M, Fletcher D. The analgesia nociception index: tailoring opioid administration. *Anesth Analg*. 2017;125:15-17.
17. De Leon-Casasola OA, Myers DP, Donaparthi S, et al. A comparison of postoperative epidural analgesia between patients with chronic cancer taking high doses of oral opioids versus opioid-naive patients. *Anesth Analg*. 1993;76(2):302-307.

30

Management of Acute Pain in Amputation

Joel Castellanos, Christopher Reid, and John J. Finneran

Introduction

Amputation is a common procedure with ~185 000 people undergoing amputations annually in the United States alone. Adequate pain management can be difficult with patients who have undergone amputations because of the extent of tissue injury altering the perception not only at the peripheral level but also at the central level as well. The combination of direct tissue (peripheral nerves, soft tissue, and bone) injury as well as central sensitization results in a varied nociceptive and neuropathic pain presentation that requires a multimodal and individualized treatment protocol for optimal pain management.

Epidemiology

Amputees Per Year

Every year, ~185 000 people undergo amputations in the United States.[1] The main causes of lower extremity amputations are vascular disease (including diabetes and peripheral arterial disease) and trauma, which when combined account for almost 98% of amputations. Cancer follows these two causes as the third leading cause of lower extremity amputations. Trauma accounts for the overwhelming majority of upper limb amputations (77%) followed by congenital limb deformities and cancer (6%).[1]

Total Amputees

There are currently ~2 million people who are living with an amputation in the United States. Most patients suffer from postoperative residual limb pain, and ~10% of patients having persistent limb pain.[2] In the postoperative period, incidence of phantom sensation is 84% and 90% at 6 months. The incidence of phantom limb pain is higher in patients undergoing an upper extremity amputation compared to a lower extremity amputation.[2] A study done in the Netherlands in upper limb amputees found significant associations between phantom limb pain and phantom sensations as well as between phantom pain and residual limb pain.[3]

Classification of Postamputee Pain

Residual Limb Pain

Residual limb pain, or "stump pain," refers to pain in the remaining parts of the amputated extremity. The residual limb pain can be accompanied by hyperalgesia, an increased sensitivity to painful stimulus, and/or allodynia, pain elicited from nonpainful stimuli. There are several possible etiologies of residual limb pain, which will be covered in this section.

Postoperative pain

Immediately after an amputation, postsurgical wound pain is most prevalent. The pain is often described as constant, aching, throbbing pain with associated erythema and edema; this reflects the postsurgical inflammatory process that is occurring. This pain is primarily a nociceptive process; however, it can coexist with neuropathic pain processes as well.

In general, acute postoperative pain gradually dissipates over 14-21 days. In some patients, this pain transforms into a persistent residual limb pain. This occurs in ~10% of patients.[2] This transition from acute to chronic pain in the residual limb can occur for a variety of reasons. These include infection, vascular claudication secondary to inadequate blood supply; wound failure; heterotopic ossification; seroma, hematoma, or neuroma formation; and/or poorly fitting prosthesis.

Infection

Infection is not uncommon after amputation, especially in patients who are undergoing amputation secondary to vascular complications. Risk factors for infection after an amputation include below vs above knee amputation, presence of diabetes or vascular disease, and poor nutrition status.[4] Differentiating infection from routine postoperative inflammation can be difficult, but the presence of worsening pain, purulent exudate, wound failure, and prolonged erythema and edema are clinical signs that suggest infection. Uncontrolled residual limb infections can quickly become life-threatening with the development of sepsis and requirement for debridement, surgical revision, and potentially loss of more residual limb to preserve life. Following complete blood count, inflammatory markers (eg, erythrocyte sedimentation rate and C-reactive protein levels), blood and wound cultures, and imaging should also be used to help differentiate postoperative inflammation from developing infection.

Neuroma

After a peripheral nerve is injured through trauma, ischemia, or transection, an inflammatory response occurs. Although the exact pathophysiology of neuroma formation is not well understood, neuroma formation occurs as the proximally cut nerve ends are inhibited from reconnecting to their distal end organs by scarring and fascicular escape.[5] A neuroma develops from uncontrolled axonal growth and is intertwined with support cells such as myofibroblasts, Schwann cells, and endothelial cells. Up to 60% of patients who[6] have suffered a peripheral nerve injury may develop a painful neuroma.

Phantom limb pain

Phantom limb pain is a neuropathic pain that occurs in 45%-85% of patients who undergo amputation.[4,7] The pain is located in the area of the limb that is no longer present and may become a disabling condition in many patients. The exact pathophysiology of phantom limb pain is yet to be discovered but likely is caused by a combination of damage to the peripheral nerves as well as maladaptive neuroplasticity of the spinal cord and somatosensory cortex.

Management of Postamputation Pain

Optimal pain control is best achieved through multimodal analgesia. This concept was originated by Kehlet and Dahl for postoperative pain control, but now is the underpinning of both acute and chronic pain management.[8] This approach may consist of interventional approaches and/or infusions targeted neuraxial or peripherally, medications of differing classes, physical therapy, and other adjunct treatment approaches.

Presurgical Counseling and Pain Psychology, Rehab Counseling

Undergoing an amputation has a profound effect on not only a persons' function but also psychosocial status. When able, presurgical amputation counseling by certified prosthetist or physiatrist to help set reasonable postoperative expectations regarding pain as well as postoperative timeline to prosthesis. In the case of traumatic or unplanned amputation, these issues should also be addressed postoperatively. Pain psychology consultation should be in place as well provide the patient coping mechanisms to help manage pain as well as to help with adjustment to limb loss.[9]

Postoperative Pain Management

Acute postoperative management of patient undergoing an amputation surgery begins with intravenous patient-controlled analgesia. This allows patients to titrate the dose of opioid medication, typically fentanyl or hydromorphone, to adequate pain control. As acute postsurgical inflammation begins to subside, calculating the daily oral morphine equivalents required for adequate pain control through the intravenous patient-controlled analgesia can be converted to oral opioids. Oral opioids can be supplemented with neuropathic pain medications such as anticonvulsants (gabapentin, pregabalin, valproate) and antidepressants (amitriptyline, nortriptyline, duloxetine). Modalities can also be used to help with pain control. These include ice, heat, soft tissue mobilization, and transcutaneous electrical nerve stimulation. Physical therapy and occupational therapy can also help with pain control with progressive mobility, motor imagery, and mirror box therapy, which has been shown to help with both residual and phantom limb pain.[10]

Regional Anesthesia

Postoperatively, amputee patients have both peripherally and centrally acting pain processes caused by nociceptive pain input from the site of surgery as well as the dissonance between the physical body and the still existing motor and sensory cortex of that respective limb that was amputated.[11] Regional anesthesia may interfere with the propagation of the peripheral painful stimuli to the brain and therefore is a potential prophylactic and therapeutic modality.[12]

Various regional anesthesia techniques have been studied for the treatment of pain related to amputation surgery. An early tenet was the use of epidural analgesia preoperatively. This modality initially was found to decrease phantom limb pain incidence, but the effect has proven to be inconsistent.[13] The use of epidural analgesia does have utility in improved pain control in the acute postoperative phase. A recent study examined the effect of preemptive epidural anesthesia (bupivacaine and fentanyl) 48 hours prior to surgery, intraoperative epidural anesthesia, and postoperative epidural analgesia for 48 hours after surgery. This long duration epidural analgesia reduced the incidence of phantom limb pain at 6 months.[14]

Perineural Analgesia

The need for systemic anticoagulation often prevents use of neuraxial analgesia in amputee patients.[15] Further, epidural infusions are not commonly used as outpatient. In contrast, continuous peripheral nerve blocks are not contraindicated in anticoagulated patients, are frequently provided as ambulatory infusions, and therefore, may provide a duration of analgesia that is more aligned with the time scale of the postoperative pain.[15]

Perineural infusions also avoid the hemodynamic perturbations associated with epidural and spinal anesthesia.[16-18] Studies have also demonstrated a benefit in preoperative intervention in the realm of peripheral nerve targeted approaches with effectiveness of preemptive analgesia was correlated with initiation of therapy at least 24 hours or more preoperatively.[19,20]

This has led to an increased interest in preoperative analgesia in a preventative manner where blunting both peripheral and central sensitization to painful stimuli occurs throughout the entire continuum of care starting before surgery in a multimodal approach.[20,21] There currently is no evidence from large randomized trials to demonstrate a benefit of continuous peripheral nerve blocks as prophylactic treatment for phantom pain; however, such trials are currently taking place and may provide this evidence in the future.

Once established, there are few therapeutic modalities that have been shown to reliably reduce the frequency and severity of phantom pain. Small case series have demonstrated a benefit of single injection peripheral nerve blocks for treating existing phantom pain. Additionally, the improvement in phantom pain symptoms following peripheral nerve block is reflected in a rapid reversal of the reorganization of somatosensory cortex that occurs in these patients.[22] Unfortunately, the benefit provided by single injection nerve blocks is typically transient, with the phantom pain returning with the resolution of the block.

In contrast to single injection nerve blocks, which have a during measured in hours, continuous peripheral nerve blocks have a duration measured in days or weeks.[23] Continuous peripheral nerve blocks can also be administered as an outpatient therapy, in contrast to epidural infusions, which generally requires hospital admission. As mentioned above, the reorganization of the somatosensory cortex that occurs in phantom pain is reversed by single injection nerve blocks. Given that this reorganization is reversible, it has been suggested that extended duration nerve blocks may lead to a long-term or permanent reversal of this reorganization. In such a way, an extended duration continuous peripheral nerve block could improve phantom pain for much longer than the duration of the infusion.[24] One case series suggests such an effect, while large randomized trials are currently being conducted.[24]

Regenerative Peripheral Nerve Interface and Other Intraoperative Surgical Approaches

A large portion of amputees experience disabling sensory experiences related to the loss of their limb and the management of the transected nerves. This can impact their quality of life as well as their ability to utilize a prosthesis.[25,26] Two main problems arise from transecting nerves at the time of amputation. The first is phantom limb pain, and the second is residual limb pain. The former is a noxious neurocognitive response to the absence of normal nerve signaling. Residual limb pain may be the result of direct postsurgical changes that could be mechanical (ie, compression against bone) or more commonly a result from neuroma. Both forms of postamputee pain are incredibly common and may occur in the majority of amputees.[27-29]

The concept of the regenerative peripheral nerve interface (RPNI) was initially developed in the laboratory as a means to control myoelectric prosthesis. Incidentally, it was noted that there was an absence of neuroma formation in RPNI-treated nerves.[30-33] The technique involves isolating major group fascicles of transected peripheral nerves and then securely wrapping the transected end with an autogenous free muscle graft (Fig. 30.1). The mechanism by which this is purported to create benefit is through providing a multitude of available motor end plate receptors in the deinnervated free muscle graft to allow for ample sites for the transected axons to find a home. Experts have stated the importance of and coined the phrase, "...giving nerves somewhere to go and something to do." In other words, if transected nerves do not have a sensory organ or motor end plate, they are at risk of aberrant signaling, which results in postamputation pain.

Initially, this treatment was targeted at treating existing neuroma pain. Woo et al. retrospectively reviewed their RPNI patients over a 2-year period who were treated for symptomatic neuromas in either the upper or lower extremity. Seventy-one percent of patients noted a reduction in neuroma pain and 53% noted a reduction in phantom pain.[30]

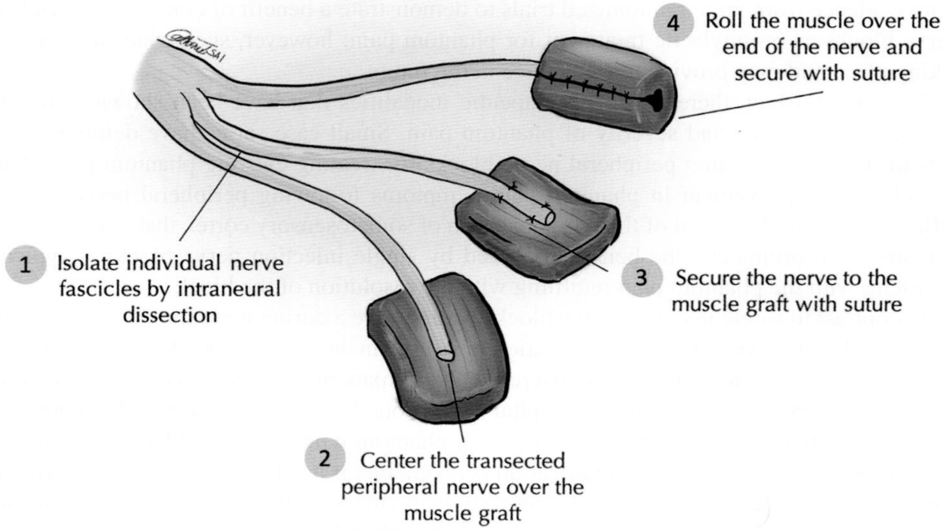

FIGURE 30.1 Depiction of creating a regenerative peripheral nerve interface (RPNI). (Courtesy of Catherine Tsai.)

The same group then evaluated the impact of performing RPNI at the time of amputation and compared outcomes between patients receiving RPNI and those without (control patients).[32] On a minimum of 4 weeks of follow-up, zero RPNI patients and 13% of the control patients developed symptomatic neuromas. Phantom limb pain developed in 51% of the RNPI patients compared to 91% of control patients.

Despite the absence of long-term follow-up or acceptance as standard of care, RPNI shows early promise in mitigating the significant pain issues related to transecting nerves at the time of amputation. The procedure is not labor or time intensive and has minimal additive risk.

Peripheral Nerve Stimulation

Electric current used to stimulate nerves and modulate the activity is referred to as "neuromodulation" and has been employed for more than a century.[34] Early peripheral nerve stimulators required open surgical procedures to implant leads adjacent to target nerves. However, the advent of ultrasound guidance and percutaneously inserted stimulator leads has allowed for precise stimulation of peripheral nerves without the need for surgery or hospital admission and has been successfully employed for both acute and chronic pain.[35,36] The physiologic mechanism by which peripheral nerve stimulation produces analgesia has not been fully elucidated; however, it has been proposed that the "Gate Control Theory" of pain control is responsible. This theory, put forth by Melzack and Wall in 1965, suggests that stimulation of large diameter afferent fibers produces an inhibitory effect or "Gate" for smaller diameter afferent fibers.[37] Thus, the electrical stimulation activates large diameter sensory afferents, which in turn inhibit the painful afferent signaling via smaller diameter afferent nerves.

Percutaneous peripheral nerve stimulation has been proposed as a treatment for established phantom limb pain. Several case reports and one pilot study have demonstrated benefit of femoral and sciatic nerve stimulation in lower extremity amputation patients.[38] A single case report suggests that brachial plexus stimulation may provide relief of upper extremity phantom pain. Peripheral nerve stimulation has the theoretical benefit in phantom pain patients of providing nonpainful sensory afferent signaling to the somatosensory cortical regional associated with the phantom limb. Further randomized, controlled trials evaluating the effectiveness of peripheral nerve stimulation for treatment of phantom pain are underway.

Conclusion

Postamputation pain management should be multimodal and individualized. Ideally, the postamputation pain management plan should be initiated preoperatively and include both preoperative counseling as well as a well-defined treatment plan. This treatment plan should include a combination of oral/intravenous opioids for nociceptive surgical pain, oral neuropathic medications for neuropathic (neuroma and phantom) limb pain, the use of peripheral nerve interventions, surgical techniques to limit the incidence of phantom limb pain, along with a comprehensive rehabilitation approach. This comprehensive multimodal approach gives patients who have undergone an amputation the best chance at managing their acute pain and preventing chronic neuropathic pain related to their amputation.

REFERENCES

1. Ziegler-Graham K, et al. Estimating the prevalence of limb loss in the United States: 2005 to 2050. *Arch Phys Med Rehabil*. 2008;89(3):422-429.
2. Jensen TS, et al. Phantom limb, phantom pain and stump pain in amputees during the first 6 months following limb amputation. *Pain*. 1983;17(3):243-256.
3. Kooijman CM, et al. Phantom pain and phantom sensations in upper limb amputees: an epidemiological study. *Pain*. 2000;87(1):33-41.
4. Neil M. Pain after amputation. *BJA Education*. 2015;16(3):107-112.
5. Watson J, et al. Neuromas of the hand and upper extremity. *J Hand Surg Am*. 2010;35(3):499-510.
6. Peters BR, et al. Targeted muscle reinnervation for the management of pain in the setting of major limb amputation. *SAGE Open Med*. 2020;8:2050312120959180.
7. Sherman RA, Sherman CJ. Prevalence and characteristics of chronic phantom limb pain among American veterans. Results of a trial survey. *Am J Phys Med*. 1983;62(5):227-238.
8. Kehlet H, Dahl JB. The value of "multimodal" or "balanced analgesia" in postoperative pain treatment. *Anesth Analg*. 1993;77(5):1048-1056.
9. Desmond D, MacLachlan M. Psychological issues in prosthetic and orthotic practice: a 25 year review of psychology in Prosthetics and Orthotics International. *Prosthet Orthot Int*. 2002;26(3):182-188.
10. Smurr LM, et al. Managing the upper extremity amputee: a protocol for success. *J Hand Ther*. 2008;21(2):160-175; quiz 176.
11. Flor H, et al. Phantom-limb pain as a perceptual correlate of cortical reorganization following arm amputation. *Nature*. 1995;375(6531):482-484.
12. D'Mello R, Dickenson AH. Spinal cord mechanisms of pain. *Br J Anaesth*. 2008;101(1):8-16.
13. Bach S, Noreng MF, Tjéllden NU. Phantom limb pain in amputees during the first 12 months following limb amputation, after preoperative lumbar epidural blockade. *Pain*. 1988;33(3):297-301.
14. Karanikolas M, et al. Optimized perioperative analgesia reduces chronic phantom limb pain intensity, prevalence, and frequency: a prospective, randomized, clinical trial. *Anesthesiology*. 2011;114(5):1144-1154.
15. Horlocker TT, et al. Regional anesthesia in the patient receiving antithrombotic or thrombolytic therapy: American Society of Regional Anesthesia and Pain Medicine Evidence-Based Guidelines (Fourth Edition). *Reg Anesth Pain Med*. 2018;43(3):263-309.
16. Fisher A, Meller Y. Continuous postoperative regional analgesia by nerve sheath block for amputation surgery—a pilot study. *Anesth Analg*. 1991;72(3):300-303.
17. Wiegel M, et al. Complications and adverse effects associated with continuous peripheral nerve blocks in orthopedic patients. *Anesth Analg*. 2007;104(6):1578-1582, table of contents.
18. Chelly JE, Ghisi D, Fanelli A. Continuous peripheral nerve blocks in acute pain management. *Br J Anaesth*. 2010;105(Suppl 1):i86-i96.
19. Hsu E, Cohen SP. Postamputation pain: epidemiology, mechanisms, and treatment. *J Pain Res*. 2013;6:121-136.
20. Vadivelu N, et al. Preventive analgesia for postoperative pain control: a broader concept. *Local Reg Anesth*. 2014;7:17-22.
21. Katz J, Clarke H, Seltzer Z. Review article: preventive analgesia: quo vadimus? *Anesth Analg*. 2011;113(5):1242-1253.

22. Birbaumer N, et al. Effects of regional anesthesia on phantom limb pain are mirrored in changes in cortical reorganization. *J Neurosci*. 1997;17(14):5503-5508.
23. Ilfeld BM. Continuous peripheral nerve blocks: an update of the published evidence and comparison with novel, alternative analgesic modalities. *Anesth Analg*. 2017;124(1):308-335.
24. Ilfeld BM, et al. Treating intractable phantom limb pain with ambulatory continuous peripheral nerve blocks: a pilot study. *Pain Med*. 2013;14(6):935-942.
25. McFarland LV, et al. Unilateral upper-limb loss: satisfaction and prosthetic-device use in veterans and service members from Vietnam and OIF/OEF conflicts. *J Rehabil Res Dev*. 2010;47(4):299-316.
26. Sinha R, van den Heuvel WJ, Arokiasamy P. Factors affecting quality of life in lower limb amputees. *Prosthet Orthot Int*. 2011;35(1):90-96.
27. Ehde DM, et al. Chronic phantom sensations, phantom pain, residual limb pain, and other regional pain after lower limb amputation. *Arch Phys Med Rehabil*. 2000;81(8):1039-1044.
28. Soroush M, et al. Neuroma in bilateral upper limb amputation. *Orthopedics*. 2008;31(12).
29. Sehirlioglu A, et al. Painful neuroma requiring surgical excision after lower limb amputation caused by landmine explosions. *Int Orthop*. 2009;33(2):533-536.
30. Woo SL, et al. Regenerative peripheral nerve interfaces for the treatment of postamputation neuroma pain: a pilot study. *Plast Reconstr Surg Glob Open*. 2016;4(12):e1038.
31. Kung TA, et al. Regenerative peripheral nerve interface viability and signal transduction with an implanted electrode. *Plast Reconstr Surg*. 2014;133(6):1380-1394.
32. Kubiak CA, et al. Prophylactic regenerative peripheral nerve interfaces to prevent postamputation pain. *Plast Reconstr Surg*. 2019;144(3):421e-430e.
33. Kubiak CA, Kemp SWP, Cederna PS. Regenerative peripheral nerve interface for management of postamputation neuroma. *JAMA Surg*. 2018;153(7):681-682.
34. Gildenberg PL. History of electrical neuromodulation for chronic pain. *Pain Med*. 2006;7(suppl_1):S7-S13.
35. Huntoon MA, Burgher AH. Review of ultrasound-guided peripheral nerve stimulation. *Tech Reg Anesth Pain Manag*. 2009;13(3):121-127.
36. Ilfeld BM, et al. Ultrasound-guided percutaneous peripheral nerve stimulation: neuromodulation of the suprascapular nerve and brachial plexus for postoperative analgesia following ambulatory rotator cuff repair. A proof-of-concept study. *Reg Anesth Pain Med*. 2019;44:310-318.
37. Melzack R, Wall PD. Pain mechanisms: a new theory. *Science*. 1965;150(3699):971-979.
38. Gilmore C, et al. Percutaneous peripheral nerve stimulation for the treatment of chronic neuropathic postamputation pain: a multicenter, randomized, placebo-controlled trial. *Reg Anesth Pain Med*. 2019;44(6):637-645.

SECTION IV

Treatment Modalities

31

Opioid Agonists

Lisa To and Juan Gabriel Garcia

Introduction

Opioids are a group of natural, synthetic, or semisynthetic chemicals that interact with opioid receptors on nerve cells in the body and reduce the intensity of pain signals. They are one of the most prescribed medications among medical professionals and are used ubiquitously in a variety of settings. Their effectiveness has resulted in opioids becoming a target for recreational abuse leading to a worldwide public health burden. Data obtained from the CDC suggest that, in the past 5 years, more than 17% of Americans had at least one opioid prescription filled, with an average of 3.4 opioid prescriptions dispensed per patient.[1] Natural and synthetic opioids continue to be a mainstay in medicine for the foreseeable future, used in every facet of medicine, and as such, it is imperative that providers understand the utility of this drug as well as its global effects.

Terminology

The terms opioids and opiates are often used interchangeably, though there is a distinction. For completeness, the term opiate analgesic primarily describes naturally occurring opium products such as heroin, morphine, and codeine, obtained from the juice of the poppy. An opioid is an all-encompassing term that includes natural or synthetic compounds that act like morphine and binds to the same receptors.

History

Organic opioids were first identified by the Sumerians in Mesopotamia around 3400 BC. This was the first group to cultivate the poppy plant, calling it Hul Gil or "joy plant," which subsequently led to the isolation of opium for its euphoric effect. The opium poppy is botanically classified as *Papaver somniferum*. The genus is named after a Greek noun for poppy, the species derived from a Latin word meaning "sleep inducing." Soon after this isolation, its use became widely spread throughout Europe, the Middle East, and North Africa. In the 7th century BC, doctors considered opium a cure for almost every ailment, sometimes mixing it with licorice or balsam.[2]

Morphine is commonly considered to be the archetypal opioid analgesic and the standard to which all other opioids and opiates are compared. Morphine was first isolated from opium in 1806 by Friedrich Sertürner, a German scientist who studied alkaloid chemistry and was able to describe the isolation, crystallization, and pharmacological properties of what is considered the first modern opioid.[3] He named the pure alkaloid after Morpheus, the Greek god of dreams. This discovery, in conjunction with the invention of hypodermic needles by Charles Pravaz and Alexander Wood, led to widespread clinical use of morphine.[4]

Four chemical groupings of natural, synthetic, and semisynthetic opioid alkaloids have been characterized as derivatives from the parent *P somniferum*. These groupings are morphinan, phenylpiperidine, diphenlyheptane, and benzomorphan derivatives.

Morphinan derivatives, also known as phenanthrenes, include the most common opioids and are the most widely used among practitioners. This group includes oxycodone, hydrocodone, hydromorphone, morphine, codeine, nalbuphine, buprenorphine, and butorphanol. Phenylpiperidine derivatives include fentanyl, alfentanil, sufentanil, and meperidine. This group is also widely used, though in a smaller clinical setting when compared to morphinan derivatives. Diphenlyheptane derivatives include propoxyphene and methadone. Benzomorphan derivatives consist of only pentazocine. This drug is a partial agonist that is characterized by high incidence of dysphoria and is not commonly used in clinical practice.

Pharmacology

Since pain is a sensory and emotional experience, the transmission of pain is multifactorial and complex.[5] However, in the simplest depiction, pain is transmitted as a noxious stimulus along a three-neuron system that originates at the periphery and terminates at the cerebral cortex. The first is a nociceptor, which is a primary afferent neuron with a peripheral terminal at the site of stimulation. The second is a neuron in the spinal cord or dorsal horn that receives input from the nociceptor and then projects to the thalamus. The final, third neuron projects from the thalamus to the sensory cortex.[6,7] The integration of this noxious stimuli in the supraspinal region then leads to the perception of pain, which has many components—sensory, emotional, and physiologic.

Noxious sensations can be categorized into two components: a fast, sharp, and well-localized sensation, which is conducted by A-δ fibers, and a slow, dull, poorly localized sensation, which is conducted by C fibers.

Opioids inhibit the sensation of nociceptive pain by blocking the transmission at every step along this pathway. They do so by binding to a variety of G-coupled receptors that in turn attenuate nociceptive transmission.

Clinically important effects of opioids are mediated by three receptors known as μ, κ, and δ. The nomenclature has since evolved, and internationally, these receptors are known as MOP, KOP, and DOP. A fourth receptor, NOP, may also be involved in pain processing. The three classes of receptors share significant gene sequence homologies and belong to the rhodopsin family of GPCRs.[8] These receptors in humans have been mapped to chromosome 1p355-33 (DOP), chromosome 8q11.23-21 (KOP), and chromosome 6q25-26 (MOR).[9] These opioid receptors are widely distributed and are found in neuronal cells at the periphery, dorsal horn of the spinal cord, brainstem, thalamus, and cortex, as well as nonneuronal cells in the GI tract. All opioid receptors couple to G_i/G_o proteins—this binding of an agonist receptor causes membrane hyperpolarization. Immediate opioid effects are mediated by inhibition of adenylyl cyclase and activation of phospholipase C. These intracellular events inhibit voltage-gated Ca^{2+} channels causing downstream reduction of neurotransmitter release from presynaptic terminals and activate inwardly rectifying of K^+ channels, which hyperpolarizes and inhibits postsynaptic response to excitatory neurotransmitters.[10]

The clinical effects of a particular opioid depend on which receptor that it binds (Table 31.1). Opioids are often characterized by the differences in affinity for specific receptors and their functional response. MOP is ubiquitous and seen throughout the CNS. All MOP receptors are encoded by a single gene, OPRM1, found on chromosome 6q24-a25. There have been over 20 MOP receptor variants that have been identified, which may account for the variability in efficacy and toxicity with MOP agonists.[11] The effects of MOP involve analgesia, euphoria, respiratory depression, sedation, tolerance, physical dependence, decreased gastrointestinal motility, biliary spasm, and miosis. DOP receptors are widely distributed, and they are

TABLE 31.1 **OPIOID RECEPTORS**

Receptors	Primary Effect
MOP	Analgesia, euphoria, respiratory depression, sedation, tolerance, dependence, decreased GI motility, biliary spasm, mitosis
DOP	Analgesia
KOP	Spinal analgesia, sedation, respiratory depression
NOP	Stress, anxiety, learning, memory, reward/addiction, tolerance

primarily responsible for mediating the analgesic effects of endogenous opioids. KOP receptors share several effects with MOP, including analgesia, sedation, and respiratory depression. The KOP receptors have been further divided into several subclasses that are relevant to opioid pharmacology. κ_1 receptor mediates spinal analgesia, whereas κ_3 mediates supraspinal analgesia, sedation, and respiratory depression.[12] NOP is a relatively newer class of receptors that act in a similar fashion to the classical receptors. NOP receptors are thought to effect locomotion, stress, anxiety, feeding, learning and memory, reward/addiction, and urogenital activity. It is believed that the NOP system may be involved in development of tolerance to opioids. The characterization of this receptor is ongoing and may prove useful in reducing tolerance and providing analgesia in the future.[13]

Mechanism of Action

Many drugs are characterized by their clinical effect that results from the potentiation or inhibition of the receptor they bind. When discussing the pharmacodynamic interaction of opioid receptor ligands, they can be classified as agonists, partial agonists, and antagonists at the receptor. A full agonist binds to its selective opioid receptor and undergoes conformational change to produce maximal downstream effect of that receptor. Nearly all opioid agonists target the MOP receptor. Partial agonists bind to their receptor in a similar fashion; however, the conformational change is less pronounced resulting in limited intrinsic activity. A unique characteristic of partial opioid agonist is that the analgesic effect of these medications will plateau despite increases in dosage. An antagonist is a compound that has high affinity of binding to the receptor, though it produces no efficacy.

Morphine and Structurally Related Opioid Agonists

Morphine

Powdered opium is derived from the dried milky juice of unripe seed capsules of the poppy plant and contains a number of alkaloids, including morphine, codeine, and papaverine. These alkaloids are divided into two distinct chemical classes, phenanthrenes (morphine, codeine, thebaine) and benzylisoquinolines (papaverine, noscapine).

Morphine is the prototypical MOP receptor ligand and is characterized as a relatively long-acting opioid with a relatively safe side effect profile. Morphine is metabolized by demethylation and glucuronidation producing two major metabolites, morphine-6-glucuronide and morphine-3-glucuronide. While both metabolites are active, M6G occurs in a higher concentration with a greater affinity for MOR and is thus largely responsible for analgesic effects, while M3G is believed to be responsible for the excitatory effects of morphine.[14,15] M6G is excreted by the kidney through glomerular filtration and can accumulate in patients with renal dysfunction.

Additionally, morphine is metabolized in small amounts to codeine and hydromorphone. Very little morphine is excreted unchanged. Its effect on the nucleus accumbens results in respiratory depression and decreased response to arterial carbon dioxide tension. Histamine release often results in a small degree of hypotension and bronchospasm. Additionally, there is a decrease in sympathetic tone causing venous pooling and orthostatic hypotension. A commonly recognized side effect of morphine is related to its effect on the GI tract, most commonly, decreased intestinal motility and biliary smooth muscle spam. Most potent inhibitors of morphine metabolism include tamoxifen, diclofenac, naloxone, carbamazepine, TCAs, and benzodiazepines.

Codeine

Codeine was first isolated in 1832 and has weak MOP receptor affinity making it ~60% as potent as morphine. It is a pro-drug and must be metabolized into morphine by CYP2D6 to have clinical effects. Its half-life is estimated to be between 2 and 4 hours but can vary due to heterogeneity of the population's cytochrome P-450 enzyme CYP2D6. Once absorbed, codeine is metabolized by the liver. Codeine plays a role in treatment of mild-moderate pain and has been effective in the management of cough. The most common adverse effect of codeine is constipation that is usually seen when initiating therapy or increasing the dosage. Nausea and vomiting are often reported with initial dosing but often resolve after continued exposure. A unique feature of codeine is that it may be ineffective in 10% of the Caucasian population with CYP2D6 polymorphisms. Other polymorphisms may also lead to ultrarapid metabolism, resulting in increased sensitivity to the drug, due to higher than expected serum concentrations.[16,17]

Papaverine

Papaverine was discovered in 1848 by Georg Merck, a German chemist. It is an opioid derivative that inhibits phosphodiesterase resulting in elevated cAMP levels. The most common clinical use of papaverine is related to its action as a direct smooth muscle vasodilator that affects both coronary and peripheral circulation, as such, it is utilized for treatment of vasospasm in a variety of settings. Most commonly, it is used in the treatment of acute mesenteric ischemia and erectile dysfunction.

Heroin

Heroin was one of the first synthetic alkaloids and was developed by Bayer Pharmaceuticals in 1898 as an antitussive. It is found to act agonistically on a variety of central nervous system opioid receptors and is estimated to be twice as potent as morphine. Heroin is metabolized in the CNS into monoacetylmorphine, which is a potent MOP receptor agonist. In the peripheral tissues, it is metabolized to 6-monoacetylmorphine (6-MAM) and subsequently hydrolyzed to morphine. Heroin and 6-MAM are highly lipophilic and rapidly crosses the blood-brain barrier. Peak serum levels are seen within 10 minutes subcutaneously, 5 minutes intranasally and intramuscularly, and <1 minute intravenously. Respiratory depression and extreme physiologic dependence are the most concerning adverse effects and are often seen with misuse. Heroin is excreted in the urine, largely as free, conjugated morphine. There are currently no FDA-approved medical indications for its use, making it a schedule I controlled substance.[18]

Hydrocodone

Hydrocodone is a moderately potent semisynthetic opioid that produces its analgesic effects by activating MOP receptors in the CNS. It is made from codeine and is equivalent to oxycodone in potency. It is metabolized by the liver via CYP2D6 and CYP3A4 to the active metabolite hydromorphone and inactive metabolite norhydrocodone. Clinical uses include management of acute or chronic pain in which an nonopioid treatment is inadequate.

Hydromorphone

Hydromorphone is a semisynthetic opioid that has all the opioid characteristics of morphine. It is more lipophilic than morphine, subsequently has a faster onset of action, and significantly more potent. It is metabolized to hydromorphone-3-glucoronide in the liver.

Oxycodone

Oxycodone is a semisynthetic opioid with potent agonist activity. Oxycodone is metabolized by cytochrome CYP3A4 and CYP2D6 into oxymorphone and noroxycodone, which subsequently are excreted via the kidneys. Presently, it is one of the most commonly abused opioid medications in the United States. Because of its potency and ease of distribution, there is high misuse potential thus providers are urged to initiate therapy at the lowest dosage and for the shortest duration of time. The side effect profile of oxycodone is equivalent to that of other common opioids.[19]

Oxymorphone

Oxymorphone is a semisynthetic opioid, derived from thebaine, with potent agonist activity. Oxymorphone is extensively metabolized by the liver and eliminated as 3- and 6-glucuronides.

Morphine and its derivatives have a variety of side effects that correlate to the wide distribution of MOP, DOR, KOP receptors, which include nausea, vomiting, dizziness, respiratory depression, pruritus, constipation, urinary retention, delayed gastric emptying, hypotension, confusion, muscle rigidity, and withdrawal. Opioids should be used carefully in patients with decreased pulmonary function, such as COPD, and obesity, as opioids can further compromise their pulmonary function through increased respiratory depression. Although opioids can release histamine, an allergic response is not common.[20]

Morphinan Derivatives

Levorphanol

Levorphanol is an opioid agonist that closely mirrors morphine. It is seven times more potent and produces less side effects such as nausea and vomiting. Levorphanol has a long half-life, 12-16 hours, and repeated administration can lead to elevated concentrations of active drug. The D-isomer is dextrorphan and possesses inhibitory effects at NMDA receptors.[21]

Meperidine

Meperidine is a strong MOP agonist but also possesses local anesthetic properties. Meperidine has been useful in the treatment of postanesthetic shivering. Meperidine is metabolized by the liver, creating *N*-demethyl, normeperidine and merperidinic acid. Meperidine can cause CNS excitation, which is concerning for development of seizures and tremors, due to accumulation of the metabolite normeperidine, which has a long half-life of 15-20 hours.[22]

Fentanyl, Remifentanil, Sufentanil

These synthetic opioids are phenylpiperidine derivatives, which are highly lipid soluble and rapidly cross the blood-brain barrier. These drugs are widely used as anesthetic adjuvants due to their quick onset and quick termination effect during bolus dosing. Fentanyl can be administered transdermally, intravenously, transbuccally, and epidurally; therefore, it has widespread utility for acute and malignant pain states. Fentanyl is 100 times more potent than morphine, and sufentanil is 1000 times more potent than morphine.

Remifentanil has a faster onset, when compared to fentanyl and sufentanil, and is unique in that it is metabolized by plasma esterases and is not dependent on the liver or kidneys for metabolism and elimination. Due to its short duration of action, it is most efficiently utilized as a continuous intravenous infusion. The context sensitive halftime of remifentanil allows for recovery of respiratory function within 3-5 minutes, and full recovery within 15 minutes.[23]

Methadone

Methadone is a long-acting opioid agonist. Methadone is a racemic mixture made up of a potent L-methadone and its isomer D-methadone; however, most of its pharmacological activity is due to L-methadone. The half-life of this medication is 15-40 hours, so it is important to note that repeated administration over several days will result in drug accumulation. On the other hand, when the medication is abruptly stopped, slow release of methadone from tissue will result in withdrawal symptoms. It is commonly used in a variety of settings—opioid detoxification, opioid maintenance in addiction, and chronic pain states.[24]

Tramadol

Tramadol is a synthetic codeine analogue that possesses weak MOP agonist activity and inhibition of NE and 5HT reuptake. Tramadol is a racemic mixture; the positive enantiomer inhibits 5HT reuptake, while the negative enantiomer inhibits NE reuptake and stimulates $\alpha 2$ receptors. Tramadol is effective in the treatment of mild to moderate pain. The side effects are similar to other opioids but also include dry mouth, seizures, and increased risk for serotonin syndrome when used with other MAOI and SSRI medications due to impaired 5HT metabolism.[25]

Tapentadol

Tapentadol has a similar structure to tramadol. It is a weak inhibitor of monoamine reuptake and strong agonist at MOP receptors. Like tramadol, serotonin syndrome is a risk, especially when tapentadol is used with SSRIs, SNRIs, TCA, or MAOI. Tapentadol is metabolized by glucuronidation.

Partial Agonists

Nalbuphine

Nalbuphine acts as a competitive antagonist at MOP receptors and agonists at KOP receptors. Unlike other opioids, it does not cause respiratory depression or euphoria. It is used to produce analgesia and to treat morphine-induced pruritus.[26]

Buprenorphine

Buprenorphine is partial MOR agonist, derived from thebaine. It is highly lipophilic and, therefore, 50 times more potent than morphine. It is metabolized in the liver to its active metabolite, norbuprenorphine, which has only weak activity. The partial opioid receptor binding pattern allows buprenorphine to possess a ceiling effect. Buprenorphine can safely treat acute pain, chronic pain, and opioid dependence.[27]

Concerns With Therapeutic Use

In acute pain states, opioids can be very effective in treating pain. However, its use in chronic pain states are concerning for the development of tolerance, hyperalgesia, and dependence.

Tolerance and dependence will largely depend on the type of opioid utilized, amount prescribed, frequency, and confounding psychosocial comorbidities. It is well documented that there is a concerning opioid epidemic in the United States, which consumes nearly 80% of the world's supply of prescription opioids due to recreational drug use. When treating chronic pain, it is important to optimize conservative options and nonopioid coanalgesics.

REFERENCES

1. "Understanding the Epidemic." *Centers for Disease Control and Prevention*. March 17, 2021. www.cdc.gov/drugoverdose/epidemic/index.html
2. Booth M. *Opium: a History*. St. Martin's Press; 1998.
3. Pathan H, Williams J. Basic opioid pharmacology: an update. *Br J Pain*. 2012;6(1):11-16. doi:10.1177/2049463712438493
4. Blakemore PR, White JD. Morphine, the Proteus of organic molecules. *Chem Commun*. 2002;(11):1159-1168.
5. Charlton JE, ed. *Opioids: Core Curriculum for Professional Education in Pain*. IASP Press; 2005.
6. Vrooman BM, Rosenquist RW. Chronic pain management. In: Butterworth JF IV, Mackey DC, Wasnick JD, eds. *Morgan & Mikhail's Clinical Anesthesiology*. 6th ed. McGraw-Hill; 2018.
7. Liu Q, Gold MS. Neurobiologic mechanisms of nociception. In: Hadzic A, ed. *Hadzic's Textbook of Regional Anesthesia and Acute Pain Management*. 2nd ed. McGraw-Hill; 2017.
8. Stevens CW. The evolution of vertebrate opioid receptors. *Front Biosci*. 2009;14:1247-1269.
9. Dreborg S, et al. Evolution of vertebrate opioid receptors. *Proc Natl Acad Sci U S A*. 2008;105:15487-15492.
10. Shang Y, Filizola M. Opioid receptors: structural and mechanistic insights into pharmacology and signaling. *Eur J Pharmacol*. 2015;763:206-213.
11. Law PY, Loh HH, Wei L-N. Insights into the receptor transcription and signaling: implications in opioid tolerance and dependence. *Neuropharmacology*. 2004;47(suppl 1):300-311.
12. Rosow C, Dershwitz M. Opioid analgesics. In: Longnecker DE, Mackey SC, Newman MF, Sandberg WS, Zapol WM, eds. *Anesthesiology*. 3rd ed. McGraw-Hill; 2017.
13. Gear RW, Bogen O, Ferrari LF, Green PG, Levine JD. NOP receptor mediates anti-analgesia induced by agonist-antagonist opioids. *Neuroscience*. 2014;257:139-148.
14. Smith MT. Neuroexcitatory effects of morphine and hydromorphone: evidence implicating the 3-glucuronide metabolites. *Clin Exp Pharmacol Physiol*. 2000;27:524-528.
15. Osborne R, et al. The analgesic activity of morphine-6-glucuronide. *Br J Clin Pharmacol*. 1992;34:130-138.
16. Eichelbaum M, Evert B. Influence of pharmacogenetics on drug disposition and response. *Clin Exp Pharmacol Physiol*. 1996;23:983-985.
17. Caraco Y, et al. Impact of ethnic origin and quinidine coadministration on codeine's disposition and pharmacodynamic effects. *J Pharmacol Exp Ther*. 1999;290:413-422.
18. Rook EJ, et al. Pharmacokinetics and pharmacokinetic variability of heroin and its metabolites: review of the literature. *Curr Clin Pharmacol*. 2006;1:109-118.
19. Yaksh T, Wallace M. Opioids, analgesia, and pain management. In: Brunton LL, Hilal-Dandan R, Knollmann BC, eds. *Goodman & Gilman's: The Pharmacological Basis of Therapeutics*. 13th ed. McGraw-Hill; 2017.
20. Baldo BA, Pham NH. Histamine-releasing and allergenic properties of opioid analgesic drugs: resolving the two. *Anaesth Intensive Care*. 2012;40(2):216-235.
21. Prommer E. Levorphanol: revisiting an underutilized analgesic. *Palliat Care*. 2014;8:7-10.
22. Latta KS, et al. Meperidine: a critical review. *Am J Ther*. 2002;9:53-68.
23. Stroumpos C, et al. Remifentanil, a different opioid: potential clinical applications and safety aspects. *Expert Opin Drug Saf*. 2010;9:355-364.
24. Fredheim OM, et al. Clinical pharmacology of methadone for pain. *Acta Anaesthesiol Scand*. 2008;52:879-889.
25. Grond S, Sablotzki A. Clinical pharmacology of tramadol. *Clin Pharmacokinet*. 2004;43:879-923.
26. Schmidt WK, et al. Nalbuphine. *Drug Alcohol Depend*. 1985;14:339-362.
27. Elkader A, Sproule B. Buprenorphine: clinical pharmacokinetics in the treatment of opioid dependence. *Clin Pharmacokinet*. 2005;44:661-680.

32

Acute Pain Management in Patients on Medication Maintenance Therapy—Buprenorphine, Methadone, or Naltrexone

Sameer K. Goel, Shilen P. Thakrar, Tina S. Thakrar, Caitlin E. Martin, Dharti Patel, and Savitri Gopaul

Introduction

Besides dulling pain and suffering, the μ-opioid receptor is associated with side effects ranging from mild tolerance and hyperalgesia to respiratory depression and death.[1] From 1999 to 2018, the opioid overdose epidemic has killed close to half a million Americans; ~128 people die from an opioid overdose daily,[2] with opioid overdose accounting for 46 800 total deaths in 2018, exceeding the total number of deaths caused by motor vehicle crashes. Additionally, an estimated 1.7 million Americans suffer from opioid use disorder (OUD).[3] This significant public health implication does not appear to be improving, as recent evidence suggests new persistent opioid use to be common and underappreciated after both major and minor surgeries.[4]

With the increasing number of Americans suffering from OUD, the FDA has approved three medications to target and treat OUD—buprenorphine (μ-opioid receptor partial agonist), methadone (μ-opioid receptor full agonist), and naltrexone (μ-opioid receptor antagonist). Due to their favorably long half-lives, buprenorphine and methadone decrease physiologic cravings that are known to drive aberrant drug-seeking behavior.[5] Naltrexone, on the other hand, is an opioid antagonist that may help reset the ventral tegmental area, nucleus accumbens (with projections to the prefrontal cortex), and dopaminergic reward pathways,[5,6] which play a role in persistent OUD. These individual medications for opioid use disorder (MOUD) have shown to result in significant reductions in illicit drug use and overdose deaths, criminal offenses, and concomitant infectious diseases including HIV and hepatitis C.[5] These treatments have improved health and well-being as well as daily functioning for individuals affected with OUD.

As a result of effective public health approaches aimed at dampening the increasing morbidity and mortality of the opioid overdose crisis, MOUD use is on the rise, and consequently, clinicians can expect to encounter patients receiving buprenorphine, methadone, or naltrexone.[6] OUD, as with other substance use disorders (SUDs), is a type of addiction; addiction is a chronic medical disease with a neurobiological basis shaped by one's environment where individuals continue to use opioids despite adverse consequences.[5-7] Due to the chronic nature of OUD, even if people are engaged in treatment with OUD, substance use recurrence is not uncommon, just as for other chronic diseases such as hypertension and diabetes. Pain, stress, mood with a combination of medical and surgical conditions are common incident factors for substance use recurrence that require effective treatment strategies and increased support from health care providers to mitigate harm.[8,9] Patients on MOUD generally exhibit opioid tolerance, requiring escalating doses of opioids to achieve the same analgesic effect.[10-12] Interestingly, these patients also exhibit increased sensitivity to pain and comorbid chronic pain conditions.[12-14] Additionally, development of opioid-induced hyperalgesia, an increase in pain sensitivity from opioids as a result of neuroplastic changes in pain perception, and psychosocial issues are common in patients receiving MOUD.[10,13] Thus, the management of acute pain in this patient population is challenging and requires specific considerations and planning. This chapter provides a review of the management of patients on MOUD and clinical suggestions for the optimal care for this patient population.

Medications for Opioid Use Disorder

Buprenorphine: Pharmacology

Buprenorphine is a thebaine derivative originally developed in the 1970s as an analgesic.[15,16] Due to its unique pharmacologic profile, it was later discovered to have the potential for treatment in OUD.[16] Buprenorphine is a partial agonist at the μ-opioid receptor and a full antagonist at the κ-opioid receptor.[16] It also binds the delta and opioid-receptor-like 1 (ORL-1) receptors.[16] As an ORL-1 receptor agonist, buprenorphine has a distinct interaction with pain processing.[17] Activating the ORL-1 receptor in the dorsal horn is analgesic, but as illustrated in animal models, cerebral activation of ORL-1 blunts antinociception.[17] Antagonism at the κ-opioid receptor reduces opioid misuse and has been implicated in the treatment of depressive symptoms.[16,18,19] Many of buprenorphine's clinical attributes come from its partial agonism at the μ-opioid receptor. Buprenorphine is a lipophilic compound that dissociates very slowly from the μ-opioid receptor; this along with its long half-life is both thought to play a role in its extended duration of action.[18,20] In addition to its dissociative properties, buprenorphine has a high affinity for the μ-opioid receptor and will not be readily displaced by either μ-opioid receptor full agonists or antagonists, such as naloxone.[18,21] Conversely, because of its heightened affinity, buprenorphine will compete for binding at the receptor site and displace receptor-bound opioid agonists precipitating withdrawal when taken by individuals physically dependent on opioids.[16]

Once absorbed, buprenorphine is metabolized primarily by the CYP3A4 enzymes in the liver into the metabolite norbuprenorphine.[15] At therapeutic doses, buprenorphine and its metabolites do not inhibit cytochromes resulting in few drug-drug interactions.[20] The clearance of buprenorphine is largely via the gastrointestinal tract, and its elimination is not impacted by renal function making it safe to use in those with renal failure or on hemodialysis.[17] Buprenorphine has been shown to provide effective analgesia at low to moderate doses and on average is 30 times more potent than morphine.[18,21] Unlike other opioids, buprenorphine has a dose-ceiling effect on respiratory depression but not on analgesia.[17] The respiratory depression associated with buprenorphine is found to be related to its metabolite and not the parent compound itself.[17]

Buprenorphine comes in sublingual, transdermal, subcutaneous, and intravenous formulations. Sublingual buprenorphine is typically taken once daily, but some patients may split their dosing into twice (BID) or three (TID) times a day dosing to maintain its therapeutic effect throughout the day and night. For the treatment of OUD, the combination product of buprenorphine with naloxone as a sublingual film is most commonly used. Naloxone, an opioid antagonist, is active parenterally; however, it has limited oral and sublingual bioavailability. Therefore, the naloxone component is solely a diversion and misuse deterrent.[22] Specifically, if the combination product of buprenorphine with naloxone is injected, the naloxone component becomes active within 20 minutes, which would initiate withdrawal with opiates present[22] and would attenuate any "rush" that could occur, decreasing the risk of misuse.[22] Most patients on buprenorphine for OUD are on doses between 8 and 24 mg. Based on clinical studies with small sample sizes, the percentage of μ-opioid receptors occupied by buprenorphine is <50% at a dose of 2 mg/day and >80% at a higher dose of 16 mg/day.[21,23] From empirical data, the higher dose of buprenorphine has been shown to decrease withdrawal symptoms and displace or block full opioid agonists such as hydromorphone.[24] However, clinically, there is extensive individual variation in the daily dosages required to achieve stability for patients. For example, some patients only require 8 mg daily to not have any withdrawal or craving symptoms throughout a 24-hour period, while other patients may require 24 mg daily to achieve the same clinical effect.

Buprenorphine: Management

The implementation of the Drug Addiction Treatment Act (DATA) in 2000 has allowed more providers to prescribe MOUD, resulting in more adults who are prescribed buprenorphine present for surgery and procedural interventions. Controversy has ensued as there are limited guidelines on the management of acute pain in patients on buprenorphine; therefore, achieving effective analgesia during this period can be difficult due to its pharmacological predominance as a partial μ-receptor agonist. Based on early case reports and expert opinion, initial management was to stop buprenorphine 72 hours prior to an anticipated procedure or intervention that results in acute pain.[25] The thought behind this recommendation was based on the potential interference of buprenorphine with full μ-opioid receptor agonists. Because buprenorphine has a high affinity to its receptors, maintaining a patient on buprenorphine preprocedure would require higher and more frequent dosing of opioid agonists to manage pain. However, Kornfeld and Manfredi reported potential complications, including acute withdrawal, which can worsen pain from abruptly discontinuing buprenorphine prior to surgery.[26] Moreover, a recent retrospective cohort and other observational studies have concluded that continuing buprenorphine perioperatively and adding opioid analgesics along with multimodal adjuncts (Table 32.1) for breakthrough pain after surgery is an effective management strategy.[9,14] Further, splitting a patient's buprenorphine total daily dose into split dosing, such as three- or four-times daily dosing, is a useful strategy to continue a patient on their dose of buprenorphine that ensures OUD and recovery stability (no withdrawal, craving) with additional analgesic benefits from the buprenorphine itself. At our institution, this is a common method we use for patients in the perioperative period.

Another strategy (but not preferred) for acute pain control involves converting buprenorphine to a methadone regimen with the thought that better analgesia can be achieved using a full opioid agonist over a partial agonist[27]; the data on this specific regimen, however, are limited. Additionally, this method lends to complex postprocedure management for restarting patients on buprenorphine given methadone's long half-life; this delayed restart of a patient's

TABLE 32.1 RECOMMENDATIONS FROM CASE SERIES, OBSERVATIONAL STUDIES, AND EXPERT PANEL OPINION—SPECIFICALLY FOR PERIOPERATIVE PAIN MANAGEMENT OF BUPRENORPHINE

- Continue buprenorphine therapy in all combinations—SL, TD[a]
- Maximize nonopioid analgesics (eg, acetaminophen, gabapentinoids, NSAIDs, muscle relaxants)
- Consider regional and/or neuraxial analgesia
- Utilize opioids with higher μ-opioid receptor affinity when indicated (eg, hydromorphone/fentanyl)
- Consider other adjuvant therapeutic options including heat/cold treatment, acupuncture, massage, transcutaneous electrical nerve stimulation (TENS)

Note: Patients should be closely monitored for adequate analgesia and adverse effects such as excess sedation and respiratory depression.
[a]SL, sublingual; TD, transdermal; NSAIDs, nonsteroidal anti-inflammatory drugs.

medication for OUD can place the patient at risk of instability and substance use recurrence. Lastly, some experts suggest that the κ-antagonist effect of buprenorphine may help reduce opioid-induced hyperalgesia, which is commonly seen in patients receiving MOUD.[25] Thus, continuation of buprenorphine through the perioperative period with the use of an individualized multimodal pain management plan may be the optimal strategy for many patients. Discontinuation of buprenorphine in stabilized OUD or chronic pain patients without appropriate periprocedural pain management presents medical risks and burdens patients, prescribers, and the health system as a whole.

Methadone: Pharmacology

In 1972, the Food and Drug Administration (FDA) approved the use of methadone, a long-acting synthetic μ-opioid receptor agonist, for the treatment of OUD.[28] It is the most widely used and studied pharmacotherapy for OUD in the world. Methadone is highly bound to plasma proteins making it very bioavailable; additionally, it is a racemic mixture with R and S enantiomers having *N*-methyl-D-aspartate antagonist activity.[5,29] The R enantiomer is also responsible for the opioid effect.[5,29] Methadone has long been the treatment of choice due to its long half-life, cross-tolerance to other opioid agonists, and μ-opioid receptor agonist activity, thus lessening risk of misuse and blunting the euphoric effects of illicit opioids.[5,29]

The peak plasma levels of orally administered methadone are achieved within 2-4 hours.[5,29] However, the half-life of methadone varies significantly from 8 to 59 hours.[3] It is metabolized in the liver, primarily by the CYP450 3A4 enzyme, and eliminated through renal and fecal route.[3] This also leads to substantial individual variability in the total daily dose required for patients to achieve stability with regard to their OUD and recovery (eg, no cravings or withdrawal).[30] Methadone dosages used for OUD range typically from ~50 to 200 mg.[30] Intriguingly, methadone undergoes a biphasic elimination pattern explaining its potential clinical uses and resultant misconceptions (see *Methadone: Management Recommendations*). The α-elimination (8-12 hours) is associated primarily with analgesia and β-elimination (30-60 hours) is associated with withdrawal suppression in chronic OUD.[5,29] The importance of the biphasic elimination arises in the dosing regimen. The analgesic component of methadone will wear off within 8 hours leaving acute pain untreated for the remainder of the day unless re-dosed at more frequent intervals compared to outpatient dosing for OUD.[31] This is important to emphasize for patients with comorbid pain and OUD as methadone is typically dosed on a daily basis where patients go to a licensed OUD outpatient treatment program, or "methadone clinic," to receive their medication daily.

Methadone can prolong the QTc interval and has been associated with torsades de pointes and sudden cardiac death with QTc intervals >500 ms.[5] The potential for QTc prolongation and the development of life-threatening arrhythmias appear to be related to the dose and chronicity of methadone use.[32] Due to the interindividual variability in methadone's bioavailability, clearance, and half-life, clinicians need to be vigilant of any hepatic insult or administration of concomitant medications that may impact the cytochrome P-450 system and thereby significantly change the methadone serum concentration.[33]

Methadone: Management Recommendations

Patient anxiety related to fear of discrimination due to profound existing stigma with regard to OUD and MOUD are not inconsequential. Equally, fears regarding a patient's inadequate treatment of their pain with their maintenance MOUD are profound. This, in addition to clinicians' misconception or simply lack of knowledge may cause distrust, in turn, complicating delivery of adequate pain relief. That a once daily maintenance dose of methadone provides adequate analgesia for acute pain in addition to MOUD is a common misconception. Generally, methadone should be continued uninterrupted through the acute phase of illness or surgery after the dose and frequency have been verified with the patient's methadone provider or program.[33] To alleviate anxiety, patients must be reassured that their methadone will be continued and possibly split dosed at more frequent intervals unless clinically contraindicated (eg, no less than a patient's total daily dose of methadone either given in a single dose or split into smaller doses). Moreover, side effects such as sedation, euphoria, opioid-induced constipation, and respiratory depression should be monitored and treated. Additionally, their acute pain should be aggressively treated with multimodal agents. For example, utilization of regional and neuraxial anesthesia, as well as nonopioid and nonpharmacological agents as part of the pain management regimen, can be beneficial. If the patient is strictly nil per os (NPO), the methadone dose can be given intravenously (IV). Converting the dose from oral to IV can be difficult, especially at higher doses, and conversion may warrant involvement of a pharmacist or the primary methadone prescriber to determine the appropriate dosing. In general, the oral dose should be reduced by half or two-thirds and then given by IV in divided doses every 6-8 hours.[5,31] In addition to the patient's daily methadone maintenance dose, opioid analgesics can be utilized when indicated. However, in patients on daily methadone for maintenance, partial opioid agonists (ie, butorphanol and nalbuphine) should be avoided as they can precipitate withdrawal.[28]

Additional Important Buprenorphine and Methadone Management Considerations

The perioperative period can be an especially vulnerable time for patients with OUD with regard to adequate pain control and stabilizing OUD recovery. Thus, close coordination between pain management and addiction medicine teams is paramount to ensure that the patient receives adequate pain control and is centrally involved in this decision-making process. Close outpatient follow-up pre- and postoperatively must be established. There is a common misperception that providing patients in OUD recovery with acute pain medications, like short-acting opioids, leads to recurrence of substance use.[9] In fact, stress and anxiety associated with unrelieved pain is more likely to trigger recurrence of substance use.[9]

In addition to dose and frequency verification, the patient's MOUD prescriber should be notified of any changes to a patient's condition, including any hospitalizations or surgeries, changes in medications, and information regarding any controlled substances prescribed to the patient, as they may be detectable by drug testing. Most importantly, close outpatient follow-up with all teams should be arranged before discharge to ensure that the patient is followed closely in a recovery promoting manner (eg, no more than 1 week postdischarge follow-up with MOUD prescriber, pill counts at visits, inclusion of and educating family members involved in medication administration at home, and use of pill lock boxes). In addition, discharge with opioid analgesics should include a taper plan. A multidisciplinary team approach and patient-centric care to formulate and implement a plan is essential to delivering consistent, high-quality care.

Buprenorphine and Methadone: In Pregnancy

Opioid use disorder is a chronic disease, and like other chronic diseases, it continues into pregnancy. Just as it is preferred to continue medical treatments and optimize chronic diseases, like diabetes and hypertension, MOUD is no exception. Both buprenorphine and methadone are safe medications for OUD in pregnancy, and for women who are on MOUD at the start of pregnancy or desire to start MOUD during pregnancy, this is highly recommended given their proven benefits to reduce overdose risk and improve both maternal and fetal outcomes.[34,35] In 2018, the Substance Abuse and Mental Health Administration published a guidance document outlining recommendations for MOUD treatment during pregnancy and postpartum care.[34,36] Recommendations from this document include (1) medically supervised withdrawal or detoxification during pregnancy and postpartum care is not recommended[37]; (2) switching from methadone to buprenorphine during pregnancy is not recommended and should only be considered on an individual basis; and (3) withdrawal of the neonate, or neonatal abstinence syndrome, is a temporary condition without high-quality evidence indicating long-term ill effects for children from the withdrawal itself and should be treated with both nonpharmacologic and pharmacologic interventions as indicated.[38] Lastly, it is common for patients to need increased total daily dosing of buprenorphine and methadone during pregnancy to maintain stability due to changes in maternal physiology[39]; the dose of MOUD is not correlated with neonatal withdrawal risk or severity.[40] Overall, providing comprehensive and compassionate care to the mother-infant dyad affected by OUD is of paramount importance. Optimizing maternal health and supporting a healthy family living environment are the most significant drivers of long-term positive outcomes.[41]

The same recommendations outlined above apply to acute pain management during labor and delivery for patients receiving MOUD. First, patients should continue their MOUD at their prescribed dosages throughout the intra-and postpartum periods, no matter the planned delivery method (vaginal vs cesarean delivery). Careful consultation between addiction medicine, obstetrics, and anesthesia providers should be conducted prenatally to devise an individualized pain management plan.[42] It has been shown that birthing parents on buprenorphine therapy have more pain with vaginal delivery and postpartum compared to those not on any opioid therapy.[43] This finding supports the idea that birthing parents on MOUD are hyperalgesic at baseline and require uniquely tailored pain management regimen.[44] As expected, many parturients on buprenorphine or methadone need significantly more pain medication compared to opioid naive pregnant women. Seventy percent of women required more opioid analgesia 24 hours after a cesarean section compared to non–opioid-dependent pregnant women.[45,46] Common management decisions for these patients include planning an early epidural during labor and leaving the epidural catheter *in situ* post cesarean delivery for up to 24 hours.[39]

Breastfeeding is recommended for women receiving MOUD given its health benefits for the newborn in addition to decreasing neonatal withdrawal risk and severity.[36,47] While buprenorphine and its metabolite norbuprenorphine are found in breast milk, there are no clinically significant adverse side effects to neonates or children.[47] Buprenorphine is excreted into breast milk in a 1:1 ratio and has minimal effects on the neonatal abstinence scoring in infants.[45] Receipt of additional opioids for pain control, such as after a cesarean delivery, is not a contraindication for breastfeeding. In general, women with OUD should be encouraged to breast-feed and be supported in doing so.

Naltrexone: Pharmacology

Naltrexone is an opioid antagonist that competitively binds μ-opioid receptors, blocking the effects of both endogenous and exogenous opioids.[28] Naltrexone has both an oral as well as a monthly intramuscular (IM) extended-release (XR) formulation. It was initially approved for the treatment of alcohol dependence. Orally, naltrexone is readily absorbed in the gastrointestinal tract with peak concentrations achieved at 1 hour after undergoing first-pass metabolism.[5] The XR naltrexone, introduced in 2010 for treatment of OUD, is a 380 mg suspension. It is embedded in a biodegradable microsphere matrix that undergoes hydrolysis when it absorbs water and yields opioid antagonism for 28 days.[5] The XR formulation of naltrexone circumvents first-pass hepatic metabolism. It reaches peak blood levels 2 hours after IM injection, then transiently again 2-3 days after injection. The concentrations, and thus the effects of naltrexone's μ-opioid receptor antagonism, begin to gradually decline ~14 days after injection. Both formulations are metabolized by the liver and renally excreted. Oral naltrexone has a half-life of 4 hours as opposed to the XR naltrexone, which has an elimination half-life of ~10 days.[5]

Naltrexone: Management Recommendations

Pain management is clinically challenging for patients with OUD receiving naltrexone. Naltrexone should be discontinued prior to any acute management of pain in close coordination with the prescribing physician. For instance, in the setting of a scheduled surgery, oral naltrexone should be discontinued at least 2 days prior to the day of surgery due to its 10-hour half-life.[5] Unfortunately, less guidance is available for naltrexone XR. Although successful pain management has been reported in the 4th week of naltrexone XR and onwards, close monitoring and caution should be utilized, in coordination with the prescribing physician due to the variation in responses.[5] This variability arises from the upregulation of the μ-opioid receptors; combined with the coadministration of opioids and variable levels of naltrexone XR over the course of the month, serious side effects range from risk of overdose to precipitated withdrawal.[28] If surgery is performed while the patient is within 4 weeks of the last injection of naltrexone XR, routine doses of opioids may be ineffective and higher doses may be necessary. Unlike opioid agonists, naltrexone by itself will not cause withdrawal when discontinued. However, due to the upregulation of μ-opioid receptors after naltrexone is no longer present, opioid analgesics can elicit an exaggerated response.[28] Weighing the benefits against the risks and maximizing opioid-sparing techniques, including regional anesthesia and nonopioid agents, is paramount. An individualized approach involving the patient and the prescriber in the decision-making process helps to manage acute pain and prevent substance use recurrence.

Evaluating Patients Receiving MOUD

A thorough evaluation of a patient with OUD in an acute setting begins with a pain history (Table 32.2). Baseline pain scores and daily function helps to set goals and expectations. Identifying pain generator(s) allows one to have a targeted approach to pain management interventions. In addition, a medication reconciliation is essential to identify potential drug-drug interactions and identify medications whose cessation may lead to withdrawal. Referring to the state prescription drug monitoring program is a must to verify controlled substances and find contact information of prescribers and pharmacies. It is important to note that methadone may not be listed on the prescription drug monitoring program if dispensed by a methadone program.

Social determinants of health and patient values are just as important as the provision of medical care. Patients with diagnosis of OUD often have coexisting psychiatric and SUD comorbidities. Screening tools such as depression screens and pain catastrophizing scales can help guide perioperative pain management. Chronic pain patients as well as those with SUDs with a history of pain-related anxiety (or generalized anxiety disorder), major depressive disorder, and/or posttraumatic stress disorder along with significant pain catastrophizing have a higher risk of opioid misuse.[28] Pain catastrophizing scales can be utilized to identify patients with feelings of helplessness and levels of catastrophizing thought processes regarding their acute pain and may assist with making informed decisions regarding their pain management plan.[28] Furthermore, the opioid risk tool can be utilized to identify patients with acute or chronic pain at risk of non-prescribed substance use and can assist in the guidance of formulating an acute pain management plan that would limit those risks.[5]

Diagnostic laboratory studies, including a comprehensive metabolic panel, can help identify any changes in hepatic and renal function from baseline as well as any aberrancy in electrolytes that will need correcting. An electrocardiogram can assess the QTc interval and can be an essential part of a workup for any cardiopulmonary disease. Caution should be used in continuing methadone concomitantly with other QT prolonging medications.

Pain management of patients with OUD is challenging, and the use of MOUD in patients with OUD is an important part of modern medical treatment. Multimodal analgesia including,

TABLE 32.2 CLINICAL SUGGESTIONS FOR OPTIMAL CARE OF PATIENTS ON MOUD

History • Pain generator(s) • Baseline pain score, for example, Visual Analog Scale • Baseline function (physical therapy, occupational therapy, activities of daily living [ADLs], instrumental activities of daily living [IADLs]) • Review of prescription drug monitoring program and/or records from prescribers
Associated comorbidities/general review of systems (ROS) • Cardiac—coronary disease, heart failure, endocarditis from injection drug use • Pulmonary—preexisting disease (asthma, COPD), acute exacerbation (pneumonia), sleep apnea and use of CPAP or BIPAP • Gastrointestinal/hepatic—hepatitis, cirrhosis and sequelae, constipation, nausea/vomiting • Renal—baseline function, dialysis • Nutrition—Perioperative Nutrition Screen (PONS) or American Society of Parenteral and Enteral Nutrition (ASPEN) criteria for malnutrition • Neurologic—seizures, stroke, neuropathy, sleep disturbances • Endocrine/metabolic—diabetes/insulin management, thyroid function, osteopenia, erectile dysfunction, menstrual irregularity • Catastrophizing score, depression and anxiety screen, opioid-risk tool (ORT)
Social • History of tobacco, alcohol, and non-prescribed substance use • Other social determinants of health and well-being including access to providers and other aspects of care including family relationships, housing status, work/career status
Medications • Reconciliation, verification of dose and frequency • Review of prescription drug monitoring program and/or records from prescribers • Review drug interactions
Physical examination • Baseline vital signs suggestive of toxicity or withdrawal • Mental status findings—speech, memory, mood, alertness
Labs/diagnostics • Complete metabolic panel (baseline renal and hepatic function, electrolytes, albumin) • EKG/QTc • Urine drug screen • Urine pregnancy test • HIV/hepatitis serology if indicated

but not limited to, nonopioid adjuncts and utilizing regional or neuraxial analgesia along with nonpharmacological approaches is ideal. Use of multimodals begins with preemptive analgesia, which is defined as pain treatment preventing altered central processing from afferent nerve fibers associated with inflammation and tissue injury.[48,49] Preemptive analgesia includes the use of acetaminophen, nonsteroidal inflammatory drugs, gabapentinoids, clonidine, and dexamethasone. Many of these drugs are becoming implemented into standardized perioperative surgical protocols at institutions focused on Enhanced Recovery After Surgery (ERAS).[49] Moreover, combining different pain medications targeting different receptors reduces overall dosage of any one particular medication thereby reducing potential side effects. Nonsteroidal inflammatory drugs have been proven to reduce perioperative opioid requirement by 20%-30%.[50] Interestingly, the use of pregabalin has been shown to reduce pain intensity and the use of breakthrough opioids.[51] The use of lidocaine infusion in the perioperative setting has been reported to reduced morphine requirements within the first 24 hours after bariatric surgery[52]; while the use of intravenous lidocaine in the perioperative setting remains controversial, the theoretical benefits of disrupting additional pain conduction pathways may benefit the patient on MOUD. Additionally, analgesic adjuncts such as the $\alpha 2$ agonist, dexmedetomidine,[53] and the *N*-methyl-D-aspartate antagonist, ketamine,[54] have been shown to reduce opioid requirement postoperatively. While most of these drugs were studied in the opioid naive patient, they play an even more important role in patients on MOUD.

When opioids are necessary, it should be noted that patients with OUD may require higher doses of opioid analgesics due to tolerance, hyperalgesia, and increased pain sensitivity. This can be done with appropriate monitoring and a patient-centric treatment plan that involves shared decision-making with multidisciplinary coordination of care. Lastly, due to the risk of side effects, non-prescribed substance use and adverse events of opioids, patients and their families should receive opioid analgesic safe use, storage, and disposal education. Close monitoring is important to ensure that patients continue their OUD treatment and receive necessary support from their primary care pain specialists and/or addiction treatment providers.

REFERENCES

1. Shafer SL. Opioids. Opioids!! Opioids??? *ASA Monitor*. 2020;84(2):4-5.
2. Opioid Overdose: Understanding the Epidemic. Centers for Disease Control and Prevention. Published March 19, 2020. Accessed August 13, 2020. https://www.cdc.gov/drugoverdose/epidemic/index.html
3. Medications for Opioid Use Disorder—SAMHSA. store.samhsa.gov/sites/default/files/SAMHSA_Digital_Download/PEP20-02-01-006_508.pdf
4. Brummett CM, Waljee JF, Goesling J, et al. New persistent opioid use after minor and major surgical procedures in US adults. *JAMA Surg*. 2017;152(6):e170504. doi:10.1001/jamasurg.2017.0504
5. Harrison TK, Kornfeld H, Aggarwal AK, Lembke A. Perioperative considerations for the patient with opioid use disorder on buprenorphine, methadone, or naltrexone maintenance therapy. *Anesthesiol Clin*. 2018;36(3):345-359. doi:10.1016/j.anclin.2018.04.002
6. DCD. 5-Point Strategy To Combat the Opioid Crisis. Reviewed August 30, 2020. Accessed October 14, 2020. https://www.hhs.gov/opioids/about-the-epidemic/hhs-response/index.html
7. American Society of Addiction Medicine. ASAM Definition of Addiction. Published 2019. Accessed October 14, 2020. https://www.asam.org/Quality-Science/definition-of-addiction
8. Griffin ML, McDermott KA, McHugh RK, Fitzmaurice GM, Jamison RN, Weiss RD. Longitudinal association between pain severity and subsequent opioid use in prescription opioid dependent patients with chronic pain. *Drug Alcohol Depend*. 2016;163:216-221. doi:10.1016/j.drugalcdep.2016.04.023
9. Macintyre PE, Russell RA, Usher KA, Gaughwin M, Huxtable CA. Pain relief and opioid requirements in the first 24 hours after surgery in patients taking buprenorphine and methadone opioid substitution therapy. *Anaesth Intensive Care*. 2013;41(2):222-230. doi:10.1177/0310057X1304100212
10. Hayhurst CJ, Durieux ME. Differential opioid tolerance and opioid-induced hyperalgesia: a clinical reality. *Anesthesiology*. 2016;124(2):483-488. doi:10.1097/ALN.0000000000000963
11. White JM. Pleasure into pain: the consequences of long-term opioid use. *Addict Behav*. 2004;29(7):1311-1324. doi:10.1016/j.addbeh.2004.06.007
12. The use of opioids for the treatment of chronic pain. A consensus statement from the American Academy of Pain Medicine and the American Pain Society. *Clin J Pain*. 1997;13(1):6-8.
13. Morasco BJ, Turk DC, Donovan DM, Dobscha SK. Risk for prescription opioid misuse among patients with a history of substance use disorder. *Drug Alcohol Depend*. 2013;127(1–3):193-199. doi:10.1016/j.drugalcdep.2012.06.032
14. Goel A, Azargive S, Weissman JS, et al. Perioperative Pain and Addiction Interdisciplinary Network (PAIN) clinical practice advisory for perioperative management of buprenorphine: results of a modified Delphi process. *Br J Anaesth*. 2019;123(2):e333-e342. doi:10.1016/j.bja.2019.03.044
15. Miller PM. Buprenorphine for opioid dependence. *Interventions for Addiction*. Academic Press/Elsevier; 2013.
16. Coe MA, Lofwall MR, Walsh SL. Buprenorphine pharmacology review: update on transmucosal and long-acting formulations. *J Addict Med*. 2019;13(2):93-103. doi:10.1097/ADM.0000000000000457
17. Davis MP. Twelve reasons for considering buprenorphine as a frontline analgesic in the management of pain. *J Support Oncol*. 2012;10(6):209-219. doi:10.1016/j.suponc.2012.05.002
18. Quaye AN, Zhang Y. Perioperative management of buprenorphine: solving the conundrum. *Pain Med*. 2019;20(7):1395-1408. doi:10.1093/pm/pny217
19. Thakrar S, Lee J, Martin CE, Butterworth J IV. Buprenorphine management: a conundrum for the anesthesiologist and beyond - a one-act play. *Reg Anesth Pain Med*. 2020;45(8):656-659. doi:10.1136/rapm-2020-101294
20. Johnson RE, Fudala PJ, Payne R. Buprenorphine: considerations for pain management. *J Pain Symptom Manage*. 2005;29(3):297-326. doi:10.1016/j.jpainsymman.2004.07.005

21. Roberts DM, Meyer-Witting M. High-dose buprenorphine: perioperative precautions and management strategies. *Anaesth Intensive Care*. 2005;33(1):17-25. doi:10.1177/0310057X0503300104
22. Comer SD, Sullivan MA, Vosburg SK, et al. Abuse liability of intravenous buprenorphine/naloxone and buprenorphine alone in buprenorphine-maintained intravenous heroin abusers. *Addiction*. 2010;105(4):709-718. doi:10.1111/j.1360-0443.2009.02843.x
23. Greenwald M, Johanson CE, Bueller J, et al. Buprenorphine duration of action: mu-opioid receptor availability and pharmacokinetic and behavioral indices. *Biol Psychiatry*. 2007;61(1):101-110. doi:10.1016/j.biopsych.2006.04.043
24. Chen ZR, Irvine RJ, Somogyi AA, Bochner F. Mu receptor binding of some commonly used opioids and their metabolites. *Life Sci*. 1991;48(22):2165-2171. doi:10.1016/0024-3205(91)90150-a
25. Anderson TA, Quaye ANA, Ward EN, Wilens TE, Hilliard PE, Brummett CM. To stop or not, that is the question: acute pain management for the patient on chronic buprenorphine. *Anesthesiology*. 2017;126(6):1180-1186. doi:10.1097/ALN.0000000000001633
26. Kornfeld H, Manfredi L. Effectiveness of full agonist opioids in patients stabilized on buprenorphine undergoing major surgery: a case series. *Am J Ther*. 2010;17(5):523-528. doi:10.1097/MJT.0b013e3181be0804
27. Alford DP, Compton P, Samet JH. Acute pain management for patients receiving maintenance methadone or buprenorphine therapy. *Ann Intern Med*. 2006;144(2):127-134. doi:10.7326/0003-4819-144-2-200601170-00010
28. Ward EN, Quaye AN, Wilens TE. Opioid use disorders: perioperative management of a special population. *Anesth Analg*. 2018;127(2):539-547. doi:10.1213/ANE.0000000000003477
29. Lugo RA, Satterfield KL, Kern SE. Pharmacokinetics of methadone. *J Pain Palliat Care Pharmacother*. 2005;19(4):13-24.
30. Crist RC, Clarke TK, Berrettini WH. Pharmacogenetics of opioid use disorder treatment. *CNS Drugs*. 2018;32(4):305-320. doi:10.1007/s40263-018-0513-9
31. Oral Methadone Dosing Recommendations for the Treatment of Chronic Pain. Accessed September 5, 2020. https://www.pbm.va.gov/PBM/clinicalguidance/clinicalrecommendations/Methadone_Dosing_Recommendations_for_the_Treatment_of_Chronic_Pain_July_2016.pdf
32. Murphy GS, Szokol JW. Intraoperative methadone in surgical patients: a review of clinical investigations. *Anesthesiology*. 2019;131(3):678-692. doi:10.1097/ALN.0000000000002755
33. Garrido MJ, Trocóniz IF. Methadone: a review of its pharmacokinetic/pharmacodynamic properties. *J Pharmacol Toxicol Methods*. 1999;42(2):61-66. doi:10.1016/s1056-8719(00)00043-5
34. National Institute on Drug Abuse. *Treating Opioid Use Disorder During Pregnancy*. National Institute on Drug Abuse; 2020. Accessed August 25, 2020. https://www.drugabuse.gov/publications/treating-opioid-use-disorder-during-pregnancy
35. Klaman SL, Isaacs K, Leopold A, et al. Treating women who are pregnant and parenting for opioid use disorder and the concurrent care of their infants and children: literature review to support National guidance. *J Addict Med*. 2017;11(3):178-190. doi:10.1097/ADM.0000000000000308
36. Clinical Guidance for Treating Pregnant and Parenting Women With Opioid Use Disorder and Their Infants—SAMHSA. https://store.samhsa.gov/product/Clinical-Guidance-for-Treating-Pregnant-and-Parenting-Women-With-Opioid-Use-Disorder-and-Their-Infants/SMA18-5054
37. Terplan M, Laird HJ, Hand DJ, et al. Opioid detoxification during pregnancy: a systematic review. *Obstet Gynecol*. 2018;131(5):803-814. doi:10.1097/AOG.0000000000002562
38. Jones HE, Kraft WK. Analgesia, opioids, and other drug use during pregnancy and neonatal abstinence syndrome. *Clin Perinatol*. 2019;46(2):349-366. doi:10.1016/j.clp.2019.02.013
39. Martin CE, Shadowen C, Thakkar B, Oakes T, Gal TS, Moeller FG. Buprenorphine dosing for the treatment of opioid use disorder through pregnancy and postpartum. *Curr Treat Options Psychiatry*. 2020;7(3):375-399. doi:10.1007/s40501-020-00221-z
40. Jones HE, Kaltenbach K, Heil SH, et al. Neonatal abstinence syndrome after methadone or buprenorphine exposure. *N Engl J Med*. 2010;363(24):2320-2331. doi:10.1056/NEJMoa1005359
41. Johnson E. Models of care for opioid dependent pregnant women. *Semin Perinatol*. 2019;43(3):132-140. doi:10.1053/j.semperi.2019.01.002
42. Martin CE, Terplan M, Krans EE. Pain, opioids, and pregnancy: historical context and medical management. *Clin Perinatol*. 2019;46(4):833-847. doi:10.1016/j.clp.2019.08.013
43. Meyer M, Paranya G, Keefer Norris A, Howard D. Intrapartum and postpartum analgesia for women maintained on buprenorphine during pregnancy. *Eur J Pain*. 2010;14(9):939-943. doi:10.1016/j.ejpain.2010.03.002
44. Jones HE, Heil SH, Baewert A, et al. Buprenorphine treatment of opioid-dependent pregnant women: a comprehensive review. *Addiction*. 2012;107(Suppl 1):5-27. doi:10.1111/j.1360-0443.2012.04035.x
45. Sen S, Arulkumar S, Cornett EM, et al. New pain management options for the surgical patient on methadone and buprenorphine. *Curr Pain Headache Rep*. 2016;20(3):16. doi:10.1007/s11916-016-0549-9

46. Vilkins AL, Bagley SM, Hahn KA, et al. Comparison of post-cesarean section opioid analgesic requirements in women with opioid use disorder treated with methadone or buprenorphine. *J Addict Med*. 2017;11(5):397-401. doi:10.1097/ADM.0000000000000339
47. Jansson LM; Academy of Breastfeeding Medicine Protocol Committee. ABM clinical protocol #21: guidelines for breastfeeding and the drug-dependent woman. *Breastfeed Med*. 2009;4(4):225-228. doi:10.1089/bfm.2009.9987
48. Devin CJ, McGirt MJ. Best evidence in multimodal pain management in spine surgery and means of assessing postoperative pain and functional outcomes. *J Clin Neurosci*. 2015;22(6):930-938. doi:10.1016/j.jocn.2015.01.003
49. Weibel S, Jelting Y, Pace NL, et al. Continuous intravenous perioperative lidocaine infusion for postoperative pain and recovery in adults. *Cochrane Database Syst Rev*. 2018;(6):CD009642. doi:10.1002/14651858.CD009642.pub3
50. Dahl V, Raeder JC. Non-opioid postoperative analgesia. *Acta Anaesthesiol Scand*. 2000;44(10):1191-1203. doi:10.1034/j.1399-6576.2000.441003.x
51. Khurana G, Jindal P, Sharma JP, Bansal KK. Postoperative pain and long-term functional outcome after administration of gabapentin and pregabalin in patients undergoing spinal surgery. *Spine (Phila Pa 1976)*. 2014;39(6):E363-E368. doi:10.1097/BRS.0000000000000185
52. Sakata RK, de Lima RC, Valadão JA, et al. Randomized, double-blind study of the effect of intraoperative intravenous lidocaine on the opioid consumption and criteria for hospital discharge after bariatric surgery. *Obes Surg*. 2020;30(4):1189-1193. doi:10.1007/s11695-019-04340-2
53. Chilkoti GT, Karthik G, Rautela R. Evaluation of postoperative analgesic efficacy and perioperative hemodynamic changes with low dose intravenous dexmedetomidine infusion in patients undergoing laparoscopic cholecystectomy—A randomised, double-blinded, placebo-controlled trial. *J Anaesthesiol Clin Pharmacol*. 2020;36(1):72-77. doi:10.4103/joacp.JOACP_184_17
54. Nielsen RV, Fomsgaard JS, Siegel H, et al. Intraoperative ketamine reduces immediate postoperative opioid consumption after spinal fusion surgery in chronic pain patients with opioid dependency: a randomized, blinded trial. *Pain*. 2017;158(3):463-470. doi:10.1097/j.pain.0000000000000782

33

Patient-Controlled Drug Delivery Systems (ie, PCA)

Nellab Yakuby, Lindsey Cieslinski, Kelsey De Silva, and Caroline Galliano

Introduction

In 1963, Roe[1] was the first to manage postoperative pain by titrating small intermittent intravenous (IV) boluses of morphine at intervals of 10-30 minutes, until it was apparent that adequate relief was obtained.[2] He found that small IV doses of opioids provide more effective pain relief than conventional intramuscular (IM) injections. Roe described the widely differing analgesic requirements among postoperative patients. The first attempt at patient controlled analgesia (PCA) was described by Sechzer in 1968.[3] Sechzer, known as the true pioneer of PCA, evaluated the analgesic response to small IV doses of opioid administered according to patient demand by a nurse in 1968 and then by machine in 1971.[2] Though theoretically a great study, it was impractical for clinical practice to provide multiple and frequent administration of IV doses of opioid by nurses to large numbers of patients. Since that time, PCA devices have evolved enormously in technological sophistication.

PCA is a conceptual framework for administration of analgesics[2] (Fig. 33.1). The broader concept of PCA is applicable to any analgesic given by any route of delivery; it can be considered PCA if administered on immediate patient demand in sufficient quantities.[2] An ideal PCA system has many advantages[4] and demonstrates efficacy for a variety of surgeries, ease of preparation, maintenance, and administration, with minimal technology-related complication. Additionally important is the safety profile of the analgesic given while optimizing patient comfort and satisfaction.[5] An ideal system minimizes analgesic gaps by providing immediate dosing upon patient activation, providing uniform analgesia, and thereby reducing painful waiting periods.[5] Less commonly discussed, yet still desirable, is the compatibility with overall current clinical care–encompassing treatments like physician therapy and antithrombotic therapy.[5]

PCA systems offer advantages over traditional intermittent dosing approaches of postoperative pain management.[4] PCA methods optimize analgesic efficacy by allowing the patients to determine their need and dose frequency offering an inherent level of comfort and safety in the form of a physiologic negative feedback loop.[5] A patient who is sedated will not choose to deliver additional doses of medication, thus, minimizing overdoses. PCA doses are typically smaller than bolus doses administered by nurses, which may improve the side effect to benefit ratio.[5] Interestingly, PCA is associated with a higher total dose of opioid, yet it is not associated with increased risks of dangerous side effects.[6]

In general, PCA improves pain control and patient overall satisfaction.[6]

New PCA technologies include "smart" IV-PCA infusion pumps, needle-free options, such as the fentanyl HCl iontophoretic transdermal system (ITS), and PCA devices made for intranasal delivery.[5] The sufentanil sublingual tablet system is another example of a newer PCA system that works by buccal delivery of opioids. Newer technologies like smart IV infusion

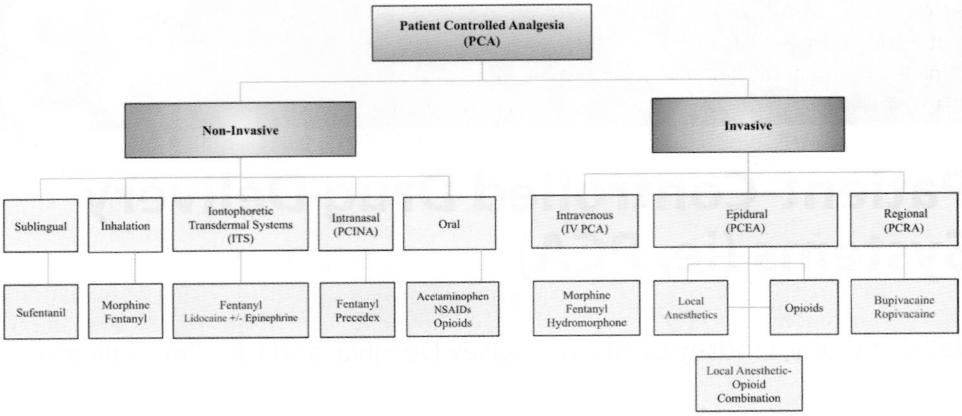

FIGURE 33.1 Patient-Controlled Analgesia (PCA).

pumps can help reduce the incidence of medication errors by providing decision support to assist with proper dosing.[5]

The most common PCA system is administered intravenously; however, an analgesic can be delivered by other routes (epidural, peripheral nerve catheter, subcutaneous, intranasal, or transdermal) under patient control.[4] The combination of multiple nonopioid analgesics with opioids delivered by PCA presents advantages over opioids alone.[4] Morphine, hydromorphone, and fentanyl are some of the most common agents for PCA.[6] This chapter will cover all of the current modalities of PCA and drug combinations available as well as the ongoing areas of research for future methods of PCA to better treat acute pain.

Intravenous Patient-Controlled Analgesia

Austin deserves credit for first elucidating the pharmacologic principles that are the basis for intravenous patient-controlled analgesia (IV-PCA).[2] To demonstrate the steepness of the concentration-effect curve from opioid analgesics, they administered small increments of meperidine, measured plasma concentrations, and assessed patient pain scores[2] until the minimum effective analgesic concentration (MEAC) is achieved, which marks the difference between severe pain and analgesia.[2] Two prerequisites for effective opioid analgesia were thus established: (1) individualize dosage and titrate to pain relief response to achieve the MEAC and establish analgesia, and (2) maintain constant plasma opioid concentrations to avoid peaks and troughs.[2] These requirements cannot be achieved with as-needed or around-the-clock IM injections. After titrating to achieve the MEAC and establish analgesia, patients use PCA to maintain plasma opioid concentrations at or just above their individual MEAC, also known as the "optimal plasma concentration."[2]

The benefits of IV-PCA in comparison to intermittent IM injection delivery of opioids have been best summarized in two published systematic reviews.[2] Both of these evidence-based reviews concluded that IV-PCA offers better analgesic efficacy, as well as superior patient satisfaction to IM injection. Although there is no evidence to support reduced opioid consumption or a difference in opioid-related side effects, Walder et al.[7] concluded that PCA reduces postoperative pulmonary complications.[2]

In an IV-PCA system, the patient initiates an activation button attached by a cord to a PCA pump. A small dose of opioid is delivered to the patient from the IV line to an indwelling catheter.[5] Dosing is controlled by a staff-programmed PCA pump. For all modes of PCA, there are the following basic variables: initial loading dose, demand dose, lockout interval, background infusion rate, and 1-hour and 4-hour limits. The two most common modes of PCA are demand dosing, which is a fixed-size dose that is intermittently self-administered, and continuous infusion plus demand dosing, a constant-rate fixed background infusion supplemented by patient on-demand dosing.[2] The latter is also known as a basal infusion rate, which is a constant infusion rate regardless of whether the patient activates demand doses. Basal infusion PCA is generally not appropriate due to increased risk of overdose and respiratory depression. Additionally, when a background infusion is used with IV-PCA in opioid-naive patients, the incidence of respiratory depression is frequent.[2] However, a basal infusion can be implemented in those opioid-dependent or opioid-tolerant patients to replace a patient's baseline opioid requirement. The basal dose can be calculated based on the opioid equivalence of the patient's total daily chronic opioid and then is reduced by 30%-50%.[6] Dosing is controlled by a programmed PCA pump, which is adjustable by trained staff and a lockout interval enforced to prevent excessive dosing.[5]

The initial loading dose allows for titration of medication when activated by the programmer prior to initiation of the medication to the patient. It can be used by postanesthesia care unit staff to titrate opioids to the MEAC or to give "breakthrough" doses. To prevent overdose by continual demand, all PCA devices use a lockout interval (or delay), which is the length of time the device will not administer another demand dose after a successful patient demand dose has been delivered, even if the patient continues to push the demand button.[2] The lockout interval is designed to prevent overdose. Ideally, it should be long enough for the patient to experience the maximal effect of one dose before another is permitted. Therefore, speed of onset of analgesia is paramount in setting the lockout interval. Based on this rationale, one might consider using a slightly shorter lockout interval when using the "fentanyl family of opioids" compared to morphine or hydromorphone.[2] Whichever opioid is chosen for IV-PCA, knowledge of its pharmacology is a prerequisite for setting the dosing variables of the PCA device. Individual patient characteristics such as age, gender, and body weight are often assumed to be important factors influencing any pharmacologic therapy. Age affects opioid dosing, whereas gender and body weight do not.

Generally speaking, IV-PCA offers rapid analgesia, without the effects of first-pass metabolism with the goal of adequate titration in order to minimize the peaks and troughs in serum concentrations associated with clinician-controlled analgesia.[5] Morphine, fentanyl, and hydromorphone are the most common agents used for IV-PCA.[5] Tramadol is used extensively for IV-PCA in some European countries.[2] Although meperidine was the initial drug used to discover PCA, modern medicine has concluded meperidine for IV-PCA invites adverse outcomes in some patients while offering no advantage over alternative opioids.[2] Meperidine metabolites have greater seizure potential when combined with certain drugs. Hydromorphone and morphine IV-PCA remain the "gold standard" as the most studied and most commonly used IV-PCA drugs in the United States. It is important to note that morphine has an active metabolite via glucuronidation—morphine-6-glucuronide (M6G) and morphine-3-glucuronide (M3G). M6G produces analgesia, sedation, and respiratory depression. Prolonged and delayed onset of respiratory depression has been reported in patients with renal failure receiving parenteral morphine.[2] Therefore, it is recommended to avoid morphine for IV-PCA in patients with serum creatinine 2.0 mg/dL.[2] The more potent hydromorphone may have the best pharmacologic profile with similar onset and duration of action to morphine, but with decreased pruritus and nausea, and the absence of active metabolites.[2] Because of its lipophilicity, fentanyl has a quicker onset than morphine, perhaps making it better suited for IV-PCA; however, the rapid redistribution half-life of fentanyl results in a short duration of effect.[2,6]

Overall, IV-PCA is associated with high patient satisfaction.[5] PCA is used to sustain comfort, allowing the patient to self-administer enough drugs to achieve a balance between analgesia and side effects.[5] The common side effects of IV-PCA are the same side effects seen with opioid administration by any route or method of delivery; specifically, nausea and vomiting, constipation, pruritus, sedation, and, less commonly, respiratory depression and confusion.[2] Postoperative nausea and vomiting (PONV) are the most common and most bothersome side effects of IV-PCA.[2] Anesthesia & Analgesia has published Consensus Guidelines for identifying and managing patients at risk of PONV associated with IV-PCA.[8] Overall, small doses of pure opioid antagonists appear to be effective in reducing IV-PCA-related PONV and pruritus.[2] Although PONV is the most bothersome side effect to patients, respiratory depression is the most concerning for clinicians due to the potential sequelae of hypoxic injury as a result of opioid overdose.[2] An overall incidence for respiratory depression with IV-PCA can be estimated as 0.25%.

Nonpharmacologic drawbacks to IV-PCA involve the modality requiring an invasive indwelling catheter. The pump apparatus and accessories may limit patient mobility and thereby limit a patient's level of comfort and access to performing activities of daily living while recovering in the hospital setting. IV line occlusions can lead to gaps in medication administration, catheter infiltration, needle-related injuries, and staff errors in programming administration are all potential downfalls associated with IV-PCA administration.[5]

There are significant benefits of a multimodal approach to acute pain management and IV-PCA should not be considered a stand-alone therapy. Scheduled administration of NSAIDs clearly improves analgesia and reduces IV-PCA opioid requirements. Local wound infiltration, peripheral nerve blocks, and continuous catheter techniques can all be used effectively in conjunction with IV-PCA. Interestingly, a number of investigators have examined adding analgesic drugs directly to the IV-PCA mixture. These trials separately added ketamine and magnesium to morphine PCA and found that it significantly improved pain relief and reduced 24-hour cumulative morphine consumption.[2] These same investigators also found that adding small amounts of ketamine or magnesium to tramadol IV-PCA improved pain relief and reduced the amount of tramadol required after major abdominal surgery.[2] Ketamine clearly has an evolving role in acute pain management. However, caution and consideration of potential medication error should be evaluated before routinely adding it to an IV-PCA mixture.

Despite these disadvantages, IV-PCA is an accepted standard for acute postoperative pain management.[5] Even though IV-PCA has a very acceptable safety profile, life-threatening mishaps do occur. Furthermore, there is no evidence to support a decrease in morbidity and mortality with IV-PCA, except perhaps some mild decrease in pulmonary complications.[2] It is clear that IV-PCA is inferior to epidural analgesia and other peripheral nerve block techniques for pain relief after severely painful surgical procedures.[2] Next, we will discuss the other modalities of PCA pain relief.

Nontraditional Invasive PCA Delivery Systems

Though the traditional route of PCA delivery has been IV, patient-controlled epidural analgesia (PCEA) and patient-controlled regional analgesia (PCRA) are other modalities of PCA utilizing neuraxial routes that have been developed more recently.[9]

Patient-Controlled Epidural Analgesia

Patient-controlled epidural analgesia (PCEA) has most extensively been studied and used in the obstetric patient, as epidural analgesia is the most common modality and a highly effective way of providing safe labor analgesia.[9-11] A multicenter, randomized controlled trial found that IV-PCA and PCEA had the same rates of cesarean delivery or instrumental vaginal delivery, yet patients in the PCEA group reported better pain relief and satisfaction.[11,12] Patients receiving IV-PCA had more adverse effects such as more sedation, more likelihood of antiemetic therapy, and more neonates requiring naloxone when compared to the PCEA group.[11,12] In addition to labor analgesia, this mode of analgesia has also been effective in managing postoperative pain, including but not limited to patients who have undergone major operations such as abdominal, thoracic, or spinal surgery.

PCEA allows for individualization of analgesic requirements and a reduction in total opioid consumption with subsequent decrease in associated adverse systemic effects, a particularly attractive benefit in the setting of a current opioid crisis. Additionally, several studies suggest that PCEA compares favorably with use of traditional epidural analgesia delivered at a fixed rate, or continuous epidural infusion (CEI); with the added benefit of reduction in total local anesthetic dosing and attendant motor block.[9]

In variable scenarios, epidural analgesia has consistently demonstrated to be superior to IV-PCA and systemic opioids.[13] A meta-analysis demonstrated that for all types of surgery and pain assessments, epidural analgesia including PCEA, provided superior postoperative analgesia when compared with IV-PCA.[14] This was further supported in a systematic review of the analgesic efficacy of epidural analgesia.[11] Moreover, though satisfaction is a complex concept and difficult to measure, the improvement in postoperative analgesia and its benefits may contribute to greater patient satisfaction.[15] PCEA is also regarded as a relatively safe and effective technique.[15]

Despite numerous investigations, the optimal PCEA analgesic solution and delivery parameters are not clearly defined. There are many combinations of PCEA parameters that can be classified using the following framework: (1) the type of infusion rate and (2) the infusion drug class. The type of infusion rate can be specified as a demand-dose alone, a continuous background infusion alone or a combination of both. This can be further classified by the infusion drug class as local anesthetic alone, opioid alone or a local anesthetic-opioid combination.

In contrast to IV-PCA, the use of a continuous infusion in addition to the demand dose, otherwise known as a background infusion, is routinely used for PCEA. It may provide analgesia superior to that of the use of a demand dose alone, particularly when a local anesthetic is used, to maintain a continuous segmental sensory block.[16] Epidural infusion of local anesthetic alone may be warranted for postoperative analgesia as it has been shown to minimize opioid consumption and its related side effects; however, this method also has adverse effects.[5] The use of local anesthetic alone in epidural analgesia is associated with significant failure rates, relatively high incidence of motor block and blockage of sympathetic fibers contributing hypotension.[2,15] Generally, lower concentrations of bupivacaine or ropivacaine are used to avoid these issues due to their differential and preferential clinical sensory blockade with minimal impairment of motor function.[15]

Conversely, opioids may be used alone for postoperative epidural infusion yet are also not without their own adverse side effects.[15] Pruritus is one of the most common side effects of epidural administration of opioids.[17] Nausea and vomiting is associated with neuraxial opioids and may be related to the cephalad migration of opioids within the CSF to the area postrema in the medulla. Urinary retention also occurs more frequently with opioid epidural administration than with systemic opioid delivery, which may be attributed to spinal cord opioid receptors decreasing the strength of detrusor muscle contractions.[15]

Though respiratory depression has always been an area of major concern regarding opioid use regardless of which route it is administered, neuraxial opioids used in appropriate doses are not associated with higher rates of respiratory depression than systemic administration. Risk factors that do increase respiratory depression with neuraxial opioids include increasing dose, increasing age, concomitant use of systemic opioids or sedatives, possibility of prolonged or extensive surgery, and the presence of comorbid conditions.[18]

Myriad adverse effects of epidural analgesia can be attributed to side effects of administering drugs through the neuraxial route. Fortunately, the rates of side effects for PCEA are favorable and comparable to those reported with CEI; their incidence is 1.8%-16.7% for pruritus, 3.8%-14.8% for nausea, 13.2% for sedation, 4.3%-6.8% for hypotension, 0.1%-2% for motor block, and 0.2%-0.3% for respiratory depression.[19] Despite many studies, the optimal local anesthetic and opioid dose for providing the lowest pain scores along with the fewest medication-related side effects is unknown and further investigation is needed. However, general consensus of many acute pain specialists is toward a combination of low-concentration local anesthetic plus an opioid in an attempt to improve analgesia while minimizing aforementioned side effects, as it can provide analgesia superior to that of either analgesic alone.[15] A lipophilic opioid is commonly used secondary to its rapid analgesic onset and shorter duration of action that is more suitable for use with PCEA.[15] With the onset of analgesia also comes the potential for respiratory depression more quickly seen with lipophilic opioids in PCEA over hydrophilic agents.

Other elements of PCEA have received particular attention over the years. The use of clonidine as an adjuvant medication when used in a local anesthetic-opioid combination PCEA demonstrated a reduction in incidence of opioid rescue without negatively affecting hemodynamics.[11] Additionally, consideration should be made as to the location of insertion of the epidural catheter. Epidural catheters inserted at a site congruent with the dermatome level of the incision infuse analgesics to the appropriate region, thus, providing superior analgesia, minimizing drug requirements with their associated side effects and decreasing morbidity.[15] Of note, there is an increased risk associated with placement of an epidural in the thoracic region.

Epidural analgesia has the potential benefits of decreased morbidity, such as fewer cardiopulmonary complications, less thromboembolism, better mental status, earlier restoration of gastrointestinal function, enhanced functional exercise capacity, and earlier discharge from the hospital.[11] A large database study further supports the conclusion that mortality is lower for patients who receive perioperative epidural analgesia, especially with a local anesthetic-based analgesic solution that attenuates the pathophysiologic response to surgery.[11,15] Meta-analysis of randomized data from 141 trials found that this overall reduction in mortality was by ~30%, though these results were primarily in orthopedic patients.[15]

Use of epidural analgesia can decrease the incidence of a variety of postoperative complications, such as gastrointestinal, pulmonary, and possibly cardiac-related issues.[15] By inhibiting sympathetic outflow, minimizing total opioid consumption, and mitigating spinal reflex inhibition gastrointestinal system, postoperative thoracic epidural analgesia can help propagate return of gastrointestinal motility without compromising bowel vessel anastomosis.[15] Overall, PCEA use is associated with earlier fulfillment of discharge criteria when compared to those who receive opioid epidural analgesia.[15]

In patients undergoing abdominal and thoracic surgery, epidural use for postoperative analgesia has shown decreased postoperative pulmonary complications, likely by preserving postoperative pulmonary function via adequate analgesia, therefore, reducing "splinting" behavior and attenuating the spinal reflex inhibition of diaphragmatic function.[15,20] In a recent meta-analysis, thoracic epidural analgesia with a local anesthetic-based regimen also had a lower rate of incidence of pulmonary infections and complications.[15,21]

Furthermore, postoperative thoracic epidural analgesia may decrease the incidence of postoperative myocardial infarction. This may be due to attenuation of both the stress response and hypercoagulability, superior postoperative analgesia, and favorable redistribution of coronary blood flow. These findings are in alignment with the known physiologic benefits of thoracic epidural analgesia, such as a reduction in the severity of myocardial ischemia or size of infarction and attenuation of sympathetically mediated coronary vasoconstriction.[21]

There may also be an association between the use of neuraxial anesthesia and immune function. It is possible that cancer recurrence and metastasis may be lower in patients who receive paravertebral or epidural analgesia vs receiving conventional systemic opioids after mastectomy or prostatectomy.[11] In a recent meta-analysis of 14 studies including a range of cancer types, a positive association between epidural analgesia and overall survival was demonstrated.[11] Additionally, epidural analgesia for total hip or knee replacement may decrease the risk of surgical site infections compared with general anesthesia.[15]

We have discussed many of the benefits of the use of PCEA thus far; however, it is important to note that PCEA is not suitable or advantageous for every type of surgery or patient.

Hansdottir et al. demonstrated in their randomized control study that with regards to elective cardiac surgery, thoracic PCEA offers no major advantage with respect to hospital length of stay, quality of recovery, or morbidity when compared with IV-PCA.[22] In general, the overall potential benefits of PCEA must be weighed against the potential risks associated with placement of a catheter, which include epidural hematoma, infection, or neurological injury.[22]

The concurrent use of anticoagulants and neuraxial analgesia has been topic of much debate over the years with the advent of more potent anticoagulants for thromboprophylaxis, further limiting the use of PCEA because of an increased incidence of spinal hematoma.[23] The American Society of Regional Anesthesia and Pain Medicine has a series of guidelines based on the available literature for administration of neuraxial techniques in the presence of various anticoagulants and antiplatelet therapy. Still, the literature is constantly changing and no definitive conclusions have been reached despite numerous investigating studies.[24]

As for neuraxial associated neurologic injury, one review revealed that the rate of neurologic complications after central neuraxial blockade is <0.04% and after a peripheral nerve block is <3%.[15] Overall, permanent neurologic injury after any type of neuraxial blockade is rare in contemporary anesthetic practice.[15]

Though there may be a positive correlation with immunity associated with epidural placement as discussed previously, direct infection from postoperative epidural analgesia placement may result from exogenous or endogenous sources.[15] Central infection such as meningitis and spinal abscess associated with epidural analgesics are rare, <1 in 10 000.[25] However, a more frequent incidence has also been observed, 1 in 1000, in patients who had a longer duration of epidural analgesia or coexisting immunocompromising or complicating diseases.[15,25] There may also be a relatively higher rate of superficial inflammation or cellulitis (4%-14%) with longer duration of catheterization.[15] With that said, epidural analgesia in the general surgical population is typically limited to short-term catheter use of <4 days.[15]

There is also the risk of possible migration of the epidural catheter out of the epidural space and into the intrathecal, intravascular, or subcutaneous space, which can decrease the effectiveness or cause further lethal complications. The failure rate of epidural catheter analgesia ranges from ~6% to 30% and a higher failure rate with thoracic epidural catheters than lumbar catheters. Regardless of this less frequent occurrence of migration into intravascular and intrathecal space, precautions such as use of an epinephrine-containing test dose may prevent further potential complications such as a high or total spinal, seizures, and neurotoxicity.[15]

Finally, advances in technology create a new cohort of potential limitations and risks associated with patient-controlled analgesia. As with IV-PCA, one issue with PCEA is reliance on a pump that requires advanced qualifications of hospital staff for programming and administration. Additionally, the manual programming of PCEA pumps introduces the risk of programming errors with potential for very serious complications.[5]

Patient-Controlled Regional Analgesia (PCRA)

Recent advances in patient-controlled drug delivery systems have led to the development of more intricate and efficient delivery mechanisms.[6] Patient-controlled regional analgesia (PCRA) uses a variety of techniques to provide postoperative pain relief via placement of an indwelling catheter in various regions of the body, thus, limiting systemic exposure to opioids. Using PCRA, patients can initiate the delivery of small doses of local anesthetics, most frequently ropivacaine or bupivacaine, directly congruent with a specific region of the body necessitating analgesia postoperatively.[5] Similar to other PCA modalities, PCRA allows the patient to individualize and modify the intensity and duration of postoperative pain, while minimizing bothersome motor and sensory blockade associated with neuraxial analgesia administration.[2] The most common technique used is a continuous infusion of local anesthetic; though in some cases, a combination of local anesthetic and opioid is administered.[2]

These infusions are administered through either a staff-programmed electronic pump or a disposable elastomeric pump. An elastomeric pump is a device that consists of a distensible bulb within an outer protective bulb that stores analgesic medications via a built-in filling port.[2,15] It can dispense analgesics to the desired postoperative site via a delivery tube with a bacterial filter, which further connects to an indwelling catheter within the patient. The rate of infusion of analgesics within the elastomeric pump can be adjusted by a dial, or another type of modulating apparatus, controlled by the patient. These elastomeric pumps are typically portable ambulatory pumps that introduce a new avenue of convenience as they may be used at home or on an outpatient basis.[15]

PCRA catheter techniques are increasingly being used to manage postoperative pain in hospitalized and ambulatory surgery patients.[2] The use of peripheral regional analgesic techniques can provide site-specific analgesia superior to that with systemic opioids and may result in favorable outcomes.[15] Randomized control trials suggest that the use of peripheral regional analgesia may facilitate postoperative rehabilitation through the accelerated resumption of passive joint range-of-motion and earlier actual discharge from the hospital or rehabilitation center.[15] Minimizing opioids with continuous regional anesthesia techniques allows for an alert patient who is free of pain and without the common systemic side effects of opioid medications; thus, it is recommended to avoid the opioid tolerance observed with IV administration of opioids.[23,26] Peripheral regional techniques also have advantages over neuraxial techniques, such as less hemodynamic instability and decreased risk for spinal hematoma.[15] In general, there is less concern for interaction with anticoagulants than with neuraxial analgesia.[11]

There is a high patient satisfaction rate with PCRA, likely related to the use of elastomeric infusion pumps and their ability to deliver effective postoperative analgesia in the comfort of one's own homes as an outpatient.[15,27] In the setting of discharging a patient to utilize PCRA at home, clinicians must ensure that the patient and their caregivers receive proper instruction and that a physician is readily available at all times to address potential issues.[9] If the patient is not in a monitored setting, the risk may increase for complications such as infection, leaking or disconnection of indwelling catheters, or potential injury to the numb limb. Despite being an invasive procedure, PCRA displays the safety, efficacy, individualization, and patient satisfaction congruent with an optimal PCA system, particularly in orthopedic surgery patients.[5]

As with most PCA modalities, the optimal parameters for peripheral regional analgesia have yet to be elucidated. With the evolution of ultrasound-guided technology and new block techniques, peripheral nerve blocks are becoming more popular and integrated into new clinical pathways.[15] Unlike PCEA, the inclusion of opioids in PNC PCA solutions is unnecessary, as peripheral opioids may increase side effects without improving analgesia.[11] Typically, a continuous infusion of local anesthetics alone is used as it has shown to provide superior analgesia compared with bolus dosing only. For PNC PCA, ropivacaine may be associated with reduction of complete motor and sensory block, compared with bupivacaine.[11] Common concentrations of local anesthetic for PNC PCA include ropivacaine, 0.2%-0.3%, and bupivacaine, 0.12%-0.25%.[11] A combination of low-dose continuous infusion along with a demand dose generally provides a favorable outcome, as it reduces local anesthetic consumption without reducing analgesia.[11] In one study evaluating perineural interscalene catheter infusion rates for moderately painful shoulder surgery, decreasing the basal rate of ropivacaine 0.2% infusion from 8 mL/h to 4 mL/h demonstrated similar analgesia effect; however, there was a higher incidence of breakthrough pain and sleep disturbance.[11] The duration of action of postoperative analgesia via local anesthetic peripheral nerve blocks may last up to 24 hours after injection, but it depends on many variables. Thus, the introduction of adjuvant drugs to PCRA that can help prolong the duration of action of local anesthetics and improve the quality of nerve blocks, such as dexamethasone, clonidine, and dexmedetomidine.[15]

Different subtypes of PCRAs have been developed over the years, which include incisional PCRA, intra-articular PCRA, and perineural PCRA. Intra-articular (IA PCRA) and incisional PCRA provide direct wound infiltration analgesia, within an incision or joint, such

first and at which point the device shuts off and can be replaced. This allows patients to safely titrate analgesia to comfort.[40] The fentanyl ITS is activated and an audible beep occurs when the patient double-clicks the recessed, on-demand dosing button. A red light from a light-emitting diode remains illuminated during the 10-minute dose delivery period; during this time, the system is unresponsive to additional doses of fentanyl.[40] An LCD display informs the patient when the next dose is available for demand and quantifies the number of doses delivered.[5]

Fentanyl ITS system offers the advantage of portable convenience, eliminates the risk of needlestick injuries, as well as infection risk associated with invasive venous access. The self-contained unit allows for enhanced patient mobilization without tubing, or IV poles. In addition, the elimination of multiple system components and the minimal time that is expected to be required for system setup may translate into cost savings.[10] Although no studies have quantified the exact value of monetary gain, studies do find a cost reduction benefit to PCINA and transdermal PCA when compared to IV-PCA. This cost reduction is partially attributed to lower staffing and labor costs, as PCINA and transdermal PCA may reduce both nursing time requirements and acquired staff expertise. Additionally, studies report patient and nursing satisfaction with assessment of ease of use and convenience.[41] Lastly, the simple and easy design of both PCINA and fentanyl ITS eliminates the many costly medication errors and potentially life-threatening PCA programming errors associated with mistakes in traditional PCA pump programming.[41]

The fentanyl ITS has also demonstrated efficacy and safety similar to a standard regimen of morphine IV-PCA for the management of acute postsurgical pain in a number of large active-controlled clinical studies.[41] The incidence of overall opioid-related adverse events in each treatment group was similar in the subgroups divided by age and was similar to those observed in the overall population. The most common reported symptoms were nausea, fever, anemia, and headache. However, the incidence of nausea and vomiting is reported to be >10% in chronic treatment with transdermal fentanyl.[33] The most common treatment-related adverse events in patients receiving fentanyl ITS were skin application site reactions, which resolved spontaneously upon removal.[41]

As technological advances allow our patient population to live longer, it is important to point out that no unique safety concerns were uncovered in elderly patients.[42] Studies do highlight the concern of patient self-administration of opioids and the association of opioids with respiratory depression. Importantly, no patient in the fentanyl ITS group experienced clinically relevant respiratory depression; however, five cases reported in the morphine IV-PCA group.[42] Although there are no reports of cases of an iontophoretic fentanyl overdose, it is important to note that any compromise to the delivery mechanism may result in the administration of supratherapeutic doses without patient awareness.[41]

Although there are plenty of advantages to fentanyl ITS, there are patient circumstances in which this would not be the best treatment modality. One potential limitation is the fixed single dosage that cannot be adjusted to meet individual opioid requirements, as with opioid-tolerant or opioid-dependent patients that may need a basal infusion, or to administer additional bolus doses; this system might not be enough to adequately manage their pain. However, the current data analysis demonstrated that the system provided effective pain control for patients, regardless of age or BMI.[41] Additionally, the fentanyl ITS may only be used for a maximum of 24 hours before it must be discarded and replaced with a new system, which has the potential to result in analgesic gaps if a patients is not administered a new system in a timely fashion, and may also result in unnecessary cost if a system is applied and not used within 24 hours.[41]

Fentanyl ITS has been demonstrated to be safe and effective for postoperative pain management in several large, randomized clinical trials, with efficacy equal to that of a standard regimen of morphine IV-PCA after a broad range of major surgical procedures and across multiple patient subpopulations.[41]

Three large clinical studies analysis of pooled data comparing fentanyl ITS and morphine IV-PCA for safety and efficacy is also notable as the first of its kind, for the development of relative dosing ratios between the two opioid analgesics.[40] The mean number of doses activated in the first 24 hours by patients who received fentanyl ITS was lower compared with patients who received morphine IV-PCA during that same time period and did not approach the maximum of 80 doses that may be delivered by each 24-hour fentanyl ITS.[42] Relative dosing ratios varied around 30:1 over 6, 12, and 24 hours, suggesting that ~30 μg fentanyl provided an equianalgesic dose compared with 1 mg morphine.[42] Additionally, this overall dosing ratio remained at ~30:1, regardless of age or BMI.[42]

This is an important step in translating study data into everyday clinical practice enabling clinicians who are more comfortable with morphine IV-PCA to use fentanyl ITS safely and effectively.[42]

Acute Pain Service

Development and incorporation of an Acute Pain Service (APS) in clinical settings has improved the management of postoperative analgesia and helped minimize complications or adverse effects related to PCA.[22] An APS is based on the concept that a team of physicians and nurses who are well-educated about PCA can improve management of postoperative analgesia and promote PCA safety with training and appropriate patient selection.[22] A study comparing PCA management by an APS vs managed by the surgical staff demonstrated that patients in the former group had significantly fewer side effects, were more likely to have appropriate modifications made to their regimen for inadequate analgesia or side effects, and were more likely to transition to oral opioids instead of IM after PCA.[43] Thus, APS may better tailor PCA regimens to suit individual patients' needs through their specialized training and knowledge of postoperative analgesia management.

New PCA Modalities

New modalities for PCA delivery are being explored to improve treatment of pain, both acute and chronic. The invasive nature, decreased mobility, and complicated dosing regimen associated with IV-PCA and epidural PCA have been a major concern in regard to PCA use. In response, new developing routes for analgesic delivery have been a focus of PCA delivery. Current modalities of study include sublingual, inhalation, and oral. These emerging technologies aim to address the major issues of PCA and show potential in reducing the postoperative recovery time. The newer modalities have shown a reduction in invasiveness and the preprogramming shows promise in reducing the risk of programming errors and the PCA preparation time.

Sublingual

The current method of sublingual analgesia for PCA is a sufentanil tablet that sits under the tongue. Sufentanil's highly lipophilic nature allows for sublingual administration and rapid analgesic onset.[44] Though IV sufentanil is associated with a short half-life due to rapid redistribution, sublingual sufentanil has been shown to have a longer plasma time and a lower concentration maximum, making it a safer and more effective analgesic alternative to IV sufentanil.[44] The PCA formulation of the sublingual sufentanil tablet consists of 40 tablets dosed at 15 μg that have a 20-minute lock out period between doses over a period of 72 hours, which is the maximum duration of treatment.[45] The device also has a security method in place to ensure single-user administration with radiofrequency identification, an adhesive thumb tag that specifically pairs the patient to the device.[45]

Most adverse effects, interactions, and contraindications of sublingual sufentanil are similar to those of other opiates. The most common side effects associated with sufentanil sublingual tabs are nausea, vomiting, and fever, while the most common adverse effect of the drug being respiratory depression.[46] Controlled studies showed that after administration of the sublingual PCA, 46.9% of patients experienced nausea vs 36.4% of the placebo, 17.7% of patients experienced fever (experienced by 11.1% of the placebo), and 11.7% of patients experienced vomiting (experienced by 6.2% of the placebo).[46] Recent studies have shown that sublingual PCA is associated with less discontinuation due to adverse events than IV morphine PCA.[46]

Three randomized control trials aimed to assess analgesic control with sublingual sufentanil have shown that the sublingual PCA patient group had pain control that was statistically more adequate than the placebo group.[47-49] During these trials, sublingual sufentanil was found to be noninferior to morphine IV-PCA.[46] The study suggested enhanced pain control with sublingual sufentanil than IV morphine PCA, with a statistically significant 12.9% difference in treatments.[46] Additionally, nurses and patients involved with the sufentanil sublingual PCA trial suggested that the system was easy to use.[46] However, more evidence is needed to further corroborate the findings of the study.

Though most of the current clinical studies performed have limited generalizability due to healthy populations undergoing elective procedures, sublingual sufentanil shows promise as a PCA that is safer and associated with less adverse outcomes than IV morphine PCA. Additionally, sublingual administration of analgesia provides an option to patients unable to swallow pills or patients that have trouble with IV access. Limitations of sublingual PCA include the potential for inadequate pain relief in patients with chronic opioid therapy due to the low doses of the drug and a maximum of 72 hours for post-operative pain management.[45] Sublingual sufentanil PCA is currently not FDA-approved and further evaluation of the drug's efficacy and proper usage of the device should be assessed.

Inhalation

Inhalation of morphine or fentanyl has been studied as possible PCA alternatives to IV analgesia. The mechanism of administration uses aerosolized liquid drug formulations as a vehicle for analgesia delivery.[50] Whereas nebulizers and metered dose inhalers target the more proximal anatomy of the lung, the inhaled analgesia delivery systems aim to target the more distant portions of the lung, increasing systemic drug delivery.[50] The side effects associated with inhaled morphine and fentanyl are similar to those of IV morphine, such as sleeping, dizziness, nausea, vomiting, and rash, with respiratory depression being the most severe side effect.

Though most current studies do not specifically address inhalation analgesia related to PCA devices, the trials do convey the increased efficacy of inhaled analgesia in comparison to traditional IV analgesia in acute settings.[50] A study measuring the acute posttrauma pain in the emergency department found that a 20 mg nebulized morphine bolus was more effective and had less side effects than titrated IV morphine.[50] Aerosolized fentanyl PCA has shown promise as an alternate modality of analgesia as preliminary studies suggest it adequately manages pain postoperatively. Importantly, aerosolized fentanyl PCA shows limited effects on respiratory rates, oxygen saturation, and hemodynamics after drug administration. This makes a compelling argument for increased utilization of aerosolized PCA as a primary method of pain management.[51] However, there have been limited developments within this subcategory of analgesia and more research is needed to fully grasp the implications of inhaled PCA.

Oral

Oral pain medications have been widely used and their analgesic effects thoroughly studied, but recent innovations have applied this recognized form of analgesia to PCA devices. This emergence of oral PCA attempts to directly combat the underestimation of pain and undermedication for which acute pain patients frequently encounter. Evidence has shown that oral PCA in comparison to medications administered by health care workers provides better analgesic effects, less sedation, and decreases patient anxiety.[52] Additionally, the variety of analgesic oral PCA medications available allow for more pain control options than the other emerging PCA modalities. A huge area of concern with oral PCA is the security methods put in place to ensure a safe, easy method of medication delivery with no potential for errors or inappropriate dispersal of medication. Oral PCA dispensers address potential issues providers and patients face by employing the following measures[52]:

- Use original medication packaging for easy integration of PCA into patient care routines.
- Direct administration of medication into that patient's mouth allowing the device to verify consumption and allow strict control of pill consumption.
- Locked safe for dispersal of high-risk narcotic drugs.
- Use personal identification through radiofrequency identification wristbands to disperse only to the patient.
- Enable remote monitoring and management with alerts and reminders for providers.
- Allow for data collection and management to assess a patient's clinical status.

Using an oral PCA device that abided by the measures listed above, a pilot study conducted on patients in an acute postoperative care setting confirmed the safety, efficacy, and usability of the oral PCA delivery system.[52] Safety was adequate throughout the duration of the study with no reported severe adverse events, pill dispensing during lockout periods, overdoses, or pill malformations.[52] The efficiency of the system was shown through 67% more pills being dispensed to the test group than the control, significantly reduced pain scores in the test group in comparison to control, and a reduction in pill intake time with the test group in comparison to the control group.[52] Usability of the device was confirmed by a 90% satisfaction by all study participants, including medical staff and patients.[52] Despite the overwhelming evidence in support of oral PCA in this study, similar to the other emerging PCA modalities, more research needs to be done to further verify the efficacy and safety of the oral PCA delivery system.

Cost Considerations

Though PCA provides a great alternative to current methods of acute pain management, cost-effectiveness should be considered to determine the feasibility of incorporating these systems into hospital settings. Although exact monetary data are limited, some investigators have concluded that IV-PCA is more costly when compared to IM injections.[5] The costs associated with PCA modalities are both direct and indirect medical expenses divided into four categories: cost of technology, drugs, staff, and adverse events, including side effects.[5,53] While there is no way to uniformly assess these factors across different health care environments, studies have been done in the United States in an attempt to quantify the total cost of PCA implementation and care.[53]

Upon analysis of PCA usage in over 500 hospitals, data found that the cost breakdown of IV-PCA consists of the PCA opioids, equipment, bacteremia, phlebitis, health care worker needlestick injury, and IV-PCA errors, the majority of the cost coming from the medication and equipment.[53] There is a pharmacoeconomic burden associated with partially used PCA drug cassettes.[5] The study concluded that the average cost of IV-PCA in a US hospital setting in the first 48 hours of a major surgery ranged from $342-$389. The cost breakdown shows a range in the cost of equipment and opioid drugs ($196-$243) that stems from differences found in postoperative opioid consumption; less opioid consumption was found in surgeries that utilized nerve blocks. Another large portion of the cost associated with IV-PCA is the management of bacteremia ($106.76) due to the PCA catheter acting as a nidus for infection. Though not included in the total IV-PCA cost, there are also expenses associated with the limited mobility that occur with IV-PCA use in addition to the medical complications frequently associated with limited mobility following major surgery, such as deep venous thrombosis ($18.17), pulmonary embolism ($43.19), and postoperative pneumonia ($265.02). Although IV-PCA probably reduces nursing time allocated to analgesia administration in comparison with IM injections, nursing time is still a considerable expense in the overall cost of IV-PCA.

All-encompassing cost analyses must be performed with specific time-motion studies to more accurately quantify total time devoted to the PCA system in order to make conclusions regarding the financial cost-effectiveness of PCA.[2]

Consideration of cost-effectiveness in PCA is not to relegate adequate postoperative pain management to a matter of hospital finances, but to fully comprehend the implications of PCA implementation and the feasibility of this system in the modern health care system. Though the drugs and technology associated with IV-PCA came out to a total of $196-$243, the hazards associated with IV-PCA use account for a significant portion of the total cost.[53] As developing research continues to make advancements in reducing adverse effects and improving PCA technology, PCA's have the potential to become the cost-effective standard of care in managing pain in acute postoperative settings.

Summary

IV-PCA is the current standard of care for management of postoperative pain. There has been significant evidence showing the enhanced analgesic effect of IV administration of opioids in comparison to IM opioid administration.[54] Despite an overall improvement in achieving optimal analgesia, IV-PCA has not been shown to reduce the adverse effects associated with opioids or the total opioid consumption.[55] There are also life-threatening mistakes that occur with IV-PCA technologies and the invasive nature of administration puts the patient at risk for infections and limits mobility.[56]

Epidural delivery of opiates has been shown to have greater potency and provides better analgesia than IV administration.[5] There are less systemic opioid effects associated with epidural administration. There is earlier mobilization and less gastrointestinal side effects in patients with PCEA in comparison to IV-PCA.[14] Additionally, when local anesthetics are used instead of opioids in PCEAs, postoperative opioid intake is significantly decreased.[57] Though a beneficial option over traditional IV-PCA methods, PCEAs are not without serious potential risk of complications such as epidural hematomas and neurological injury.[5]

PCRA incorporates a localized perineural, intra-articular, or incisional approach to analgesia by using small doses of local anesthetics, primarily ropivacaine and bupivacaine. Though traditionally used for single bolus or continuous infusions, regional techniques have expanded to incorporate PCA technologies. Some studies have shown superiority in analgesia and lower anesthetic consumption in regional PCA compared to continuous infusions.[58] As with any PCA that employs an indwelling catheter, there is an increased risk of infection and limited mobility, but beneficially, there is a significant reduction in opiate intake when PCRAs are used in a postoperative setting.[58]

The iontophoretic transdermal system is a recent technological advancement that incorporates iontophoresis, which uses a low-intensity electrical field to transfer medication from a gel reservoir across intact skin.[5] The fentanyl ITS uses this technology to deliver 40 μg fentanyl over a 10-minute period. It is a noninvasive on-demand delivery PCA that offers logistic advantages for patients and nursing staff, eliminating potential medication errors and the need for venous access. It allows for rapid delivery of analgesia, uniquely different from the historically slower onset analgesia of the transdermal patches.[5] As a noninvasive PCA, it provides a reduction in infection risk and allows for greater patient mobility due to the self-contained, needle-free, compact system design. Several large, randomized clinical trials studies have shown that fentanyl ITS provides equivalent analgesia to morphine IV-PCA, the current standard of care for postoperative pain.[41] Limitations associated with transdermal PCA are the fixed preprogrammed dosing of the system without the ability to alter dosages and potential dermal reactions at the site of placement.[41] The intranasal route for analgesia has shown rapid onset, avoidance of first-pass metabolism, high patient satisfaction, and ease in administration making it a viable pain- management alternative.[5] Intranasal fentanyl PCA has been shown to have analgesic effects in the postoperative setting that are comparable to IV-PCA.[33] Some noted disadvantages of intranasal fentanyl include side effects related specifically to intranasal or inhalation route of administration as well as shorter half-life, slower onset compared with IV administration of fentanyl.[5,33] However, only a small number of trials have evaluated this promising route of administration. Some authors suggest management of postoperative pain relief with PCINA plays a role in acute pain in children and patients for whom IV access is difficult rather than become a standard route.[5]

Sublingual, inhalation, and oral are all routes of delivery that are being explored for PCA utilization. These three emerging modes are still in various stages of development and have not been cleared by the FDA for acute pain management. These modes continue to undergo investigations and have thus far provided promising research as future noninvasive options for PCA.

PCA has proven to be better at pain management and has higher rates of patient satisfaction than non-PCA.[59] The initial modality of IV-PCA has spurred the development of various routes of administration, expanding the field to include innovative applications of analgesia. Though a strong foundation has been developed since its origin in the mid-1960s, PCA has yet to be established as the safest and most efficacious option for analgesia. Further PCA research and development is needed in technology, pharmaceuticals, and system processes.[59]

The current PCA technologies need further development toward ensuring patient safety, reducing the invasive nature of the technologies and reducing contamination. Additional safety device features are needed to ensure appropriate administration of medication, proper drug dosing, and adequate lockout periods to reduce side effects and adverse patient outcomes.[59] The catheters associated with IV-PCA, PCEA, and PCRA serve as a nidus for infection, potentially further complicating a patient's postoperative course. Continued research into noninvasive alternatives will provide more patient mobility simultaneously reducing the complications associated with indwelling catheter placement.

IV-PCA, the most commonly used PCA, employs opioids to combat analgesia. Opioids have been associated with adverse side effects that can hinder postoperative recovery and are known to be extremely addictive.[59] Alternate, nonopioid medications for pain control that have the same onset time and pain relief as opioids should continue to be applied to PCA technologies to minimize side effects and adverse outcomes. There have been some studies that suggest drug combinations may be a promising area of study to potentiate analgesic effects and duration.[59]

The processes associated with PCA refer to the education and feasibility of application in the health care setting.[59] PCA should continue to focus on a user-friendly interface that appropriately communicates with the patient as well as the health care provider. In order for health care institutions to be receptive to incorporating PCA, the implementation of these systems should leave little room for human error by providing thorough education and training of PCA management. Additionally, a reduction in the amount of supervision and maintenance needed to support PCA will enhance the efficacy of timely pain relief along with safety.[59]

PCA is an effective and safe approach to patient-centered care in acute pain management. Over the years, there have been significant advancements in the field with many prospective potential options to come as there are still areas requiring improvement to ensure the best patient outcomes.

REFERENCES

1. Roe BB. Are postoperative narcotics necessary? *Arch Surg*. 1963;87:912-915.
2. Grass JA. Patient-controlled analgesia. *Anesth Analg*. 2005;101(5 Suppl):S44-S61. doi:10.1213/01.ane.0000177102.11682.20
3. Sechzer PH. Objective measurement of pain. *Anesthesiology*. 1968;29:209-210.
4. Hadzic A. Chapter 70: Intravenous Patient-controlled analgesia. *Hadzic's Textbook of Regional Anesthesia and Acute Pain Management*. 2nd ed. McGraw-Hill Education; 2017.
5. Viscusi ER. Patient-controlled drug delivery for acute postoperative pain management: a review of current and emerging technologies. *Reg Anesth Pain Med*. 2008;33(2):146-158. doi:10.1016/j.rapm.2007.11.005. PMID: 18299096
6. Kaye AD, Ali SIQ, Urman RD. Perioperative analgesia: ever-changing technology and pharmacology. *Best Pract Res Clin Anaesthesiol*. 2014;28(1):3-14.
7. Walder B, Schafer M, Henzi I, Tramer MR. Efficacy and safety of patient-controlled opioid analgesia for acute postoperative pain: a quantitative systematic review. *Acta Anaesthesiol Scand*. 2001;45:795-804.

8. Gan TJ, Meyer T, Apfel CC, et al. Consensus guidelines for managing postoperative nausea and vomiting. *Anesth Analg*. 2003;97:62-71.
9. Elliot JA. Patient controlled analgesia. In: Smith HS, ed. *Current Therapy in Pain*. 1st ed. Saunders/Elsevier; 2009:73-77.
10. Halpern SH, Muir H, Breen TW, et al. A multicenter randomized controlled trial comparing patient-controlled epidural with intravenous analgesia for pain relief in labor. *Anesth Analg*. 2004;99:1532-1538.
11. Soffin EM, Liu SS. Patient controlled analgesia. In: *Essentials of Pain Medicine*. 4th ed. Elsevier; 2018:117-122.
12. Halpern SH, Breen TW, Campbell DC. A multicenter, randomized, controlled trial comparing bupivacaine with ropivacaine for labor analgesia. *Anesthesiology*. 2003;98:1431-1435.
13. Wheatley RG, Schug SA, Watson D. Safety and efficacy of postoperative epidural analgesia. *Br J Anaesth*. 2001;87:47-61.
14. Wu CL, Cohen SR, Richman JM, et al. Efficacy of postoperative patient-controlled and continuous infusion epidural analgesia versus intravenous patient-controlled analgesia with opioids: a meta-analysis. *Anesthesiology*. 2005;103:1079-1088.
15. Hurley RW, Wu CL. Acute postoperative pain. In: Elkassabany NM, ed. *Miller's Anesthesia*. 9th ed. Elsevier; 2020:2614-2638.
16. Liu SS, Wu CL. Effect of postoperative analgesia on major postoperative complications: a systematic update of the evidence. *Anesth Analg*. 2007;104:689-702.
17. Dolin SJ, Cashman JN. Tolerability of acute postoperative pain management: nausea, vomiting, sedation, pruritus, and urinary retention. Evidence from published data. *Br J Anaesth*. 2005;95:584-591.
18. Lehmann KA. Recent developments in patient-controlled analgesia. *J Pain Symptom Manage*. 2005;29(5 Suppl):S72-S89. doi:10.1016/j.jpainsymman.2005.01.005
19. Halpern SH, Carvalho B. Patient-controlled epidural analgesia for labor. *Anesth Analg*. 2009;108:921-928.
20. Liu SS, Wu CL. The effect of analgesic technique on postoperative patient-reported outcomes including analgesia: a systematic review. *Anesth Analg*. 2007;105:789-808.
21. Popping DM, Elia N, Marret E, Remy C, Tramer MR. Protective effects of epidural analgesia on pulmonary complications after abdominal and thoracic surgery: a meta-analysis. *Arch Surg*. 2008;143:990-999. discussion 1000.
22. Momeni M, Crucitti M, Kock MD. Patient-controlled analgesia in the management of postoperative pain. *Drugs*. 2006;66(18):2321-2337. doi:10.2165/00003495-200666180-00005
23. Horlocker TT, Vandermeulen E, Kopp SL, Gogarten W, Leffert LR, Benzon HT. Regional anesthesia in the patient receiving antithrombotic or thrombolytic therapy. *Reg Anesth Pain Med*. 2018;43(3):263-309. doi:10.1097/aap.0000000000000763
24. Bateman BT, Mhyre JM, Ehrenfeld J, et al. The risk and outcomes of epidural hematomas after perioperative and obstetric epidural catheterization: a report from the multicenter perioperative outcomes group research consortium. *Anesth Analg*. 2013;116(6):1380-1385.
25. Practice advisory for the prevention, diagnosis, and management of infectious complications associated with neuraxial techniques: a report by the American Society of Anesthesiologists Task Force on infectious complications associated with neuraxial techniques. *Anesthesiology*. 2010;112:530-545.
26. Rawal N, Allvin R, Axellson K, et al. Patient-controlled regional analgesia (PCRA) at home. *Anesthesiology*. 2002;96(6):1290-1296.
27. Axelsson K, Nordenson U, Johanzon E, et al. Patient-controlled regional analgesia (PCRA) with ropivacaine after arthroscopic subacromial decompression. *Acta Anaesthesiol Scand*. 2003;47(8):993-1000. doi:10.1034/j.1399-6576.2003.00146.x
28. Rasouli MR, Viscusi ER. Adductor canal block for knee surgeries: an emerging analgesic technique. *Arch Bone Jt Surg*. 2017;5(3):131-132.
29. Andersen LO, Kehlet H. Analgesic efficacy of local infiltration analgesia in hip and knee arthroplasty: a systematic review. *Br J Anaesth*. 2014;113:360-374.
30. Scheffel PT, Clinton J, Lynch JR, Warme WJ, Bertelsen AL, Matsen FA. Glenohumeral chondrolysis: a systematic review of 100 cases from the English language literature. *J Shoulder Elbow Surg*. 2010;19:944-949.
31. Fredman B, Shapiro A, Zohar E, et al. The analgesic efficacy of patient-controlled ropivacaine instillation after cesarean delivery. *Anesth Analg* 2000;91:1436-1440.
32. Zohar E, Fredman B, Phillipov A, Jedeikin R, Shapiro A. The analgesic efficacy of patient-controlled bupivacaine wound instillation after total abdominal hysterectomy with bilateral salpingo-oophorectomy. *Anesth Analg*. 2001;93:482-487.
33. Prommer E, Thompson L. Intranasal fentanyl for pain control: current status with a focus on patient considerations. *Patient Prefer Adherence*. 2011;5:157-164. doi:10.2147/PPA.S766
34. Riediger C, Haschke M, Bitter C, et al. The analgesic effect of combined treatment with intranasal S-ketamine and intranasal midazolam compared with morphine patient-controlled analgesia in spinal surgery patients: a pilot study. *J Pain Res*. 2015;8:87-94. https://doi.org/10.2147/JPR.S75928
35. Bouida W. Ali KBH, Soltane BH, et al. Effect on opioids requirement of early administration of intranasal ketamine for acute traumatic pain. *Clin J Pain*. 2020;36(6):458-462. doi:10.1097/AJP.0000000000000821

36. Seppänen S-M, Kuuskoski R, Mäkelä KT, Saari TI, Uusalo P. Intranasal dexmedetomidine reduces postoperative opioid requirement in patients undergoing total knee arthroplasty under general anesthesia. *J Arthroplasty*. 2021;36(3):978-985.e1.
37. Viscusi ER, Siccardi M, Damaraju CV, Hewitt DJ, Kershaw P. The safety and efficacy of fentanyl iontophoretic transdermal system compared with morphine intravenous patient-controlled analgesia for postoperative pain management: an analysis of pooled data from three randomized, active-controlled clinical studies. *Anesth Analg*. 2007;105(5):1428-1436. doi:10.1213/01.ane.0000281913.28623.fd
38. Sheikh NK, Dua A. Iontophoresis analgesic medications. [Updated 2020 Jun 23]. In: *StatPearls* [Internet]. StatPearls Publishing; 2020. https://www.ncbi.nlm.nih.gov/books/NBK553090/
39. Roustit M, Blaise S, Cracowski JL. Trials and tribulations of skin iontophoresis in therapeutics. *Br J Clin Pharmacol*. 2014;77(1):63-71. doi:10.1111/bcp.12128
40. Bakshi P, Vora D, Hemmady K, Banga Iono AK. Iontophoretic skin delivery systems: success and failures. *Int J Pharm*. 2020;586:119584. https://doi.org/10.1016/j.ijpharm.2020.119584
41. Poplawski S, Johnson M, Philips P, Eberhart LH, Koch T, Itri LM. Use of fentanyl iontophoretic transdermal system (ITS) (IONSYS®) in the management of patients with acute postoperative pain: a case series. *Pain Ther*. 2016;5(2):237-248. doi:10.1007/s40122-016-0061-2
42. Minkowitz HS, Rathmell JP, Vallow S, Gargiulo K, Damaraju CV, Hewitt DJ. Efficacy and safety of the fentanyl iontophoretic transdermal system (ITS) and intravenous patient-controlled analgesia (IV PCA) with morphine for pain management following abdominal or pelvic surgery. *Pain Med*. 2007;8(8):657-668. doi:10.1111/j.1526-4637.2006.00257.x
43. Stacey BR, Rudy TE, Nelhaus D. Management of patient-controlled analgesia: a comparison of primary surgeons and a dedicated pain service. *Anesth Analg*. 1997;85(1):130-134. doi:10.1097/00000539-199707000-00023
44. Van de Donk T, Ward S, Langford R, Dahan A. Pharmacokinetics and pharmacodynamics of sublingual sufentanil for postoperative pain management. *Anaesthesia*. 2018;73(2):231-237.
45. Giaccari LG, Coppolino F, Aurilio C, et al. Sufentanil sublingual for acute postoperative pain: a systematic literature review focused on pain intensity, adverse events, and patient satisfaction. *Pain Ther*. 2020;9(1):217-230.
46. Melson TI, Boyer DL, Minkowitz HS, et al. Sufentanil sublingual tablet system vs. intravenous patient-controlled analgesia with morphine for postoperative pain control: a randomized, active-comparator trial. *Pain Pract*. 2014;14(8):679-688.
47. Minkowitz HS, Leiman D, Melson T, Singla N, DiDonato KP, Palmer PP. Sufentanil Sublingual Tablet 30 mcg for the management of pain following abdominal surgery: a randomized, placebo-controlled, phase-3 study. *Pain Pract*. 2017;17(7):848-858.
48. Ringold FG, Minkowitz HS, Gan TJ, et al. Sufentanil sublingual tablet system for the management of postoperative pain following open abdominal surgery: a randomized, placebo-controlled study. *Reg Anesth Pain Med*. 2015;40(1):22-30.
49. Jove M, Griffin DW, Minkowitz HS, Ben-David B, Evashenk MA, Palmer PP. Sufentanil sublingual tablet system for the management of postoperative pain after knee or hip arthroplasty: a randomized, placebo-controlled study. *Anesthesiology*. 2015;123(2):434-443.
50. Grissa, MH, Boubaker H, Zorgati A, et al. Efficacy and safety of nebulized morphine given at 2 different doses compared to IV titrated morphine in trauma pain. *Am J Emerg Med*. 2015;33(11):1557-1561.
51. Clark A, Rossiter-Rooney M, Valle-Leutri F. Aerosolized liposome-encapsulated fentanyl (AeroLEF) via pulmonary administration allows patients with moderate to severe post-surgical acute pain to self-titrate to effective analgesia. *J Pain*. 2008;9(4):42-42.
52. Wirz S, Conrad S, Shtrichman R, Schimo K, Hoffmann E. Clinical evaluation of a novel technology for oral patient-controlled analgesia, the *PCoA® Acute* device, for hospitalized patients with postoperative pain, in pilot feasibility study. *Pain Res Manag*. 2017;2017:7962135.
53. Palmer P, Ji X, Stephens J. Cost of opioid intravenous patient-controlled analgesia: results from a hospital database analysis and literature assessment. *Clinicoecon Outcomes Res*. 2014;6:311-318.
54. Tveita T, Thoner J, Klepstad P, Dale O, Jystad A, Borchgrevink PC. A controlled comparison between single doses of intravenous and intramuscular morphine with respect to analgesic effects and patient safety. *Acta Anaesthesiol Scand*. 2008;52(7):920-925.
55. Hudcova J, McNicol E, Quah C, Lau J, Carr DB. Patient controlled opioid analgesia versus conventional opioid analgesia for postoperative pain. *Cochrane Database Syst Rev*. 2006;(4):CD003348.
56. Yi Y, Kang S, Hwang B. Drug overdose due to malfunction of a patient-controlled analgesia machine—a case report. *Korean J Anesthesiol*. 2013;64(3):272-275.
57. Winacoo JN, Maykel JA. Operative anesthesia and pain control. *Clin Colon Rectal Surg*. 2009;22(1):41-46. doi:10.1055/s-0029-1202885
58. Vadivelu N, Mitra S, Narayan D. Recent advances in postoperative pain management. *Yale J Biol Med*. 2010;83(1):11-25.
59. Nardi-Hiebl S, Eberhart L, Gehling M, et al. Quo Vadis PCA? A review on current concepts, economic considerations, patient-related aspects, and future development with respect to patient-controlled analgesia. *Anesthesiol Res Pract*. 2020;2020:1-7.

34

NSAIDs and COX-2 Inhibitors

Matthew R. Eng and Kapil Anand

Introduction

Non–steroidal anti-inflammatory drugs (NSAIDs) and selective cyclooxygenase 2 (COX-2) inhibitors have become valuable anti-inflammatory and analgesic medications in the perioperative environment for their effectiveness and low side effect profile. With increasing economic pressures, patient satisfaction demands, and unfavorable adverse effects of opioids, multimodal techniques in pain management has become increasingly important. Commonly utilized NSAID medications for acute pain management include paracetamol, ibuprofen, ketorolac, diclofenac, and naproxen (Table 34.1). Commonly utilized COX-2 inhibitor drugs include rofecoxib, valdecoxib, and celecoxib (see Table 34.1).

Mechanism of Action

NSAIDs inhibit an enzyme in the prostaglandin synthesis pathway called cyclooxygenase. Prostaglandins are released during local tissue injury and decrease the pain threshold at the site of injury as well as local surrounding tissue. The inflammation and hyperalgesic state of the tissue notifies the nociceptors of increased pain and inflammation. NSAIDs prevent the production of prostaglandins at the periphery and spinal cord by inhibition of the cyclooxygenase enzyme.

NSAIDs are nonspecific in their inhibition of the cyclooxygenase enzyme. Consequently, the blockade of the cyclooxygenase 1 isoenzyme results in gastrointestinal adverse events and platelet inhibition. COX-1 isoenzymes and COX-2 isoenzymes in a reduced effect are associated with gastrointestinal bleeding, ulceration, and perforation. The production of arachidonic acid metabolites including the gastric protective prostacyclin PGI2 is likely responsible. COX-2 isoenzyme inhibiting medications present the ability to block prostaglandin synthesis conferring analgesic and anti-inflammatory benefits with reduced gastrointestinal side effects. The reversible inhibition of thromboxane A2 production causes inhibition of platelet aggregation. Compared with placebo, in patients undergoing tonsillectomy, a higher risk of rebleeding was present when administering conventional NSAIDs. Platelet inhibition has not been demonstrated in COX-2 inhibitor medications.

Analgesic and Anti-inflammatory Properties

As acute pain management has become increasingly more important, the benefits of NSAIDs and COX-2 inhibitors should be well understood. A multimodal approach to acute pain management utilizing opioid sparing analgesics has been associated with faster resumption of daily activities, faster discharge times, improved patient satisfaction, and a reduction in complications. Further, the reduction of postoperative acute pain has been associated with a reduction in the development of chronic pain.

TABLE 34.1 COMMON PERIOPERATIVE NSAIDs

NSAID	Mechanism of Action	Half Life (h)
Paracetamol	Nonselective COX inhibition	1.5-2.5
Ketorolac	Nonselective COX inhibition	5.2-5.6
Ibuprofen	Nonselective COX inhibition	2
Diclofenac	Nonselective COX inhibition	1-2
Naproxen	Nonselective COX inhibition	12-17
Celecoxib	COX-2 selective inhibition	11
Rofecoxib	COX-2 selective inhibition	17
Valdecoxib	COX-2 selective inhibition	8-11

COX-2 inhibitors and NSAIDs have been demonstrated to be effective in a wide variety of surgical procedures for acute pain management.

Ketorolac

One of the older NSAID medications, ketorolac, has been used in practice since 1976. Ketorolac may be used for moderate to severe pain and may be used in a wide variety of surgical operations for acute pain management. Ketorolac has been demonstrated to be effective in patients undergoing ambulatory outpatient procedures, orthopedic procedures, and major abdominal operations.[1-3] Either 30 mg or 60 mg has been demonstrated to be effective in patients undergoing outpatient or abdominal surgery in reducing acute pain.[3] The potency of ketorolac is impressively equivalent to morphine 4 mg as demonstrated when administered 10 mg or 30 mg for postsurgical pain.[1] In a review of patients receiving ketorolac between 1986 and 2001, the authors found that the potent analgesic ketorolac reduced opioid consumption by 36%.[4] Over 90% of the medication is metabolized in the kidney, and it has been associated in kidney failure in patients with a predisposition to kidney failure. Further, theoretical risks remain regarding the NSAID platelet inhibition properties and gastrointestinal side effects.

Ibuprofen

Ibuprofen is an NSAID medication commonly used in oral formulation without a prescription to treat fever, headaches, and mild/moderate inflammatory conditions. When used perioperatively, ibuprofen can offer analgesia for acute pain management to spare opioid consumption. Ibuprofen has been demonstrated to improve analgesia in oral surgery, hand surgery, total knee and hip replacement surgery, thyroid surgery, and laparoscopic surgery.[5-10] In patients undergoing laparoscopic cholecystectomy operations, a single dose of ibuprofen was associated with a reduction in opioid consumption by 45% within the first 24 hours as compared to placebo.[7] Similar to ketorolac, chronic use or high dosages may contribute to kidney impairment. The nonselective cyclooxygenase enzyme activity of ibuprofen also inhibits the production of thromboxane A2, which may impair platelet aggregation.

Naproxen

Similar to ibuprofen, naproxen is a nonprescription NSAID used to treat fever, headaches, and mild/moderate inflammatory conditions. When used as an analgesic adjuvant on the day of surgery and in the immediate postoperative period, naproxen 500-1000 mg daily has been demonstrated to reduce pain severity as well as opioid consumption. In patients undergoing knee arthroscopy, the patients administered naproxen sodium 550 mg demonstrated an improvement in pain level as well as the functional ability of the operative knee and leg at 10 days as compared to placebo.[11] The same side effects with platelet inhibition and kidney impairment are found with naproxen.

COX-2 Inhibitors

Because of the risks to gastrointestinal bleeding and platelet inhibition, there has been much interest in the use of COX-2 inhibitors. Celecoxib is the most commonly used medication in this class. There were some initial concerns regarding this class of medication because of cardiovascular complications and an increase in wound infections.[12] Consequently, rofecoxib and valdecoxib were removed from the market. However, the safety of COX-2 inhibitors following noncardiac operations in short-term usage has been demonstrated to be safe without complication.[12] COX-2 inhibitor medications offer analgesic benefit to ambulatory surgery procedures, orthopedic procedures, laparoscopic procedures, and more.[13-15] When administered either preoperatively or postoperatively, COX-2 inhibitors have demonstrated analgesic benefit leading to earlier resumption of daily activities, decreased postoperative complications, and improved patient satisfaction. COX-2 inhibitors have less gastrointestinal side effects and do not cause platelet inhibition.[13,16-19]

Conclusion

Acute pain management with NSAIDs and COX-2 inhibitors should be considered in most postsurgical patients as part of a multimodal approach. With limited side effects and contraindications, this class of medications can contribute to a multimodal approach with great analgesic benefit. Patients undergoing ambulatory surgery or major inpatient surgery may all benefit from NSAIDs and COX-2 inhibitors. Adoption of ERAS protocols and clinical pathways have demonstrated value in standardizing the utilization of this class of medication. Few side effects have been attributed to NSAIDs in at-risk populations and with chronic use, and cardiovascular risks have been controversial with COX-2 inhibitors. Improvement in patient satisfaction, reduction in opioid consumption, and reduction in postoperative complications is associated with the administration of NSAIDs and COX-2 inhibitors for acute pain.

REFERENCES

1. White PF, Raeder J, Kehlet H. Ketorolac: its role as part of a multimodal analgesic regimen. *Anesth Analg.* 2012;114:250-254. doi:10.1213/ANE.0b013e31823cd524
2. Ding Y, White PF. Comparative effects of ketorolac, dezocine, and fentanyl as adjuvants during outpatient anesthesia. *Anesth Analg.* 1992;75(4):566-571. doi:10.1213/00000539-199210000-00018
3. Parker RK, Holtmann B, Smith I, White PF. Use of ketorolac after lower abdominal surgery: effect on analgesic requirement and surgical outcome. *Anesthesiology.* 1994;80(1):6-12. doi:10.1097/00000542-199401000-00005
4. Macario A, Lipman AG. Ketorolac in the era of cyclo-oxygenase-2 selective nonsteroidal anti-inflammatory drugs: a systematic review of efficacy, side effects, and regulatory issues. *Pain Med.* 2001;2(4):336-351. doi:10.1046/j.1526-4637.2001.01043.x
5. Merry AF, Gibbs RD, Edwards J, et al. Combined acetaminophen and ibuprofen for pain relief after oral surgery in adults: a randomized controlled trial. *Br J Anaesth.* 2010;104(1):80-88. doi:10.1093/bja/aep338
6. Lawhorn CD, Bower CM, Brown RE, et al. Topical lidocaine for postoperative analgesia following myringotomy and tube placement. *Int J Pediatr Otorhinolaryngol.* 1996;35(1):19-24. doi:10.1016/0165-5876(95)01275-3
7. Ahiskalioglu EO, Ahiskalioglu A, Aydin P, Yayik AM, Temiz A. Effects of single-dose preemptive intravenous ibuprofen on postoperative opioid consumption and acute pain after laparoscopic cholecystectomy. *Medicine (United States).* 2017;96(8):e6200. doi:10.1097/MD.0000000000006200
8. Weinheimer K, Michelotti B, Silver J, Taylor K, Payatakes A. A prospective, randomized, double-blinded controlled trial comparing ibuprofen and acetaminophen versus hydrocodone and acetaminophen for soft tissue hand procedures. *J Hand Surg Am.* 2019;44(5):387-393. doi:10.1016/j.jhsa.2018.10.014

9. Ilyas AM, Miller AJ, Graham JG, Matzon JL. Pain management after carpal tunnel release surgery: a prospective randomized double-blinded trial comparing acetaminophen, ibuprofen, and oxycodone. *J Hand Surg Am.* 2018;43(10):913-919. doi:10.1016/j.jhsa.2018.08.011
10. Mutlu V, Ince I. Preemptive intravenous ibuprofen application reduces pain and opioid consumption following thyroid surgery. *Am J Otolaryngol.* 2019;40(1):70-73. doi:10.1016/j.amjoto.2018.10.008
11. Rasmussen S, Thomsen S, Madsen SN, Rasmussen PJS, Simonsen OH. The clinical effect of naproxen sodium after arthroscopy of the knee: a randomized, double-blind, prospective study. *Arthroscopy.* 1993;9(4):375-380. doi:10.1016/S0749-8063(05)80309-3
12. Nussmeier NA, Whelton AA, Brown MT, et al. Complications of the COX-2 inhibitors parecoxib and valdecoxib after cardiac surgery. *N Engl J Med.* 2005;352(11):1081-1091. doi:10.1056/nejmoa050330
13. Ekman EF, Wahba M, Ancona F. Analgesic efficacy of perioperative celecoxib in ambulatory arthroscopic knee surgery: a double-blind, placebo-controlled study. *Arthroscopy.* 2006;22(6):635-642. doi:10.1016/j.arthro.2006.03.012
14. White PF. Role of non-opioid analgesic techniques in the management of pain after ambulatory surgery. *Anesth Analg.* 2002;94(3):577-585.
15. Khan AA, Dionne RA. COX-2 inhibitors for endodontic pain. *Endod Top.* 2002;3(1). doi:10.1034/j.1601-1546.2002.30104.x
16. Recart A, Issioui T, White PF, et al. The efficacy of celecoxib premedication on postoperative pain and recovery times after ambulatory surgery: a dose-ranging study. *Anesth Analg.* 2003;96(6):1631-1635. doi:10.1213/01.ANE.0000062526.60681.7B
17. White PF, Sacan O, Tufanogullari B, Eng M, Nuangchamnong N, Ogunnaike B. Effect of short-term postoperative celecoxib administration on patient outcome after outpatient laparoscopic surgery. *Can J Anesth.* 2007;54(5):342-348. doi:10.1007/BF03022655
18. Issioui T, Klein KW, White PF, et al. The efficacy of premedication with celecoxib and acetaminophen in preventing pain after otolaryngologic surgery. *Anesth Analg.* 2002;94(5):1188-1193. doi:10.1097/00000539-200205000-00025
19. Watcha MF, Issioui T, Klein KW, White PF. Costs and effectiveness of rofecoxib, celecoxib, and acetaminophen for preventing pain after ambulatory otolaryngologic surgery. *Anesth Analg.* 2003;96(4):987-994. doi:10.1213/01.ANE.0000053255.93270.31

35

Meloxicam: Pharmacology and Role in the Management of Acute Pain

Carley E. Boyce, Luke Mosel, Sarahbeth R. Howes, Benjamin Cole Miller, Victoria L. Lassiegne, Mark R. Alvarez, Jake Huntzinger, Alan David Kaye, Varsha D. Allampalli, Elyse M. Cornett, and Jonathan S. Jahr

Introduction

The International Association for the Study of Pain (IASP) defines pain as: "an unpleasant sensory and emotional experience associated with actual or potential tissue damage, or described in terms of such damage."[1] Adequate postoperative pain control is not only of utmost importance to patients but also to physicians as well, because of the correlation to worse outcomes impacting patients' health and quality of life, and in severe cases of poorly treated postoperative pain, degradation to severe chronic pain syndromes. Some adverse effects (AEs) that have been associated with inadequate pain control include delirium, chronic pain, and impairments in social and physical function.[2,3]

The current management of postoperative pain and recovery from painful procedures is considered unsatisfactory by many and continues to be an important clinical problem and an opportunity for improvement. Opioids have been a staple in the management of postoperative care and recovery; however, they are frequently associated with AEs such as nausea, vomiting, constipation, ileus, pruritus, and respiratory depression along with dependence, misuse, and over-reliance.[4] These constraints have driven the search for an adequate method of pain control with an emphasis on nonopioid analgesics. A valuable method is intravenous lidocaine; a Cochrane retrospective review reported low to moderate evidence that this intervention impacted pain scores when compared to placebo.[5] Another intervention is a multimodal technique for pain management. This approach involves the administration of two or more analgesics with different mechanisms of action via the same or different routes to optimize effectiveness while minimizing AEs. The American Society of Anesthesiologists Task Force recommends a regimen that includes acetaminophen, nonselective non–steroidal anti-inflammatory drug (NSAID), or cyclooxygenase-2 (COX-2) selective NSAIDs unless contraindicated.[6]

Meloxicam is an example of a long-acting preferential COX-2 inhibitor nonsteroidal NSAID with analgesic, antipyretic, and anti-inflammatory activities through reduction of prostaglandin biosynthesis. The use of oral meloxicam is limited by its slow onset of action due to its poor aqueous solubility. The peak plasma concentration is not reached until 9-11 hours after oral administration of a 30-mg dose and is thus not an ideal treatment for acute pain; however, intravenous meloxicam in its nanocrystal formulation is currently available due to its shorter time to peak plasma concentration.[4]

Related to the role of COX-1 constitutive enzyme activity facilitating platelet aggregation, vasoconstriction, and gastrointestinal and renal homeostasis, the safety concerns associated with intravenous meloxicam are similar to those of any NSAID or Coxib, including oral meloxicam and incorporating concerns of bleeding, cardiovascular, and renal events.[7,8] In one study, pooled data from a phase II/phase III clinical program exhibited low incidence of treatment-emergent adverse events (TEAEs). The intravenous meloxicam was reportedly tolerated well in subjects with moderate-to-severe postoperative pain, with most commonly reported TEAEs being nausea, vomiting, and headache. In this study, intravenous meloxicam also reduced need for postoperative opioid use when monitored, suggesting that IV meloxicam may represent a beneficial and suitable replacement of current postoperative pain management.[8] This review, therefore, aims to delineate the medical research surrounding pain management and describe the safety and tolerability of intravenous meloxicam in the treatment of acute pain.

Pharmacokinetics and Pharmacodynamics

Pharmacokinetics

While meloxicam has long been prescribed and administered by mouth for numerous types of pain, its use for acute pain has only recently become widely accepted due to the development of an intravenous formulation. This is primarily related to the shortened time to peak plasma concentrations.[7,9]

Absorption

Meloxicam administered intravenously achieved maximum plasma concentration within minutes (Tmax –0.12 hours) after a single 30 mg dose. Following administration of 30 mg meloxicam orally, maximum plasma concentrations (Cmax) were achieved in 9-11 hours (Tmax).[10,11]

Distribution

Meloxicam given intravenously is more than 99% bound to albumin within the therapeutic dose range, and the fraction of protein binding is independent of drug concentration. Due to this extensive albumin binding, the steady state volume of distribution was found to be between 0.15 and 0.2 L/kg. Synovial fluid concentrations approach 40%-45% of plasma concentration.[7,9,12]

Metabolism/Elimination

Meloxicam is eliminated primarily in the liver via Phase 1 by P450 (CYP) 2C9 with no active metabolites. Excretion is via urine and feces with very small amounts left unchanged.[9,13,14] Elimination half-life is 20-24 hours, which makes it an ideal drug for once-daily dosing. Age, race, gender, and mild to moderate hepatic impairment have little clinical impact on meloxicam pharmacokinetics. Mild renal impairment made only small changes to maximum plasma concentrations with no changes in dosing required. Meloxicam is not recommended for patients with moderate-to-severe renal dysfunction.[7,9,13,15] Drugs that interact significantly with meloxicam include methotrexate, cyclosporine, NSAIDs, salicylates, pemetrexed, angiotensin-converting enzyme inhibitors, angiotensin receptor blockers, beta-blockers, aspirin, and lithium. Dosage reduction of meloxicam IV should be considered in patients receiving concomitant CYP2C9 inhibitors.[9,13]

Pharmacodynamics

The mechanism of action of meloxicam is via inhibition of the cyclooxygenase pathway where it inhibits the conversion of arachidonic acid to prostaglandins. COX-1 enzyme produces prostaglandins that have gastrointestinal, renal, and platelet effects. The COX-2 enzyme produces prostaglandins that mediate pain perception. Meloxicam preferentially inhibits the COX-2 pathway but does have some COX-1 effects as well.[16] Meloxicam thus displays less gastrointestinal and platelets effects than other less selective COX inhibitors and has no additional renal risk associated.[7,13,16,17]

Anti-inflammatory/Analgesic/Antipyretic

Various animal and human studies have evaluated the anti-inflammatory effects of meloxicam with a suppression in inflammation shown in animal models with a single dose. Human studies used a decrease in erythrocyte sedimentation rate, C-reactive protein, and aquaporin-1 expression to monitor effects on inflammation. Meloxicam administration has been common in the treatment of chronic arthritis and musculoskeletal pain for many years.[7,9] Analgesic effects are well documented, and in one study, a 50% reduction in analgesic effects was not found until 18 hours after dosing.[7,9,14,16] Similar to other NSAIDs, meloxicam does not have any direct effect on the thermoregulatory center in the hypothalamus in normothermic individuals. The anti-inflammatory effect is responsible for its effectiveness in pyrogen-induced fever.[9,18]

Safety and Efficacy

The safety of meloxicam IV has been evaluated across a wide range of both postoperative and perioperative pain management strategies. The full range of the pain spectrum is explored through numerous major surgeries, including, but not limited to, elective abdominal hysterectomy, bunionectomy, total knee arthroplasty (TKA), and spinal surgery. Meloxicam IV is a more selective COX-2 inhibitor, but like all NSAIDs, it carries the same black box warnings analogous to other NSAIDs, such as gastrointestinal bleeding, hepatorenal events, and thrombotic injury.[7] These side effects were specifically explored in addition to others through various safety measures like vital signs, physical examination, laboratory values (hemoglobin and hematocrit), 12-lead EKGs, accessory medications (ie, multimodal analgesic protocol or standard of care), and supplemental medications (rescue opioid consumption) in both Phase II and Phase III trials.[8] In a Phase II blinded, single-dose study exploring meloxicam IV at doses 5-60 mg after elective abdominal hysterectomy, only mild to moderate adverse events were reports and no serious adverse events were related to the study medication. Adverse events of special interest, specifically hepatic and anemic events, did not increase in incidence with increasing dosage.[19] In a pooled analysis comparing 1426 adult subjects from seven postoperative studies, there was a higher association of side effects reported from the placebo groups vs meloxicam IV groups.[8] Overall safety evaluations for meloxicam IV shows a lower incidence of adverse events compared with placebo and known adverse events with opioid use.[20]

With the formulation of meloxicam for IV use, utilization in the acute pain setting is now possible due to its' faster onset of action than its' oral counterpart.[9] IV meloxicam shows a rapid onset of analgesia, which is evident as early as 15-30 minutes after administration of a single dose of meloxicam IV 30 mg.[4] The analgesic effect is also sustained over its 24-hour dosing interval.[4] IV meloxicam has demonstrated analgesic efficacy in a variety of surgical settings, including orthopedic, abdominal, and colorectal surgeries.[7] In comparison to placebo, all meloxicam IV doses showed statistically significant postoperative pain intensity relative to a placebo.[19] Meloxicam was then compared to one of the common opioid analgesics, morphine, and was showed to produce statistically significant reductions in pain intensity at doses of meloxicam IV 60, 30, and 15 mg.[19] In trials where opioid use was monitored, meloxicam reduced postoperative rescue opioid, which suggest that IV meloxicam may represent a useful alternative to current postoperative management options.[8] With IV meloxicam, overall opioid consumption was significantly decreased postoperatively and was associated with quicker time for first dose to first ambulation and a first dose to discharge when compared to placebo.[20] Additionally, recent evidence suggests that IV meloxicam has also shown the ability to reduce postoperative pain if it is administered preoperatively in patients.[7]

Important Clinical Studies and Improvements for IV Meloxicam (See Table 35.1)

A 2021 randomized, double-blind, placebo-controlled study investigated the safety and efficacy of IV meloxicam in 55 patients who underwent colorectal surgery with bowel resection with or without anastomosis for relief of postoperative pain. This study demonstrated that patients who received IV meloxicam consumed fewer opioids, reported lower sum of pain intensity differences over 24 hours ($SPID_{24}$), and had a decreased length of stay and shorter length of time to first bowel sound, flatus, and bowel movement after surgery.[21] Overall, these data suggest that use of meloxicam IV postoperatively may effectively reduce opiate use and expenditure of health care resources and possibly increase functional benefit. Another 2018 randomized control trial (RCT) with 200 patients who suffered moderate-to-severe pain after bunionectomy and were treated with IV meloxicam vs placebo resulted in a primary end point $SPID_{48}$ that was lower for meloxicam than it was for placebo, indicating that the drug was more effective than placebo for postoperative pain.[4] Secondary end points, such as SPID at differing time intervals and time to first use of rescue analgesia, were also investigated and were lower and longer, respectively, for patients treated with IV meloxicam.[4]

One might question the benefit of such information above, considering that patients in these studies were treated for pain control with either meloxicam or placebo and conclude that something given for pain is better than nothing at all. This highlights the importance of comparing standard postoperative pain control with this new approach of using IV meloxicam. A 2019 phase II RCT including 486 women with moderate-to-severe pain following total abdominal hysterectomy compared the efficacy of placebo vs IV meloxicam vs morphine with the primary end point being $SPID_{24}$ and total pain relief (TOTPAR24) through 24 hours postadministration. The results of this trial revealed statistically significant differences for morphine and IV meloxicam compared to placebo, with those receiving morphine and meloxicam reporting lower $SPID_{48}$ and higher TOTPAR24 values.[19] The study also found that meloxicam IV doses ≥15 mg also significantly enhanced $SPID_{48}$ and TOTPAR24 relative to morphine.[19]

Several other recent RCTs supported the data collected in the above studies, suggesting that IV meloxicam is highly effective compared to placebo when offering patients postoperative acute pain relief. For instance, a 2018 RCT in which 230 patients underwent surgery for dental impaction and two other RCTs in which patients underwent TKA and abdominoplasty, respectively, all revealed that IV meloxicam is superior to placebo for postsurgical moderate-to-severe pain relief.[20,22,23] These studies also addressed the side effect profile of meloxicam, and all suggest that the most common AEs of this medication experienced include GI side effects (nausea, vomiting, constipation) and headaches and dizziness. A 2020 review in a peer reviewed pain management journal studied results from pooled Phase II and III trials, most discussed in this section, included 910 subjects who underwent diverse surgeries and reported similar findings to the first research trial reported. The pooled results demonstrated that IV meloxicam had similar rates of AEs in meloxicam and placebo-treated groups.[7] This article summarized many of the previously discussed results in order to reiterate how once daily IV meloxicam decreased opioid consumption, decreased reported pain on the SPID scale, decreased the length of hospital stay, and increased functional improvement.[7]

TABLE 35.1 CLINICAL SAFETY AND EFFICACY

Study Name	Groups Studied and Intervention	Results and Findings	Conclusions
Silinsky et al.[21]	55 subjects who underwent colorectal surgery with bowel resection were treated with IV meloxicam for postoperative pain	Those who received IV meloxicam required fewer opioids, reported a lower sum of pain intensity differences (SPID) over 24 h, and demonstrated a quicker time to first bowel sound, flatus, and bowel movement.	The data suggest prescribing IV meloxicam postoperatively may effectively reduce opiate use and result in a reduction of health care system expenditures.
Pollak et al.[4]	200 subjects who suffered from moderate-to-severe pain following bunionectomy were treated with either IV meloxicam or placebo.	SPID over 48 h was lower for meloxicam than placebo. Secondary end points of SPID at differing intervals and time to first use of rescue analgesia for those receiving IV meloxicam were lower and longer, respectively.	IV meloxicam was more effective than placebo for postoperative pain.
Rechberger et al.[19]	486 women with moderate-to-severe pain following total abdominal hysterectomy compared the pain management achieved by placebo vs IV meloxicam vs morphine.	Unsurprisingly, those receiving IV meloxicam or morphine demonstrated lower $SPID_{24}$ and higher total pain relief from 0 to 24 h (TOTPAR24) relative to placebo. The meloxicam group receiving ≥15 mg significantly enhanced $SPID_{48}$ and TOTPAR24 relative to morphine.	At higher doses, IV meloxicam demonstrates a greater degree of pain control than standard doses of morphine. These results suggest a viable nonopioid alternative for postoperative pain control.
Christensen et al.[22]	230 subjects following dental impaction surgery were treated with IV meloxicam vs ibuprofen and placebo for management of postoperative pain.	$SPID_{24}$ results favored both the IV meloxicam and ibuprofen groups relative to placebo, with both doses of IV meloxicam studied outperforming ibuprofen. Additionally, patients subjectively rated IV meloxicam best among the treatment options, and those receiving IV meloxicam were least likely to use rescue analgesia.	Results favored active treatment vs placebo and suggested IV meloxicam offered patients better postoperative pain control relative to ibuprofen.
Berkowitz et al.[20]	181 subjects following elective total knee arthroplasty were treated with IV meloxicam vs placebo to track the cumulative use of opioids during the postoperative period.	Those treated with IV meloxicam demonstrated both a statistically significant reduction in opioid use and a lower degree of adverse effects relative to the placebo group. Additionally, $SPID_{24}$ values demonstrated the superiority of IV meloxicam for postoperative pain control.	IV meloxicam represents an opportunity to reduce the overall usage of opioids for the management of postoperative pain in the setting of total knee arthroplasty.
Singla et al.[23]	219 subjects were treated with IV meloxicam vs placebo to analyze postoperative pain control following abdominoplasty.	Meloxicam treatment groups exhibited statistically significant differences in $SPID_{24}$ relative to placebo, with these patients demonstrating a higher degree of pain control. Those in the meloxicam treatment arm also required fewer opioid rescue medications relative to placebo.	In the setting of postoperative abdominoplasty, meloxicam resulted in a reduction of overall opioid use while also demonstrating a higher degree of pain control.

IV Meloxicam and Platelet Function, and Network Meta-analysis to Evaluate IV Meloxicam vs Other Intravenous Nonopioid Medications for Moderate-to-Severe Postoperative Pain

Platelet Function Study

Non–steroidal anti-inflammatory drugs (NSAIDs) are an integral part of the World Health Organization (WHO) Pain Ladder, which has been applied across acute and chronic pain settings, as a first-line defense to prevent or treat pain.[17] Intravenous (IV) meloxicam (meloxicam IV) is a novel formulation of NanoCrystal Colloidal Dispersion meloxicam being developed for the management of moderate-to-severe pain. A concern of NSAID use in the peri- or postoperative setting is the potential for platelet dysfunction and risk of bleeding-related events.[17] However, research has demonstrated that the association of NSAID use with increased bleeding risk is primarily related to reductions in thromboxane associated with inhibition of cyclooxygenase-1 (COX-1) by nonselective NSAIDs and that a lower risk of events has been observed with the use of COX-2–selective NSAIDs. Meloxicam IV, with its higher affinity for COX-2 inhibition, is anticipated to have a lower risk for platelet dysfunction–related events while maintaining a prolonged duration of analgesic action.[17] See Table 35.2 for COX Selectivity of Common NSAIDs. One method of evaluating the effects of drugs or other conditions on platelet function is in analyzing blood samples using the platelet function analyzer (PFA-100; Siemens Healthcare Diagnostics, Deerfield, IL, USA), a device that determines a closure time (CT) by simulating the platelet adhesion and aggregation that would occur following a vascular injury. Analysis can be performed using two different testing reagent cartridges, collagen with epinephrine (CEPI) and collagen with adenosine diphosphate (CADP). The CEPI cartridges are known to be sensitive to aspirin-induced platelet abnormalities, while the CADP cartridges are primarily sensitive to various thrombocytopathies with lower sensitivity to aspirin effects.[17]

This study underwent institutional review board (IRB) review and approval, and all subjects (blood donors) provided informed consent prior to participation. Healthy volunteers provided a single whole blood sample (~20 mL) for analysis. Each whole blood sample was

TABLE 35.2 COX SELECTIVITY OF COMMON NSAIDs (COX-2/COX-1 IC_{80} RATIO)

	Agent	COX-2/COX-1 IC_{80} Ratio
Greater COX-1 selectivity	Ketorolac	294
	Aspirin	3.8
	Naproxen	3
	Ibuprofen	2.6
	Diclofenac	0.23
	Celecoxib	0.11
	Meloxicam	0.091
Greater COX-2 selectivity	Rofecoxib	<0.05

Network meta-analysis
COX, cyclooxygenase; IC, inhibitory concentration; NSAID, non–steroidal anti-inflammatory drug.
Adapted and modified from Jahr JS, Searle S, McCallum S, et al. Platelet function: meloxicam intravenous in whole blood samples from healthy volunteers. *Clin Pharmacol Drug Dev*. 2020;9(7):841-848.

aliquoted to allow analysis under negative control (1 condition), positive control (2 conditions), and meloxicam IV (4 conditions) test conditions, using both the CEPI and CADP cartridges. Whole blood aliquots were treated according to the test condition and incubated for ~10 minutes prior to analysis in the PFA-100. All blood samples were to be analyzed within 2.5 hours of collection. Subject/donor eligibility criteria were 18- to 40-year-old male and female nontobacco users, no recent medication use; prescription, OTC, or vitamin/nutritional supplement; no known medical history affecting coagulation or platelet function (ie, anemia, thrombocytopenia); negative control (untreated sample) CT within normal range; and CEPI < 150 second and CADP < 110 seconds. Testing conditions included negative control: untreated whole blood and positive control ketorolac IV 2.5 and 5 μg/mL, reflecting approximate Cmax following a 15 and 30 mg ketorolac IV bolus, respectively. Meloxicam IV doses were 5, 10, 15, and 20 μg/mL, reflecting approximate Cmax following a 30 mg meloxicam IV dose (5 μg/mL), along with additional concentrations exceeding the exposure at the planned therapeutic dose. Statistical analysis test results were evaluated for quality control (QC) based on a repeat sample analysis from a single meloxicam IV test condition, with an acceptance criterion of ≤20% variance from the original result. Treatment effect on CT was analyzed using an analysis of variance (ANOVA) to assess treatment effect with and without controlling for covariates.

Results revealed that whole blood samples were analyzed from 13 eligible subjects (7 male, 6 female). The statistical analyses included data from 8 subject samples (2 male, 6 female); 5 subject samples were excluded, 1 due to instrument malfunction and 4 due to out of range QC sample result. Data were reported for the statistical analysis set unless otherwise noted.

CADP analysis: sample analysis using the CADP reagent cartridge did not demonstrate a significant overall treatment effect on CT ($P = .5715$). No individual treatment demonstrated a significant change in CT vs untreated control ($P \geq .0907$). No significant prolongation in CT was observed in meloxicam IV–treated whole blood samples at concentrations reflecting therapeutic and supratherapeutic exposure levels compared with untreated control. In contrast, significant prolongations in CT were observed in samples reflecting therapeutic ketorolac concentrations compared with untreated control. When compared with ketorolac, meloxicam IV therapeutic exposure levels were observed to have numerically shorter CTs. These results suggest a potential clinical benefit of meloxicam IV over ketorolac with regard to a decreased risk of platelet dysfunction.

The study concluded that no significant prolongation in CT was observed in meloxicam IV–treated whole blood samples at concentrations reflecting therapeutic and supratherapeutic exposure levels compared with untreated control. In contrast, significant prolongations in CT were observed in samples reflecting therapeutic ketorolac concentrations compared with untreated control. When compared with ketorolac, meloxicam IV therapeutic exposure levels were observed to have numerically shorter CTs. These results suggested a potential clinical benefit of meloxicam IV over ketorolac with regard to a decreased risk of platelet dysfunction.

IV meloxicam had not yet been compared to other nonopioid IV analgesics. A network meta-analysis was conducted to assess the safety and efficacy of MIV relative to other IV nonopioid analgesics for moderate-to-severe postoperative pain.[24] This study adhered to best practices guidelines and was conducted according to a prespecified, publicly-registered protocol (PROSPERO).[24] The scope was updated to focus on studies without preemptive administration, which reflects the clinical scenario in which MIV has been evaluated.

For the systematic literature review, PubMed, Medline, EBSCO, Web of Science, Scopus, ClinicalTrials.gov, and Cochrane CENTRAL were searched for RCTs published between January 2000 and February 2019 (excluding nonhuman studies and studies with solely pediatric cohorts). Inclusion criteria included open abdominal surgery, joint arthroplasty, hysterectomy, or bunionectomy; treated with IV nonopioid analgesics; administered postoperatively after patients reached a moderate-to-severe pain level; pain measured objectively; and follow-up was ≥12 hours postoperatively. Studies were assessed independently by three reviewers and discrepancies were adjudicated by consensus. Data were double abstracted centrally in Covidence.

Outcomes were evaluated postoperatively and compared IV meloxicam compared to other nonopioid IV analgesics based on sum of pain intensity difference (SPID), morphine milligram equivalents (MMEs) consumed, and adverse events (AEs) and opioid-related AEs (ORADEs). Procedures were grouped as abdominal (hysterectomy, abdominoplasty, and C-sections), bunionectomy, and orthopedic (predominantly joint arthroplasties). Bayesian random effects in network meta-analysis generated standardized mean differences and odds ratios (OR) for continuous and dichotomous outcomes. Surface under the cumulative ranking curve (SUCRA) was used to generate treatment rankings for each outcome. Risk of bias and evidence certainty were assessed using the Cochrane Handbook and the GRADE frameworks, respectively.

The literature search yielded 2303 unduplicated studies from which we retained 17 RCTs for analysis in the network meta-analysis. Pooled analysis of pain outcomes across time points demonstrated the following probabilities that IV meloxicam produced the largest SPID, which is consistent with SUCRA rankings. IV meloxicam was associated with a pooled 18% reduction in MMEs (range 26%-12%) vs acetaminophen: 14% reduction, vs ketorolac: 16% reduction. IV meloxicam offered no relative benefits with respect to non-ORADEs but was associated with lower pooled odds of gastrointestinal ORADEs (OR = 0.72; 95% credible interval [Crl] 0.66-0.78) and respiratory ORADEs (OR = 0.51; 95% Crl 0.59-0.42). IV meloxicam was associated with lower pain, MME utilization, and ORADEs postoperatively for a number of clinical comparisons. The quality of our outcomes was moderate overall. This reflects an expected lack of head-to-head studies for IV meloxicam, which is investigational at this time. Key limitations include sparse networks, extrapolation of IV meloxicam abdominoplasty data to other abdominal procedures, and no direct comparisons for IV meloxicam.

Conclusion

Meloxicam, historically prescribed for chronic pain, has recently been developed into an intravenous formulation that creates value in management of acute postoperative pain.

Postoperative pain management continues to be a challenge and focus for medical providers. Opioids have long been the mainstay treatment, but while effective in managing pain, they demonstrate a number of undesirable side effects limiting the recovery of the patient. While many alternatives to opioids have been explored, The American Society of Anesthesiologists Task Force currently recommends a multimodal technique to pain management. This recommendation includes the utilization of acetaminophen and either a nonselective, or COX-2 selective NSAID.[6]

Meloxicam preferentially inhibits the COX-2 pathway, which reduces prostaglandins involved in inflammation and pain perception. Meloxicam has less inhibition of the COX-1 enzyme than nonselective NSAIDs possess, leading to less untoward gastrointestinal, renal, and platelet side effects.[7,13,16,17] The pharmacokinetics of intravenous meloxicam makes it an ideal drug for the treatment of acute pain compared to the oral version. When 30 mg is administered intravenously, the mean time to peak plasma concentration is around 7 minutes allowing relatively quick pain relief.[10,11] In addition to its quick onset, meloxicam can be conveniently dosed daily as a result of its elimination half-life of 20-24 hours.[9,13,15]

Intravenous meloxicam has proven to be an efficacious treatment for acute postoperative pain with demonstrating superiority of meloxicam for pain reduction over placebo, ibuprofen, and even routine doses of morphine.[19,22] In addition to effective pain control, the use of IV meloxicam reveals a statistically significant reduction in opioid use.[7] One study of patients who underwent colorectal surgery reported that with meloxicam, there was a faster return to bowel function suggesting intravenous meloxicam may improve functional recovery in certain patient populations.[21]

The studies reviewed in this chapter suggest that intravenous meloxicam is a safe option for pain management, having been studied in several different types of surgeries. In a pooled analysis of seven postoperative studies, there was a greater association of side effects reported from the placebo groups vs intravenous meloxicam groups.[8] Safety evaluations for intravenous meloxicam also show a lower incidence of adverse events compared with opioid use.[20] The most common side effects that were associated with meloxicam use were GI effects, headaches, and dizziness. IV meloxicam is metabolized by the liver, so dosages should be decreased accordingly in use with other CYP 2C9 inhibitors.[9,13] Meloxicam may be used in patients with mild renal impairment but should be avoided in patients with moderate-to-severe renal dysfunction.[7,9,13,15]

While intravenous meloxicam is a novel formulation, the efficacy and safety illustrated in this chapter make a strong case for its use in acute postoperative pain management, compared to current alternatives. The selective COX-2 inhibitor's desirable pharmacokinetics, safety profile, and proven efficacy make it a valuable tool in a multimodal pain management approach.

REFERENCES

1. Raja SN, Carr DB, Cohen M, et al. The revised International Association for the Study of Pain definition of pain: concepts, challenges, and compromises. *Pain*. 2020;161(9):1976-1982.
2. Sinatra R. Causes and consequences of inadequate management of acute pain. *Pain Med*. 2010;11(12):1859-1871.
3. Morrison RS, Magaziner J, Gilbert M, et al. Relationship between pain and opioid analgesics on the development of delirium following hip fracture. *J Gerontol A Biol Sci Med Sci*. 2003;58(1):M76-M81.
4. Pollak RA, Gottlieb IJ, Hakakian F, et al. Efficacy and safety of intravenous meloxicam in patients with moderate-to-severe pain following bunionectomy: a randomized, double-blind, placebo-controlled trial. *Clin J Pain*. 2018;34(10):918-926.
5. Weibel S, Jelting Y, Pace NL, et al. Continuous intravenous perioperative lidocaine infusion for postoperative pain and recovery in adults. Cochrane Anaesthesia, Critical and Emergency Care Group, editor. *Cochrane Database Syst Rev* [Internet]. 2018[cited 2021 Apr 30];6(6):CD009642. http://doi.wiley.com/10.1002/14651858.CD009642.pub3
6. Practice guidelines for acute pain management in the perioperative setting. *Anesthesiology*. 2012;116(2):248-273.
7. Berkowitz RD, Mack RJ, McCallum SW. Meloxicam for intravenous use: review of its clinical efficacy and safety for management of postoperative pain. *Pain Manag*. 2021;11(3):249-258.
8. Viscusi ER, Gan TJ, Bergese S, et al. Intravenous meloxicam for the treatment of moderate to severe acute pain: a pooled analysis of safety and opioid-reducing effects. *Reg Anesth Pain Med*. 2019;44(3):360-368.
9. Bekker A, Kloepping C, Collingwood S. Meloxicam in the management of post-operative pain: narrative review. *J Anaesthesiol Clin Pharmacol*. 2018;34(4):450-457.
10. Türck D, Busch U, Heinzel G, Narjes H. Clinical pharmacokinetics of meloxicam. *Arzneimittelforschung*. 1997;47(3):253-258.
11. Distel M, Mueller C, Bluhmki E, Fries J. Safety of meloxicam: a global analysis of clinical trials. *Br J Rheumatol*. 1996;35(Suppl 1):68-77.
12. Davies NM, Skjodt NM. Clinical pharmacokinetics of meloxicam. *Clin Pharmacokinet*. 1999;36(2):115-126.
13. Safety & Tolerability [Internet]. Anjeso. [cited 2021 May 2]. https://www.anjeso.com/safety-tolerability
14. Gottlieb IJ, Tunick DR, Mack RJ, et al. Evaluation of the safety and efficacy of an intravenous nanocrystal formulation of meloxicam in the management of moderate-to-severe pain after bunionectomy. *J Pain Res*. 2018;11:383-393.
15. Del Tacca M, Colucci R, Fornai M, Blandizzi C. Efficacy and tolerability of meloxicam, a COX-2 preferential nonsteroidal anti-inflammatory drug. *Clin Drug Investig*. 2002;22(12):799-818.
16. Bacchi S, Palumbo P, Sponta A, Coppolino MF. Clinical pharmacology of non-steroidal anti-inflammatory drugs: a review. *Antiinflamm Antiallergy Agents Med Chem*. 2012;11(1):52-64.
17. Jahr JS, Searle S, McCallum S, et al. Platelet function: meloxicam intravenous in whole blood samples from healthy volunteers. *Clin Pharmacol Drug Dev*. 2020;9(7):841-848.
18. Engelhardt G, Homma D, Schlegel K, Utzmann R, Schnitzler C. Anti-inflammatory, analgesic, antipyretic and related properties of meloxicam, a new non-steroidal anti-inflammatory agent with favourable gastrointestinal tolerance. *Inflamm Res*. 1995;44(10):423-433.

19. Rechberger T, Mack RJ, McCallum SW, Du W, Freyer A. Analgesic efficacy and safety of intravenous meloxicam in subjects with moderate-to-severe pain after open abdominal hysterectomy: a phase 2 randomized clinical trial. *Anesth Analg*. 2019;128(6):1309-1318.
20. Berkowitz RD, Steinfeld R, Sah AP, et al. Safety and efficacy of perioperative intravenous meloxicam for moderate-to-severe pain management in total knee arthroplasty: a randomized clinical trial. *Pain Med.* 2021;22(6):1261-1271.
21. Silinsky JD, Marcet JE, Anupindi VR, et al. Preoperative intravenous meloxicam for moderate-to-severe pain in the immediate post-operative period: a Phase IIIb randomized clinical trial in 55 patients undergoing primary open or laparoscopic colorectal surgery with bowel resection and/or anastomosis. *Pain Manag*. 2021;11(1):9-21.
22. Christensen SE, Cooper SA, Mack RJ, McCallum SW, Du W, Freyer A. A randomized double-blind controlled trial of intravenous meloxicam in the treatment of pain following dental impaction surgery. *J Clin Pharmacol*. 2018;58(5):593-605.
23. Singla N, Bindewald M, Singla S, et al. Efficacy and safety of intravenous meloxicam in subjects with moderate-to-severe pain following abdominoplasty. *Plast Reconstr Surg Glob Open*. 2018;6(6):e1846.
24. Carter JA, Black LK, Sharma D, Bhagnani T, Jahr JS. Efficacy of non-opioid analgesics to control postoperative pain: a network meta-analysis. *BMC Anesthesiol*. 2020;20:272. https://doi.org//10.1186. S12871-020-01147-y

36

Skeletal Muscle Relaxants, Antidepressants, Antiepileptics, Gabapentinoids

Anand M. Prem, Maryam Jowza, and Dominika James

Introduction

While the prevalence of chronic pain in the adult population averages about 20% in the United States, the prevalence of acute pain is poorly understood. Thirty to fifty percent of patients in the hospital setting report pain of moderate to severe intensity. Over the past 20 years, the United States has seen a dramatic increase in deaths from opioid overdose that coincided with increases in the prescribing of opioids for pain management.[1] The escalation of overdose deaths from illicit opioids (including heroin and synthetic opioids such as fentanyl) seen in the past decade was driven in part by a growing number of people whose use began with prescription opioids.[1] According to the National Center for Drug Abuse Statistics, in 2017, more than 11 million Americans misused prescription opioids with 19 000 deaths involving prescription opioids in 2016 alone.

The liberal use of opioids in pain management was brought on by a combination of factors beyond the scope of this chapter, but central to the opioid crisis was the belief that addiction is rare as long as opioids were used to treat pain.[1] Recent studies however have shown that even a relatively brief exposure to opioids can increase the risk for chronic opioid use, opioid use disorder, and addiction. In many of these opioid-related overdose deaths, the initial exposure to opioids started with an opioid prescription for the management of acute pain, either in the immediate postoperative period or in the outpatient setting.[1] To address the ongoing opioid crisis, while adequate pain control is still a priority, every effort must be made to minimize opioid use in the perioperative period and increase the use of multimodal pain regimens. Enhanced recovery after surgery protocols focus on regimens that include nerve blocks, nonsteroidals, muscle relaxants, gabapentinoids, lidocaine, acetaminophen, and ketamine to decrease postoperative opioid consumption and reduce hospital stays. This chapter reviews the role of other nonopioid adjuvants such as antidepressants, muscle relaxants, antiepileptics as well as gabapentinoids as a component of a multimodal regimen for the treatment of acute pain (Table 36.1).

Antidepressants

The need to find safer, nonopioid agents to control pain is getting renewed attention, and antidepressants can play a significant role in pain treatment, improving the pain experience and reducing the need for opioids. Although antidepressants have ample evidence to support their efficacy in chronic pain over the past 50 years, they are often underutilized in the management of acute and postoperative pain.[2]

TABLE 36.1 NONOPIOID ADJUNCTS USED IN PAIN MANAGEMENT

Class	Mechanism of Action	Common Pain Indication	Notes
Skeletal muscle relaxants	Variety of agents with heterogeneous mechanisms of action on CNS	Limited evidence in support of use in acute back pain	Most agents have sedating side effects
Antidepressants	Of the various classes, TCAs and SNRIs most effective for pain; thought to strengthen descending inhibitory pain pathways at level of the spinal cord	Used most commonly in neuropathic pain states, fibromyalgia	Treatment of pain does not depend on treatment of mood
Antiepileptics	Heterogeneous compounds with various mechanisms of action, many agents act as inhibitors of voltage-gated Na channels	Neuropathic pain	More studies are needed to determine effectiveness in acute pain
Gabapentinoids	Inhibits the $\alpha 2$ delta subunit of the presynaptic voltage-gated calcium channels	Neuropathic pain	May have opioid-sparing effect in acute pain

CNS, central nervous system; TCA, tricyclic antidepressant; SNRI, selective norepinephrine serotonin reuptake inhibitor.

The antidepressant classes used in pain include the following (Table 36.2):

1. Tricyclic antidepressants (TCAs): amitriptyline, nortriptyline, imipramine, desipramine, clomipramine, maprotiline
2. Serotonin noradrenaline (norepinephrine) reuptake inhibitors (SNRIs): duloxetine, venlafaxine, milnacipran
3. Selective serotonin reuptake inhibitors (SSRIs): fluoxetine, paroxetine, citalopram, sertraline
4. Dopamine noradrenaline reuptake inhibitors: bupropion

Tricyclic antidepressants are antagonists of peripheral sodium channels and spinal *N*-methyl-D-aspartate (NMDA) receptors, which helps prevent central sensitization, a crucial component in the pathophysiology of acute postoperative pain.[3] Although supported by a large body of evidence, the use of older TCAs in the management of pain is restricted by their numerous undesirable side effects.[2,4] The SSRIs though have a better safety profile with fewer serotonin receptor-mediated side effects, but their use in pain has not been studied as extensively as they are less effective than traditional TCAs.[2] The newer class of serotonin (5-HT)-norepinephrine (NE) reuptake inhibitors such as venlafaxine inhibit the reuptake of both 5-HT and NE, similar to the TCAs but without affecting other nontherapeutic receptors, leading to fewer side effects and better patient tolerance.[2] They also minimally interact with the cytochrome P-450 system leading to minimal interaction with other drugs making them a useful component of any multimodal pain treatment regimen.

Evidence for Antidepressants in the Treatment of Acute Pain

In a 2014 review of 15 studies involving 985 participants with acute postoperative pain who were treated with antidepressants, 8 trials demonstrated superiority to placebo for early reduction of pain.[4] However, methodological concerns in these studies led the authors to conclude that there was insufficient evidence supporting the use of antidepressants in the treatment of acute pain as well as prevention of chronic postoperative pain. Future trials conducted in

TABLE 36.2 SUMMARY OF ANTIDEPRESSANTS

Class	Examples	Mechanism	Side Effects	Notes
Tricyclic antidepressants (TCAs)	Amitriptyline Nortriptyline Desipramine	Serotonin reuptake inhibition, norepinephrine reuptake inhibition, peripheral sodium channel antagonist, spinal *N*-methyl-D-aspartate (NMDA) receptor antagonist, anticholinergic, antihistaminic	Anticholinergic: xerostomia, tachycardia, urinary retention, constipation, amblyopia, and memory disturbances. Antihistaminic: sedation, drowsiness, weight gain. QT prolongation	Use limited by side effects
Selective serotonin receptor reuptake inhibitors (SSRIs)	Fluoxetine Paroxetine Citalopram Sertraline	Presynaptic serotonin reuptake blocker increases concentration of serotonin in the synaptic cleft	Nausea, diarrhea, tremor, headache, sedation, sexual side effects	Little analgesics efficacy
Selective norepinephrine serotonin reuptake inhibitors (SNRIs)	Duloxetine Venlafaxine Milnacipran	Serotonin (5-HT) and norepinephrine (NE) reuptake inhibition	Nausea, diarrhea, fatigue, somnolence, sexual dysfunction, hypertension	Well tolerated in neuropathic pain, fibromyalgia
Dopamine noradrenaline reuptake inhibitors	Bupropion	Noradrenergic and dopaminergic reuptake inhibition	Insomnia, nervousness, headache, irritability, lowered seizure threshold	Evidence for analgesic efficacy is mixed

carefully selected patients should evaluate the indications and contraindications for antidepressants in the acute perioperative setting as well as the potential for adverse drug interactions and increased risk for perioperative bleeding.[4] Targeting patients particularly at high risk for developing chronic postsurgical pain may justify the risk of adverse effects from antidepressant use.[4]

As the analgesic effects of antidepressant drugs in chronic pain are typically seen days to weeks after initiation of treatment and escalation of doses, antidepressants may need to be initiated and titrated for days to weeks before surgery to optimize results in postoperative pain. In the absence of a clear time frame during which acute postoperative pain transitions to chronic postsurgical pain, antidepressants may need to be continued for several days or even weeks after postsurgical hospital discharge.[4]

Initiation of Treatment

Antidepressants typically need to be initiated at ¼ to ½, the recommended dose and titrated up gradually over 2-3 weeks to the full dose, to minimize side effects and improve patient tolerance. This is especially key in the elderly population. Pain patients are often on other medications that can potentiate the side effects of antidepressants, and this must be taken to account while titrating the dose. Frequent reassessments every 2-4 weeks is ideal before dose increases.

Mechanism of Action of Antidepressants as Analgesics

While there is consensus regarding the therapeutic benefits of antidepressants such as amitriptyline and duloxetine in the treatment of neuropathic pain, the mechanism by which they exert these actions is still poorly understood.[2-4]

Antidepressants in chronic pain act via several different postulated mechanisms. Reinforcement of the descending inhibitory pain pathways by increasing the amount of norepinephrine and serotonin in the synaptic cleft at both the supraspinal and spinal levels is one of the major mechanisms. Relief of underlying depression that adversely alters the affective component of pain is another. In acute pain, the primary mechanisms by which antidepressants act include blockage of sodium channels, NMDA receptor antagonism,[3,4] blockade of central substance P receptors, and neuromodulation of the endogenous opioid systems.[2]

Within each class of antidepressant, there are again considerable differences in the extent of pain relief each drug provides in different populations. This was evident in one cross over study that looked at 31 patients with postherpetic neuralgia treated with amitriptyline and nortriptyline. While five patients had good pain relief with amitriptyline, they continued to experience moderate to severe pain with nortriptyline, and four other patients had good pain relief with nortriptyline but none with amitriptyline.

Painful Conditions That Respond to Antidepressants

While a variety of pain syndromes have been treated with antidepressants, neuropathic pain appears to be the most responsive to this class of drugs. Peripheral neuropathy from compressive, diabetic, postherpetic or HIV-related etiology, postradiation or chemotherapy neuritis, deafferentation pain, central pain syndromes, plexopathies, and postlaminectomy pain syndrome respond well to antidepressants,[2,3,5] while their role in purely nociceptive pain is less impressive.

Tricyclic Antidepressants

This oldest class of antidepressants have the most evidence for their efficacy in the treatment of acute neuropathic and chronic pain. Their analgesic properties are independent of their antidepressant actions.[2,3] However, they also act on multiple other neuroreceptors, which account for their numerous side effects, often limiting their use in the chronic pain patient.[2] The choice of a TCA to treat depression is primarily based on the patient's tolerance of their anticholinergic and antihistaminic side effects, as they are all equally effective as antidepressants. Amitriptyline and imipramine are associated with more sedation, orthostatic hypotension, and weight gain. Nortriptyline has fewer anticholinergic side effects, and desipramine is the least of all TCAs.[4]

Role in the treatment of pain

TCAs have independent analgesic effects unrelated to their antidepressant effect, unlike SSRIs.[2,3] They are superior to SNRIs as analgesics likely due to NMDA receptor antagonism and sodium channel blockade, in addition to their serotonin and norepinephrine reuptake inhibition.[2-4] They are effective in pain from diabetic neuropathy, postherpetic neuralgia, complex regional pain syndrome, radicular pain, poststroke pain, and chronic headaches.[5] They have opioid-sparing properties and can be used effectively as preemptive analgesics in the management of acute perioperative pain. The usual analgesic doses (25-75 mg) are lower than the typical antidepressant dose (75-150 mg).[5,6]

Adverse effects

TCAs block the muscarinic receptors producing anticholinergic effects such as xerostomia, tachycardia, urinary retention, constipation, amblyopia, and memory disturbances. Sedation, drowsiness, weight gain, and potentiation of other central nervous system (CNS) depressants are attributed to histamine (H1) receptor blockade.[3-6] They block Alpha 1 adrenergic receptors leading to drowsiness and postural hypotension, while Alpha 2 adrenergic receptor blockade can cause priapism and interfere with the antihypertensive properties of Alpha 2 agonists such as clonidine and methyldopa, if given simultaneously. Some TCAs block dopaminergic receptors causing extrapyramidal symptoms, rigidity, tremor, akinesia, tardive dyskinesia, neuroleptic malignant syndrome, as well as increased prolactin production. All TCAs decrease the seizure threshold.

Initiation of treatment

Routine laboratory screening of blood urea nitrogen, creatinine, electrolytes, and liver function tests is recommended before starting treatment with TCAs. As they are arrhythmogenic and can prolong the QT interval, all patients above 40 years of age or with preexisting cardiac disease should get a baseline EKG to ensure that the corrected QT (QTC) interval is <450 ms. TCAs should be initiated at the lowest dose possible, especially in the elderly and gradually titrated up to therapeutic doses based on tolerance to side effects.

Discontinuation of TCAs: Abrupt discontinuation can lead to a withdrawal syndrome manifested by fever, sweating, headache, dizziness, nausea, and akathisia.

Overdose with TCAs: Unlike with SSRIs, overdose with TCAs can be lethal, and this is a leading cause of drug overdose deaths, usually a result of the anticholinergic and arrhythmogenic effects. TCAs have a narrow therapeutic range, requiring periodic blood level monitoring, as 3-5 times the therapeutic dose can be potentially lethal.

Selective Serotonin Reuptake Inhibitors

Selective serotonin reuptake inhibitors are the most widely prescribed antidepressants due to their efficacy and low side effect profile. They block the presynaptic serotonin reuptake pump in the CNS increasing the concentration of serotonin in the synaptic cleft and facilitating neurotransmission.

Role in pain treatment

There is little evidence to support SSRIs as sole analgesics.[4-7] In conjunction with other analgesics in the patient with depression, pain reduction is seen due to improvement in the affective component of pain from its antidepressant properties. Case reports of sustained pain relief in patients with diabetic neuropathy are not supported by double-blind placebo-controlled trials.

Initiation of therapy

Prior to initiating therapy with SSRIs, no additional lab work is required. A thorough review of the patient's medical history and concurrent medications will determine suitability. Titration of dose is based on clinical response and tolerance of side effects. Typically started at ½ the recommended dose and titrated up over the course of a week.

Paroxetine is more sedating and a stronger anxiolytic due to its anticholinergic effects and given at night. It has a shorter half-life than other SSRIs, with potential for withdrawal symptoms, if discontinued abruptly. Fluoxetine is more stimulating and given in the morning. Sertraline and citalopram are less sedating and usually prescribed in the mornings.

SSRIs induce or inhibit various cytochrome P-450 (CYP450) enzymes, increasing the serum levels of TCAs and benzodiazepines. They can also alter the levels of other drugs metabolized by the liver such as antipsychotics, lithium, carbamazepine, and analgesics methadone, oxycodone, and fentanyl. Paroxetine, fluoxetine, fluvoxamine to a lesser extent, and sertraline at higher doses inhibit cytochrome C2D6 increasing the blood levels of some opioid metabolites. Citalopram and escitalopram have minimal CYP450 enzyme inhibition.

Adverse effects

Nausea, diarrhea, tremor, headache, sedation, and overstimulation are common side effects. Sexual side effects like impotence, ejaculatory dysfunction, decreased libido, and inability to attain orgasm are seen in about 75% patients on SSRIs, especially with advanced age.[8]

Rarer side effects include akathisia, dystonia, syndrome of inappropriate antidiuretic hormone, and palpitations.[3-7] Osteoporosis and increased risk for bleeding have been reported with all SSRIs. Other medications the patient is on such as anticoagulants, antiplatelet agents and non–steroidal anti-inflammatory drugs (NSAIDs) can increase this risk, particularly in the high-risk population.

Serotonin syndrome is a significant risk when SSRIs are coadministered with SNRIs, TCA, triptans, monoamine oxidase inhibitors (MAOIs), antiemetics as well as several common analgesics such as tramadol, fentanyl, meperidine, and pentazocine. Use with tramadol can also lower seizure threshold. Overdosing on SSRIs is rarely fatal. Discontinuing SSRIs must include a gradual taper to avoid withdrawal symptoms such as nausea, diarrhea, headache, or myalgias.

Serotonin and Norepinephrine Reuptake Inhibitors

This class of antidepressants are increasingly being recognized as useful adjuvants in the treatment of musculoskeletal pain, fibromyalgia, and chronic pain.[9] They bind to both the Serotonin (5-HT) and Norepinephrine (NE) transporters inhibiting their reuptake. They however differ in their affinity to these receptors and consequently their potency. They are also weak inhibitors of alpha-1, cholinergic and histamine receptors, accounting for their better side effect profile in comparison to TCAs. Unlike SSRIs, they typically have an ascending dose-response curve leading to increased effect with higher doses.[10] When used in conjunction with MAOIs or tramadol, these medications can cause serotonin syndrome.

Venlafaxine (brand name: Effexor)

Pharmacokinetics: Venlafaxine is a relatively weak 5-HT and an even weaker NE uptake inhibitor with an almost 30-fold difference in binding of the two transporters.[10] At lower doses, it primarily binds to the serotonin transporter and as the dose is increased, it increasingly binds to the NE transporter. Venlafaxine is primarily metabolized by the cytochrome P2D6 (CYP2D6) enzyme to the active metabolite *O*-desmethylvenlafaxine (desvenlafaxine).[10] Venlafaxine has a half-life of 5 hours, while desvenlafaxine has a half-life of 12 hours. This is further prolonged in patients with renal and hepatic impairment, requiring dose reduction by 50% in the presence of significant hepatic and renal dysfunction.[10] Both have low protein binding and minimally interact with the cytochrome P450 system minimizing any potential for drug-drug interactions.

Initiation of treatment

Start low at 37.5 mg 2-3 times a day for a week and then titrate up to 150-225 mg/day based on clinical response and tolerance of side effects. Extra caution is required in hypertensive patients due to elevation of blood pressure at higher doses.

Adverse effects

Typical side effects include nausea, diarrhea, fatigue, somnolence, and sexual dysfunction, while higher doses produce mild increases in blood pressure, tachycardia, tremors, diaphoresis, and anxiety. Due to the inhibition of NE reuptake, dose-dependent elevation in blood pressure can occur, though rarely seen at doses below 225 mg/day.

Evidence for role in pain

Venlafaxine is structurally like tramadol and in mice has been shown to provide opioid receptor–mediated analgesia reversed by naloxone. Medical literature supports the use of venlafaxine in multiple pain states including fibromyalgia, headaches, and neuropathic pain conditions such as peripheral neuropathy, postherpetic neuralgia, intercostal neuralgia, complex regional pain syndrome, post-stroke pain, and atypical facial pain in multiple sclerosis.[5-10] Its antinociceptive effect is independent of its antidepressant activity. Tolerance by patients is significantly better than with TCAs or SSRIs with minimal reported adverse events. Venlafaxine retains its efficacy with long-term maintenance therapy, unlike prolonged therapy with SSRIs.

Duloxetine (brand name: Cymbalta)

Duloxetine is a more potent 5-HT and NE reuptake inhibitor than venlafaxine. Duloxetine's binding affinity is about 10:1 for the 5-HT and NE transporter. It is also a moderate inhibitor of CYP2D6, requiring caution when administered with other drugs that are preferentially metabolized by CYP2D6. This may require dose reductions as well as careful monitoring for adverse effects.[10]

Adverse effects

Nausea, dry mouth, constipation, insomnia, dizziness, asthenia, and hypertension are common side effects.[5,10]

Indications

Duloxetine is indicated for treatment of major depressive disorder, generalized anxiety disorder, pain from diabetic peripheral neuropathy, fibromyalgia, and musculoskeletal pain. As the only FDA-approved antidepressant for use in pain and psychiatric conditions, it is the preferred choice for neuropathic pain in patients with psychiatric disorders.[10]

Milnacipran (brand name: Savella)

Milnacipran is an SNRI that is marketed in the United States primarily as a treatment for fibromyalgia and not as an antidepressant.[10] It is metabolized by CYP3A4, while direct conjugation and renal elimination account for majority of its clearance. It has minimal pharmacokinetic and pharmacodynamic interactions with other drugs. Its half-life is about 10 hour requiring twice a day dosing.[10] Dysuria is a common dose-dependent adverse effect seen in up to 7% of patients. Higher doses can cause blood pressure and pulse elevations.[10]

Antidepressants and Risk of Bleeding

Both SSRIs and SNRIs have intermediate to high degrees of serotonin reuptake inhibition and are associated with increased bleeding risk due to inhibition of serotonin-mediated platelet aggregation.[3,5,11] Other proposed mechanisms include decreased platelet binding affinity, inhibition of calcium mobilization, and decreased NSAID metabolism increasing their blood levels and antiplatelet effects. However, nonserotonergic antidepressants such as bupropion, mirtazapine, and some TCAs do not inhibit serotonin reuptake and are not associated with increased intraoperative bleeding risk. SSRI-induced increases in gastric acid secretion can add to the risk of GI bleed associated with NSAIDs, especially in patients with liver failure.[11]

Other Antidepressants

Bupropion (brand names: Wellbutrin, Zyban)

Bupropion is an inhibitor of both noradrenergic and dopaminergic reuptake with independent analgesic efficacy in the treatment of neuropathic pain. Unlike other antidepressants, it a psychostimulant.[6]

Indications

Indications for buproprion include depression, neuropathic pain, attention deficit hyperactivity disorder, and smoking cessation. It be used to offset the sedative effects of opioids in the treatment of pain.

Role in pain treatment

Evidence for its analgesic efficacy is mixed with two studies supporting its use in a wide variety of neuropathic pain conditions, while a randomized controlled trial (RCT) in 44 patients with chronic low back pain (LBP) showed no significant analgesic effect.

Initiation of treatment

Starting dose is 75-100 mg/day given in the mornings. Night-time dosing may cause insomnia. Over a week, dose is titrated up to 100-150 mg twice daily.

Adverse effects

Common side effects are insomnia if given at night, nervousness, headache, and irritability and lowered seizure threshold at higher doses, in the range of 450-600 mg/day. This necessitates caution when coprescribed with tramadol, as lowering of seizure threshold can be additive. It is prudent to avoid bupropion in patients who take MAOIs and have eating disorders or seizures.[6]

Mirtazapine (brand name: Remeron)

Mirtazapine has a novel mechanism of action. It enhances noradrenaline and serotonin neurotransmission by its direct action on various alpha-adrenergic and serotonergic receptors.[6,12] It is a highly effective antidepressant with effects seen sooner than most other antidepressants, as early as in the first week of treatment but with limited analgesic potential.

Adverse effects

There are no significant anticholinergic effects. Serotonergic and antihistaminic effects are seen at low doses of 15-30 mg/day leading to weight gain, sedation, and antianxiety effects, while noradrenergic effects are seen with higher doses 45-60 mg/day accounting for anxiety and excitation.[6] It decreases the release of cortisol and corticotrophin. Neutropenia and agranulocytosis can occur occasionally.

Trazodone (brand name: Desyrel)

Trazodone is a serotonin-2 antagonist/reuptake inhibitor (SARI) used for both insomnia and depression. Its sedative properties limit one's ability to increase the dose enough to be effective as an antidepressant.[6] It is often the preferred choice for insomnia in patients with pain.[6] Typical dose for insomnia is 25-100 mg at bedtime and for depression it is 50-600 mg/day.

Common side effects are dry mouth, constipation, dizziness, orthostatic hypotension, and headache. Priapism occurs in 1:1000 to 1:10 000 cases.[6]

As an analgesic, there is little evidence to support it, though it can help by its antidepressant effect improving the affective component of pain perception.[6]

Skeletal Muscle Relaxants

Skeletal muscle relaxants are often prescribed for a variety of musculoskeletal conditions including LBP, neck pain, myofascial pain syndrome, fibromyalgia, and tension headache, though evidence of their clinical efficacy and tolerability is limited, at best.[13] The goal of prescribing muscle relaxants is to alleviate pain from muscle spasms and restore function, allowing the patient to return to their activities of daily living. They act either centrally within the brain or at the level of the spinal neurons.

Evidence of Effectiveness in Acute Pain

Back and neck pain

Most of the evidence supporting their efficacy comes from poorly designed studies. Several meta-analyses and systematic reviews support the short-term use of muscle relaxants to treat acute LBP when acetaminophen or NSAIDs are ineffective, contraindicated or not tolerated.[13] There is no evidence to suggest muscle relaxants are superior to these over-the-counter medications, though they may be more effective than placebo.[13-16] Studies comparing different muscle relaxants have not shown that any one is superior to another. Cyclobenzaprine has been shown to be effective in a variety of painful musculoskeletal conditions and is the most studied drug in this class.[13,15] The sedative effect of cyclobenzaprine and tizanidine is especially beneficial in patients with insomnia due to muscle spasms. The evidence to support the efficacy of less sedating muscle relaxants such as methocarbamol and metaxalone is even more limited.[13] The use of muscle relaxants in the treatment of acute pain is limited by their side effects, with drowsiness and dizziness commonly reported with all of them.[13-15]

In a 2016 review of 15 RCT involving 3362 participants, only 5 trials that involved 496 participants provided high quality evidence of clinically significant pain relief from muscle relaxants for the short-term relief of acute LBP.[17] No information was provided on long-term outcomes, and their efficacy for chronic LBP is unknown. There was no evidence to support the use of benzodiazepines in LBP. The median adverse event rate for muscle relaxants in these clinical trials was like placebo.[6,13,17]

There is some evidence supporting the use of nonbenzodiazepine skeletal muscle relaxants, like carisoprodol, cyclobenzaprine, orphenadrine, and tizanidine for moderate short-term relief of acute LBP, compared to placebo.[13] Evidence for use in chronic LBP is limited.

In a meta-analysis of 14 low quality studies comparing cyclobenzaprine with placebo for back and neck pain, it was found to be moderately more effective than placebo for the first few days of treatment but not at 2 weeks and with more CNS side effects.[13,15]

Evidence points to the use of muscle relaxants more as adjunctive therapy to analgesics in treating acute LBP, than first-line agents. In an open-label study of 20 patients, the cyclobenzaprine in addition to naproxen provided a statistically significant decrease in muscle spasm and tenderness compared with naproxen alone.[6,13] A cochrane review of three high-quality trials involving 560 total patients showed tizanidine plus NSAIDs provided more effective relief of pain and muscle spasm than analgesics alone.[13] There is reasonable evidence for combination therapy in quicker recovery, with minimal overall side effects.[13]

Fibromyalgia

In a meta-analysis of five trials with poor blinding and a high drop-out rate involving 312 patients with fibromyalgia, the authors reported that cyclobenzaprine moderately improved sleep and pain, but the long-term benefits were unknown.[13]

Comparison Data

There are limited data comparing skeletal muscle relaxants to one another. In a systematic review of 46 trials with methodological shortcomings on LBP or neck pain, involving cyclobenzaprine, tizanidine, carisoprodol, and orphenadrine, all were shown to have some benefit. One study showed carisoprodol to be better than diazepam at relief of muscle spasm and functional status in patients with LBP. while another comparing tizanidine with chlorzoxazone (Parafon Forte) did not show any significant difference.[13]

Another systematic review that included a few higher quality studies revealed no difference in outcomes among cyclobenzaprine vs carisoprodol; chlorzoxazone vs tizanidine; or diazepam vs tizanidine.[13,14]

Low back pain or fibromyalgia patients may benefit from cyclobenzaprine at half of its manufacturer-recommended dose (5 mg), with fewer adverse effects. Higher doses of cyclobenzaprine or tizanidine are reserved for patients with severe discomfort or muscle spasm, where sedation may be beneficial.[13] Ideal candidates are younger patients with limited or no comorbidities. While metaxalone and methocarbamol have limited evidence to support their use, they benefit patients who are unable to tolerate the more sedating muscle relaxants.[13]

Adverse Effects

Although there is limited evidence for the effectiveness of skeletal muscle relaxants in musculoskeletal pain, strong evidence exists for increased total adverse effects (RR = 1.50; 95% CI, 1.14-1.98) and CNS adverse effects (RR = 2.04; 95% CI, 1.23-3.37) with muscle relaxant use compared to placebo (RR = 0.95; 95% CI, 0.29-3.19) in 8 different acute LBP trials.[13,15] Gastrointestinal adverse effects were no different in the two groups. CNS side effects such as drowsiness, dizziness, and headache are common to most drugs in this class. Respiratory depression when used in combination with other sedatives is not uncommon.[6,13-18] In one study, muscle relaxant use in acute LBP was associated with slower recovery of function.[19]

The choice of a muscle relaxant in an individual patient should ultimately be based on patient preference, side effect profile, cost, insurance coverage, as well as potential for abuse and drug interactions, in the absence of comparable efficacy data.

Skeletal Muscle Relaxants Are Broadly Divided Into Two Subclasses

1. Antispastic—baclofen and dantrolene often prescribed for conditions like cerebral palsy and multiple sclerosis.
2. Antispasmodic—carisoprodol, cyclobenzaprine, metaxalone, methocarbamol are among the commonest agents prescribed for acute musculoskeletal pain.

Despite their popularity, the American Pain Society and American College of Physicians do not recommend routine use of muscle relaxants as first-line agents in the treatment of pain but are considered if acetaminophen or NSAIDs are ineffective, contraindicated, or not tolerated.[14]

Cyclobenzaprine (Brand Name: Flexeril)

Structurally like TCAs, cyclobenzaprine inhibits norepinephrine reuptake in the locus coeruleus, and in the spinal cord, it inhibits the descending serotonergic pathways. This has an inhibitory effect on alpha motor neurons in the spinal cord and decreased firing, resulting in a reduction of spinal reflexes, both monosynaptic and polysynaptic.[6,14] A meta-analysis evaluating the efficacy of cyclobenzaprine showed superiority to placebo in the treatment of fibromyalgia but inferior to antidepressants. There is strong evidence for cyclobenzaprine use in cervical and lumbar spinal pain and muscle spasm and moderate evidence for use in temporomandibular joint disorder with myofascial pain.[6]

Dose: 5 mg three times daily, increased as tolerated to 10 mg thrice daily

Adverse effects: Anticholinergic side effects such as drowsiness, dry mouth, urinary retention, increased intraocular pressure. Rarely seen are arrhythmias, seizures, myocardial infarction.

Precautions: Avoid use in hepatic impairment.[13]

FDA Pregnancy Category C

Tizanidine (brand name: Zanaflex)

Tizanidine is an antispastic agent, a weak agonist at alpha-2 adrenergic receptors and enhances presynaptic inhibition of spinal motor neurons.

Dose: start with 4 mg every 6-8 hours. Increase as tolerated up to 36 mg daily. Taper before discontinuation to avoid withdrawal symptoms and rebound hypertension.[13]

Adverse effects: Dose-related hypotension, dry mouth, and sedation. Hepatotoxicity requiring liver function tests at 1, 3, and 6 months after initiation.

Decreased effectiveness is seen with oral contraceptives.

FDA Pregnancy Category C

Carisoprodol (brand name: Soma)

Carisoprodol blocks interneuronal activity in the descending reticular formation and spinal cord to produce muscle relaxation and is metabolized to a class III controlled substance, **meprobamate**, which is a sedative that can produce psychological and physical dependence.[6,13,18] Discontinuation may lead to withdrawal symptoms and must be done gradually.

Dose: 350 mg four times daily. Not recommended in children below 12 years of age.

Adverse effects: Idiosyncratic (brief visual loss, transient quadriplegia, mental status changes) and allergic type reactions can occur at the start of treatment. Respiratory depression is seen when used in combination with other sedatives such as benzodiazepines, barbiturates, and other muscle relaxants. It is contraindicated in acute intermittent porphyria.[13,18]

Due to their abuse potential and lack of superiority to other muscle relaxants, carisoprodol and diazepam should be last choice agents reserved for patients that fail to respond to other agents.

FDA Pregnancy Category: C

Diazepam (brand name: Valium)

A centrally acting antispastic agent that increases inhibitory GABA transmission. It has a long elimination half-life and should be avoided in the elderly and in patients with significant cognitive or hepatic impairment. Complete blood count and liver function tests must be monitored regularly. Studies show strong evidence for use in spasticity of spinal origin and moderate evidence in tension-type headache and orofacial pain.

Dose: 2-10 mg three to four times daily.

Adverse effects: It has abuse potential and can interact with CYP450 inhibitors.

FDA Pregnancy Category: D

Must be avoided especially in the first trimester. Older studies showed an increased chance (1%) of cleft lip/palate anomalies, but this has since been refuted.[20]

Baclofen (brand name: Lioresal)

Baclofen is a centrally acting antispastic agent that reduces the release of excitatory neurotransmitters in the brain and spinal cord by activating the GABA-B receptors and inhibits the release of substance P in the spinal cord.[6,14] There is strong evidence for baclofen use in spasticity of spinal origin and moderate evidence for use in cervical dystonia, upper motor neuron disease, stiff person syndrome and acute back pain.[6,14] It is FDA approved for use in intrathecal pumps for spasticity.[6,14]

Dose: 5 mg thrice daily, titrated up slowly to 80 mg/day.

Adverse effects: Confusion, ataxia, constipation, hypotension, and weight gain. Withdrawal syndrome with increased spasticity, seizures, and hallucinations occurs with abrupt discontinuation of higher doses.[14] Use in caution with impaired renal function.

FDA Pregnancy Category: C

Metaxalone (brand name: Skelaxin)

Dizziness and drowsiness are seen less often than with other muscle relaxants. It should be used with caution in liver failure. Can lead to respiratory depression when used with other sedatives.

Adverse effects: Leukopenia, rarely hemolytic anemia, paradoxical muscle cramps.[13,18]

Dose: 800 mg three times daily. Not recommended in children below 12 years of age.

FDA Pregnancy Category: C

Methocarbamol (brand name: Robaxin)

Is a centrally acting relaxant, though exact mechanism is not known. There is moderate quality evidence for its use in acute muscle spasm and nocturnal leg cramps.[13]

Dose: 1500 mg four times daily for first 3 days, then titrated down to 750 mg four times daily.

Adverse effects: Can cause exacerbation of myasthenia gravis symptoms and may cause black, brown, or green urine.[13]

FDA Pregnancy Category: C

Few reports of fetal abnormalities.

Chlorzoxazone (brand name: Parafon Forte)

Chlorzoxazone is centrally acting likely through inhibition of polysynaptic reflex pathways, though exact mechanism of action is unknown. There is moderate evidence for its use in acute back pain, acute lumbosacral muscle strain, and musculoskeletal pain.[6]

Dose: 250 mg three to four times daily.

Adverse effects: Red or orange urine. Gastrointestinal irritation and rarely bleeding. Avoid in patients with hepatic impairment. Hepatotoxicity is rare.

FDA Pregnancy Category: C

Orphenadrine (brand name: Norflex)

Has a long elimination half-life requiring reduced dosages in the elderly.[13]

Dose: 100 mg twice daily.

Adverse effects: Anticholinergic effects, GI irritation, confusion, tachycardia, and hypersensitivity reactions are seen with higher doses. Aplastic anemia is rare. Avoid in patients with glaucoma, cardiospasm, and myasthenia gravis.[13]

FDA Pregnancy Category: C

Summary

Overall, there is limited evidence to support the use of skeletal muscle relaxants in musculoskeletal pain. They are not preferred first-line agents and should be considered only for short-term pain relief, often as an adjunct with other pain treatment modalities that include physical therapy, over the counter analgesics, NSAIDs, opioids, and trigger point injections.[13,14] They may also be used as an alternative to NSAIDs in patients with renal and gastrointestinal dysfunction. Chronic daily use of muscle relaxants is not evidence based.[13]

Antiepileptic Drugs

Antiepileptic drugs (AEDs), also known as membrane stabilizers, are frequently used in chronic pain management especially for treatment of neuropathic pain states. Neuropathic pain encompasses a variety of clinical entities such as diabetic peripheral neuropathy, trigeminal neuralgia, and spinal cord injury pain. AEDs have been used in treatment of these conditions for years; however, it is only within the last decade that these medications have gained popularity for use in the acute perioperative setting. In the following section, we will cover AEDs commonly used in pain management, discuss pertinent mechanisms of action, and present data regarding use for acute pain states.

Notably, AEDs all share a common side effect of an increase in risk of suicidal thoughts or behaviors regardless of the indication for use. As such, patients placed on AEDs ought to be monitored for mood changes, depression, or suicidal thoughts.[21,22]

Gabapentinoids

Gabapentin and pregabalin are collectively classified as "gabapentinoids." While the name "gabapentin" suggests a mechanism of action involving γ-aminobutyric acid (GABA) neurotransmission or receptor, these drugs act as inhibitors at the alpha 2 delta subunit of the presynaptic voltage-gated calcium channels reducing calcium influx in presynaptic terminals. Although these agents are structurally like the neurotransmitter GABA, they lack any action at the GABA receptor.[5,23]

Gabapentin was originally approved for seizure disorder but has since been utilized for a number of other neurological conditions including neuropathic pain, restless leg syndrome, alcohol withdrawal, and anxiety.[24] As of this writing, gabapentin is approved by the United States Food and Drug Administration (FDA) for treatment of seizures and postherpetic neuralgia.[5]

The pharmacologic action of gabapentin is due to the activity of the parent compound rather than its metabolites. Its oral bioavailability is not dose proportional as absorption is dependent on active transport receptors in the gut. Bioavailability decreases with increase in dose. For example, a dose of 900 mg divided in three times per day dosing is 60% absorbed, 3600 mg administered three times per day is 33% absorbed, and 4800 mg is 27% absorbed. Peak plasma concentration occurs 3 hours after ingestion. Elimination is by renal excretion of the unchanged drug. The half-life ranges from 5 to 7 hours in those with normal renal function. The dose should be adjusted in patients with renal insufficiency and those on hemodialysis.[5]

Pregabalin has a mechanism of action like gabapentin. It is currently approved for use in seizure disorders, diabetic peripheral neuropathy, pain related to spinal cord injury, fibromyalgia, and post herpetic neuralgia. Compared with gabapentin, pregabalin has higher oral bioavailability with >90% absorption, and peak plasma levels are noted within an hour after ingestion. Unlike gabapentin, absorption is independent of dose. Pregabalin is eliminated by renal excretion as unchanged drug with a mean elimination half-life of 6.3 hours when renal function is normal. As with gabapentin, the dose must be adjusted in those with renal failure.[23]

Despite differences in pharmacokinetics and absorption, gabapentin and pregabalin are often used interchangeably because of their similar molecular structure and mode of action. Unfortunately, there are no trials with head-to-head comparison of the two drugs for pain. Anecdotally, however, patients often report responding differently to each of these medications both in terms of efficacy as well as related side effects.

The side effect profiles of gabapentin and pregabalin are similar. The most common adverse reactions in adults are dizziness, somnolence, dry mouth, peripheral edema, blurred vision, and weight gain. Peripheral edema is more common in patients concurrently taking thiazolidinediones. A more serious, but less common side effect is angioedema which may lead to airway compromise. This may be more common in patients taking angiotensin receptor inhibitors (ACE inhibitors).[5,23] Further, as both agents are antiepileptics, there is a risk of seizure activity with abrupt discontinuation.

With growing popularity of multimodal perioperative pain control, enhanced recovery after surgery protocols, and increasing attention to opioid sparing techniques, gabapentinoid use has gained popularity in the perioperative period.[24] These agents are used in diverse surgical populations and in various dose ranges and frequencies. The concept at the center of use of these agents is their believed synergism with other analgesics leading to opioid sparing effects. Early studies suggested that a single dose of gabapentin or pregabalin administered before surgery was associated with a decrease in postoperative pain and opioid use though the most favorable dosing regimen was not clear.[25-31] Studies also emerged suggesting the potential of these drugs as "preemptive analgesics." Preemptive analgesia is a treatment that is initiated prior to surgical incision in order to reduce peripheral and central sensitization.[25] In theory, a preemptive analgesic will decrease acute postoperative pain and also decrease the likelihood for development of chronic pain after surgery. Currently, cumulative evidence does not support the theory of preemptive analgesia, which has now been, and this has been replaced with the concept of "preventative analgesia." As opposed to "preemptive analgesia," which claims analgesic benefits solely from a treatment delivered prior to surgical insult, "preventive analgesia" focuses on longitudinal analgesic treatment, such that the time course for intervention is longer and includes preoperative, intraoperative, and postoperative time periods.[32]

More recent studies and rigorous meta-analysis have not been as favorable toward the use of gabapentinoids in the perioperative period. While these studies may show a statistically significant difference in postoperative acute pain and an opioid-sparing effect, these results do not reach clinical significance.[33,34] Similarly, there are no differences in the incidence of postoperative chronic pain regardless of the dosing regimen. These studies do find increase in side effects such as dizziness, sedation, and visual disturbances. The studies favor a decrease in postoperative nausea and vomiting in patients receiving gabapentinoids. This decrease is unrelated to a decrease in opioid use.[34,35]

Despite this, gabapentinoids remain a popular mainstay for multimodal analgesia in the perioperative period, which is likely influenced by the widespread interest in use of opioid-sparing agent and due to concern for opioid addiction. Clinicians tend to view gabapentinoids to be relatively safe, without risk for abuse and with limited drug interactions.

With increase in gabapentinoid use and prescribing, reports of misuse of these agents are also increasing. The overall prevalence of misuse and abuse of gabapentinoids is reported to be about 1%, with rates as high as 68% among patients with prior history of opioid use disorder.[36,37] This is likely related to the reported amplification of euphoria experienced with concurrent opioid use. Recent studies also find that the odds of respiratory depression and death increase with concomitant opioid and gabapentinoid use.[37]

Reports of recreational use and diversion of gabapentinoids is also increasing. Pregabalin is classified to a schedule V substance by the Drug Enforcement Administration indicating potential for abuse. In the United States, some states have either reclassified gabapentin as controlled substance or require its reporting on the prescription drug monitoring systems. In the United Kingdom, both gabapentin and pregabalin were reclassified to controlled medicines, requiring stricter legal controls.[38,39]

Topiramate

Topiramate is approved for use in seizure disorder and for migraine prophylaxis, though it is also used off-label to treat neuropathic pain and chronic LBP.[40,41] The exact mechanism of action is not known, but evidence points to various mechanisms including blockade of voltage-dependent sodium channels, augmentation of GABA activity, antagonism of AMPA/kainate subtype of the glutamate receptor, and inhibition of carbonic anhydrase enzyme.[40]

Topiramate is rapidly absorbed after oral ingestion, and peak plasma concentration occurs 2 hours after ingestion. Absorption is not affected by food. The elimination half-life is 21 hours and steady state occurs after 4 days of treatment in those with normal renal function. Topiramate is eliminated unchanged renally. The dose must be decreased in those with renal dysfunction.[40]

The most common side effects of topiramate are paresthesias, anorexia, change in taste, weight loss, memory impairment, and difficulty with concentration/attention.[40] Given high comorbidity of pain and obesity, some providers use topiramate as an analgesic with a concomitant benefit of weight loss.[42] Other precautions include use in those with glaucoma as it can cause elevation in intraocular pressure and in those with a history of kidney stones and/or use of carbonic anhydrase inhibitors.

In addition to off-label use for neuropathic pain conditions and fibromyalgia, topiramate is also more recently used for treatment of alcohol use disorder.[43] There are currently no studies investigating its utility in acute perioperative pain states.

Carbamazepine/Oxcarbazepine

Carbamazepine is an anticonvulsant, which is also approved for treatment of trigeminal neuralgia. It modulates voltage-gated sodium channels inhibiting action potentials and decreasing synaptic transmission. Carbamazepine is thought to be the gold standard for treatment of trigeminal neuralgia, but its use is limited by side effects. The most common side effects include dizziness, drowsiness, ataxia, and nausea. It also comes with a black box warning for severe skin reactions toxic epidermal necrolysis (TEN) and Stevens-Johnson syndrome (SJS). The risk for these reactions is high in patients of Han Chinese ancestry, and there is an association between the HLA-B*1502 gene and Steven Johnson syndrome/toxic epidermal necrolysis (SJS/TEN). As such, patients who belong to genetically high-risk ethnic groups should be tested for the HLA-B*1502 allele prior to initiating therapy. In addition to a black box warning for fatal skin reactions, carbamazepine also has a black box warning for agranulocytosis and aplastic anemia. Patients should have hematologic testing prior to initiation of therapy and remain monitored throughout its course.[44]

Carbamazepine has an 80% absorption rate and about 80% of the drug is protein bound. Another complicating factor in its clinical use is that it stimulates the cytochrome P-450 system and induces its own metabolism making dose adjustments necessary. Because it is an enzyme inducer, it enhances metabolism of other medications by the liver.[44]

Oxcarbazepine is a structural analog of carbamazepine. It has a similar mechanism of action to carbamazepine, but because of differences in pathways involved for metabolism, it has a more favorable side effect profile. Side effects include hyponatremia and allergic rash. About 25%-30% of patients with hypersensitivity reaction to carbamazepine also experience a hypersensitivity to oxcarbazepine.[45]

While oxcarbazepine is not approved for use in pain conditions, some clinicians prefer this agent to carbamazepine because of its more favorable side effect profile. To date, there are no data regarding use of either carbamazepine or oxcarbazepine for acute surgical pain. One study suggests limited effectiveness in carbamazepine use in acute herpes zoster.[46] Data for both agents are more robust for use in chronic neuropathic pain conditions.[47]

Lamotrigine

Lamotrigine acts primarily via inhibition of voltage-gated calcium channels as well as sodium channels leading to decreased presynaptic release of excitatory neurotransmitters such as glutamate, which is thought to be responsible for its antinociceptive properties. It is well absorbed with 100% bioavailability. Lamotrigine can have side effects including SJS/TEN.[48]

Lamotrigine has been evaluated in treatment of chronic neuropathic pain, but the data in terms of its use in treatment of acute perioperative pain are largely lacking.[49] Benefits of lamotrigine in treatment of chronic neuropathic conditions such as diabetic neuropathy have been demonstrated in animal studies and then successfully applied in human clinical research.[50]

In their study, Shah et al. evaluated preincisional use of lamotrigine, comparing its preemptive analgesic effects to those of diclofenac for patients undergoing various major surgeries under spinal anesthesia. In this study, lamotrigine was found to be superior to diclofenac and placebo in terms of postoperative pain scores, analgesic use, and PACU stay.[51] Another small RCT by the same group also found statistically significant lower pain score, shorter PACU stay, and less postoperative analgesic requirement in patients who received a single preoperative dose of lamotrigine compared with topiramate.[52] Further studies are needed to determine use of lamotrigine in the perioperative setting.[53]

Antiepileptic drugs have therapeutic benefit in treatment of neuropathic pain states, but more studies are needed to determine effectiveness for acute pain. These medications are not without risk, and this must be balanced with analgesic benefit.

REFERENCES

1. Kolodny A, Courtwright DT, Hwang CS, et al. The prescription opioid and heroin crisis: a public health approach to an epidemic of addiction. *Annu Rev Public Health*. 2015;36(1):559-574.
2. Barkin RL, Fawcett J. The management challenges of chronic pain: the role of antidepressants. *Am J Ther*. 2000;7(1):31-47.
3. Dharmshaktu P, Tayal V, Kalra BS. Efficacy of antidepressants as analgesics: a review. *J Clin Pharmacol*. 2012;52(1):6-17. doi:10.1177/0091270010394852
4. Wong K, Phelan R, Kalso E, et al. Antidepressant drugs for prevention of acute and chronic postsurgical pain: early evidence and recommended future directions. *Anesthesiology*. 2014;121:591-608. doi:10.1097/ALN.0000000000000307
5. Finnerup NB, Attal N, Haroutounian S, et al. Pharmacotherapy for neuropathic pain in adults: a systematic review and meta-analysis. *Lancet Neurol*. 2015;14:162-173.
6. Benzon HT, et al. *Essentials of Pain Medicine*. 4th ed. Elsevier; 2018. Accessed July 14, 2019. https://www.clinicalkey.com
7. Fishbain D. Evidence-based data on pain relief with antidepressants. *Ann Med*. 2000;32(5):305-316. doi:10.3109/07853890008995932
8. Hoyt Huffman L, et al. Medications for acute and chronic low back pain: a review of the evidence for an American Pain Society/American College of Physicians Clinical Practice Guideline. *Ann Intern Med*. 2007;147:505-514.
9. Arbuck D. The use of antidepressants in multimodal pain management. *Pract Pain Manag*. 2019.
10. Shelton RC. Serotonin and norepinephrine reuptake inhibitors. *Handb Exp Pharmacol*. 2019;250:145-180. doi:10.1007/164_2018_164
11. Bixby AL, VandenBerg A, Bostwick JR. Clinical management of bleeding risk with antidepressants. *Ann Pharmacother*. 2019;53(2):186-194.
12. Boer T, Ruigt G, Berendsen H. The α_2-selective adrenoceptor antagonist Org 3770 (mirtazapine, Remeron®) enhances noradrenergic and serotonergic transmission. *Hum Psychopharmacol Clin Exp*. 1995;10:S107-S118.
13. See S, Ginzburg R. Choosing a skeletal muscle relaxant. *Am Fam Physician*. 2008;78(3):365-370.
14. Witenko C, Moorman-Li R, Motycka C, et al. Considerations for the appropriate use of skeletal muscle relaxants for the management of acute low back pain. *P T*. 2014;39(6):427-435.
15. van Tulder MW, Touray T, Furlan AD, et al. Muscle relaxants for nonspecific low back pain: a systematic review within the framework of the cochrane collaboration. *Spine*. 2003;28(17):1978-1992. doi:10.1097/01.BRS.0000090503.38830.AD
16. Abdel Shaheed C, Maher C, Williams K, McLachlan A. Efficacy and tolerability of muscle relaxants for low back pain: systematic review and meta-analysis. *Eur J Pain*. 2017;21:228-237. doi:10.1002/ejp.907
17. Bhatia A, Engle A, Cohen SP. Current and future pharmacological agents for the treatment of back pain. *Expert Opin Pharmacother*. 2020;21(8):857-861. doi: 10.1080/14656566.2020.1735353
18. Toth PE, Urtis J. Commonly used muscle relaxant therapies for acute low back pain: a review of carisoprodol, cyclobenzaprine hydrochloride, and metaxalone. *Clin Ther*. 2004;26(9):1355-1367. doi:10.1016/j.clinthera.2004.09.008
19. Bernstein E, Carey TS, Garrett, JM. The use of muscle relaxant medications in acute low back pain. *Spine*. 2004;29(12):1346-1351. doi:10.1097/01.BRS.0000128258.49781.74
20. Bellantuono C, Tofani S, Di Sciascio G, Santone G. Benzodiazepine exposure in pregnancy and risk of major malformations: a critical overview. *Gen Hosp Psychiatry*. 2013;35(1):3-8. doi:10.1016/j.genhosppsych.2012.09.003
21. Perucca P, Gilliam FG. Adverse effects of antiepileptic drugs. *Lancet Neurol*. 2012;11(9):792-802.
22. U.S. Food and Drug Administration, Center for Drug Evaluation and Research. Gabapentin Approved Labeling Text dated 03/01/2011. https://www.accessdata.fda.gov/drugsatfda_docs/label/2011/020235s036,020882s022,021129s022lbl.pdf
23. U.S. Food and Drug Administration, Center for Drug Evaluation and Research. Pregabalin Label. https://www.accessdata.fda.gov/drugsatfda_docs/label/2012/021446s028lbl.pdf
24. Goodman CW, Brett AS. A clinical overview of off-label use of gabapentinoid drugs. *JAMA Intern Med*. 2019;179(5):695-701.
25. Møiniche S, Kehlet H, Dahl JB. A qualitative and quantitative systematic review of preemptive analgesia for postoperative pain relief: the role of timing of analgesia. *Anesthesiology*. 2002;96(3):725-741.
26. Hurley RW, Cohen SP, Williams KA, Rowlingson AJ, Wu CL. The analgesic effects of perioperative gabapentin on postoperative pain: a meta-analysis. *Reg Anesth Pain Med*. 2006;31(3):237-247.

27. Buvanendran A, Kroin JS, Della Valle CJ, Kari M, Moric M, Tuman KJ. Perioperative oral pregabalin reduces chronic pain after total knee arthroplasty: a prospective, randomized, con-trolled trial. *Anesth Analg*. 2010;110:199-207.
28. Burke SM, Shorten GD. Perioperative pregabalin improves pain and functional outcomes 3 months after lumbar discectomy. *Anesth Analg*. 2010;110:1180-1573.
29. Clarke H, Bonin RP, Orser BA, Englesakis M, Wijeysundera DN, Katz J. The prevention of chronic postsurgical pain using gabapentin and pregabalin: a combined systematic review and meta-analysis. *Anesth Analg*. 2012;115(2):428-442.
30. Mishriky BM, Waldron NH, Habib AS. Impact of pregabalin on acute and persistent postoperative pain: a systematic review and meta-analysis. *Br J Anaesth*. 2015;114(1):10-31.
31. Katz J, Clarke H, Seltzer Z. Review article: preventive analgesia: quo vadimus? *Anesth Analg*. 2011;113(5):1242-1253.
32. Hah J, Mackey SC, Schmidt P, et al. Effect of perioperative gabapentin on postoperative pain resolution and opioid cessation in a mixed surgical cohort: a randomized clinical trial. *JAMA Surg*. 2018;153(4):303-311.
33. Fabritius ML, Strøm C, Koyuncu S, et al. Benefit, and harm of pregabalin in acute pain treatment: a systematic review with meta-analyses and trial sequential analyses. *Br J Anaesth*. 2017;119(4):775-791.
34. Verret M, Lauzier F, Zarychanski R, et al. Canadian Perioperative Anesthesia Clinical Trials (PACT) Group: perioperative use of gabapentinoids for the management of postoperative acute pain: a systematic review and meta-analysis. *Anesthesiology*. 2020;133:265-279.
35. Fabritius ML, Wetterslev J, Mathiesen O, Dahl JB. Dose-related beneficial and harmful effects of gabapentin in postoperative pain management: Post hoc analyses from a systematic review with meta-analyses and trial sequential analyses. *J Pain Res*. 2017;10:2547-2563.
36. Mersfelder TL, Nichols WH. Gabapentin: abuse, dependence, and withdrawal. *Ann Pharmacother*. 2016;50(3):229-233.
37. Evoy KE, Morrison MD, Saklad SR. Abuse and misuse of pregabalin and gabapentin. *Drugs*. 2017;77:403-426.
38. Peckham AM, Ananickal MJ, Sclar DA. Gabapentin use, abuse, and the US opioid epidemic: the case for reclassification as a controlled substance and the need for pharmacovigilance. *Risk Manag Healthc Policy*. 2018;11:109-116.
39. Throckmorton DC, Gottlieb S, Woodcock J. The FDA and the next wave of drug abuse: proactive pharmacovigilance. *N Engl J Med*. 2018;379(3):205-207.
40. U.S. FDA, Center for Drug Evaluation and Research. Topiramate Label. https://www.accessdata.fda.gov/drugsatfda_docs/label/2017/020505s057_020844s048lbl.pdf
41. Muehlbacher M, Nickel MK, Kettler C, et al. Topiramate in treatment of patients with chronic low back pain: a randomized, double-blind, placebo-controlled study. *Clin J Pain*. 2006;22(6):526-531.
42. Smith SM, Meyer M, Trinkley KE. Phentermine/topiramate for the treatment of obesity. *Ann Pharmacother*. 2013;47(3):340-349.
43. Manhapra A, Chakraborty A, Arias AJ. Topiramate pharmacotherapy for alcohol use disorder and other addictions: a narrative review. *J Addict Med*. 2019;13(1):7-22.
44. U.S. FDA, Center for Drug Evaluation and Research. Carbamazepine Label. https://www.accessdata.fda.gov/drugsatfda_docs/label/2009/016608s101,018281s048lbl.pdf
45. U.S. FDA, Center for Drug Evaluation and Research. Oxcarbazepine Label. https://www.accessdata.fda.gov/drugsatfda_docs/label/2017/021014s036lbl.pdf
46. Wiffen PJ, Derry S, Moore RA, Kalso EA. Carbamazepine for chronic neuropathic pain and fibromyalgia in adults. *Cochrane Database Syst Rev*. 2014;(4):CD005451.
47. Stefano G, Cesa S, Truini A, Cruccu G. Natural history, and outcome of 200 outpatients with classical trigeminal neuralgia treated with carbamazepine or oxcarbazepine in a tertiary centre for neuropathic pain. *J Headache Pain*. 2014;15:34.
48. U.S. Food and Drug Administration, Center for Drug Evaluation and Research. Lamotrigine Label. https://www.accessdata.fda.gov/drugsatfda_docs/label/2015/020241s045s051lbl.pdf
49. Vinik AI, Tuchman M, Safirstein B, et al. Lamotrigine for treatment of pain associated with diabetic neuropathy: results of two randomized, double-blind, placebo-controlled studies. *Pain*. 2007;128:169-179.
50. Paudel KR, Bhattacharya S, Rauniar G, Das B. Comparison of antinociceptive effect of the antiepileptic drug gabapentin to that of various dosage combinations of gabapentin with lamotrigine and topiramate in mice and rats. *J Neurosci Rural Pract*. 2011;2:130-136.
51. Shah P, Bhosale UA, Gupta A, Yegnanarayan R, Sardesai S. A randomized double-blind placebo-controlled study to compare preemptive analgesic efficacy of novel antiepileptic agent lamotrigine in patients undergoing major surgeries. *N Am J Med Sci*. 2016;8(2):93-99.
52. Bhosale UA, Yegnanarayan R, Gupta A, Shah P, Sardesai S. Comparative pre-emptive analgesic efficacy study of novel antiepileptic agents gabapentin, lamotrigine and topiramate in patients undergoing major surgeries at a tertiary care hospital: a randomized double-blind clinical trial. *J Basic Clin Physiol Pharmacol*. 2017;28(1):59-66.
53. Wiffen PJ, Derry S, Moore RA. Lamotrigine for acute and chronic pain. *Cochrane Database Syst Rev*. 2013;(12):CD006044.

37

Local Anesthetics and Topical Analgesics

Ashley Wong and Naum Shaparin

Introduction

Local anesthetics have been used since the 19th century for their anesthetic properties.[1] Local anesthetics are drugs that bind to sodium channels on nerves and reversibly block propagation of action potentials. The first discovered anesthetic, cocaine, was used by indigenous people living in the Andes mountains who noted a numbing sensation when they chewed on coca leaves.[2] Years later, cocaine was isolated from the coca plant and refined for use in ophthalmic surgeries. Since then, several synthetically derived local anesthetics have been developed to be used in the clinical setting. There is a wide range of uses for local anesthetics, therapeutically and diagnostically. Local anesthetics are used in multiple clinical settings including for peri-op anesthesia and to treat a variety of acute or chronic pain syndromes. This chapter will provide a description of the mechanism of action, pharmacokinetics, clinical use, and potential toxicity associated with local anesthetics.

Mechanism of Action

The mechanism underlying all local anesthetics is their capacity to reversibly bind to sodium (Na^+) channels on nerves. This allows inhibition of neuronal impulse propagation and generation of action potentials that are responsible for nerve conduction and ultimately can lead to abolished sensation and motor function.

Action Potential Physiology

Consistent with all biological cell membranes, the neuronal membrane is made up of an amphipathic phospholipid bilayer. Dispersed throughout this bilayer are embedded protein channels that span the thickness of the membrane. These channels create a conduit between the intracellular and extracellular environments and allow efficient passage of essential molecules across the layer when polarity, gradient, or size impede natural diffusion. Voltage-gated Na^+ channels play a critical role in triggering nerve action potentials and local anesthetic mechanism of action.

The electrical resting potential of a neuron is around −70 mV, where the negative implies an overall negative intracellular environment compared to the extracellular environment. As a stimulus reaches the target cell, the permeability of the Na^+ channel increases, which allows an influx of Na^+ into the cell. If the electrical differential reaches a threshold, which is usually around −55 mV, an action potential is created and an increase amount of Na^+ influx into the cell occurs. This allows further propagation of the signal down a nerve. Local anesthetics work by binding to these Na^+ channels to block action potential creation.

The Na^+ channel is made up of specific protein subunits and functional domains. Local anesthetics reversibly bind to the inner protein subunit of the Na^+ channel and prevent the channel from opening.[3] Once a local anesthetic binds to the Na^+ channel, a change in membrane permeability to Na^+ occurs, impeding the influx of more sodium through the channel and inhibiting the generation of action potentials. There is no change in overall resting membrane potential or sodium concentration gradient.[4] Clinically, we use this to our advantage to block impulse conduction of sensation and create local anesthesia. Local anesthetics can exert this function on any type of nerve, in any part of the body.

Differential Nerve Blockade

Different nerve fiber types have varying sensitivity to local anesthetics. Generally, small diameter nerve fibers are more susceptible to nerve blockade compared to larger diameter fibers. Small sympathetic nerve fibers are blocked first followed by the small, myelinated A-delta fibers that mediate pain and temperature. Then, large myelinated A-gamma, A-alpha, and A-beta nerves, which contribute to touch, pressure, and motor function, are blocked last.[5] This is the general mechanism behind differential nerve block using local anesthetics. Typically, upon administration of local anesthetic, sympathetic function is impaired first. Therefore, vasodilation and its clinical manifestations are the first marker of a successful local anesthetic block. As the local anesthetic block progresses, patients will then feel a loss of pain sensation, followed by the loss of temperature, touch, pressure, vibration, and then lastly, motor function. Clinically, this becomes relevant in situations where preferential blockade of sensory nerve fibers over motor fibers are desired, such as during labor.

Local Anesthetic Pharmacology

Most local anesthetics consist of a hydrophilic tertiary amine that attaches to a hydrophobic aromatic ring. These moieties are connected by an intermediate chain. Local anesthetics that are an exception to this include prilocaine, which lacks a tertiary amine and has a secondary amine instead, and benzocaine, which has a primary amine.[6] The intermediate chain contains either an ester or an amide link, which defines the two classifications of local anesthetics into aminoesters or aminoamides (further discussed later in this chapter). The duration of onset, action, and potency of each local anesthetic is based on multiple factors including pH of surrounding tissue, local anesthetic lipid solubility, concentration, ionization, and pKa.

Lipid solubility and concentration of the local anesthetic determines potency of the anesthetic. The term "hydrophilic" describes greater affinity to water, and therefore, "hydrophobic" describes substances that tend to repel water. Local anesthetics that are highly hydrophobic cross nerve cell membranes easier and can produce a more potent and longer acting blockade than less hydrophobic anesthetics.[6] Accordingly, increased hydrophobicity will also increase the adverse effects of local anesthetics.

The onset of action is determined by the local anesthetic pKa and the pH of the surrounding tissue. All local anesthetics exist in protonated (ionized) and uncharged (nonionized) forms when placed in physiologic pH conditions (7.35-7.45).[7] The pKa is used to define the acidity of each local anesthetic in solution. The nonionized forms of local anesthetics are able to penetrate and cross cell membranes easier, resulting in a faster onset of action. The proportion of ionized to nonionized form changes with the pH of the environment it is delivered in. The pH of the surrounding tissue influences the local anesthetic activity by altering the percentage of the base and protonated forms. In inflamed/infected tissue that has a lower pH than normal tissue, local anesthetics become more protonated and penetrate the tissues slower, causing slower onset of action. Addition of sodium bicarbonate to local anesthetics in these situations may raise the pH and allow faster onset of action.

Specific Local Anesthetics

Local anesthetics are typically divided into aminoamides and aminoesters. Aminoamides are much more stable in solution compared to aminoesters. The anesthetics that are classified as aminoamides are lidocaine, mepivacaine, prilocaine, bupivacaine, and ropivacaine. Aminoesters include cocaine, procaine, tetracaine, chloroprocaine, benzocaine. Procaine is known as the prototypic aminoester, and lidocaine is the prototypic aminoamide. An easy way to remember the anesthetics in each group is to know that aminoamides contain letter "i" twice in their name and so does "aminoamides." A summary of the particular properties of each local anesthetic is detailed in Table 37.1.

Clinical Use

Local anesthetics have numerous uses in clinical practice such as for peripheral nerve blockade for diagnostic and therapeutic purposes, local infiltration, regional anesthesia in perioperative management, neuraxial administration, or topical preparation for analgesia.

TABLE 37.1 LOCAL ANESTHETIC PROPERTIES

	Local Anesthetic Properties				
	Classification	Duration of Action	Recommended Max Dosage	Typical Concentrations	Misc.
Lidocaine	Amide	0.5-2 h	400-500 mg	0.5%-2%	The most commonly used LA
Mepivacaine	Amide	1-1.5 h	300-400 mg	0.5%-2%	Typically used in epidural blocks and regional anesthesia
Prilocaine	Amide	0.5-1.5 h	350 mg	0.5%-3%	Often used in dentistry or in combination with lidocaine in EMLA formulation
Ropivacaine	Amide	2-5 h	225 mg	0.2%-0.75%	Long duration but less cardiotoxic than bupivacaine
Cocaine	Ester	Up to 1.5 h	300 mg	4% or 10%	Available in solution for ENT/ophthalmic use
Procaine	Ester	0.5 h	500 mg	1%-2%	Slow onset, short duration
Tetracaine	Ester	2-3 h	20 mg topical	0.25%-1%	Available in solution for ENT/ophthalmic use
Chloroprocaine	Ester	0.25-0.5 h	800 mg	1%-2%	Fast onset, short duration
Benzocaine	Ester	Varies	Varies	Varies	Available in topical cream, ointment, or spray

This table details local anesthetic properties including classification, duration of action, recommended maximum dosing, typical concentrations used, and specific miscellaneous drug facts.

When deciding which local anesthetic to use, there are certain factors to consider including concentration, volume, and addition of adjuvant medications. With increasing dosage of local anesthetic, the duration of action and density of anesthesia increases. Dosage can be increased by increasing concentration of the local anesthetic solution. Increasing volume of local anesthetic will increase the amount of spread from initial site of administration. When larger areas need to be anesthetized, diluted solutions of local anesthetics can be used to increase volume while limiting toxicity from the local anesthetic.

Adjuvant medications can be mixed with local anesthetics to enhance duration of action or efficacy of anesthesia. Local anesthetics have vasodilating activity, which can lead to rapid absorption into the bloodstream.[8] Addition of epinephrine, which is a vasoconstrictor, to local anesthetics will lead to longer duration of action of the local anesthetic at the injection site. Sodium bicarbonate is another commonly used adjuvant that is added to local anesthetic solutions. By increasing pH (creating a more basic solution), sodium bicarbonate decreases time to onset and increases potency of the local anesthetic. Other adjuvants such as dexamethasone and dexmedetomidine have also been added in an effort to prolong analgesic effects of local anesthetics.[9,10] A short-acting local anesthetic can also be combined with a long-acting one to provide immediate procedural analgesia with acting pain control.

Local Infiltration

All of the local anesthetics can be used for local subcutaneous or intradermal infiltration. The onset of action for most local anesthetics is immediate and therefore decision regarding what local anesthetic to use is based on duration of action and potential adverse effects.

Peripheral Nerve Blockade

Deposition of local anesthetic near a specific nerve or nerves constitutes a peripheral nerve block. Peripheral nerve block techniques have greatly improved over time with the addition of ultrasound guidance. The advantage of using ultrasound is that it allows for more accurate localization of the nerve of interest, decreased need for a larger volume of anesthetic, and avoidance of intravascular administration.[11,12]

Central Neuraxial Blockade

Epidural or spinal techniques can be used to administer local anesthetics to the neuraxial space to cause central blockade. Spinal anesthesia is indicated for surgeries and manipulation below the umbilicus including the lower abdominal, pelvic, and lower extremity area. Typically, spinal anesthesia only requires a single shot without catheter placement. Since the local anesthetic is given directly into the cerebral spinal fluid, it can produce a dense motor block along with a sensory block. In an epidural block, the local anesthetic must diffuse through the epidural space and into the cerebral spinal fluid area. Therefore, onset of analgesia is longer than with a spinal block and a dense motor block is rare. Epidural administration of a local anesthetic is often given for labor and delivery with catheter placement to allow for administration of anesthesia over a longer period of time.

Tumescent Local Anesthesia

Tumescent anesthesia is a technique that was initially developed by plastic surgeons to perform liposuction procedures using only local anesthesia. A large volume of diluted local anesthetic is mixed with epinephrine and injected subcutaneously into the area of interest. This creates a swollen, firm, fully anesthetized area of tissue that can be manipulated surgically. Typical total doses range from 35 to 55 mg/kg during these procedures.[13,14] Close monitoring for toxicity effects for at least 18 hours after administration must be done due to the slow absorption from subcutaneous tissue to blood circulation.

Intravenous Administration

A Bier block is an intravenous regional anesthesia procedure that provides surgical anesthesia and pain control to an upper or lower extremity. Local anesthetic is injection intravenously to the upper or lower extremity of interest that has been tied off by tourniquet to allow for an isolated, distal extremity blockade.

Intravenous (IV) infusion of local anesthetic has been used for many years to treat various pain states, particularly neuropathic pain. IV infusion for several hours to several days for pain control has been practiced.[15] IV lidocaine is the most commonly used local anesthetic in these situations. Studies have shown benefit in abdominal surgery, spinal surgery, trauma surgery, and hysterectomies where perioperative administration of IV lidocaine decreased analgesic consumption and pain scores.[16] IV lidocaine infusion has also been shown to ameliorate chronic neuropathic pain.[17] Caution must be taken with dose-related adverse effects of IV local anesthetic infusions. More research needs to be done to evaluate long-term results of IV local anesthetic infusions.

Topical Administration

The topical formulation of lidocaine 5% patches and cream has been proven to be beneficial for pain relief in postherpetic neuralgia and other painful peripheral neuropathies.[15,18] The combination of prilocaine and lidocaine, marketed as EMLA cream, is also effective for topical analgesia.[19] This is often used prior to venipuncture in the pediatric population. Lidocaine and tetracaine are also available in spray form, which is often used in endoscopic and bronchoscopy procedures.

Adverse Effects

Local anesthetics are generally considered safe to use; however, with high doses and prolonged administration, serious adverse effects may develop. The amount of toxicity is proportional to the amount of local anesthetic in the circulatory system. All local anesthetics cause similar adverse effects; however, there are some idiosyncratic effects with specific local anesthetics.

Systemic Toxicity

Systemic toxicity can be caused by high volume and/or concentration of local anesthetics, particularly with inadvertent intravascular administration. Initially, neurotoxic stimulation is seen including muscle twitching, irritability, and eventual clonic-type convulsions with increasing amounts of local administration. Local anesthetics can work directly on nerves that control myocardial tissues causing decreased electrical excitability and force of contraction. Cardiovascular excitation is then followed by depression and respiratory failure if not reversed. Signs of neurotoxic effects include sedation, altered mental status, and most critically, coma. Although all local anesthetics can cause cardiovascular adverse effects, bupivacaine has been shown to be uniquely cardiotoxic compared to other local anesthetics. A study that compared bupivacaine to ropivacaine noted significantly longer atrioventricular delay with toxic levels of bupivacaine and therefore special attention should be paid when using bupivacaine in large doses.[20]

Other manifestations of systemic toxicity include general decrease in smooth muscle motility leading to decreased bowel contractions and relaxation of vascular and bronchial smooth muscle.

Hypersensitivity

Allergy to local anesthetic is relatively rare.[21] If a person experiences an allergy to local anesthetics, it is more commonly due to the aminoesters local anesthetic type. The aminoesters are metabolized to *p*-aminobenzoic, which is the usual culprit for hypersensitivity reactions.[21] A hypersensitivity reaction can vary from allergic dermatitis or an asthma attack.

Alternatively, it is possible to have a hypersensitivity reaction to the preparation that the local anesthetic is suspended in. Sulfite preparation and methylparaben are common preservatives used with local anesthetics that can cause hypersensitivity reactions.

Methemoglobinemia

A rare potential side effect of using local anesthetics is methemoglobinemia. The build-up of metabolites of local anesthetics, in particular prilocaine and benzocaine, can cause the iron in hemoglobin to conform to the Fe^{3+} form, which is unable to bind to oxygen. This leads to cyanosis and tissue hypoxia. Therefore, prilocaine and benzocaine should be avoided in patients with known genetic forms of methemoglobinemia.

REFERENCES

1. Ruetsch Y, et al. From cocaine to ropivacaine: the history of local anesthetic drugs. *Curr Top Med Chem.* 2001;1(3):175-182. doi:10.2174/1568026013395335
2. Mofenson HC, Caraccio TR. Cocaine. *Pediatr Ann.* 1987;16(11):864-874. doi:10.3928/0090-4481-19871101-06
3. Fozzard H, et al. Mechanism of local anesthetic drug action on voltage-gated sodium channels. *Curr Pharm Des.* 2005;11(21):2671-2686. doi:10.2174/1381612054546833
4. Strichartz G. Molecular mechanisms of nerve block by local anesthetics. *Anesthesiology.* 1976;45(4):421-441. doi:10.1097/00000542-197610000-00012
5. Nathan PW, Sears TA. Some factors concerned in differential nerve block by local anaesthetics. *J Physiol.* 1961;157(3):565-580. doi:10.1113/jphysiol.1961.sp006743
6. Tetzlaff JE. The pharmacology of local anesthetics. *Anesthesiol Clin North Am.* 2000;18(2):217-233. doi:10.1016/s0889-8537(05)70161-9
7. Covino BG, Giddon DB. Pharmacology of local anesthetic agents. *J Dent Res.* 1981;60(8):1454-1459. doi:10.1177/00220345810600080903
8. Becker DE, Reed KL. Essentials of local anesthetic pharmacology. *Anesth Prog.* 2006;53(3):98-109. doi:10.2344/0003-3006(2006)53[98:eolap]2.0.co;2
9. Hussain N, et al. Equivalent analgesic effectiveness between perineural and intravenous dexamethasone as adjuvants for peripheral nerve blockade: a systematic review and meta-analysis. *Can J Anesth.* 2017;65(2):194-206. doi:10.1007/s12630-017-1008-8
10. Hussain N, et al. Investigating the efficacy of dexmedetomidine as an adjuvant to local anesthesia in brachial plexus block. *Reg Anesth Pain Med.* 2017;42(2):184-196. doi:10.1097/aap.0000000000000564
11. Abrahams MS, et al. Ultrasound guidance compared with electrical neurostimulation for peripheral nerve block: a systematic review and meta-analysis of randomized controlled trials. *Br J Anaesth.* 2009;102(3):408-417. doi:10.1093/bja/aen384
12. Koscielniak-Nielsen ZJ. Ultrasound-guided peripheral nerve blocks: what are the benefits? *Acta Anaesthesiol Scand.* 2008;52(6):727-737. doi:10.1111/j.1399-6576.2008.01666.x
13. Ostad A, et al. Tumescent anesthesia with a lidocaine dose of 55 mg/kg is safe for liposuction. *Dermatol Surg.* 1996;22(11):921-927. doi:10.1111/j.1524-4725.1996.tb00634.x
14. Klein JA. The tumescent technique for liposuction surgery. *Am J Cosmet Surg.* 1987;4(4):263-267. doi:10.1177/074880688700400403
15. Rowbotham MC, et al. Lidocaine patch: double-blind controlled study of a new treatment method for post-herpetic neuralgia. *Pain.* 1996;65(1):39-44. doi:10.1016/0304-3959(95)00146-8
16. Eipe N, et al. Intravenous lidocaine for acute pain: an evidence-based clinical update. *BJA Educ.* 2016;16(9):292-298. doi:10.1093/bjaed/mkw008
17. Tremont-Lukats IW, et al. A randomized, double-masked, placebo-controlled pilot trial of extended iv lidocaine infusion for relief of ongoing neuropathic pain. *Clin J Pain.* 2006;22(3):266-271. doi:10.1097/01.ajp.0000169673.57062.40
18. O'connor AB, Dworkin RH. Treatment of neuropathic pain: an overview of recent guidelines. *Am J Med.* 2009;122(10):S22-S32. doi:10.1016/j.amjmed.2009.04.007

19. Maunuksela E-L, Korpela R. Double-blind evaluation of a lignocaine-prilocaine cream (EMLA) in children. *Br J Anaesth*. 1986;58(11):1242-1245. doi:10.1093/bja/58.11.1242
20. Graf BM, et al. Differences in cardiotoxicity of bupivacaine and ropivacaine are the result of physicochemical and stereoselective properties. *Anesthesiology*. 2002;96(6):1427-1434. doi:10.1097/00000542-200206000-00023
21. Eggleston ST, Lush LW. Understanding allergic reactions to local anesthetics. *Ann Pharmacother*. 1996;30(7-8):851-857. doi:10.1177/106002809603000724

38

Peripheral Nerve Blocks

Aimee Pak

Peripheral Nerve Block: Background

Interest in regional anesthesia (RA) has renewed since the turn of the 21st century due to the changing landscape of American health care, greater awareness of pain management and its health effects, and the societal consequences from the opioid crisis.

Benefits of Regional Anesthesia

Poorly controlled acute pain may cause multisystem morbidity, negatively affect sleep, disturb mood, impair physical functionality, and worsen overall quality of life.[1] Acute pain may lead to chronic pain after surgery and has a high incidence (10%-60%) after common surgical procedures: hernia repair (6.2%), abdominal hysterectomy (9.9%), and thoracotomy (19.1%) at 12 months postoperatively.[1] Poorly controlled pain on the day of surgery is a risk factor for opioid use beyond 6 months,[1] which contributes to the U.S. opioid epidemic.

Therefore, potential benefits of RA programs have been investigated. One study that analyzed 13 897 regional anesthetics at an orthopedic ambulatory surgery center reported that 94% of patients had no or mild postoperative pain on the day of surgery, 67% by the first postoperative day, and 76% by the second postoperative day.[2] In contrast, a U.S. survey of 300 ambulatory patients reported 29% having mild pain in the immediate postoperative period.[3]

Mechanism of Peripheral Nerve Blockade

The peripheral nerve contains cablelike neural fibers within multiple bundling levels. The outermost epineurium is the layer surrounding connective and adipose tissue, extrinsic blood vessels, and fascicles.[4,5] Each fascicle has a perineurium encasing a longitudinal collection of axons, intrinsic blood vessels, and surrounding endoneurium.[4] The axon is the cytoplasmic projection of a neuron and is associated with myelin from Schwann cells.[5] Axons may divide and join neighboring fascicles.[4] The number of fascicles and the nonneural to neural tissue ratio increases when moving distally along a peripheral nerve.[4]

Local anesthetics (LA) block sodium channels to interrupt axonal impulse propagation.[4] Pharmacological factors contribute to differences in individual LA clinical properties: (1) P_{ka} (inversely related to onset of action), (2) protein binding (inversely related to duration), and (3) lipid solubility (directly related to potency).

After equilibrating with the surrounding tissue and penetrating the thick vascular perineurium, a significantly reduced amount of the LA will ultimately reach its effector site.[4] LA volume and concentration will affect its diffusion and perineurium penetration, respectively.[4] Both are important as a high-volume, low concentration solution may result in an incomplete conduction blockade.[4,5] Thicker peripheral nerves with greater neural tissue density require higher concentration but lower volume.[4] Additional factors contribute to variations in conduction blockade but are beyond the scope of this chapter.

Peripheral Nerve Block: Complications

Unfortunately, several general complications may occur with peripheral nerve blocks (PNBs). Complications specific to a certain nerve block procedure will be addressed in the next section.

- *Peripheral nerve injury (PNI)* is an uncommon complication that is reported to occur 2-4 per 10 000 blocks.[6] Transient postoperative neurologic symptoms, however, are common though with good prognosis.[6] The degree of axonal disruption determines severity and long-term prognosis of PNI: neuropraxia (damage limited to myelin sheath; recovery within weeks to months), axonotmesis (axonal injury; prolonged and potentially incomplete recovery), and neurotmesis (complete nerve transection; requires surgical intervention with uncertain recovery).[5]
- The mechanism of PNI are broadly categorized as: mechanical (traumatic or injection), vascular (ischemic), and chemical (neurotoxic).[5,6] Direct needle-to-nerve trauma or trauma from a high-pressure intraneural injection may occur, particularly if the perineurium or fascicle is disrupted.[5,6] Fortunately, the perineurium may be difficult to penetrate with short-beveled, blunt tipped needles,[7] such as with commercially available PNB needles. Ischemia from direct vascular injury, occlusion of the vasa nervorum feeding arteries, or compression from hematoma formation within the nerve sheath may cause PNI.[5] Chemical injury from PNB injectate may cause an acute inflammatory reaction or chronic fibrosis.[5] LA concentration, duration of exposure, and injection proximity to a fascicle all may affect LA neurotoxicity.[5]
- Avoidance of intraneural injection and careful evaluation of RA performance under heavy sedation or general anesthesia are advised.[5] However, PNB have not been found to be an independent risk factor for PNI.[6] There are multiple other etiologies for perioperative PNI: surgical factors (positioning, traction, stretch, transection, compression injuries) and patient factors (metabolic derangements, hereditary conditions, vascular disease, entrapment neuropathies, preexisting neural compromise [ie, "double crush"]).[5,6]
- *Local anesthetic systemic toxicity (LAST)* is a rare but potentially fatal complication with a reported incidence ranging from 0.04 to 0.37 per 1000 PNB based on registry data.[8] Acute toxicity occurs when LA inhibits sodium, calcium, and potassium movement through their channels in central nervous system cells and cardiac myocytes. Thus, its classical presentation involves rapidly progressing neurological and cardiovascular symptoms that are initially excitatory (eg, agitation, auditory changes, metallic taste, seizures; tachycardia, hypertension, arrhythmias) then inhibitory (eg, respiratory arrest, coma; bradycardia, depressed cardiac conduction, cardiac arrest).[7] However, nearly two-thirds of cases from 2014 to 2016 have atypical presentations (only cardiovascular or central nervous system symptoms) or delayed presentations beyond 5 minutes after injection (up to 12 hours after injection).[8]
- While no RA technique or single factor can prevent LAST occurrence, risk mitigation strategies are critical: avoidance of vascular injection, minimizing LA systemic uptake, utilizing ultrasound guidance (USG), and recognition of susceptible populations.[8] Additionally, rapid recognition of prodromal signs and initiation of appropriate management, which may include lipid rescue therapy, is important.
- *Pneumothorax* is a potential complication of thoracic nerve blocks (eg, paravertebral nerve block) and with certain approaches to the brachial plexus (ie, interscalene and supraclavicular). Based on the International Registry of Regional Anesthesia (IRORA) data, there is an incidence of 6.6 per 10 000 blocks.[9]
- *Infection* caused by PNB appear to be uncommon (0.86 per 10 000).[9] It may occur more frequently with indwelling peripheral nerve catheter, despite aseptic techniques, with reported bacterial colonization rates from 7.5% to 57% depending on location (highest

with femoral and axillary catheters) and number of colonies used to define colonization.[7] Needle puncture though active infectious sites should be avoided.[10]

- *Vascular puncture and hematoma formation* may occur with any invasive procedure. Larger-bore needles (such as for nerve catheter placement), number of attempts, and any coagulopathy may increase the risk for blood loss or hematoma development.[10] IRORA data reported block-related hematoma, including retroperitoneal hematoma, formation at 12 per 10 000 and arterial puncture at 39 per 10 000.[9] Injection site compressibility should be taken into consideration, particularly with concurrent anticoagulation therapy.[10] The 2018 fourth edition guidelines by the American Society of Regional Anesthesia (ASRA) address this concern specifically and recommend applying neuraxial anticoagulation guidelines similarly for any perineuraxial, deep plexus, or deep peripheral block.[11]

Preparation and Technique

Monitoring and Sedation

Cardiopulmonary monitoring with intermittent or continuous blood pressure monitoring, continuous electrocardiography, and pulse oximetry is mandatory.[12] RA complications may present as conduction abnormalities, hemodynamic instability, or hypoxia. Since light sedation is commonly provided during RA procedures, oxygenation and ventilation monitoring is important. Supplemental oxygen should be administered, and capnography may be utilized.[12] Sedation should be carefully titrated, as loss of patient feedback may increase risk for nerve injury.[10] Certain patient populations (eg, pediatrics, developmentally disabled) may benefit from general anesthesia for safe RA placement despite the risk for nerve injury.[6]

Emergency and Resuscitation

Rapid access to emergency equipment, devices, and drugs is necessary at all RA locations. Oxygen source and delivery, suction capability with associated canisters and tubing, airway management devices and equipment (eg, laryngoscope handle and blades, various sizes of endotracheal tubes, mask-valve ventilation device, supraglottic airways, oral and nasal airways, stylets, gum elastic bougies), syringes and needles in multiple sizes are necessary.[13]

Patients undergoing RA must have ready intravenous access to administer resuscitative drugs and fluids. Emergency drugs should include vasopressors (eg, phenylephrine, ephedrine), vasodilators (eg, labetalol), chronotropic agents (eg, atropine, glycopyrrolate), rapid induction agents (eg, etomidate, succinylcholine), reversal agents (eg, naloxone, flumazenil), antihistamine (eg, diphenhydramine), and additional "code drugs" (eg, epinephrine, sodium bicarbonate, calcium chloride, or gluconate). A mobile "code cart" should be kept nearby.[13]

In suspected LAST-related cardiac arrests, immediate access to and administration of 20% intravenous lipid emulsion is a critical modification to the American Heart Association cardiac arrest protocol.[14] ASRA provides a checklist for LAST management (accessible online at https://www.asra.com/content/documents/asra_last_checklist_2018.pdf). An available, preassembled LAST bundle, including the ASRA checklist as a cognitive aid, is recommended.[15]

Ultrasound Machine

Ultrasound guidance has become widespread due to its efficacy and safety. Use of ultrasound (US) improves efficiency by decreasing RA performance time and onset time and increasing block success as defined by complete sensory blockade.[16] USG compared to nerve stimulation is associated with fewer vascular and skin punctures[17] and reduced risk of LAST.[18] USG has not been shown to eliminate the risks of RA[19] but may be an important component of safe RA practices.[10,20] An US machine with probes appropriate for the expected RA practice would be necessary.

RA Equipment

Common block-related materials, which may also be commercially available in customizable block kits, usually includes block needle (20- or 22-gauge blunt tipped), multiple size syringes and needles, additional sterile drapes, sterile US probe sleeve and gel, and skin disinfecting solution. Specific LA and concentration may be selected based on the desired block. A peripheral nerve stimulator may also be available. These preparations and equipment must be readied, and informed consent for RA should be obtained[21] prior to the performance of any PNB.

Common Blocks

This section will be targeted review of commonly performed USG nerve and fascial plane blocks with in-plane needle techniques and inclusion of select US images. Knowledge of certain emerging blocks and techniques may be limited, but best efforts are made to utilize current information at the time of publishing. Of note, a high-frequency (eg, 4-12 MHz) linear probe or low-frequency (eg, 6-2 MHz) curvilinear probe will be referenced.

Blocks of the Neck

Cervical plexus

Indication: The cervical plexus block (CPB) is indicated for head, neck, distal clavicle, and upper chest wall procedures. Deep CPB are applied in certain chronic pain treatments.[22]

Relevant Anatomy: The cervical plexus originates from the C1 to C4 spinal nerves. The C2-C4 anterior rami form the superficial, somatosensory branches (lesser occipital, greater auricular, transverse cervical, and supraclavicular nerves). These terminal nerves travel through the prevertebral fascia then deep cervical fascia to emerge posterior to the sternocleidomastoid muscle (SCM) at the C4 level.[22] The C1-C3 nerve roots form the deeper, motor branches (ansa cervicalis), located between the prevertebral fascia and transverse process at the C4 level. The carotid artery and internal jugular vein are located medial to the nerves, deep to the SCM.

Positioning and Approach: The patient should be sitting or semirecumbent and facing contralaterally. A high-frequency linear probe is placed in transverse orientation over the SCM at the C4 level, at the midpoint between the mastoid process and clavicle. The CPB nomenclature is inconsistently used in literature.[22] For this text, the superficial CPB refers to the subcutaneous infiltration of the superficial cervical branches, the intermediate CPB refers to the blockade of the superficial cervical branches between the prevertebral fascia and superficial layer of the deep cervical fascia (deep to SCM), and deep CPB refers to the blockade of the deep cervical nerves between the deep layer of the prevertebral fascia and transverse process.

The superficial CPB is often performed as a blind subcutaneous injection at the posterior SCM border at its midpoint at the C4 level. Using USG, the SCM posterior border may be visualized to prevent accidentally deeper injection.[22] A volume of 5-10 mL of 0.25% or 0.5% long-acting LA (eg, ropivacaine, bupivacaine, levobupivacaine) may be used.The intermediate CPB (Fig. 38.1) targets the posterior cervical space immediately deep to the SCM in a lateral to medial needle direction toward the carotid sheath.[22] A volume of 5-10 mL of 0.25% or 0.5% long-acting LA may be used.

The deep CPB (see Fig. 38.1) may be equally efficacious as superficial and intermediate blocks[23] but with higher risk for complications.[24] Using the same US view, the needle is

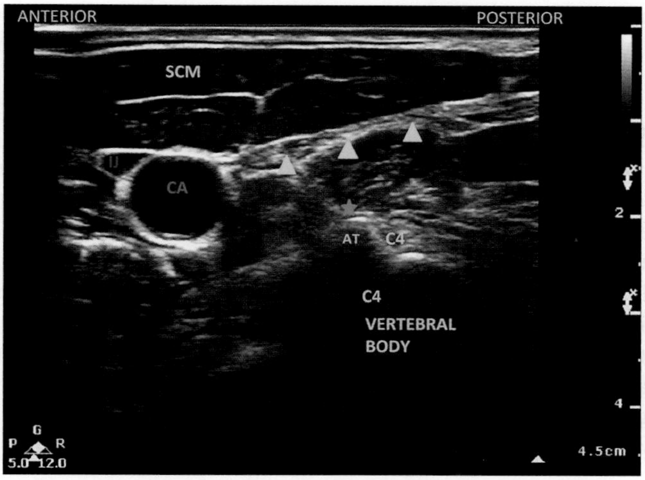

FIGURE 38.1 Intermediate and deep cervical plexus blocks. The target of the intermediate cervical plexus block is the plane deep to the sternocleidomastoid between the superficial layer of the prevertebral fascia and deep cervical fascia (*yellow triangles*). The deep cervical plexus block target is between the prevertebral fascia and C4 transverse process or at the anterior tubercle (*green star*) close to the nerve root. SCM, sternocleidomastoid muscle; IJ, internal jugular vein; CA, carotid artery; AT, anterior tubercle of C4 transverse process; C4, C4 nerve root.

advanced lateral to medial toward the C4 transverse process. A volume of 5-10 mL of 0.25% or 0.5% long-acting LA may be used.

Specific Risks and Considerations: Superficial and intermediate CPBs are easily performed and have few complications using USG, but the deep CPB is associated with several risks. The same adverse effects and complications may occur with intermediate CPB depending on the technique used (eg, paracarotid infiltration) and with larger injected volume of LA.[22]

- Phrenic nerve palsy and hemidiaphragmatic paralysis (HDP)
- The phrenic nerve (C3-C5) travels cephalad over the anterior scalene muscle surface deep to the prevertebral fascia. Not all patients develop HDP, possibly from variations in nerve root contribution (ie, higher C5 predominance) or presence of an accessory phrenic nerve.[22]
- Airway obstruction
- Bilateral deep CPBs may cause bilateral HDP, as well as vagal or hypoglossal nerve anesthesia.[22] Airway obstruction may also occur with a unilateral deep CPB in the presence of an unknown phrenic, vagal, or hypoglossal paralysis contralaterally.[22]
- Horner syndrome
- Horner syndrome has been reported with all three CPB approaches.[22]

Blocks of the Upper Extremity

The brachial plexus innervates the upper extremity and most of the shoulder. It may be blocked at different locations depending on desired target. Additional blocks, such as the CPB and intercostobrachial block, may be combined with a brachial plexus block.

Brachial plexus: interscalene approach

Indication: The interscalene block (ISB) is used for shoulder and upper arm procedures. It may be combined with a CPB for distal clavicle surgery.

Relevant Anatomy: The C5 and C6 nerve roots, and sometimes C7, are targeted between the anterior and middle scalene muscles approximately at the level of the cricoid process.

The US image appears as a three vertically stacked hypoechoic circles (stoplight sign), comprised of the C5, C6, and C7 roots or the C5 and bifid C6 roots,[25] between the scalene muscles. Notable structures include the cervical sympathetic chain cranially, vertebral artery deep to the plexus, and internal jugular and carotid sheath anteriorly.

Positioning and Approach: The patient should be placed in a supine or semirecumbent position and facing in the contralateral direction, or a lateral position may be utilized. A high-frequency linear probe should be placed in transverse orientation at the cricoid cartilage level.

The needle should be advanced in a posterior to anterior direction through the middle scalene muscle. Conventionally, the needle pierces the brachial plexus sheath between C5 and C6 (Fig. 38.2). Alternatively, the end point may be anterior to the middle scalene muscle but posterior to the C5 and C6 nerve roots without entering the plexus sheath with similar efficacy and potentially fewer side effects.[26] A 15-20 mL volume of 0.5% long-acting LA may be injected.

Specific Risks and Considerations

- Phrenic nerve palsy and HDP
- Ipsilateral phrenic nerve palsy occurs with nearly 100% incidence[27] from LA spread to the cervical roots or by direct phrenic nerve blockade over the anterior scalene muscle. Temporary HDP and reduced pulmonary function occur, with a 30% decrease in forced vital capacity.[28] Caution should be exercised in patients intolerant to decreased pulmonary volume or those with contralateral HDP. Low-volume injection (10 mL), proximal digital pressure techniques, and distal injection sites have not demonstrated reliable prevention.[28] Suprascapular and axillary blocks (see below) have been proposed as an alternative for shoulder procedures.
- Dorsal scapular nerve (DSN) and long thoracic nerve injury (LTN)
- The DSN travels within the middle scalene muscle, toward the levator scapulae and rhomboid muscles to pull the scapula medially.[29] The LTN also runs within the middle scalene muscle body close to the DSN[29] and is responsible for serratus anterior muscle

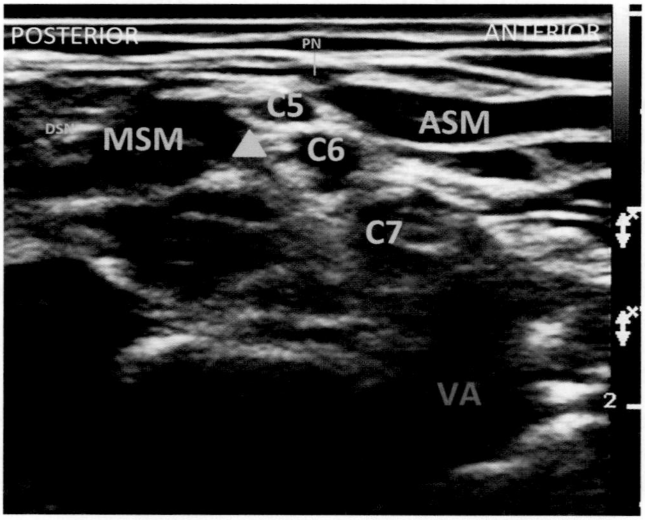

FIGURE 38.2 Interscalene brachial plexus block. The classic three cervical nerve roots are stacked between the middle and anterior scalene muscles. The needle target may be outside of the brachial plexus sheath (*yellow triangle*) or within the sheath between C5 and C6 nerve roots. MSM, middle scalene muscle; ASM, anterior scalene muscle; C5, C6, C7, cervical nerve roots; DSN, dorsal scapular nerve; PN, phrenic nerve; VA, vertebral artery.

innervation, which pulls the scapula anteriorly into the thorax. Both nerves may be injured during in-plane ISB and may develop into chronic shoulder pain syndromes.[29] DSN syndrome may also have rhomboid and levator scapulae weakness (ie, difficulty pulling scapula medially), while LTN syndrome may display a medial translation and inferior angle rotation toward the midline (ie, winged scapula).[29]

- Cervical plexus blockade
- Due to its proximity, LA diffusion to the cervical sympathetic chain and stellate ganglion may produce a benign and reversible Horner syndrome.[22,30] Hoarseness from ipsilateral recurrent laryngeal or superior laryngeal nerve blockade may occur. Emergent airway management may be necessary if a contralateral palsy exists.[30]

Brachial plexus: supraclavicular approach

Indication: The supraclavicular block (SCB) is used for upper extremity procedures distal to the shoulder. This is not a blockade of the supraclavicular nerve from the cervical plexus. An intercostobrachial block (medial aspect of upper arm) may be added for complete coverage of the upper arm distal to the shoulder or to reduce tourniquet pain.

Relevant Anatomy: The brachial plexus has formed into trunks and divisions at the level of the clavicle. Under US, the plexus appears as a hyperechoic wedge containing multiple hypoechoic circles (a "cluster of grapes") superolateral to the subclavian artery. The brachial plexus is superficially located as it is superior to the first rib, although anatomic variations exist. The pleura is deep to the first rib, and the dorsal scapular artery may be located within the trunks or branching from the subclavian or transverse cervical arteries.[31]

Positioning and Approach: The patient may be supine or semirecumbent and face toward the contralateral side or in lateral position. A high-frequency linear probe should be placed in the supraclavicular fossa posterior to the clavicle in an oblique coronal direction and directed caudally. Once the brachial plexus is identified lateral to the subclavian artery and superior to the first rib, the needle should be advanced in-plane in a posterolateral to anteromedial direction toward the inner corner pocket of the plexus (7 o'clock of the artery) (Fig. 38.3). Needle tip control should be exercised to avoid passing below the rib or advancing out-of-plane, which may risk pneumothorax. A 20-25 mL volume of 0.5% long-acting LA is commonly injected.

Specific Risks and Considerations: Like the ISB, SCB may cause phrenic nerve palsy causing HDP and Horner syndrome, though at a lower incidence of 34% and 32.1%, respectively.[32] Lower injection volume may reduce the incidence of HDP.[33] Historically, SCB was associated with a relatively high incidence of pneumothorax at 6%; however, large studies of USG SCB have reported a lower (up to 0.6 per 1000) incidence of pneumothorax.[19,34]

Brachial plexus: infraclavicular approach

Indication: The infraclavicular block (ICB) is used for upper extremity procedures distal to the shoulder. An intercostobrachial block may also be performed to provide medial upper arm coverage or to reduce tourniquet pain.

Relevant Anatomy: The brachial plexus has formed the posterior, lateral, and medial cords around the axillary artery, deep to the pectoralis muscles. The US view of the conventional lateral sagittal approach appears as three hyperechoic structures around the axillary artery, generally at the 7, 11, and 3 o'clock positions, respectively.[35] Anatomic variability frequently occurs at this point,[31,35] including multiple axillary vessels and branches.[35]

Positioning and Approach: With the conventional lateral (para) sagittal approach, the patient should be supine with the arm abducted 90° and elbow flexed to raise the clavicle,[36] while the head is turned contralaterally. Either a high- or low-frequency US probe

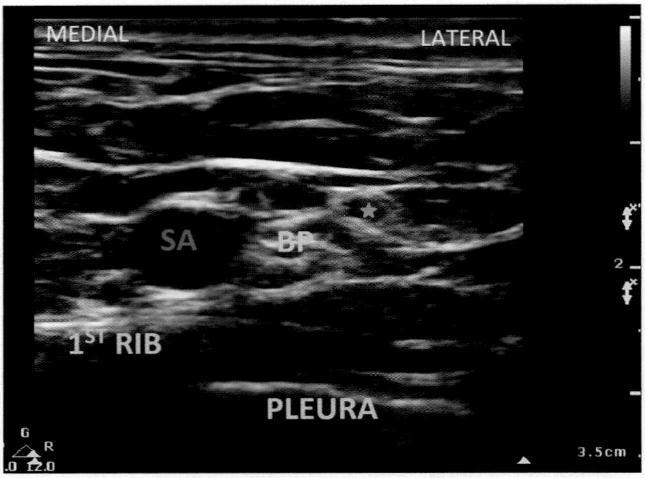

FIGURE 38.3 Supraclavicular brachial plexus block and suprascapular block (anterior approach). The trunks of the brachial plexus at the supraclavicular fossa appears lateral to the subclavian artery. The first rib and pleura are deep to the plexus. The anterior approach to the suprascapular block targets the proximal suprascapular nerve (*orange star*). BP, brachial plexus; SA, subclavian artery.

is placed longitudinally, inferior to the coracoid process, to capture the short-axis view of the axillary artery deep to the pectoralis muscles. The cords should be visualized around the artery (Fig. 38.4). The needle should be advanced in a cranial to caudal direction, at a steep angulation to the skin, to target the posterior axillary artery at the 6 o'clock position with circumferential spread if utilizing the single-injection technique. Another perivascular injection at the 9 o'clock position may be attempted if employing a double-injection technique. Needle visualization may be difficult due to the depth of the cords (usually 3-6 cm).[37] Multiple injections and larger LA volume may be needed as the cords are apart from each other and in variable locations with this approach.[37] A volume of 20-30 mL of 0.5% long-acting LA may be injected.

The costoclavicular approach is a newer approach.[38] The patient may be supine with the arms in neutral position. The linear US probe is placed transverse and slightly oblique on the anterior chest, directly inferior and parallel to the clavicle, with a cephalad tilt toward the costoclavicular space.[37] The cords are clustered together in this space at less depth than the lateral sagittal approach,[38] lateral to the axillary vessels and deep to the subclavius muscle.[37] The needle is advanced lateral to medial to target the costoclavicular space below the subclavius muscle. Needle tip control is important as the arching cephalic vein may travel directly in the needle path and the pleura lies closely inferior to the costoclavicular space.[37] As a relatively novel approach, anatomical variants, optimal technique, safety, and efficacy are still being reported. This approach may have a faster block onset than the traditional lateral sagittal approach.[39]

Another recent technique is the posterior (retroclavicular) approach. The patient may be supine with the arms in neutral position. The US probe position is similar to the lateral sagittal approach, except being 2 cm medial to the coracoid process,[40] and the US image obtained is like the lateral sagittal view. The needle entry site is superior and posterior to the clavicle and advance in a perpendicular trajectory (although initially under the acoustic shadow of the clavicle) to target the posterior wall of the axillary artery. This avoids the steep angulation needed with the conventional lateral sagittal approach, although a longer needle length may be needed.[40] More studies are needed to elucidate optimal technique, anatomical variabilities, efficacy, and safety, but early reports suggest similar efficacy compared to the coracoid approach but with more technical ease and better needle visibility due to the perpendicular angulation.[41,42]

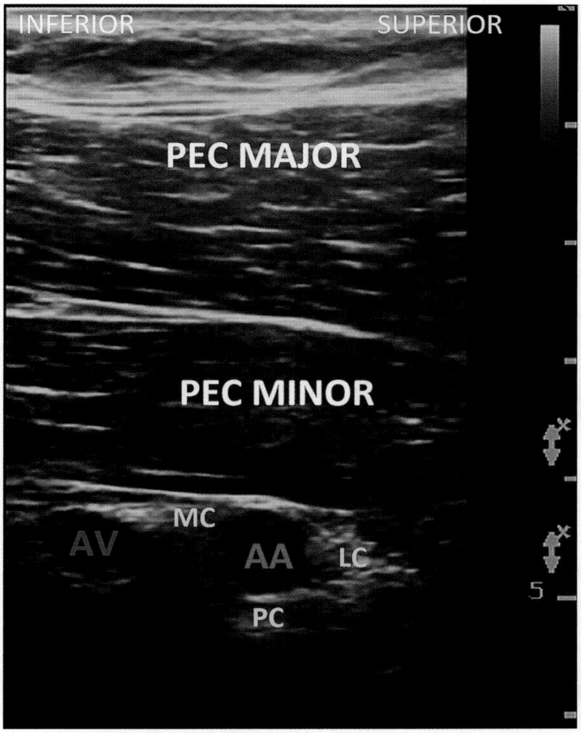

FIGURE 38.4 Infraclavicular brachial plexus block. The cords are located around the axillary artery deep to the pectoralis muscles. AA, axillary artery; AV, axillary vein; MC, medial cord; LC, lateral cord; PC, posterior cord.

Specific Risks and Considerations: Phrenic nerve palsy and HDP may also occur with the lateral sagittal ICB at a 3% incidence.[32] Horner syndrome has an occurrence rate at 3.2%.[32] Additional studies are needed to compare risk profiles of the various techniques. At this time, certain approaches may be selected based on patient comfort with positioning.

Brachial plexus: axillary approach

Indication: The axillary brachial plexus block is used for procedures distal to the elbow. This is not a blockade of the axillary nerve (see *Shoulder block: suprascapular and axillary*). For complete coverage of the anterolateral forearm, a musculocutaneous nerve block may be added.

Relevant Anatomy: The brachial plexus has formed into terminal nerves. The US image appears as three hyperechoic structures around the axillary artery: radial (posteromedial), median (anterolateral), ulnar (anteromedial).[43] The musculocutaneous nerve, which travels separately from the other terminal nerves, appears as a hyperechoic structure between the biceps brachii and coracobrachialis muscles, or through the coracobrachialis muscle only. There is anatomic variability in the exact nerve locations and axillary vessels.[43]

Positioning and Approach: The patient should be supine with the arm abducted 90°, forearm flexed, and shoulder externally rotated to expose the axillary fossa. A high-frequency linear probe should be placed in a sagittal orientation within the axillary fossa to capture a short-axis view of the axillary artery. The radial, median, and ulnar nerves should be visualized around the artery, and the musculocutaneous nerve is between the muscle bellies, posterolateral from the artery (Fig. 38.5). A double-injection technique that separately blocks the musculocutaneous nerve followed by a perivascular injection at the 6 o'clock, 12 o'clock, or both positions of the axillary artery is commonly used. Perivascular injection location or number of injections does not appear to affect efficacy

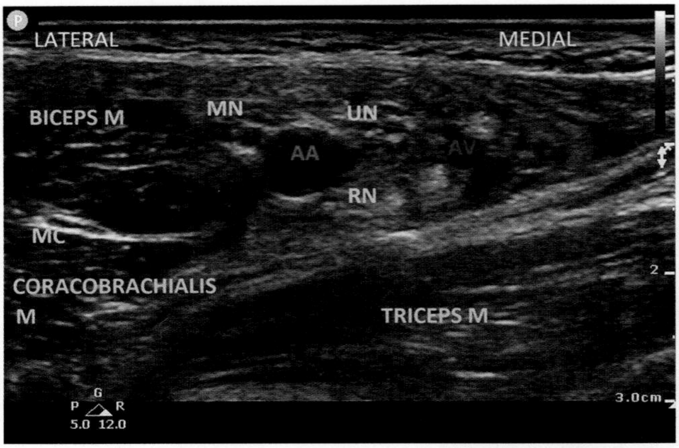

FIGURE 38.5 Axillary brachial plexus block. The median, ulnar, and radial nerves surround the axillary artery. The musculocutaneous nerve may be visualized between the biceps brachii and coracobrachialis muscles. AA, axillary artery; AV, axillary vein; MC, musculocutaneous nerve; MN, median nerve; UN, ulnar nerve; RN, radial nerve.

or onset.[44] Total volumes of 20-30 mL of 0.5% long-acting LA (5 mL for musculocutaneous) is commonly injected.

Specific Risks and Considerations: Because the vessels are superficial and easily compressible, this approach may be preferred in anticoagulated patients. Due to the distance from the phrenic nerve and pleura, this approach may be preferred for patients with poor pulmonary reserves.

Shoulder block: suprascapular and axillary

Indication: Combined suprascapular (SSNB) and axillary (ANXB) blocks have been proposed as a diaphragm-sparing alternative to ISB for shoulder procedures in 2007.[45]

Relevant Anatomy: The suprascapular and axillary nerves innervate most, but not all, of the shoulder joint. The suprascapular nerve branches from the superior trunk, which innervates most of the glenohumeral joint and most of the rotator cuff muscles.[45] Under US, the hyperechoic nerve appears within the suprascapular notch next to the suprascapular artery (posterior approach)[46] or as the lateral-most aspect of the brachial plexus inferior to the omohyoid muscle at the supraclavicular level (anterior approach).[47]

The axillary nerve is a terminal nerve from the posterior cord, which also innervates much of the glenohumeral joint, some of the rotator cuff (shared innervation of the teres minor tendon), and deltoid muscle.[45] The hyperechoic nerve may be visualized under US near the posterior circumflex humeral artery on the posterior humerus deep to the deltoid muscle.[46]

Positioning and Approach: For the anterior approach to the SSNB, the patient should be positioned as with the SCB. A high-frequency US probe should be placed in transverse orientation at the C6 level to identify the C5 nerve root.[47] As the probe moves distally, a hypoechoic nerve will leave the C5 root superior trunk, cross medially deep to the omohyoid muscle, and fuse to the superior trunk at the supraclavicular fossa[47] (see Fig. 38.3). The SSNB may be targeted at the supraclavicular fossa or as under the omohyoid muscle. Auyong et al. suggests that the anterior approach, using 15 mL of 0.5% ropivacaine, is noninferior to the traditional ISB for arthroscopic shoulder surgery and does not require AXNB.[48]

With the posterior approach to the SSNB, the patient may be positioned sitting,[45] lateral,[46] or prone.[47] The linear US probe should be placed in a transverse oblique orientation in superior to the scapular spine. A cranial tilt should visualize the suprascapular notch deep to the trapezius and supraspinatus muscles. The suprascapular artery and adjacent suprascapular nerve lie within the notch deep to the superior transverse ligament, which bridges the ends of the notch (Fig. 38.6). Injection in the supraspinatus fossa may be

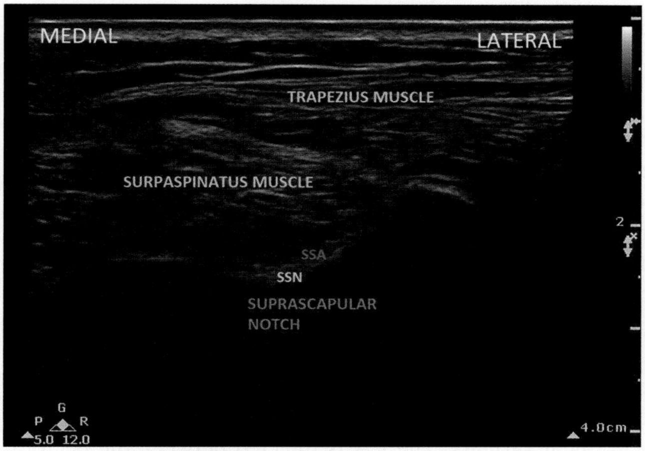

FIGURE 38.6 Suprascapular block (posterior approach). The distal suprascapular nerve travels with the suprascapular artery in the suprascapular notch of the scapula. The supraspinatus and trapezius muscles lie superficially. SSN, suprascapular nerve; SSA, suprascapular artery.

performed deep to the supraspinatus muscle.[46] A volume of 15 mL of 0.5%-0.75% ropivacaine has been reported.[45,46]

The AXNB may be performed in the sitting or lateral positions[45,46] with the shoulder in neutral position, elbow at 90°, and forearm medially rotated (ie, hands in lap). A linear US probe should be placed in the sagittal orientation parallel to the humeral shaft along the dorsal arm and immediately posterolateral to the acromion.[49] The posterior circumflex humeral artery is the vascular landmark as the axillary nerve is superior to it. In relation to the nerve, the deltoid muscle is superficial, teres minor muscle is cranial, humeral shaft is deep, and triceps muscle lies caudally[49] (Fig. 38.7). Injections of 8 mL of 20% lidocaine[49] and 15 mL of 0.5% ropivacaine[46] have been described.

Specific Risks and Considerations: An early study by Ferré et al. suggests a 40% incidence of HDP with the anterior approach, similarly to SCB and possibly by the same mechanism, while the posterior approach had a 2% incidence.[50] Additional information regarding anatomy, technique, optimal dosing and volume, and complications is likely to be produced in the future.

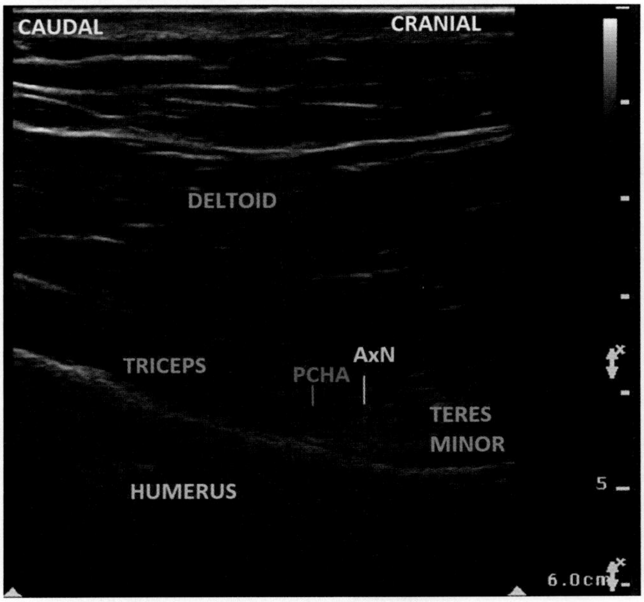

FIGURE 38.7 Axillary (nerve) block. The axillary nerve and posterior circumflex humeral artery exit the quadrilateral space, bound by the teres minor superiorly, teres major inferiorly, triceps medially, and humerus laterally, from anterior to posterior to wrap around the humerus posteroanteriorly. The nerve is superior to the artery. PCHA, posterior circumflex humeral artery; AxN, axillary nerve.

Intercostobrachial block

Indication: The intercostobrachial block may be combined with the brachial plexus block to provide more complete upper extremity blockade and may help to reduce tourniquet pain.

Relevant Anatomy: The intercostobrachial nerve originates from the second intercostal nerve, travels through the serratus anterior muscle at the midaxillary line, and into the axilla toward the posteromedial upper arm.

Positioning and Approach: A blind subcutaneous infiltration in an anteroposterior direction along the medial aspect of the upper arm distal to the axilla may be performed. US visualization may be obtained by placing a linear probe at the medial aspect of the upper arm along the humerus below the pectoralis major muscle insertion.[51] Infiltration with 5-10 mL of 0.25% long-acting LA in the anteroposterior direction from the medial upper arm to the inferior border of the triceps muscle.[51]

An USG proximal intercostobrachial approach has been described due to insufficient blockade, possibly from anatomical variants. The LA is injected between the pectoralis minor and serratus anterior muscles at the third or fourth rib at the anterior axillary line.[51]

Specific Risks and Considerations: Given the proximity to the pleura with the proximal approach, caution should be exercised to avoid causing a pneumothorax.

Blocks of the Trunk: Paravertebral and Paraspinal, Chest Wall, Abdominal Wall

Thoracic paravertebral block

Indication: The thoracic paravertebral block (TPVB) is used for unilateral thoracic or abdominal procedures. It may be used for thoracic analgesia (ie, rib fractures, anginal pain).

Relevant Anatomy: The wedge-shaped paravertebral space (PVS) contains the dorsal and ventral rami of the exiting thoracic spinal nerve and sympathetic chain from that spinal level. At each level, the space is bound by the vertebral bodies and transverse process (TP) medially, parietal pleura anteriorly, and superior costotransverse ligament (CTL) posteriorly. It continues as the intercostal space laterally.[52] The US image appears as a triangular space lateral to the transverse process between the CTL and pleura in the transverse oblique view or between two adjacent TP deep to the CTL but superficial to the pleura in the parasagittal view (Fig. 38.8).

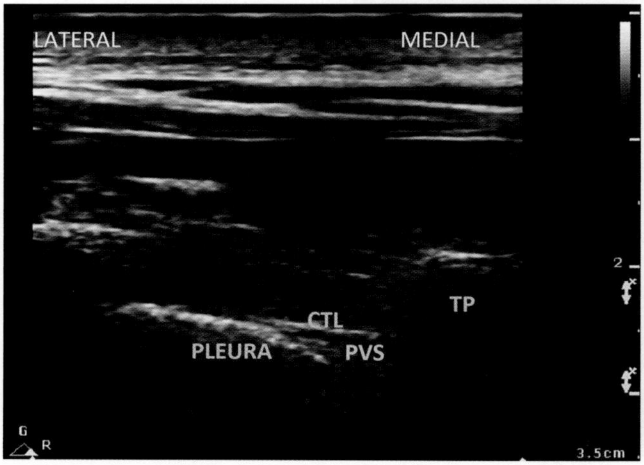

FIGURE 38.8 Thoracic paravertebral block (transverse approach). The needle target is the paravertebral space, which contain the exiting spinal nerve. The paravertebral space may be visualized lateral to the transverse process and deep to the superior costotransverse ligament. Caution is advised to avoid pleural puncture. CTL, superior costotransverse ligament; PVS, paravertebral space; TP, transverse process.

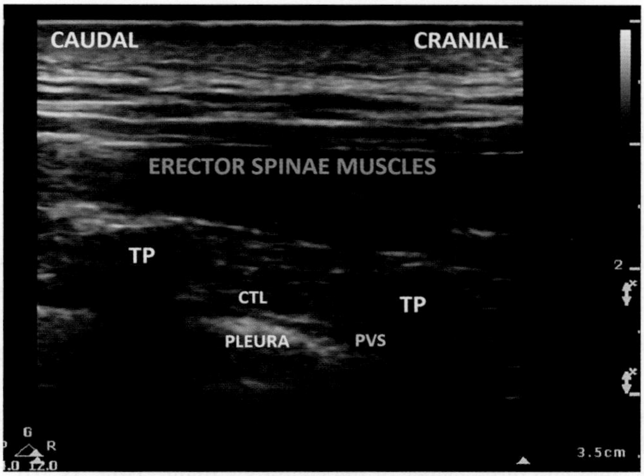

FIGURE 38.9 Thoracic paravertebral block (sagittal approach) and thoracic erector spinae plane block. The costotransverse ligament houses the paravertebral space, which may be viewed within the acoustic window between the thoracic transverse processes. The erector spinae muscles are posterior to the transverse processes. The needle target for the paravertebral block is the paravertebral space. The needle target for the erector spinae plane block is between the erector spinae muscles and transverse processes. TP, transverse process; CTL, superior costotransverse ligament; PVS, paravertebral space.

Positioning and Approach: The patient may be sitting, prone, or placed lateral. A high-frequency linear probe (or low-frequency curvilinear for deeper views) should be placed in the transverse oblique orientation between adjacent ribs at the desired vertebral level when performing the transverse approach (Fig. 38.9). As the pleura goes deeper into the thorax medially, the CTL may be visualized as a hyperechoic continuation toward the TP. The needle should be advanced in a lateral to medial trajectory and may encounter a "loss of resistance" when entering the target PVS. Injection of 20 mL of 0.5% long-acting LA should cause anterior pleural depression.[52,53]

In the parasagittal view, the probe should be placed in a longitudinal orientation between two adjacent TP. Deep to the paraspinal muscles is the hyperechoic CTL, the target hypoechoic PVS, then the sliding hyperechoic pleura. Needle direction is either superior to inferior or inferior to superior. Pleural depression will be visualized with injection.[53]

Specific Risks and Considerations:

- Anticoagulation and hematoma formation
- The PVS is an incompressible site. The same anticoagulation recommendations for neuraxial techniques are also applicable for the TPVB.[11]
- Pneumothorax
- The incidence of pneumothorax (0.9 per 1000) is low but may occur without obvious pleural puncture.[54]
- Epidural spread
- The PVS is continuous with the epidural space. A cadaver study by Seidel et al. suggests that techniques that medially direct the injectate have higher epidural spread, which may cause a more profound hypotension.[53]

Lumbar plexus (psoas compartment, lumbar paravertebral) block

Indication: The lumbar plexus block (LPB; psoas compartment, lumbar paravertebral) may be used for hip and lower extremity surgery above the knee except for the posterior compartment. A proximal sciatic nerve blockade may be combined for complete lower extremity coverage.

Relevant Anatomy: The anterior rami of L1-L3, with contributions from L4, form the lumbar plexus (LP), which supplies the anterior, medial, and lateral thigh compartments via the femoral (L2-L4), obturator (L2-L4), and lateral femoral cutaneous (L2-L3) nerves, respectively, as well as provide innervation to the hip.[55] The LP courses downward, anterior to the lumbar TP, within the psoas major muscle (PMM), and branches distal to the L5-S1 vertebral level.[55,56] The PMM lies anterior to the erector spinae muscles (ESM) and medial to the quadratus lumborum muscle (QLM). These muscular relationships will be preserved regardless of US view.

Positioning and Approach: Multiple US approaches have been described with similar efficacy.[55] The transverse approach ("Shamrock method"[57]) and paramedian sagittal approach ("trident view"[58]) will be specifically discussed. The patient should be in a lateral decubitus position, with the block side upward. A low-frequency curvilinear probe should be placed in the transverse orientation at the abdominal flank superior to the iliac crest and then moved dorsally until the QLM is visualized. The L4 TP should be visualized with the PMM anteriorly, QLM laterally, and ESM posteriorly, which creates the appearance of the stem and three leaves of the shamrock plant[57] (Fig. 38.10). The hyperechoic LP should be anterior to the TP within the PMM. Needle entry is perpendicular and ~4 cm lateral to the spine so that the anteroposterior trajectory may be visualized. Nerve stimulation may also be used in conjunction with US. This approach may be faster but equally effective as the trident view.[59] A volume of 20.4-36 mL of 0.5% ropivacaine may be optimally effective.[60] The mean skin-to-plexus depth is 74 mm, with direct correlation between depth and body mass index, so a longer block needle is recommended.[56]

With the trident view, the curvilinear US probe should be placed in a paramedian sagittal orientation to obtain the L2-L4 TP. The acoustic shadowing from the TP create a "trident" appearance. The ESM is posterior to the TP, and the PMM may be seen within the acoustic window between the TP. The hyperechoic LP may be visualized within the PMM between the L3 and L4 TP immediately deep to the ESM.[58]

Specific Risks and Considerations:

- Epidural spread
- Incidence of epidural spread varies from 3% to 27% with risk potentially related to more cephalad approach, higher injection volumes, and greater injection pressure.[55] Hemodynamic changes may potentially occur as a result.

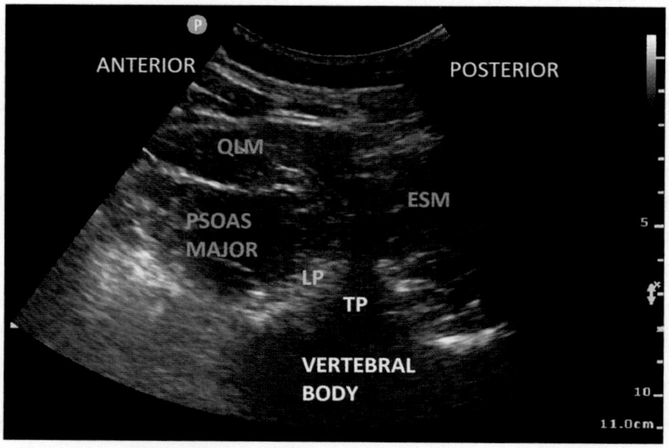

FIGURE 38.10 Posterior lumbar plexus block (Shamrock approach). The characteristic three "leaves" of the shamrock are the psoas major, quadratus lumborum, and erector spinae muscles. The "stem" of the shamrock is the transverse process of the L4 vertebral body. The needle is directed posterior to anterior toward the lumbar plexus anterior to the transverse process. QLM, quadratus lumborum muscle; ESM, erector spinae muscle; LP, lumbar plexus; TP, transverse process.

- Renal hematoma
- The inferior renal pole is at the L3 level, which may cause a renal subcapsular hematoma with cephalad needle trajectories. The L4 level may be safer.[55]
- Anticoagulation and retroperitoneal hematoma
- The LP block location is deep and incompressible. The same anticoagulation recommendations for neuraxial techniques are also applicable for the LPB.[11]
- LAST
- A higher incidence of LAST has been reported after LPB compared to other lower extremity PNB.[55] A study analyzing ropivacaine plasma concentrations after LPB found rapid LA absorption with peak levels within 10 minutes postinjection.[61] A high suspicion for LAST should be maintained due to the high LA volume and frequent combination with sciatic blockade.[61]

Paraspinal: retrolaminar block and erector spinae plane block

Indication: The retrolaminar (RLB) and recently described erector spinae plane (ESPB) blocks attempt to anesthetize the thoracic spinal nerves without entering the PVS. These blocks are less technically difficult with a lower risk profile compared to the TPVB and are not limited by coagulopathy. Both blocks may be used to provide ipsilateral, multilevel thoracic or abdominal wall analgesia with new indications being reported. Unlike the TPVB, which provides somatic and sympathetic blockade, the RLB and ESPB seem to primarily provide somatic blockade only,[62] which may be insufficient for surgical anesthesia.[63]

Relevant Anatomy: The RLB site is lateral to the spinous process and posterior to the lamina. The US image appears as a bony surface anterior to the ESM. The ESPB site is further lateral than the RLB at the TP. Under US imaging, the TP appears as tall, rectangular acoustic shadows deep to the ESM with pleura visible within the acoustic windows.

Positioning and Approach: The patient may be sitting, prone, or placed decubitus. A linear probe (or curvilinear probe for deeper views) should be placed in the parasagittal orientation lateral to the spinous processes but medial to the TP to view the laminae for the RLB. The needle target is anterior to the ESM and posterior to the laminae (Fig. 38.11).

Moving the US probe further laterally, the characteristic appearance of the TP is obtained. The needle target is anterior to the ESM and posterior to the TP for the ESPB (Fig. 38.12). The injectate should spread longitudinally within the respective plane. The ESPB may also provide multilevel intercostal analgesia[64] and potential epidural[64] and paravertebral effects.[65] Both blocks may utilize 20-30 mL of 0.25% of a long-acting LA.[63,64] The median volume needed is 3.4 mL per dermatome for the ESPB.[66]

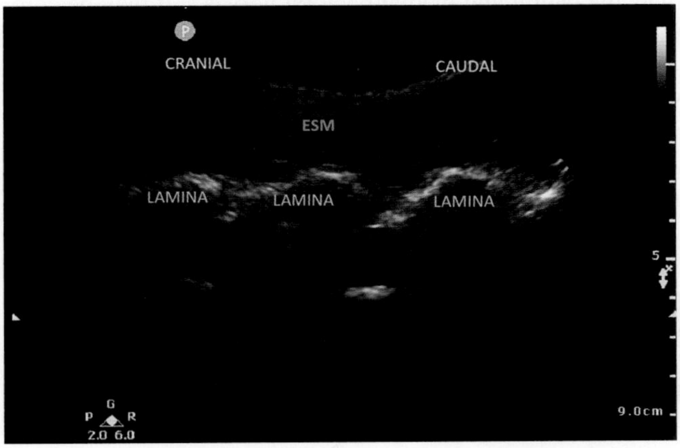

FIGURE 38.11 Thoracic retrolaminar block. The erector spinae muscles lie posterior to the vertebral laminae and medial to the transverse processes. The target of the retrolaminar block is between the erector spinae muscles and laminae. ESM, erector spinae muscles.

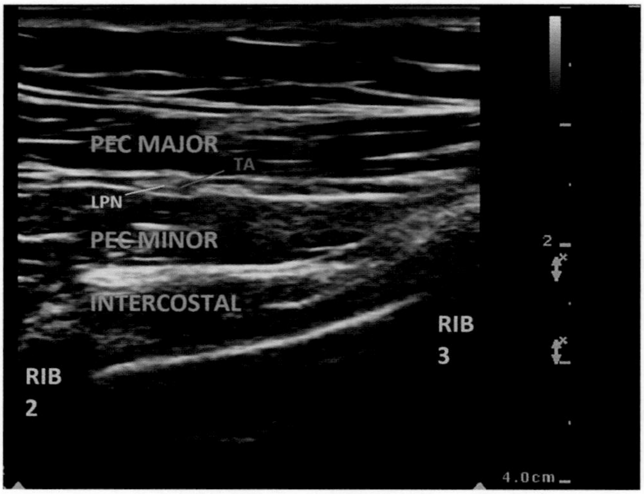

FIGURE 38.12 PECS I block. The pectoralis major and minor muscles are superficial to ribs 2 and 3. The lateral pectoral nerve and associated thoracoacromial artery lie between the pectoralis muscles. LPN, lateral pectoral nerve; TA, thoracoacromial artery.

Specific Risks and Considerations:

As both blocks are relatively new, more studies are needed to ascertain optimal dosing, anatomical mechanism, and technique as well as fully elucidate all potential complications. Currently, however, the risk profiles appear to be less than thoracic epidural or TPVB.

- Anticoagulation and hematoma formation
- RLB and ESPB injection sites are compressible, unlike the epidural and TPVB sites, and distant from major vessels. These blocks may be utilized in patients with coagulopathy or anticoagulation therapy.[67,68]
- Epidural spread
- RLB and ESPB appear to have minimal hemodynamic effect in contrast to the thoracic epidural or TPVB.[67] However, the potential for hypotension exists, possibly via epidural spread.[65,68]

Chest wall: PECS I, PECS II, and serratus anterior plane blocks

Indication: In recent years, thoracic wall fascial plane blocks have gained popularity as a technically easier, lower risk, and efficacious alternative to the TPVB.[69] PECS I, PECS II, and serratus anterior plane (SAPB) blocks have been utilized for anterolateral thoracic wall procedures (eg, breast and thoracoscopic surgery, chest tube, implantable chest wall devices) and rib fractures[69-71] with more indications being investigated. More studies are needed at this time to better understand these newer fascial plane blocks.

Relevant Anatomy: PECS I targets the lateral and medial pectoral nerves.[72] It may be combined with the PECS II block to additionally anesthetize the lateral cutaneous branches of intercostal nerves 3-6,[73] including the intercostobrachial nerve if the lateral injection approach is used,[73] and LTN.[73,74] The pectoralis major (PMaj) and minor (PMin) muscles, ribs 2 and 3, and thoracoacromial artery should be identified on US imaging for PECS I.[71] The PMaj, PMin, serratus anterior muscle (SAM), and ribs 3 and 4 should be identified for PECS II.[71] The SAPB has been reported to cover the T2-T9 dermatomes,[75] although anatomical studies suggest blockade is limited to the lateral cutaneous branches of the intercostal nerves rather than by direct intercostal nerve blockade.[76,77] The latissimus dorsi and SAM, rib 5, and pleura should be identified on US imaging for the SAPB.[75]

Positioning and Approach: The PECS I and II blocks may be performed with the patient in supine position and supine or lateral decubitus position for the SAPB. A linear US probe may be used. The PECS I block was first described by Blanco: the probe is placed in a

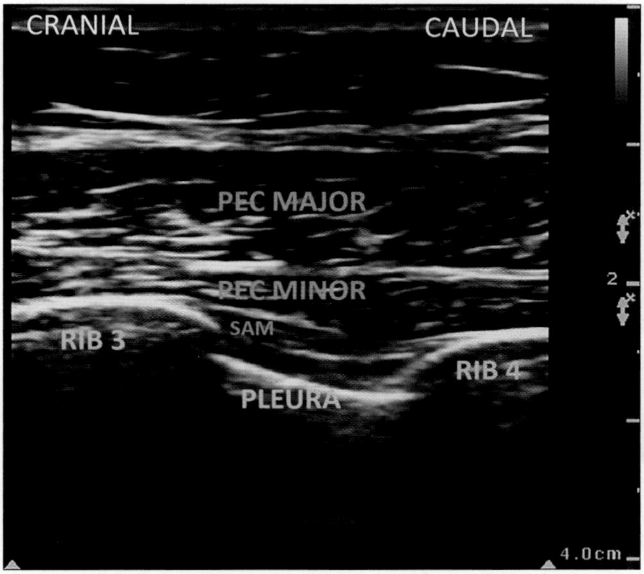

FIGURE 38.13 PECS II block. The pectoralis major, pectoralis minor, and serratus anterior muscles may be seen from superficial to deep at the anterior axillary line over ribs 3 and 4. After a PECS I injection, the needle target is the interfascial plane between the pectoralis minor and serratus anterior muscles. SAM, serratus anterior muscle.

sagittal orientation inferior to the distal clavicle to visualize ribs 2 and 3 with a cranial-to-caudal needle trajectory[72] (Fig. 38.13). Alternatively, the lateral approach by Pérez places the US probe in a transverse orientation inferior to the outer third of the clavicle at ribs 2 and 3 with a medial-to-lateral needle direction.[78] The PMaj overlies the PMin, which is superficial to the ribs. The thoracoacromial artery and adjacent lateral pectoral nerve courses between the pectoralis muscles. A volume of 10 mL of 0.25% long-acting LA is injected between PMaj and PMin.[69]

The PECS II block combines the PECS I injection with an additional injection over ribs 3 and 4 at the anterior axillary line. The linear probe is rotated to visualize the PMaj, PMin, and SAM, and the needle is advanced superomedial to inferolateral to target the interfascial plane between PMin and SAM.[74] A volume of 20 mL of 0.25% long-acting LA is injected.[69]

In the SAPB, the linear US probe is placed in a sagittal orientation at the midaxillary line over rib 5 (Fig. 38.14). The needle is advanced superoinferiorly to target the plane between the SAM and rib.[75] A volume of 20-40 mL of 0.25% long-acting LA may be injected.[69] Higher LA volume may provide a larger area of coverage.[77]

Specific Risks and Considerations:

Since these blocks are relatively novel, more studies are needed to ascertain optimal dosing, anatomical mechanism, and technique as well as elucidate all potential complications. Thus far, their risk profiles appear to be less than thoracic epidural or TPVB. As with all thoracic wall blocks near the pleura, pneumothorax may be a low risk with proper USG.

- Hematoma
- A 1.6% incidence of hematoma formation has been reported and frequently occurring in the context of anticoagulation or antiplatelet therapy.[79]

Abdominal wall: rectus sheath block

Indication: Bilateral rectus sheath block (RSB) is indicated for postoperative analgesia of midline abdominal incisions. It may be combined with transversus abdominis plane (TAP) blocks for analgesia after open and laparoscopic abdominal procedures.[80]

Relevant Anatomy: The T6-L1 ventral rami[81] pierces through the rectus abdominis muscle (RAM) in a posteroanterior direction then branches into anterior cutaneous nerves to

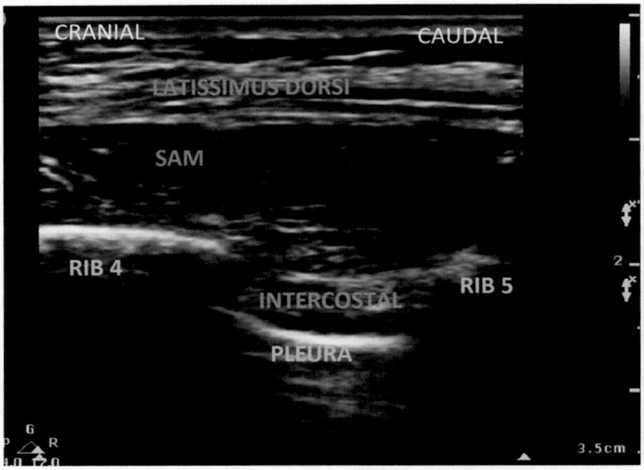

FIGURE 38.14 Serratus anterior plane block. The serratus anterior muscle is visualized over rib 4 and 5 at the midaxillary line. The needle target is the plane between the serratus anterior muscle and ribs. SAM, serratus anterior muscle.

innervate the overlying skin. There is wide communication among these nerves, which creates mixed innervation.[82] The RAM is encased by the rectus sheath anteriorly and posteriorly, the transversalis fascia is deep to the posterior rectus sheath, and the peritoneum lies deep to the transversalis fascia. A characteristic double layer appears deep to the RAM under US imaging. Deep epigastric vessels may course near or within the RAM.[83]

Positioning and Approach: The patient should be in supine position. A linear US probe (or curvilinear probe for deeper views) should be placed in transverse orientation to the abdominal midline between the xiphoid and inferior to the umbilicus. If the hyperechoic linea alba is visualized, the probe may be moved laterally to visualize the RAM. The needle target is deep to the posterior RAM but superficial to the posterior double layer (Fig. 38.15). Trauma to the deep epigastric vessels should be avoided. The block should be performed at or close to the level of the incision due to potentially limited craniocaudal spread.[82] A volume of 10-20 mL of 0.25% or 0.5% long-acting LA may be injected per side.[80]

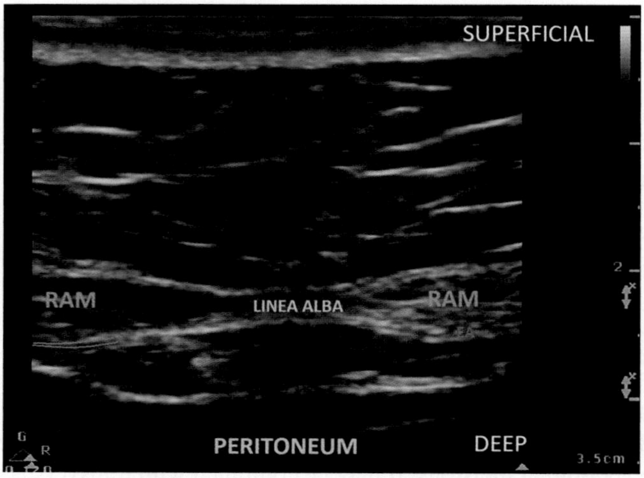

FIGURE 38.15 Rectus sheath block. The linea alba is visualized at the abdominal midline with the paired rectus abdominis muscles laterally and peritoneum deep to the abdominal wall. The (superior or inferior) epigastric artery may be visualized within or near the rectus abdominis muscle. The double layer (*green lines*) posterior to the rectus abdominis muscle is characteristic. RAM, rectus abdominis muscle; EA, epigastric artery.

Specific Risks and Considerations:

- Epigastric vascular injury and rectus sheath hematoma
- The superior or inferior deep epigastric artery and vein may be visible at different locations relative to the RAM depending on where the block is performed along the abdominal midline: anterior to the RAM within its sheath at the medial third of the muscle (at midway between the xiphoid and umbilicus), within the RAM at the middle third of the muscle (at the umbilical level), or posterior to the RAM within its sheath at the lateral third of the muscle (at the level of the anterior superior iliac spine).[83] The epigastric artery has the smallest diameter or is least likely to be encountered when the RSB is performed between the xiphoid and umbilicus, which may make this location preferable.[83,84]
- LAST
- Higher injection volume is usually necessary for compartment blocks, such as RSB. In practice, bilateral RSB are also frequently paired with bilateral TAP blocks, another compartment block. A review by Rahiri et al. found consistently reported rapid LA absorption and that LA systemic concentration may exceed acceptable thresholds.[80] Dosing limits must be considered, particularly in low weight or frail patients. Using lower injection concentration may allow for higher volume to be safely administered.

Abdominal wall: transversus abdominis plane and ilioinguinal/iliohypogastric blocks

Indication: The TAP block is indicated for many open and laparoscopic abdominal procedures, such as cesarean section, hysterectomy, appendectomy, and laparoscopic cholecystectomy. Bilateral TAP blocks have been incorporated into enhanced recovery protocols. TAP blocks are frequently combined with bilateral RSB. The ilioinguinal and iliohypogastric (II/IH) blocks are indicated for inguinal surgery. TAP blocks may provide an alternative to the thoracic epidural without issues of hypotension or coagulopathy.

Relevant Anatomy: The TAP compartment is an anterolateral abdominal plane between the internal oblique (IOM) and transversus abdominis muscles (TAM) that contains the T6-L1 nerves. Upon exiting from their respective vertebral level, the T6-T11 ventral rami continue as intercostal nerves to eventually supply the anterior abdominal wall.[82,85] The T6-T8 nerves enter the TAP at the level of the costal margin,[81] and the T9-T12 nerves enter the TAP posterior to the midaxillary line.[85] The T6-T11 lateral cutaneous branches innervate the lateral abdominal wall from the costal margin to iliac crest, while the T9-T11 and the T12 subcostal nerves provide cutaneous supply to the anterior infraumbilical abdomen.[85] L1 provides innervation to the inguinal area and medial thigh as the ilioinguinal and iliohypogastric nerves.[85] The USG view varies with the approach, but relevant anatomy includes the QLM (posterior approach), RAM (subcostal approach), and anterior superior iliac spine (II/IH block).

Positioning and Approach: Optimal patient positioning depends on the approach performed. A high-frequency linear probe (or curvilinear probe for deeper views) may be used. The patient may be placed in either supine or lateral position to perform the lateral TAP approach. The US probe should be placed in transverse orientation midway between the costal margin and iliac crest at the midaxillary line. From superficial to deep are the three visible anterolateral abdominal muscles layers—external oblique muscle (EOM), IOM, TAM—then the peritoneal space and peristaltic bowels (Fig. 38.16). The needle should be directed mediolateral into the plane between the IOM and TAM. Studies have reported a limited area of anesthesia to the T10-T11 dermatomes with a deficiency in L1 blockade.[86,87] Abdominal procedures below the umbilicus but above the inguinal area would benefit from this approach.

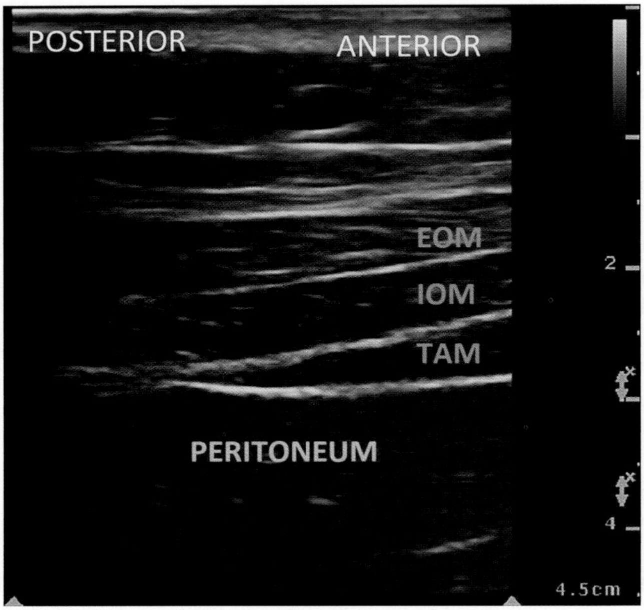

FIGURE 38.16 Transversus abdominis plane block (lateral). The three muscular layers of the anterolateral abdominal wall are visualized with the lateral transversus abdominis plane block. The needle targets the plane layer between the internal oblique muscle and transversus abdominis muscle. The peritoneum lies deep to the transversus abdominis muscle. EOM, external oblique muscle; IOM, internal oblique muscle; TAM, transversus abdominis muscle.

With the patient positioned supine, the US probe should be in an oblique transverse orientation parallel to the costal margin to visualize the plane between the RAM and TAM in the subcostal TAP approach. Needle entry is near the xiphoid with an inferolateral direction along the costal margin. This approach provided more cephalad coverage to T8 and greater dermatomal spread from T9 to T11,[88] which would be suitable for abdominal procedures above the umbilicus.

Lateral patient positioning would allow access for the posterior TAP approach. The US probe is placed in transverse orientation at the lateral abdominal wall at the midaxillary line but further posteriorly than the lateral approach. The needle trajectory is at an anteroposterior direction to target the TAP origin that is anterior to the QLM. The T9-T11 dermatomes are most reliable blocked[87] with some potential spread around the QLM and PVS.[89]

The supine position should be used for the II/IH block, which is similar to the lateral TAP but performed superior to the anterior superior iliac spine (ASIS) where the II and IH nerves travel through the TAP.[86,88] The target is the TAP between the IOM and TAM, where the nerves may be visible. This block is best for L1 anesthesia.

A volume of 10-30 mL of 0.25%-0.75% of long-acting LA is injected per side. Generally, higher volumes of dilute concentration are recommended for fascial plane blocks. Attention to total dose is critical to avoid exceeding toxic thresholds.

Specific Risks and Considerations:

- LAST
- Higher LA volume, bilateral TAP blockade, and frequent addition of bilateral RSB may risk exceeding toxic thresholds,[80] so careful dosing is important. Addition of epinephrine to the injection may lower the peak concentration and time to peak concentration for TAP blocks.[90]

Abdominal wall: quadratus lumborum block

Indication: The quadratus lumborum block (QLB) is a recently described technique that has been purported as an alternative to the TAP block for abdominal procedures as well as hip surgery. Case reports have also described its use with abdominal flaps for breast reconstruction[91] and above knee amputation.[92] Further studies are needed to clarify the anatomy, mechanism of action, indications, limitations, and optimal technique. One meta-analysis, thus far, suggests that QLB may offer better and longer analgesic duration than TAP blocks.[93]

Relevant Anatomy: The QLM lies in a craniomedial to caudolateral direction within the posterior abdominal wall with attachments at the medial border of rib 12 superiorly, posteromedial iliac crest inferiorly, and the L1-L4 TP medially. Lateral to the QLM are the anterolateral abdominal muscles. The aponeurotic sheaths of the IOM and TAM continue and ultimately connect with the thoracolumbar fascia around the QLM.[94] In relation to the QLM, the PMM lies anteromedial and the ESM are posteromedial. Of note, the kidney lies anterior to the QLM, separated by the transversalis fascia, renal fascia, and peri- and paranephric fat. The QLB may directly anesthetize the exiting spinal nerve as it crosses anterior to the QLM prior to entry into the TAP compartment; however, case reports have documented blockade from T7 to L2,[94,95] depending on approach, suggesting other mechanisms for cranial spread.

Positioning and Approach: Due to confusion in terminology throughout the literature, for the purposes of this review, the QLB approaches will be described in relation to the QLM as proposed by El-Boghdadly et al.: lateral (QL#1), posterior (QL#2), anterior or transmuscular (QL#3), and intramuscular QLB[95,96] (Fig. 38.17).

With the lateral QLB, the patient may be in supine or lateral position. A linear or curvilinear probe is placed in transverse orientation at the midaxillary line between the costal margin and iliac crest, then moved posterior to the IOM, and TAM origins to visualize the QLM. The needle is advanced in an anteroposterior direction to target the lateral aspect of the QLM within the TAM aponeurosis. At this injection site, LA may track anterior or posterior to the QLM.[96] This approach appears to have greater coverage than the lateral TAP[94] with T7-L1 anesthesia.[95]

To perform the posterior QLB, the patient may be in supine (may require support to elevate the hip) or lateral position. The same view as with the lateral QLB is obtained with the low-frequency US. The needle target is posterior to the QLM within the lumbar interfascial triangle between the QLM and ESM.[94,95] T7-L1 coverage has been reported,[95] with potential spread into the thoracic PVS.[97]

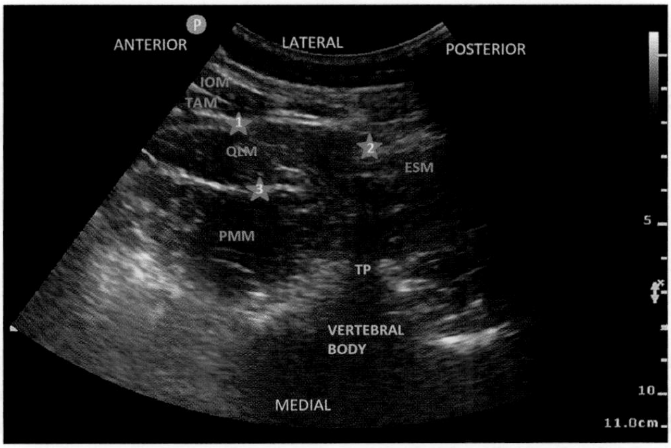

FIGURE 38.17 Quadratus lumborum block. In the lateral block (*green star*, 1), the needle targets the lateral aspect of the quadratus lumborum muscle within the transversus abdominis muscle aponeurosis. In the posterior block (*green star*, 2), the needle target is posterior to the quadratus lumborum muscle between the quadratus lumborum muscle and erector spinae muscles. In the anterior block (*green star*, 3), the needle is advanced through the quadratus lumborum muscle to target the fascial plane between the psoas major muscle and quadratus lumborum muscle. IOM, internal oblique muscle; TAM, transversus abdominis muscle; QLM, quadratus lumborum muscle; PMM, psoas major muscle; ESM, erector spinae muscle; TP, transverse process.

The patient should be positioned laterally to perform the anterior (transmuscular) QLB. The curvilinear probe is placed in transverse orientation superior to the iliac crest (to obtain the same view as with the Shamrock approach to the LPB). The needle is advanced in a posterolateral to anteromedial direction through the QLM to target the fascial plane between the PMM and QLM located anteromedially to the QLM.[95] A cadaveric study reported potential spread to the lumbar PVS,[98] which may provide T10-L4 blockade.[95]

For the intramuscular QLB, the same patient position and probe orientation as the lateral QLB should be used. The needle is advanced into the body of the QLM, and LA may be injected.[95] Lateral abdominal wall coverage from T7 to T12 has been reported[95] but without evidence of paravertebral spread.[97]

A volume of at least 20 mL per injection[93,95] and diluted concentrations such as 0.125%, 0.25%, or 0.375% of long-acting LA have been reported.

Specific Risks and Considerations:

- Organ puncture
- Anterior and lateral QLB needle end points are near the kidney.
- Hematoma
- Although rare, hematoma has been a reported complication.[99] Furthermore, due to the incompressibility of certain approaches (ie, anterior QLB), caution is recommended in coagulopathy.
- Lower extremity motor weakness
- Lumbar paravertebral spread has been reported in cadavers,[98] which may affect the LP. One report has described lower extremity weakness attributed to QLB.[100]
- Hypotension
- Hypotension has been reported as a complication, potentially through paravertebral spread.[101]
- LAST
- A study by Murouchi et al. found that though the time to peak concentration was similar, a lower peak concentration was reached after the QLB than the lateral TAP block.[102] However, careful dosing is still advised.

Blocks of the Lower Extremity

Fascia iliaca compartment block

Indication: The fascia iliaca compartment block (FICB) may provide analgesia to the hip and lower extremity above the knee with exception of the posterior compartment. The FICB has been proposed as an anterior alternative to the LPB that is simpler, safer, and more superficial.

Relevant Anatomy: The LP branches within the PMM to become the obturator nerve (ON, dorsal branch), femoral nerve (FN, ventral branch), and lateral femoral cutaneous nerve (LFCN, ventral branch) that will innervate the hip and lower extremity.[103] The FN and LFCN exit the PMM laterally and travel inferiorly in separate paths toward the inguinal ligament (IL) deep to the fascia iliaca (FI).[103] The ON continues inferomedially into the pelvis deep to the FI but exits from the FI compartment at the level of the S1 body.[103] The FI is a connective layer that attaches laterally from the inner aspect of the iliac crest, crosses closely anterior to the iliacus muscle and PMM, and medially to the psoas fascia. The potential space (FI compartment) between the FI and iliopsoas muscle may be targeted for LA injection to simultaneously block the FN and LFCN. ON blockade with the FICB is controversial and may depend on the approach: whether superior (suprainguinal approach, S-FICB) or inferior to the IL (infrainguinal approach, I-FICB).

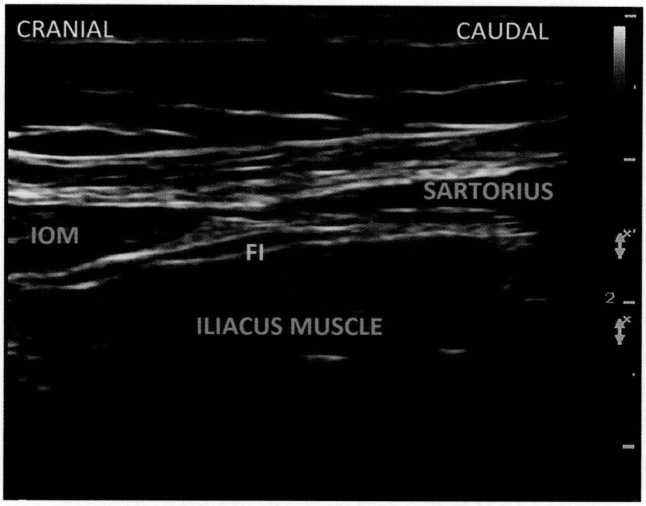

FIGURE 38.18 Fascia iliaca nerve block (suprainguinal). The "bow-tie" sign may be seen with the internal oblique muscle and sartorius muscle. The fascia iliaca overlies the iliacus muscle. The fascia iliaca should be dissected from the iliacus muscle. IOM, internal oblique muscle; FI, fascia iliaca.

Positioning and Approach: The patient should be supine. For the S-FICB approach, a high-frequency linear probe may be placed longitudinally near the ASIS over the inguinal ligament in a parasagittal orientation. Hebbard et al. initially described moving the probe inferomedially along the IL toward the FN until the deep circumflex iliac artery is visualized, then entering the needle inferior to the IL.[104] Desmet et al. modified this technique by moving the probe inferomedially then rotated clockwise to point the cranial side of the probe toward the umbilicus.[105] The "bow-tie sign" may be visualized by the IOM and sartorius muscles directly superior to the FI, which is overlying the iliacus muscle below[103,105] (Fig. 38.18). The needle is advanced in a caudal to cranial direction with LA dissecting the iliacus muscle from the FI in a cranial spread.[103-105] The S-FICB has been reported to have better, more reliable ON blockade compared to the traditional I-FICB,[106] likely from a more consistent cranial spread.[103] The S-FICB approach also appears to provide a superior blockade of the FN territory compared to the traditional I-FICB approach.[103]

For the I-FICB approach, the probe should be placed in transverse orientation caudal to the IL in the inguinal crease to visualize the iliac and sartorius muscles, FI, FN, and femoral vessels. The probe is moved laterally in the crease along the FI until the iliac and sartorius muscles intersect (Fig. 38.19). In a lateral to medial trajectory, the needle is advanced into that intersection deep to the FI so the LA dissects the FI from the muscle and spreads to the FN medially and LFCN laterally. Obturator nerve blockade with this distal injection has been unreliable,[103,106] which may be due to the distance between the ON and the FN and LFCN, or potentially from variable innervation by the ON and overlapping FN contribution.[103,106]

A volume of 20-40 mL of 0.25%-0.5% long-acting LA may be injected.[103-106] Maximum safe doses should be observed.

Specific Risks and Considerations: The FIB is considered a low-risk block.

Femoral nerve block

Indication: The femoral nerve block (FNB) is used for anterior thigh and knee analgesia. It may be combined with a sciatic nerve block (SNB) to provide below-the-knee blockade. It may be combined with sciatic, LFCN, and ON blocks for entire lower extremity anesthesia.

Relevant Anatomy: The L2-L4 spinal nerves join at the LP and give rise to the femoral nerve (FN), which descends into the inguinal region deep to the FI between the iliac muscle and PMM.[107] The FN enters the base of the femoral triangle upon crossing the IL and gives off several branches. One branch, the saphenous nerve, passes beyond the distal apex of the triangle into the adductor canal.[108] The femoral triangle is bound by the IL superiorly, sartorius muscle laterally, and adductor longus muscle medially.[108] The apex of the triangle is located at the intersection between the medial border of the sartorius muscle and medial border of the adductor longus muscle.[108] The FNB is performed at the inguinal crease. Under US imaging, the FN appears as a flat hyperechoic oval immediately lateral to the femoral artery, superficial to the iliopsoas muscle, and deep to the FI.

Positioning and Approach: With the patient supine, a high-frequency probe should be placed in the transverse orientation at the inguinal crease (see Fig. 38.19). The femoral artery should be visualized prior to its bifurcation. The femoral vein is medial, and the FN is lateral to the artery. The fascia lata extends laterally to medially above the FN and vessels, with the deeper FI overlying the FN. In a lateral to medial needle approach, LA should be deposited around the FN. Alternatively, a more lateral needle target (ie, at the groove between the iliac muscle and PMM) that is deep to the FI may offer effective blockade with a potentially safer needle-to-nerve distance.[107,109] A volume of 20 mL of 0.5% long-acting LA may be injected.

Specific Risks and Considerations:

- Quadricep muscle weakness
- Due to the nonselective sensorimotor blockade, the risks from quadricep muscle (rectus femoris and vasti muscles) weakness include prolonged reduced quadricep strength, falls, and anterior cruciate ligament reinjury have been studied by both anesthesiologists and orthopedic surgeons without achieving consensus. The adductor canal block has been compared with FNB as a potential motor-sparing alternative with similar efficacy; however, lack of standardization in evaluating motor strength and functional measures have made definitive conclusions difficult.[110,111] Compared to the FNB, the adductor canal block may have a lower fall risk in the perioperative period[112] and appears to preserve strength in the early postoperative period.[111] In contrast, another study has not found significant differences in quadricep strength between the two blocks after anterior cruciate ligament surgery.[113] FNB may increase the risk of graft rupture within the first year after anterior cruciate ligament reconstruction.[114]

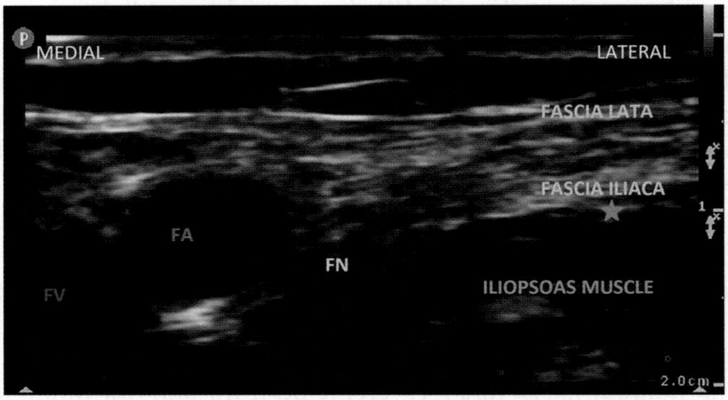

FIGURE 38.19 Fascia iliaca nerve block (infrainguinal) and femoral nerve block. The femoral vein, artery, and nerve may be visualized from medial to lateral. The femoral nerve is deep to the fascia iliaca that covers the iliopsoas muscle. The needle target of the infrainguinal fascia iliaca block (*green star*) is deep to the fascia iliaca layer to achieve its dissection from the muscle below. The needle target for the femoral nerve block is deep to the fascia iliaca near the femoral nerve, which is lateral to the femoral artery. FV, femoral vein; FA, femoral artery; FN, femoral nerve.

Adductor canal (saphenous) nerve block

Indication: The adductor canal block (ACB) of the saphenous nerve at the is performed for knee analgesia and anesthesia along the medial aspect of the lower extremity below the knee. The ACB may be preferable to the FNB if avoidance of motor blockade is desired. The ACB may be combined with other locoregional techniques for analgesia after knee surgery or combined with an SNB for lower extremity anesthesia below the knee.

Relevant Anatomy: The FN, its branches, and associated vessels travel caudally through the femoral triangle toward the distal apex and enter the adductor canal (AC; subsartorial canal, Hunter canal) as the saphenous nerve (SN). The AC ends at the adductor hiatus, which is the entry to the popliteal fossa. The SN exits the AC to continue terminally along the medial aspect of the lower extremity to the foot. While the AC is generally thought to be located at the middle third of the thigh, there is still much controversy regarding its exact anatomical location and the effects of LA injection within anatomically contiguous canals (ie, femoral triangle to AC to popliteal fossa).[115] Anatomical accuracy when performing an ACB may affect the success of knee analgesia[108] as well as potentially cause unintentional motor blockade.[115]

The AC is bound by the fascia of the vastus medialis muscle anterolaterally, fascia of the adductor longus and magnus muscles posteromedially, and the sartorius muscle and vastoadductor membrane (VAM) superiorly.[108] Under US imaging at the mid-AC, the superficial femoral artery (SFA) and vein are visible deep to the sartorius muscle, and the vastus medialis muscle lateral to the vessels and deep to the sartorius muscle. The SN is usually located deep to the sartorius muscle and its underlying VAM, and immediately superior or lateral to the SFA. The SN may be difficult to visualize.

Positioning and Approach: The patient should be positioned supine with the block-side hip externally rotated. A linear probe should be placed in transverse orientation at the medial aspect of the midthigh. The SFA should be visible deep to the sartorius muscle. Both adductor magnus and longus muscles should be seen medial to the SFA and deep to the middle of the sartorius muscle (Fig. 38.20). The needle should be advanced lateral

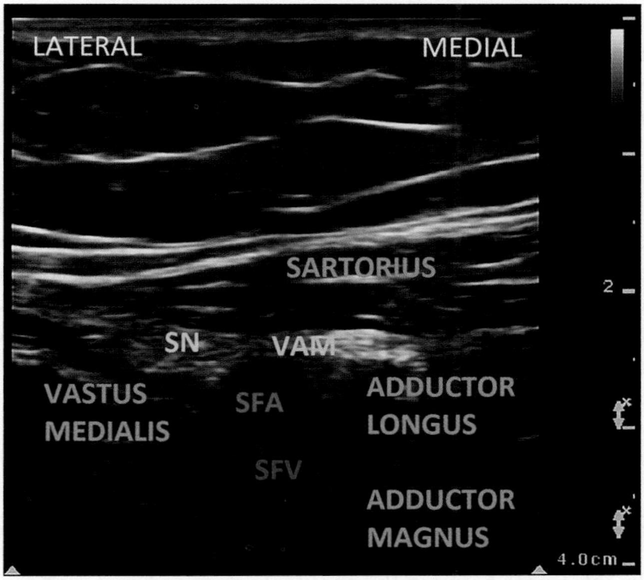

FIGURE 38.20 Adductor canal block. The superficial femoral artery and vein and saphenous nerve travel within the adductor canal. The adductor canal is bound superiorly by the sartorius muscle and underlying vastoadductor membrane, anterolaterally by the vastus medialis muscle, and posteromedially by the adductor longus and magnus muscles. The saphenous nerve is deep to the sartorius muscle and immediately superior or lateral to the SFA. SN, saphenous nerve; SFA, superficial femoral artery; SFV, superficial femoral vein; VAM, vastoadductor membrane.

to medial toward the lateral side of the SFA, deep to the VAM. A volume of 10-20 mL of 0.5% long-acting LA may be injected.

Specific Risks and Considerations:

- Inadequate analgesia
- FN branches (SN, medial vastus nerve, and medial femoral cutaneous nerve) are contained within the femoral triangle. Distal to the apex of the femoral triangle, the medial vastus nerve travels separately from the AC and the medial femoral cutaneous nerve courses between the VAM and sartorius muscle outside the AC.[108] The medial vastus nerve is responsible for the anteromedial aspect of the knee[108]; therefore, a more proximal ACB (or femoral triangle block) would provide better analgesia to the knee.[108,116] Abdallah et al. reported better analgesia with proximal, rather than distal, AC injections.[117]
- Motor weakness
- Based on anatomical models, motor weakness may occur if the femoral triangle nerves were blocked from a too proximal ACB (arguably a femoral triangle block) or by proximal LA spread from the ACB.[108] Medial vastus nerve blockade may cause vastus medialis weakness.[118] However, these concerns may not be clinically relevant as quadriceps strength was similar regardless of ACB injection site proximity[117] and larger LA volume injection did not appear to have a statistically significant effect on quadriceps strength.[119]

Lateral femoral cutaneous nerve block

Indication: The LFCN block is indicated for the lateral upper thigh and hip analgesia. It may be combined with the FN, ON, and SNBs for lower extremity anesthesia.

Relevant Anatomy: The LFCN is a sensory nerve that originates from the L2 to L3 spinal nerves, across the iliac muscle toward the ASIS. It pierces the IL medial to the ASIS and travels superficially to the sartorius muscle prior to splitting into several branches that innervate the lateral and anterolateral thigh. Variations include a branch crossing over the ASIS into the proximal thigh or over the iliac crest posterior to the ASIS.[120,121] The nerve appears as a small, flat hyperechoic structure medial to the sartorius between the fascia lata and FI.[121] A newer US view visualizes the nerve more distally within a fat-filled flat tunnel between the sartorius and tensor fasciae latae muscles and inferiorly bound by the rectus femoris muscle.[120]

Positioning and Approach: The patient should be in supine position with a linear US probe placed in transverse orientation inferomedial to the ASIS. The nerve may be visualized superficially between the fascia lata and FI, medial to the sartorius muscle.[121] The needle is advanced lateral to medial to dissect the plane between the two fasciae (Fig. 38.21). Alternatively, the US probe may be placed in transverse orientation medial to the ASIS and parallel to the IL to visualize the LFCN between the IL and sartorius muscle.[122]

The approach by Nielsen et al. similarly places a linear US probe in transverse orientation 10 cm distal to the ASIS at the proximal anterolateral thigh. The sartorius and tensor fasciae latae muscles are identified with the LFCN within the fat-filled flat tunnel. The needle is dynamically guided proximally within the tunnel in an out-of-plane trajectory.[120] A volume of 10 mL of 0.25% bupivacaine was reported.[120]

Specific Risks and Considerations: A higher success rate is associated with USG.[120]

IPACK (interspace between the popliteal artery and posterior capsule of the knee)

Indication: The interspace between the popliteal artery and posterior capsule of the knee (IPACK) injection is a relatively new motor-sparing block that is indicated for posterior knee analgesia. It may be combined with other PNB (ie, FNB, ACB) or peri-

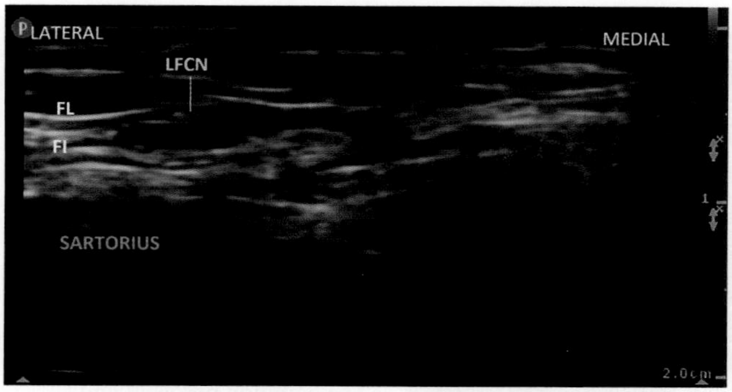

FIGURE 38.21 Lateral femoral cutaneous nerve block. The fasciae lata and iliaca are visualized inferomedial to the anterior superior iliac spine and superior to the sartorius muscle. The lateral femoral cutaneous nerve is between the two fascial layers. FL, fascia lata; FI, fascia iliaca; LFCN, lateral femoral cutaneous nerve.

articular injection for more complete knee analgesia, particularly after total knee arthroplasty.

Relevant Anatomy: While the anterior knee capsule may be relieved with FNB, femoral triangle block, or ACB, the posterior knee capsule is primarily innervated by the tibial nerve branches[123] and is a frequent source of pain.[124] Sciatic nerve or selective tibial blockade comes with associated motor weakness, which impedes ambulation during recovery.[125] The IPACK injection is thought to target the terminal sensory branches of the sciatic and posterior division of the ON that are responsible for posterior knee innervation, as well as some of the anterior knee supply.[126] Pertinent US landmarks include the popliteal vessels, femoral condyle and shaft with the proximal injection, and the popliteal vessels and the femoral condyle with the distal injection.

Positioning and Approach: Two approaches have been primarily described in literature to date. The proximal approach is performed at the anteromedial thigh inferior to the origin of the popliteal artery at the adductor hiatus and superior to the femoral condyles.[126,127] The patient should be in supine position with the block-side hip externally rotated. A high-frequency US probe should be placed in transverse orientation at the posteromedial aspect of the femur approximately one fingerbreadth above the base of the patella. The popliteal vessels are lateral to the femoral condyle. A needle is advanced in an anteromedial to posterolateral direction and LA is injected posterior to the femoral condyle toward the distal femoral shaft.[126,127] Caution to avoid injury to the saphenous nerve is warranted,[128] though the risk may be relatively low.[129]

When performing the distal approach, the patient should be positioned prone. A high-frequency US probe should be placed in transverse orientation at the popliteal crease. Once the popliteal vessels and discontinuous femoral condyles are visualized, the probe is moved cranially until the condyles transition into the continuous femoral shaft. The needle is advanced in a medial to lateral trajectory, and LA is injected at the femur (Fig. 38.22). The tibial (TN) and common peroneal nerves (CPN) should be identified to avoid injury. Kampitak et al. reported better preservation of tibial and common peroneal motor function and control of posterior knee pain after a total knee arthroplasty with the distal compared to the proximal approach.[124]

Volumes ranging from 10 to 30 mL of 0.25% long-acting LA has been reported; however, as studies are ongoing, better guidance on volume and dosing may be clarified in the future.

Specific Risks and Considerations:

- Unintentional motor blockade
- Cadaveric studies have demonstrated injectate spread to the TN and CPN with both proximal and distal injection techniques. This may cause motor blockade (eg, foot drop) that could impair ambulation.[126]

Further studies are needed to elucidate the anatomy, optimal volume and dose, technique, and complications of this new block.

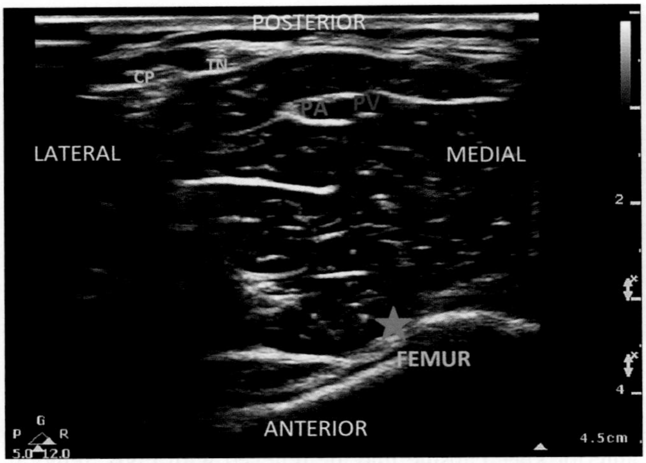

FIGURE 38.22 IPACK block (distal approach). The popliteal vessels and the continuous femoral shaft may be visualized. The needle target (*green star*) is the posterior aspect of the femur. The common peroneal and tibial nerves are identified. CP, common peroneal nerve; TN, tibial nerve; PA, popliteal artery; PV, popliteal vein.

Sciatic nerve block

Indication: The SNB may be used to provide anesthesia of the lower extremity posterior compartment or below the knee with exception of the medial aspect. It is often combined with another block, commonly an LPB, FNB, or ACB, to provide anterior coverage. A proximal SNB with an LPB or S-FICB can provide lower extremity blockade, and an FN or ACB with a popliteal SNB can provide coverage below the knee.

Relevant Anatomy: The L4-S3 ventral spinal nerves form the sciatic nerve (ScN), a composite of the TN and CPN within a common sheath.[130] From the lumbosacral plexus, it exits the pelvis, courses distally in the posterior thigh to innervate the hamstring muscles, prior to separating into its two component nerves near the popliteal fossa and supply the remainder of the lower extremity with exception of the medial SN territory.[130]

After leaving the pelvis, the ScN descends between the ischial tuberosity (IT) medially and greater trochanter (GT) laterally. At this level, the gluteus maximus muscle (GMM) is posterior and the quadratus femoris muscle (QFM) is anterior to the nerve. Under US imaging, the hyperechoic, triangular ScN[131] is sandwiched between the GMM and QFM in the anteroposterior plane and between the acoustic shadows of the GT and IT in the transverse plane. The ScN is contained within a hypoechoic subgluteal space of varying dimensions among individuals[131] between the two muscles.

At the midfemur, the ScN is medial and deep to the bone. The ScN appears as a hyperechoic, elliptical structure between the adductor magnus muscle anteriorly and biceps femoris muscle posteriorly under US imaging.[131]

At the popliteal fossa, the ScN separates into the TN and CPN; however, its bifurcation point has much variation. Bifurcation at 4.4-6.0 cm[132,133] above the popliteal crease has been reported; however, cadaveric dissections have found a high incidence of bifurcation at the lower part of the posterior thigh compartment or proximal to its exit from the gluteal region.[134] The hyperechoic ScN at the popliteal fossa is rounder than its proximal appearance under US imaging.[133] The ScN lies superficial to the popliteal vessels, between the biceps femoris muscle laterally and semimembranosus and semitendinosus muscles medially.

Positioning and Approach: The patient position depends on the selected approach. A high-frequency probe may be used for more superficial approaches, such as at the popliteal fossa. For deeper views, such as proximal sciatic approaches (eg, parasacral, transgluteal, subgluteal, infragluteal), a low-frequency probe may be preferred. Not all approaches will be discussed.

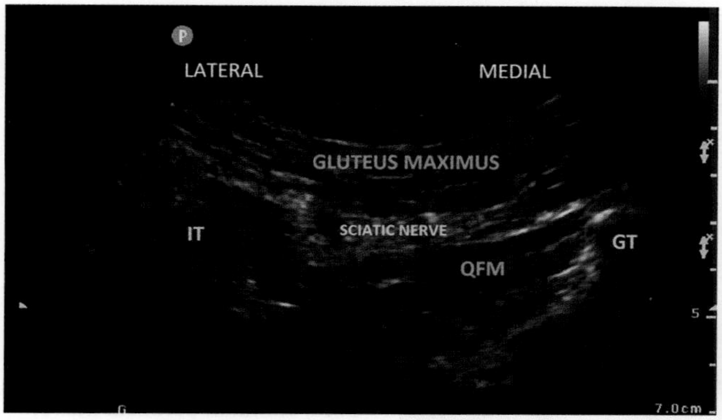

FIGURE 38.23 Posterior sciatic block (transgluteal). The sciatic nerve is identified between the gluteus maximus muscle superiorly and quadratus femoris muscle inferiorly within the subgluteal space. It is midway between the acoustic shadows created by the ischial tuberosity laterally and greater trochanter medially. IT, ischial tuberosity; QFM, quadratus femoris muscle; GT, greater trochanter.

When performing the posterior approach at the IT and GT (may be referred to as transgluteal[135] or subgluteal space[136]), the patient may be positioned prone or lateral with hip and knees flexed. The curvilinear probe is placed in transverse orientation at the midpoint of a line connecting the IT and GT. Once the ScN is identified, a needle is advanced in a lateral to medial direction into the subgluteal space where the nerve resides[136] (Fig. 38.23). A volume of 20-30 mL of 0.25%-0.5% long-acting LA may be injected.[135-137]

An anterior approach at the proximal to midfemur may be favored, particularly for patients who have difficulties with positioning. It also reduces repositioning time if either FNB or ACB is also performed; however, switching from a low-frequency to high-frequency probe may be time-consuming.[138] In supine position with the block leg externally rotated and knee flexed, the curvilinear probe is placed in transverse orientation over the anteromedial thigh at the level of the lesser trochanter.[137] The hyperechoic ScN is visualized posterolateral to the adductor magnus muscle, medial to the acoustic shadow of the lesser trochanter, and anterior to the GMM. The needle is advanced medial or lateral to the probe in a steep trajectory to target the ScN.[137,138] The high angulation to the skin may create technical challenges. An alternative entry point at the medial thigh that is perpendicular to the probe may be performed.[138] The proximity to vascular structures (eg, femoral vessels and branches) at this level may cause preference toward a more distal anterior approach at the midthigh level. At the medial thigh ~10 cm distal to the inguinal crease, the probe is moved posteromedially to visualize the hyperechoic ScN between the adductor magnus and hamstring muscles[139] and the needle is advanced in a anteromedial to posterolateral trajectory. A volume of 20 mL of 0.25%-0.5% long-acting LA may be injected.[135,137,139]

The patient may be placed prone, lateral, or supine with the lower extremity in a raised position and knee slightly flexed to access the popliteal fossa. A linear probe may be placed in transverse orientation at the popliteal crease. The TN and CPN may be identified posterior and posterolateral to the popliteal artery, respectively, and traced proximally to their bifurcation point from the ScN, commonly at the apex of the fossa (Fig. 38.24). There is debate whether injection should be pre- or postbifurcation, though the latter location appears to have a faster onset of anesthesia.[140-142] A volume of 10-30 mL of 0.5% long-acting LA may be injected.[143]

Specific Risks and Considerations:

- Incomplete popliteal blockade due to the posterior femoral cutaneous nerve (PFCN)
- The PFCN forms from the sacral plexus, exits with the ScN through the infrapiriform foramen prior to separating from the ScN at the gluteal region. The PFCN descends the posterior thigh deep to the fascia lata but superficial to the biceps femoris muscle while releasing cutaneous branches.[144] The PFCN territory was thought to be limited to the

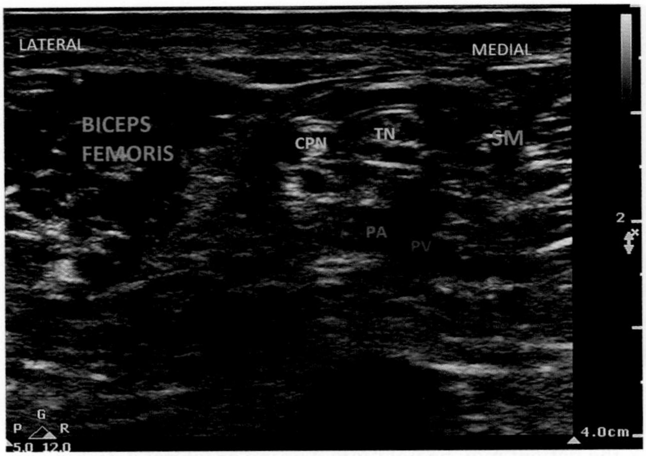

FIGURE 38.24 Popliteal block. The TN and CPN may be identified posterior to the popliteal artery between the biceps femoris muscle laterally and semimembranosus muscle medially. At their bifurcation point, they may be visualized sharing a common sheath prior to separating completely. CPN, common peroneal nerve; TN, tibial nerve; PA, popliteal artery; PV, popliteal vein; SM, semimembranosus muscle.

upper thigh with termination no further than the popliteal fossa. However, Feigl et al. published anatomical studies finding PFCN termination distal to the popliteal fossa in 44.6% of the specimens, of which nearly 20% ended within 10 cm of the medial malleolus.[144] The clinical implication is that the PFCN requires separate blockade for complete below the knee anesthesia.[144]

- Susceptibility for neural injury
- The proximal ScN appears to have a higher risk for injury compared to distal locations due to the relatively higher neural to nonneural content.[133] Mid- and subgluteal areas had a higher (2:1) ratio vs the midfemoral and popliteal region (1:1).[133]

Conclusion

Regional anesthesiology is a dynamic and evolving field that combines *in vivo* human anatomic understanding with ultrasound technology to provide targeted anesthesia and analgesia. When performed safely, the versatility and utility of peripheral nerve blockade as a nonopioid analgesic is an essential and invaluable component to acute pain management.

REFERENCES

1. Gan TJ. Poorly controlled postoperative pain: prevalence, consequences, and prevention. *J Pain Res.* 2017;10:2287-2298. doi:10.2147/JPR.S144066
2. Malchow RJ, Gupta RK, Shi Y, Shotwell MS, Jaeger LM, Bowens C. Comprehensive analysis of 13,897 consecutive regional anesthetics at an ambulatory surgery center. *Pain Med.* 2018;19(2):368-384. doi:10.1093/pm/pnx045
3. Gan TJ, Habib AS, Miller TE, White W, Apfelbaum JL. Incidence, patient satisfaction, and perceptions of post-surgical pain: results from a US national survey. *Curr Med Res Opin.* 2014;30(1):149-160. doi:10.1185/03007995.2013.860019
4. Vadhanan P, Tripaty DK, Adinarayanan S. Physiological and pharmacologic aspects of peripheral nerve blocks. *J Anaesthesiol Clin Pharmacol.* 2015;31(3):384-393. doi:10.4103/0970-9185.161679
5. Brull R, Hadzic A, Reina MA, Barrington MJ. Pathophysiology and etiology of nerve injury following peripheral nerve blockade. *Reg Anesth Pain Med.* 2015;40(5):479-490. doi:10.1097/AAP.0000000000000125
6. Neal JM, Barrington MJ, Brull R, et al. The Second ASRA Practice Advisory on neurologic complications associated with regional anesthesia and pain medicine: executive summary 2015. *Reg Anesth Pain Med.* 2015;40(5):401-430. doi:10.1097/AAP.0000000000000286
7. Jeng CL, Torrillo TM, Rosenblatt MA. Complications of peripheral nerve blocks. *Br J Anaesth.* 2010;105(suppl 1):i97-i107. doi:10.1093/bja/aeq273
8. Neal JM, Barrington MJ, Fettiplace MR, et al. The Third American Society of Regional Anesthesia and Pain Medicine Practice Advisory on local anesthetic systemic toxicity: executive summary 2017. *Reg Anesth Pain Med.* 2018;43(2):113-123. doi:10.1097/AAP.0000000000000720

9. Sites BD, Barrington MJ, Davis M. Using an international clinical registry of regional anesthesia to identify targets for quality improvement. *Reg Anesth Pain Med.* 2014;39(6):487-495. doi:10.1097/AAP.0000000000000162.
10. Helander EM, Kaye AJ, Eng MR, et al. Regional nerve blocks-best practice strategies for reduction in complications and comprehensive review. *Curr Pain Headache Rep.* 2019;23(6):43. doi:10.1007/s11916-019-0782-0
11. Horlocker TT, Vandermeulen E, Kopp SL, et al. Regional anesthesia in the patient receiving antithrombotic or thrombolytic therapy: American Society of Regional Anesthesia and Pain Medicine Evidence-Based Guidelines (Fourth Edition). *Reg Anesth Pain Med.* 2018;43(3):263-309. doi: 10.1097/AAP.0000000000000763
12. Gadsden J, McCally C, Hadzic A. Monitoring during peripheral nerve blockade. *Curr Opin Anaesthesiol.* 2010;23(5):656-661. doi:10.1097/ACO.0b013e32833d4f99
13. Tucker MS, Nielsen KC, Steele SM. Nerve block induction rooms—physical plant setup, monitoring equipment, block cart, and resuscitation cart. *Int Anesthesiol Clin.* 2005;43(3):55-68. doi:10.1097/01.aia.0000166189.91190.7d
14. Lavonas EJ, Drennan IR, Gabrielli A, et al. Part 10: special circumstances of resuscitation: 2015 American Heart Association guidelines update for cardiopulmonary resuscitation and emergency cardiovascular care. *Circulation.* 2015;132(suppl 2):S501-S518. https://www.ahajournals.org/doi/pdf/10.1161/cir.0000000000000264
15. Neal JM, Woodward CM, Harrison TK. The American Society of Regional Anesthesia and Pain Medicine checklist for managing local anesthetic systemic toxicity: 2017 version. *Reg Anesth Pain Med.* 2018;43:150-153.
16. Salinas FV. Evidence basis for ultrasound guidance for lower-extremity peripheral nerve block: update 2016. *Reg Anesth Pain Med.* 2016;41(2):261-274. doi:10.1097/AAP.0000000000000336
17. Bomberg H, Wetjen L, Wagenpfeil S, et al. Risks and benefits of ultrasound, nerve stimulation, and their combination for guiding peripheral nerve blocks: a retrospective registry analysis. *Anesth Analg.* 2018;127(4):1035-1043. doi:10.1213/ANE.0000000000003480
18. Barrington MJ, Kluger R. Ultrasound guidance reduces the risk of local anesthetic systemic toxicity following peripheral nerve blockade. *Reg Anesth Pain Med.* 2013;38(4):289-299. doi:10.1097/AAP.0b013e318292669b
19. Neal JM. Ultrasound-guided regional anesthesia and patient safety: update of an evidence-based analysis. *Reg Anesth Pain Med.* 2016;41(2):195-204. doi:10.1097/AAP.0000000000000295
20. Hadzic A, Sala-Blanch X, Xu D. Ultrasound guidance may reduce but not eliminate complications of peripheral nerve blocks. *Anesthesiology.* 2008;108(4):557-558. doi:10.1097/ALN.0b013e318168efa1
21. Wilson E. *Informed Consent and the Postoperative Pain Control Conundrum—American Society of Regional Anesthesia and Pain Medicine.* [online] ASRA.com. Accessed August 20, 2020. https://www.asra.com/asra-news/article/86/informed-consent-and-the-postoperative-p
22. Kim JS, Ko JS, Bang S, Kim H, Lee SY. Cervical plexus block. *Korean J Anesthesiol.* 2018;71(4):274-288. doi:10.4097/kja.d.18.00143
23. Ramachandran SK, Picton P, Shanks A, Dorje P, Pandit JJ. Comparison of intermediate vs subcutaneous cervical plexus block for carotid endarterectomy. *Br J Anaesth.* 2011;107(2):157-163. doi:10.1093/bja/aer118
24. Pandit JJ, Satya-Krishna R, Gration P. Superficial or deep cervical plexus block for carotid endarterectomy: a systematic review of complications. *Br J Anaesth.* 2007;99(2):159-169. doi:10.1093/bja/aem160
25. Franco CD, Williams JM. Ultrasound-guided interscalene block: reevaluation of the "Stoplight" sign and clinical implications. *Reg Anesth Pain Med.* 2016;41(4):452-459. doi:10.1097/AAP.0000000000000407
26. Palhais N, Brull R, Kern C, et al. Extrafascial injection for interscalene brachial plexus block reduces respiratory complications compared with a conventional intrafascial injection: a randomized, controlled, double-blind trial. *Br J Anaesth.* 2016;116(4):531-537. doi:10.1093/bja/aew028
27. Urmey WF, Talts KH, Sharrock NE. One hundred percent incidence of hemidiaphragmatic paresis associated with interscalene brachial plexus anesthesia as diagnosed by ultrasonography. *Anesth Analg.* 1991;72(4):498-503. doi:10.1213/00000539-199104000-00014
28. Sinha SK, Abrams JH, Barnett JT, et al. Decreasing the local anesthetic volume from 20 to 10 mL for ultrasound-guided interscalene block at the cricoid level does not reduce the incidence of hemidiaphragmatic paresis. *Reg Anesth Pain Med.* 2011;36(1):17-20. doi:10.1097/aap.0b013e3182030648
29. Saporito A. Dorsal scapular nerve injury: a complication of ultrasound-guided interscalene block. *Br J Anaesth.* 2013;111(5):840-841. doi:10.1093/bja/aet358
30. Seltzer JL. Hoarseness and Horner's syndrome after interscalene brachial plexus block. *Anesth Analg.* 1977;56(4):585-586. doi:10.1213/00000539-197707000-00033
31. Feigl GC, Litz RJ, Marhofer P. Anatomy of the brachial plexus and its implications for daily clinical practice: regional anesthesia is applied anatomy. *Reg Anesth Pain Med.* 2020;45(8):620-627. doi:10.1136/rapm-2020-101435
32. Park SK, Lee SY, Kim WH, Park HS, Lim YJ, Bahk JH. Comparison of supraclavicular and infraclavicular brachial plexus block: a systemic review of randomized controlled trials. *Anesth Analg.* 2017;124(2):636-644. doi:10.1213/ANE.0000000000001713

33. Bao X, Huang J, Feng H, et al. Effect of local anesthetic volume (20 mL vs 30 mL ropivacaine) on electromyography of the diaphragm and pulmonary function after ultrasound-guided supraclavicular brachial plexus block: a randomized controlled trial. *Reg Anesth Pain Med.* 2019;44(1):69-75. doi:10.1136/rapm-2018-000014
34. Rana MV, Desai R, Tran L, Davis D. Perioperative pain control in the ambulatory setting. *Curr Pain Headache Rep.* 2016;20(3):18. doi:10.1007/s11916-016-0550-3
35. Kumar A, Kumar A, Sinha C, Sawhney C, Kumar R, Bhoi D. Topographic sonoanatomy of infraclavicular brachial plexus: variability and correlation with anthropometry. *Anesth Essays Res.* 2018;12(4):814-818. doi:10.4103/aer.AER_140_18
36. Auyong DB, Gonzales J, Benonis JG. The Houdini clavicle: arm abduction and needle insertion site adjustment improves needle visibility for the infraclavicular nerve block. *Reg Anesth Pain Med.* 2010;35(4):403-404. doi:10.1097/AAP.0b013e3181e66ee9
37. Li JW, Songthamwat B, Samy W, Sala-Blanch X, Karmakar MK. Ultrasound-guided costoclavicular brachial plexus block: sonoanatomy, technique, and block dynamics. *Reg Anesth Pain Med.* 2017;42(2):233-240. doi:10.1097/AAP.0000000000000566
38. Karmakar MK, Sala-Blanch X, Songthamwat B, Tsui BC. Benefits of the costoclavicular space for ultrasound-guided infraclavicular brachial plexus block: description of a costoclavicular approach. *Reg Anesth Pain Med.* 2015;40(3):287-288. doi:10.1097/AAP.0000000000000232
39. Songthamwat B, Karmakar MK, Li JW, Samy W, Mok LYH. Ultrasound-guided infraclavicular brachial plexus block: prospective randomized comparison of the lateral sagittal and costoclavicular approach. *Reg Anesth Pain Med.* 2018;43(8):825-831. doi:10.1097/AAP.0000000000000822
40. Charbonneau J, Fréchette Y, Sansoucy Y, Echave P. The ultrasound-guided retroclavicular block: a prospective feasibility study. *Reg Anesth Pain Med.* 2015;40(5):605-609. doi:10.1097/AAP.0000000000000284
41. Sinha C, Kumar N, Kumar A, Kumar A, Kumar A. Comparative evaluation of two approaches of infraclavicular brachial plexus block for upper-limb surgeries. *Saudi J Anaesth.* 2019;13(1):35-39. doi:10.4103/sja.SJA_737_17
42. Blanco AFG, Laferrière-Langlois P, Jessop D, et al. Retroclavicular vs Infraclavicular block for brachial plexus anesthesia: a multi-centric randomized trial. *BMC Anesthesiol.* 2019;19(1):193. doi:10.1186/s12871-019-0868-6
43. Han JH, Kim YJ, Kim JH, Kim DY, Lee GY, Kim CH. Topographic pattern of the brachial plexus at the axillary fossa through real-time ultrasonography in Koreans. *Korean J Anesthesiol.* 2014;67(5):310-316. doi:10.4097/kjae.2014.67.5.310
44. Cho S, Kim YJ, Kim JH, Baik HJ. Double-injection perivascular ultrasound-guided axillary brachial plexus block according to needle positioning: 12 versus 6 o'clock position of the axillary artery. *Korean J Anesthesiol.* 2014;66(2):112-119. doi:10.4097/kjae.2014.66.2.112
45. Price DJ. The shoulder block: a new alternative to interscalene brachial plexus blockade for the control of postoperative shoulder pain. *Anaesth Intensive Care.* 2007;35(4):575-581. doi:10.1177/0310057X0703500418
46. Dhir S, Sondekoppam RV, Sharma R, Ganapathy S, Athwal GS. A comparison of combined suprascapular and axillary nerve blocks to interscalene nerve block for analgesia in arthroscopic shoulder surgery: an equivalence study. *Reg Anesth Pain Med.* 2016;41(5):564-571. doi:10.1097/AAP.0000000000000436
47. Siegenthaler A, Moriggl B, Mlekusch S, et al. Ultrasound-guided suprascapular nerve block, description of a novel supraclavicular approach. *Reg Anesth Pain Med.* 2012;37(3):325-328. doi:10.1097/AAP.0b013e3182409168
48. Auyong DB, Hanson NA, Joseph RS, Schmidt BE, Slee AE, Yuan SC. Comparison of anterior suprascapular, supraclavicular, and interscalene nerve block approaches for major outpatient arthroscopic shoulder surgery: a randomized, double-blind, noninferiority trial. *Anesthesiology.* 2018;129(1):47-57. doi:10.1097/ALN.0000000000002208
49. Rothe C, Asghar S, Andersen HL, Christensen JK, Lange KH. Ultrasound-guided block of the axillary nerve: a volunteer study of a new method. *Acta Anaesthesiol Scand.* 2011;55(5):565-570. doi:10.1111/j.1399-6576.2011.02420.x
50. Ferré F, Pommier M, Laumonerie P, et al. Hemidiaphragmatic paralysis following ultrasound-guided anterior vs. posterior suprascapular nerve block: a double-blind, randomised control trial. *Anaesthesia.* 2020;75(4):499-508. doi:10.1111/anae.14978
51. Moustafa MA, Kandeel AA. Randomized comparative study between two different techniques of intercostobrachial nerve block together with brachial plexus block during superficialization of arteriovenous fistula. *J Anesth.* 2018;32(5):725-730. doi:10.1007/s00540-018-2547-z
52. Krediet AC, Moayeri N, van Geffen GJ, et al. Different approaches to ultrasound-guided thoracic paravertebral block: an illustrated review. *Anesthesiology.* 2015;123(2):459-474. doi:10.1097/ALN.0000000000000747
53. Seidel R, Wree A, Schulze M. Thoracic-paravertebral blocks: comparative anatomical study with different injection techniques and volumes. *Reg Anesth Pain Med.* 2020;45(2):102-106. doi:10.1136/rapm-2019-100896
54. Niesen AD, Jacob AK, Law LA, Sviggum HP, Johnson RL. Complication rate of ultrasound-guided paravertebral block for breast surgery. *Reg Anesth Pain Med.* 2020;45(10):813-817. doi:10.1136/rapm-2020-101402

55. de Leeuw MA, Zuurmond WW, Perez RS. The psoas compartment block for hip surgery: the past, present, and future. *Anesthesiol Res Pract*. 2011;2011:159541. doi:10.1155/2011/159541
56. Awad IT, Duggan EM. Posterior lumbar plexus block: anatomy, approaches, and techniques. *Reg Anesth Pain Med*. 2005;30(2):143-149. doi:10.1016/j.rapm.2004.11.006
57. Sauter AR. The "Shamrock Method"—a new and promising technique for ultrasound guided lumbar plexus blocks. *Br J Anaesth*. 2013;111(suppl). https://doi.org/10.1093/bja/el_9814
58. Karmakar MK, Ho AM, Li X, Kwok WH, Tsang K, Ngan Kee WD. Ultrasound-guided lumbar plexus block through the acoustic window of the lumbar ultrasound trident. *Br J Anaesth*. 2008;100(4):533-537. doi:10.1093/bja/aen026
59. Strid JMC, Sauter AR, Ullensvang K, et al. Ultrasound-guided lumbar plexus block in volunteers; a randomized controlled trial. *Br J Anaesth*. 2017;118(3):430-438. doi:10.1093/bja/aew464
60. Sauter AR, Ullensvang K, Niemi G, et al. The Shamrock lumbar plexus block: a dose-finding study. *Eur J Anaesthesiol*. 2015;32(11):764-770. doi:10.1097/EJA.0000000000000265
61. Hübler M, Planitz MC, Vicent O. Early pharmacokinetic of ropivacaine without epinephrine after injection into the psoas compartment. *Br J Anaesth*. 2015;114(1):130-135. doi:10.1093/bja/aeu363
62. Costache I, Pawa A, Abdallah FW. Paravertebral by proxy—time to redefine the paravertebral block. *Anaesthesia*. 2018;73(10):1185-1188. doi:10.1111/anae.14348
63. Onishi E, Toda N, Kameyama Y, Yamauchi M. Comparison of clinical efficacy and anatomical investigation between retrolaminar block and erector spinae plane block. *Biomed Res Int*. 2019;2019:2578396. doi:10.1155/2019/2578396
64. Adhikary SD, Bernard S, Lopez H, Chin KJ. Erector spinae plane block versus retrolaminar block: a magnetic resonance imaging and anatomical study. *Reg Anesth Pain Med*. 2018;43(7):756-762. doi:10.1097/AAP.0000000000000798
65. Schwartzmann A, Peng P, Maciel MA, Forero M. Mechanism of the erector spinae plane block: insights from a magnetic resonance imaging study. *Can J Anaesth*. 2018;65(10):1165-1166. doi:10.1007/s12630-018-1187-y
66. De Cassai A, Tonetti T. Local anesthetic spread during erector spinae plane block. *J Clin Anesth*. 2018;48:60-61. doi:10.1016/j.jclinane.2018.05.003
67. Adhikary SD, Liu WM, Fuller E, Cruz-Eng H, Chin KJ. The effect of erector spinae plane block on respiratory and analgesic outcomes in multiple rib fractures: a retrospective cohort study. *Anaesthesia*. 2019;74(5):585-593. doi:10.1111/anae.14579
68. Pak A, Singh P. Epidural-like effects with bilateral erector spinae plane catheters after abdominal surgery: a case report. *A A Pract*. 2020;14(5):137-139. doi:10.1213/XAA.0000000000001164
69. Grape S, Jaunin E, El-Boghdadly K, Chan V, Albrecht E. Analgesic efficacy of PECS and serratus plane blocks after breast surgery: a systematic review, meta-analysis and trial sequential analysis. *J Clin Anesth*. 2020;63:109744. doi:10.1016/j.jclinane.2020.109744
70. Liu X, Song T, Xu HY, Chen X, Yin P, Zhang J. The serratus anterior plane block for analgesia after thoracic surgery: a meta-analysis of randomized controlled trails. *Medicine (Baltimore)*. 2020;99(21):e20286. doi:10.1097/MD.0000000000020286
71. Helander EM, Webb MP, Kendrick J, et al. PECS, serratus plane, erector spinae, and paravertebral blocks: a comprehensive review. *Best Pract Res Clin Anaesthesiol*. 2019;33(4):573-581. doi:10.1016/j.bpa.2019.07.003
72. Blanco R. The 'pecs block': a novel technique for providing analgesia after breast surgery. *Anaesthesia*. 2011;66(9):847-848. doi:10.1111/j.1365-2044.2011.06838.x
73. Versyck B, Groen G, van Geffen GJ, Van Houwe P, Bleys RL. The pecs anesthetic blockade: a correlation between magnetic resonance imaging, ultrasound imaging, reconstructed cross-sectional anatomy and cross-sectional histology. *Clin Anat*. 2019;32(3):421-429. doi:10.1002/ca.23333
74. Blanco R, Fajardo M, Parras Maldonado T. Ultrasound description of Pecs II (modified Pecs I): a novel approach to breast surgery. *Rev Esp Anestesiol Reanim*. 2012;59(9):470-475. doi:10.1016/j.redar.2012.07.003
75. Blanco R, Parras T, McDonnell JG, Prats-Galino A. Serratus plane block: a novel ultrasound-guided thoracic wall nerve block. *Anaesthesia*. 2013;68(11):1107-1113. doi:10.1111/anae.12344
76. Mayes J, Davison E, Panahi P, et al. An anatomical evaluation of the serratus anterior plane block. *Anaesthesia*. 2016;71(9):1064-1069. doi:10.1111/anae.13549
77. Kunigo T, Murouchi T, Yamamoto S, Yamakage M. Spread of injectate in ultrasound-guided serratus plane block: a cadaveric study. *JA Clin Rep*. 2018;4(1):10. doi:10.1186/s40981-018-0147-4
78. Pérez MF, Miguel JG, de la Torre PA. A new approach to pectoralis block. *Anaesthesia*. 2013;68(4):430. doi:10.1111/anae.12186
79. Ueshima H, Otake H. Ultrasound-guided pectoral nerves (PECS) block: complications observed in 498 consecutive cases. *J Clin Anesth*. 2017;42:46. doi:10.1016/j.jclinane.2017.08.006
80. Rahiri J, Tuhoe J, Svirskis D, Lightfoot NJ, Lirk PB, Hill AG. Systematic review of the systemic concentrations of local anaesthetic after transversus abdominis plane block and rectus sheath block. *Br J Anaesth*. 2017;118(4):517-526. doi:10.1093/bja/aex005
81. Rozen WM, Tran TM, Ashton MW, Barrington MJ, Ivanusic JJ, Taylor GI. Refining the course of the thoracolumbar nerves: a new understanding of the innervation of the anterior abdominal wall. *Clin Anat*. 2008;21(4):325-333. doi:10.1002/ca.20621

82. Seidel R, Wree A, Schulze M. Does the approach influence the success rate for ultrasound-guided rectus sheath blocks? An anatomical case series. *Local Reg Anesth.* 2017;10:61-65. doi:10.2147/LRA.S133500
83. Le Saint-Grant A, Taylor A, Varsou O, Grant C, Cezayirli E, Bowness J. Arterial anatomy of the anterior abdominal wall: ultrasound evaluation as a real-time guide to percutaneous instrumentation. *Clin Anat.* 2021;34(1):5-10. doi:10.1002/ca.23578
84. Bowness J, Seeley J, Varsou O, et al. Arterial anatomy of the anterior abdominal wall: evidence-based safe sites for instrumentation based on radiological analysis of 100 patients. *Clin Anat.* 2020;33(3):350-354. doi:10.1002/ca.23463
85. Tran DQ, Bravo D, Leurcharusmee P, Neal JM. Transversus abdominis plane block: a narrative review. *Anesthesiology.* 2019;131(5):1166-1190. doi:10.1097/ALN.0000000000002842
86. Hebbard PD. Cutaneous distribution of lateral transversus abdominis plane block. *Reg Anesth Pain Med.* 2017;42(2):267-268. doi:10.1097/AAP.0000000000000514
87. Furuya T, Kato J, Yamamoto Y, Hirose N, Suzuki T. Comparison of dermatomal sensory block following ultrasound-guided transversus abdominis plane block by the lateral and posterior approaches: a randomized controlled trial. *J Anaesthesiol Clin Pharmacol.* 2018;34(2):205-210. doi:10.4103/joacp.JOACP_295_15
88. Lee THW, Barrington MJ, Tran TMN, Wong D, Hebbard PD. Comparison of sensory blockade following posterior and subcostal approaches to ultrasound-guided transversus abdominis plane block. *Anaesth Intensive Care.* 2010;38:452-460.
89. Carney J, Finnerty O, Rauf J, Bergin D, Laffey JG, Mc Donnell JG. Studies on the spread of local anaesthetic solution in transversus abdominis plane blocks. *Anaesthesia.* 2011;66(11):1023-1030. doi:10.1111/j.1365-2044.2011.06855.x
90. Kitayama M, Wada M, Hashimoto H, Kudo T, Takada N, Hirota K. Effects of adding epinephrine on the early systemic absorption kinetics of local anesthetics in abdominal truncal blocks. *J Anesth.* 2014;28(4):631-634. doi:10.1007/s00540-013-1784-4
91. Spence NZ, Olszynski P, Lehan A, Horn JL, Webb CA. Quadratus lumborum catheters for breast reconstruction requiring transverse rectus abdominis myocutaneous flaps. *J Anesth.* 2016;30:506-509.
92. Ueshima H, Otake H. Lower limb amputations performed with anterior quadratus lumborum block and sciatic nerve block. *J Clin Anesth.* 2017;37:145.
93. Liu X, Song T, Chen X, et al. Quadratus lumborum block versus transversus abdominis plane block for postoperative analgesia in patients undergoing abdominal surgeries: a systematic review and meta-analysis of randomized controlled trials. *BMC Anesthesiol.* 2020;20(1):53. doi:10.1186/s12871-020-00967-2
94. Elsharkawy H, El-Boghdadly K, Barrington M. Quadratus lumborum block: anatomical concepts, mechanisms, and techniques. *Anesthesiology.* 2019;130(2):322-335. doi:10.1097/ALN.0000000000002524
95. Ueshima H, Otake H, Lin JA. Ultrasound-guided quadratus lumborum block: an updated review of anatomy and techniques. *Biomed Res Int.* 2017;2017:2752876. doi:10.1155/2017/2752876
96. El-Boghdadly K, Elsharkawy H, Short A, Chin KJ. Quadratus lumborum block nomenclature and anatomical considerations. *Reg Anesth Pain Med.* 2016;41(4):548-549. doi:10.1097/AAP.0000000000000411
97. Tamura T, Yokota S, Ito S, Shibata Y, Nishiwaki K. Local anesthetic spread into the paravertebral space with two types of quadratus lumborum blocks: a crossover volunteer study. *J Anesth.* 2019;33(1):26-32. doi:10.1007/s00540-018-2578-5
98. Adhikary SD, El-Boghdadly K, Nasralah Z, Sarwani N, Nixon AM, Chin KJ. A radiologic and anatomic assessment of injectate spread following transmuscular quadratus lumborum block in cadavers. *Anaesthesia.* 2017;72(1):73-79. doi:10.1111/anae.13647
99. Visoiu M, Pan S. Quadratus lumborum blocks: two cases of associated hematoma. *Paediatr Anaesth.* 2019;29(3):286-288. doi:10.1111/pan.13588
100. Wikner M. Unexpected motor weakness following quadratus lumborum block for gynaecological laparoscopy. *Anaesthesia.* 2017;72(2):230-232. doi:10.1111/anae.13754
101. Almeida C, Assunção JP. Hipotensão associada ao bloqueio bilateral do quadrado lombar realizado para analgesia pós-operatória em caso de cirurgia aórtica aberta [Hypotension associated to a bilateral quadratus lumborum block performed for post-operative analgesia in an open aortic surgery case]. *Rev Bras Anestesiol.* 2018;68(6):657-660. doi:10.1016/j.bjan.2018.05.003
102. Murouchi T, Iwasaki S, Yamakage M. Quadratus lumborum block: analgesic effects and chronological ropivacaine concentrations after laparoscopic surgery. *Reg Anesth Pain Med.* 2016;41(2):146-150. doi:10.1097/AAP.0000000000000349
103. Vermeylen K, Desmet M, Leunen I, et al. Supra-inguinal injection for fascia iliaca compartment block results in more consistent spread towards the lumbar plexus than an infra-inguinal injection: a volunteer study. *Reg Anesth Pain Med.* 2019;rapm-2018-100092. doi:10.1136/rapm-2018-100092
104. Hebbard P, Ivanusic J, Sha S. Ultrasound-guided supra-inguinal fascia iliaca block: a cadaveric evaluation of a novel approach. *Anaesthesia.* 2011;66(4):300-305. doi:10.1111/j.1365-2044.2011.06628.x
105. Desmet M, Vermeylen K, Van Herreweghe I, et al. A longitudinal supra-inguinal fascia iliaca compartment block reduces morphine consumption after total hip arthroplasty. *Reg Anesth Pain Med.* 2017;42(3):327-333. doi:10.1097/AAP.0000000000000543

106. Qian Y, Guo Z, Huang J, et al. Electromyographic comparison of the efficacy of ultrasound-guided suprainguinal and infrainguinal fascia iliaca compartment block for blockade of the obturator nerve in total knee arthroplasty: a prospective randomized controlled trial. *Clin J Pain*. 2020;36(4):260-266. doi:10.1097/AJP.0000000000000795
107. Fanara B, Christophe JL, Boillot A, et al. Ultrasound guidance of needle tip position for femoral nerve blockade: an observational study. *Eur J Anaesthesiol*. 2014;31(1):23-29. doi:10.1097/01.EJA.0000435016.83813.aa
108. Wong WY, Bjørn S, Strid JM, Børglum J, Bendtsen TF. Defining the location of the adductor canal using ultrasound. *Reg Anesth Pain Med*. 2017;42(2):241-245. doi:10.1097/AAP.0000000000000539
109. Vloka JD, Hadzić A, Drobnik L, Ernest A, Reiss W, Thys DM. Anatomical landmarks for femoral nerve block: a comparison of four needle insertion sites. *Anesth Analg*. 1999;89(6):1467-1470. doi:10.1097/00000539-199912000-00028
110. Smith JH, Belk JW, Kraeutler MJ, Houck DA, Scillia AJ, McCarty EC. Adductor canal versus femoral nerve block after anterior cruciate ligament reconstruction: a systematic review of level I randomized controlled trials comparing early postoperative pain, opioid requirements, and quadriceps strength. *Arthroscopy*. 2020;36(7):1973-1980. doi:10.1016/j.arthro.2020.03.040
111. Edwards MD, Bethea JP, Hunnicutt JL, Slone HS, Woolf SK. Effect of adductor canal block versus femoral nerve block on quadriceps strength, function, and postoperative pain after anterior cruciate ligament reconstruction: a systematic review of level 1 studies. *Am J Sports Med*. 2020;48(9):2305-2313. doi:10.1177/0363546519883589
112. Bolarinwa SA, Novicoff W, Cui Q. Reducing costly falls after total knee arthroplasty. *World J Orthop*. 2018;9(10):198-202. doi:10.5312/wjo.v9.i10.198
113. Runner RP, Boden SA, Godfrey WS, et al. Quadriceps strength deficits after a femoral nerve block versus adductor canal block for anterior cruciate ligament reconstruction: a prospective, single-blinded, randomized trial. *Orthop J Sports Med*. 2018;6(9):2325967118797990. doi:10.1177/2325967118797990
114. Everhart JS, Hughes L, Abouljoud MM, Swank K, Lewis C, Flanigan DC. Femoral nerve block at time of ACL reconstruction causes lasting quadriceps strength deficits and may increase short-term risk of re-injury. *Knee Surg Sports Traumatol Arthrosc*. 2020;28(6):1894-1900. doi:10.1007/s00167-019-05628-7
115. Burckett-St Laurant D, Peng P, Girón Arango L, et al. The nerves of the adductor canal and the innervation of the knee: an anatomic study. *Reg Anesth Pain Med*. 2016;41(3):321-327. doi:10.1097/AAP.0000000000000389
116. Tran J, Chan VWS, Peng PWH, Agur AMR. Evaluation of the proximal adductor canal block injectate spread: a cadaveric study. *Reg Anesth Pain Med*. 2019;rapm-2019-101091. doi:10.1136/rapm-2019-101091
117. Abdallah FW, Mejia J, Prasad GA, et al. Opioid- and motor-sparing with proximal, mid-, and distal locations for adductor canal block in anterior cruciate ligament reconstruction: a randomized clinical trial. *Anesthesiology*. 2019;131(3):619-629. doi:10.1097/ALN.0000000000002817
118. Johnston DF, Black ND, Cowden R, Turbitt L, Taylor S. Spread of dye injectate in the distal femoral triangle versus the distal adductor canal: a cadaveric study. *Reg Anesth Pain Med*. 2019;44(1):39-45. doi:10.1136/rapm-2018-000002
119. Jæger P, Koscielniak-Nielsen ZJ, Hilsted KL, Fabritius ML, Dahl JB. Adductor canal block with 10 mL versus 30 mL local anesthetics and quadriceps strength: a paired, blinded, randomized study in healthy volunteers. *Reg Anesth Pain Med*. 2015;40(5):553-558. doi:10.1097/AAP.0000000000000298
120. Nielsen TD, Moriggl B, Barckman J, et al. The lateral femoral cutaneous nerve: description of the sensory territory and a novel ultrasound-guided nerve block technique. *Reg Anesth Pain Med*. 2018;43(4):357-366. doi:10.1097/AAP.0000000000000737
121. Ng I, Vaghadia H, Choi PT, Helmy N. Ultrasound imaging accurately identifies the lateral femoral cutaneous nerve. *Anesth Analg*. 2008;107(3):1070-1074. doi:10.1213/ane.0b013e31817ef1e5
122. Bodner G, Bernathova M, Galiano K, Putz D, Martinoli C, Felfernig M. Ultrasound of the lateral femoral cutaneous nerve: normal findings in a cadaver and in volunteers. *Reg Anesth Pain Med*. 2009;34(3):265-268. doi:10.1097/AAP.0b013e31819a4fc6
123. Tran J, Peng PWH, Gofeld M, Chan V, Agur AMR. Anatomical study of the innervation of posterior knee joint capsule: implication for image-guided intervention. *Reg Anesth Pain Med*. 2019;44(2):234-238. doi:10.1136/rapm-2018-000015
124. Kampitak W, Tanavalee A, Ngarmukos S, Tantavisut S. Motor-sparing effect of iPACK (interspace between the popliteal artery and capsule of the posterior knee) block versus tibial nerve block after total knee arthroplasty: a randomized controlled trial. *Reg Anesth Pain Med*. 2020;45(4):267-276. doi:10.1136/rapm-2019-100895
125. Niesen AD, Harris DJ, Johnson CS, et al. Interspace between Popliteal Artery and posterior Capsule of the Knee (IPACK) injectate spread: a cadaver study. *J Ultrasound Med*. 2019;38(3):741-745. doi:10.1002/jum.14761
126. Tran J, Giron Arango L, Peng P, Sinha SK, Agur A, Chan V. Evaluation of the iPACK block injectate spread: a cadaveric study. *Reg Anesth Pain Med*. 2019;rapm-2018-100355. doi:10.1136/rapm-2018-100355

127. Sinha S. How I do it: infiltration between popliteal artery and capsule of knee (iPACK), 2019. Accessed August 20, 2020. https://www.asra.com/asra-news/article/158/how-i-do-it-infiltration-between-poplite
128. Sebastian MP, Bykar H, Sell A. Saphenous nerve and IPACK block. *Reg Anesth Pain Med.* 2019;rapm-2019-100750. doi:10.1136/rapm-2019-100750
129. Tran J, Chan V, Peng P, Agur A. Response to Sebastian *et al*: the saphenous nerve and iPACK blocks. *Reg Anesth Pain Med.* 2020;45(3):245-246. doi:10.1136/rapm-2019-100840
130. Vloka JD, Hadzić A, April E, Thys DM. The division of the sciatic nerve in the popliteal fossa: anatomical implications for popliteal nerve blockade. *Anesth Analg.* 2001;92(1):215-217. doi:10.1097/00000539-200101000-00041
131. Karmakar M, Li X, Li J, Sala-Blanch X, Hadzic A, Gin T. Three-dimensional/four-dimensional volumetric ultrasound imaging of the sciatic nerve. *Reg Anesth Pain Med.* 2012;37(1):60-66. doi:10.1097/AAP.0b013e318232eb92
132. Vloka JD, Hadzić A, Lesser JB, et al. A common epineural sheath for the nerves in the popliteal fossa and its possible implications for sciatic nerve block. *Anesth Analg.* 1997;84(2):387-390. doi:10.1097/00000539-199702000-00028
133. Moayeri N, van Geffen GJ, Bruhn J, Chan VW, Groen GJ. Correlation among ultrasound, cross-sectional anatomy, and histology of the sciatic nerve: a review. *Reg Anesth Pain Med.* 2010;35(5):442-449. doi:10.1097/AAP.0b013e3181ef4cab
134. Prakash, Bhardwaj AK, Devi MN, Sridevi NS, Rao PK, Singh G. Sciatic nerve division: a cadaver study in the Indian population and review of the literature. *Singapore Med J.* 2010;51(9):721-723.
135. Alsatli RA. Comparison of ultrasound-guided anterior versus transgluteal sciatic nerve blockade for knee surgery. *Anesth Essays Res.* 2012;6(1):29-33. doi:10.4103/0259-1162.103368
136. Karmakar MK, Kwok WH, Ho AM, Tsang K, Chui PT, Gin T. Ultrasound-guided sciatic nerve block: description of a new approach at the subgluteal space. *Br J Anaesth.* 2007;98(3):390-395. doi:10.1093/bja/ael364
137. Ota J, Sakura S, Hara K, Saito Y. Ultrasound-guided anterior approach to sciatic nerve block: a comparison with the posterior approach. *Anesth Analg.* 2009;108(2):660-665. doi:10.1213/ane.0b013e31818fc252
138. Dolan J. Ultrasound-guided anterior sciatic nerve block in the proximal thigh: an in-plane approach improving the needle view and respecting fascial planes. *Br J Anaesth.* 2013;110(2):319-320. doi:10.1093/bja/aes492
139. Osaka Y, Kashiwagi M, Nagatsuka Y, Miwa S. Ultrasound-guided medial mid-thigh approach to sciatic nerve block with a patient in a supine position. *J Anesth.* 2011;25(4):621-624. doi:10.1007/s00540-011-1169-5
140. Prasad A, Perlas A, Ramlogan R, Brull R, Chan V. Ultrasound-guided popliteal block distal to sciatic nerve bifurcation shortens onset time: a prospective randomized double-blind study. *Reg Anesth Pain Med.* 2010;35(3):267-271. doi:10.1097/AAP.0b013e3181df2527
141. Germain G, Lévesque S, Dion N, et al. Brief reports: a comparison of an injection cephalad or caudad to the division of the sciatic nerve for ultrasound-guided popliteal block: a prospective randomized study. *Anesth Analg.* 2012;114(1):233-235. doi:10.1213/ANE.0b013e3182373887
142. Faiz SHR, Imani F, Rahimzadeh P, Alebouyeh MR, Entezary SR, Shafeinia A. Which ultrasound-guided sciatic nerve block strategy works faster? Prebifurcation or separate tibial-peroneal nerve block? A randomized clinical trial. *Anesth Pain Med.* 2017;7(4):e57804. doi:10.5812/aapm.57804
143. Nader A, Kendall MC, De Oliveira GS Jr, et al. A dose-ranging study of 0.5% bupivacaine or ropivacaine on the success and duration of the ultrasound-guided, nerve-stimulator-assisted sciatic nerve block: a double-blind, randomized clinical trial. *Reg Anesth Pain Med.* 2013;38(6):492-502. doi:10.1097/AAP.0b013e3182a4bddf
144. Feigl GC, Schmid M, Zahn PK, Avila González CA, Litz RJ. The posterior femoral cutaneous nerve contributes significantly to sensory innervation of the lower leg: an anatomical investigation. *Br J Anaesth.* 2020;124(3):308-313. doi:10.1016/j.bja.2019.10.026

39

Neuraxial Anesthesia

Maged D. Fam and Praveen Dharmapalan Prasanna

Introduction

Neuraxial blockade is an effective method for providing anesthesia and analgesia to a variety of surgical patients. It involves accessing and depositing local anesthetics and other adjuvant drugs around the spinal cord and nerve roots. Depending on the location of placement of drugs, neuraxial blockade could be broadly discussed under subarachnoid (spinal), epidural, or caudal blocks. Although these are anatomically located closely, there are significant differences when it comes to the dosage and spread of local anesthetics. There are also differences in clinical end points such as sensory, motor, and sympathetic blockade. Among these, subarachnoid blockade typically requires the least amount of drugs compared to epidural or caudal techniques, which require a higher dose and volume of local anesthetics.

History

The presence of fluid in the subarachnoid space was known from the times of the Roman empire; however, the technique of doing a dural puncture was first described by the late 19th century. This was shortly followed by Augusta Carl Bier, a German surgeon, injecting cocaine in the subarachnoid space for patients undergoing lower lip surgery.[1] The first described incident of postural puncture headache was also described by Bier after performing a procedure upon himself. From this point onward, neuraxial anesthesia had been evolving constantly for the next hundred years. Spinal anesthesia quickly gained popularity during the dawn of the 20th century and was widely practiced in Europe and the United States by 1940s. The technique of spinal anesthesia was better understood and refined during this period, compared to the epidural blockade that was explored later. This was likely due to lack of deep understanding of the epidural anatomy, unavailability of specialized epidural needles and catheters, and the fact that spinal anesthesia produced reliable dense sensory and motor blockade in an era where muscle relaxants were not yet invented. The increasing popularity of subarachnoid block suffered a setback in the mid 1940s where case reports emerged of patients suffering permanent paraplegia following spinal anesthesia.[2] Although the real cause of permanent nerve damage in these cases were not fully understood, subsequent studies solidified the safety of spinal anesthesia, leading to its revival in the 1950s.[3] The development of the epidural technique somewhat trailed that of subarachnoid spinal block. Though the anatomy of epidural space was well studied and described by the end of the 19th century, the technique of continuous epidural blockade had to wait until the mid-20th century to be developed, by the Cuban anesthesiologist Manual Martinez Carbelo. Carbelo improvised the Tuohy needle placement with a 3.5-French catheter that was inserted into the epidural space.[4]

Advancements in pharmacology resulted in the development of safer local anesthetic agents. Moreover, the invention of less traumatic needles helped reduce common side effects such as postdural puncture headache (PDPH). Neuraxial anesthesia has matured and refined over the last century and is currently an integral part of perioperative patient care. The use of neuraxial anesthesia has gained increased attention in the last few years, as an effective tool for achieving opioid-sparing analgesia. Many of the *Enhanced Recovery After Surgery* (ERAS) pathways have integrated epidural analgesia as a key strategy.[5] A growing body of research has shown reduction in morbidity and mortality associated with the use of neuraxial blockade in patients undergoing various surgical procedures. These include reduction in cardiorespiratory complications, blood loss, and venous thromboembolism.[6]

INDICATIONS OF NEURAXIAL ANESTHESIA

- Surgery involving lower part of the body:
  - Upper/lower abdomen
  - Thoracic and chest wall pathology
  - Perineum
  - Lower extremity
- Obstetrics: vaginal delivery, cesarean section
- Painful diagnostic or therapeutic procedures below the diaphragm

Patient Selection

As with any other procedure, patient refusal is an absolute contraindication for neuraxial anesthesia. Patients with altered mental status may not be able to stay immobile during the procedure, increasing the risk of inadvertent injury to neural structures. Other absolute contraindications are confirmed severe allergy to local anesthetics or presence of active local infection at the site of injection. Spinal and epidural anesthesia should be avoided in patients with raised intracranial pressure owing to increased risk of brain herniation. One exception to this rule is intracranial hypertension due to pseudotumor cerebri syndrome also known as idiopathic intracranial hypertension.

When it comes to relative contraindications, careful risk/benefit analysis should guide the decision-making in the choice of regional anesthesia. Patients who are coagulopathic may be at increased risk of developing spinal or epidural hematoma following neuraxial blockade. Coagulopathy is considered a relative contraindication depending on the severity and the type of the underlying coagulation abnormality.

For example, thrombocytopenia is often considered a relative contraindication for neuraxial procedures; however, there is no universally accepted platelet count lower limit. Common clinical practice in the obstetric population is to not perform spinal/epidural blockade in patients with PLT count under 70 000. Recent outcome reports suggest that the risk of epidural hematoma substantially increases below the 70 000 threshold.[7] Note that not only the absolute number of platelets but the functional quality of platelets is also important for coagulation in clinical scenarios such as HELLP syndrome. The timing of these coagulation tests is also important since the levels of various coagulation factors in the cascade could fluctuate significantly within hours.

Cardiac structural and valvular conditions such as severe aortic stenosis and idiopathic hypertrophic cardiomyopathy were considered absolute contraindications to spinal anesthesia in the past. However, this is not the case anymore as current evidence indicates that neuraxial blockade can be safely performed in these patients with the use of appropriate monitoring and adequate resuscitation.[8] On a similar note, hypovolemia secondary to systemic sepsis is also a relative contraindication. Spinal or epidural anesthesia can be safely performed in these patients as long as the patient is hemodynamically stable. Many clinicians would avoid placing epidural catheters in the presence of systemic infection. When it comes to demyelinating diseases such as multiple sclerosis, the current evidence is inconclusive. Though *in vitro* studies

CONTRAINDICATIONS OF NEURAXIAL ANESTHESIA

- Absolute
  - Patient refusal
  - Infection at the site of injection
  - Raised intracranial pressure
  - Significant hemodynamic instability
  - Severe coagulopathy
- Relative
  - Spinal cord or peripheral nerve disease, for example, poliomyelitis, multiple sclerosis, demyelination
  - Severe stenotic valve lesions
  - CNS infections
  - Severe anemia
  - Uncontrolled hypertension
  - Anticoagulant/antiplatelet therapy

have demonstrated worsening of the demyelinating process following exposure to LA, human studies are inconclusive. Multiple sclerosis remains as a relative contraindication among most practitioners when it comes to spinal anesthesia.[9] Nevertheless, epidural anesthesia with lower concentration of LA is often preferred in patients with multiple sclerosis, especially in the obstetric population.

Neuroanatomy

It is important to note that the anatomical structures are highly variable depending on the age and physical characteristics of the patient. A three-dimensional understanding of the anatomy of the central nervous system is essential for successful and safe placement of spinal, epidural, and caudal anesthetic. The spinal cord is a caudal extension of the medulla oblongata and ends at L1/L2 vertebral level in most adults, and around L3 in children. The spinal cord is covered by three concentric layers of meninges. The innermost layer, pia mater, is extremely thin and closely adherent to the surface of the spinal cord. The second layer, the arachnoid membrane surrounds the pia mater to constitute the subarachnoid space in between the two membranes. The outermost protective layer, the dura matter has the highest thickness and tensile strength due to collagen fibers and is closely adherent to the arachnoid membrane. The subarachnoid space contains cerebrospinal fluid (CSF) and blood vessels that supply the spinal cord and spinal nerve roots. Arachnoid membrane and dura mater together act as a barrier to the spread of local anesthetics from epidural space into the subarachnoid space. The potential space between these two membranes is known as the subdural space and contains loose areolar tissue. Subdural space could potentially be entered during the placement of an epidural or a subarachnoid block, and this could result in the so-called subdural block, which can present as a high spinal or with a patchy sensory/motor block.[10] The primary site of action for subarachnoid block is the spinal cord itself. However, epidural local anesthetic drugs act primarily on the nerve roots. This structural difference is fundamental to the technique and the dosing of the local anesthetic used for each different type of neuro-axial blockade.

The spinal cord continues below L1 and L2 vertebrae after its termination, as a strand of fibrous tissue known as the *Filum Terminale*. The collection of spinal nerve roots that emerge from the caudal end of spinal cord, known as *Conus Medullaris*, is referred to as *Cauda Equina*. The thecal sac that contains the CSF and nerve roots ends at the level of S2 in most adults and S3 in children. The epidural space is the potential space located immediately outside dura mater. This is where the tip of the epidural needle is placed for deposition of LA. It contains loose areolar tissue, adipose tissue, a rich plexus of epidural veins and, most importantly, spinal nerve roots. The epidural space extends from the foramen magnum to the sacral hiatus and is bounded anteriorly by the posterior longitudinal ligaments, laterally by the pedicles and intervertebral foramen, and posteriorly by the ligamentum flavum. Ligamentum flavum forms an important landmark for the placement of epidural blockade. It is a dense fibroelastic connective tissue that extends caudocranially, being thicker in the low thoracic and lumbar region, and gets thinner cranially. Ligamentum flavum covers the dorsal aspect of the epidural space circumferentially, and it gains attachment to the laminae and extends from one interlaminar space to the other. Posteriorly, ligamentum flavum is formed of two folds, which fuse in the midline and fuse with the interspinous ligament. This fusion of ligamentum flavum becomes less apparent as it extends cranially especially in the upper thoracic and cervical regions. This has clinical implications while placing high thoracic or cervical epidurals where ligamentum flavum may not be appreciable in midline. The thickness of the ligamentum flavum provides tactile feedback during the placement of neuraxial blockade. Note that the thickness of ligamentum flavum is highly variable among individuals. Caudal epidural space is essentially continuation of the lumbar epidural space into the sacral hiatus. This space can be accessed through the sacrococcygeal membrane, which is continuation of the ligamentum flavum caudally.

Familiarity with the structure and anatomy of vertebrae is helpful while placing neuraxial blockade since it is essentially a blind procedure primarily guided by tactile feedback. The vertebral column extends from the occiput to the coccyx. The cervical, thoracic, lumbar, and sacral vertebrae form the protective casing for spinal cord. A typical lumbar vertebra has a vertebral body and an arch formed by the laminae. The body of the vertebra and the laminae are connected by two pedicles. The resultant central canal forms the protective case through which the spinal cord and meninges run caudally. The superior and inferior articular processes form part of the intervertebral facet joint, which is an important target for injection for patients with chronic back pain.

The midline or interspinous approach is the most common technique for neuraxial placement. The interlaminar approach, also known as the paramedian approach, is a useful technique, since the interlaminar space provides a wider area to access epidural and subarachnoid space. The paramedian approach has the advantage of not requiring the patient to hyper flex the spine. This is useful especially in patients with limited mobility of the spine. It is an approach that is also useful in patients with scoliosis in which there is a rotational and angulation deformity of the spine. Thoracic vertebrae tend to have steep and narrow spinous processes, with reduced interlaminar distance making both midline and paramedian approaches challenging. Care must be taken in the placement of thoracic epidural blockade since the spinal cord could be damaged inadvertently in case of excessive advancement of the needle.

Physiological Effects of Neuraxial Anesthesia

Cardiovascular

Perhaps the most profound and immediate effect following neuraxial blockade is on the cardiovascular system. Both spinal and epidural blocks affect the cardiovascular system in a dose-dependent manner. These changes are primarily mediated via sympathectomy and affect different components of the cardiovascular physiology such as systemic vascular resistance, venous tone, heart rate, and myocardial contractility. The most immediate response following spinal and epidural anesthesia is reduction in venous tone since most of the blood is stored in venous capacitance vessels. The reduction of venous tone results in a decrease in venous return and reduction in preload. This is considered to be the mechanism of the immediate reduction in systemic blood pressure following spinal anesthetic. The dilatory effect on arteriolar tone usually follows and is due to the sympatholytic effect. This effect is somewhat gradual and less pronounced compared to the effect on the venous capacitance vessels. The effect on heart rate is highly variable depending on the height of the blockade. Reflex tachycardia may be more pronounced in hypotensive and hypovolemic patients. Spinal anesthesia is often associated with bradycardia immediately following the placement, and this is largely due to Bezold Jarisch reflex, which results from a sudden decrease in preload from venodilation. Myocardial depression could occur with high spinal and epidural by directly affecting cardiac accelerator fibers at T1-T4 level.[11] Hypotension following epidural anesthetic is often more gradual compared to a spinal anesthetic. This could be related to the timing of incremental dosing of an epidural as opposed to a single injection of a predetermined amount of local anesthetic into the intrathecal space, in the case of spinal anesthetic. Hypotension, if goes unmanaged, will result in reduction in perfusion to all vital organs including coronary artery blood flow. Hence, it needs to be managed aggressively with fluids and vasopressors. Fluid preloading with crystalloids is no longer recommended, and co-loading is now considered the standard of care.[12,13] The choice of an intravenous vasopressor is dictated by the clinical context, with ephedrine and phenylephrine being the most commonly used first-line agents to treat hypotension secondary to neuraxial blockade. Maneuvers to enhance venous return such as placing the patient in Trendelenburg position is beneficial but need to be mindful about cranial spread of hyperbaric intrathecal local anesthetic drugs. A better approach is to flex the bed or the stretcher at the hip so that the patient sits up with the feet at the level of the heart, so as to enhance venous return without risking the cranial spread of intrathecal drugs. The commonly held belief that spinal anesthetic drops the blood pressure more profoundly compared to epidural has not been validated in clinical studies. However, clinical experience indicates that the blood pressure changes could be more gradual in case of epidural anesthesia, and this could be primarily due to the slow incremental dosing of the epidural anesthetic.

Respiratory System

Spinal or epidural anesthesia is often preferred in patients with respiratory compromise precluding the provision of safe general anesthesia. However, it needs to be noted that the spinal and epidural could result in the motor blockade of some of the accessory respiratory muscles such as anterior abdominal wall and intercostal muscles. This could be more profound in the case of a high spinal.[12] Many patients would complain of dyspnea following neuraxial placement, from the lack of sensory feedback from the chest wall muscles, and this is usually not a result of diaphragmatic dysfunction. The mechanism of apnea in a total spinal is in fact primarily due to the circulatory collapse resulting in severe hypoperfusion of the respiratory centers in the brain stem. These patients often quickly recover with aggressive resuscitation with vasopressors, inotropes, and fluids, and often resume spontaneous ventilation as blood pressure normalizes. Neuraxial blockade usually preserves the tidal volume and respiratory rate but could reduce the peak expiratory flow rate, indicating its effects on accessory respiratory muscles such as abdominal musculature.

Gastrointestinal System

The profound sympathetic blockade often results in a parasympathetic hyperactivity. This could result in increased activity of gastrointestinal smooth muscles, resulting in hyper peristalsis, nausea, and vomiting. Nausea and vomiting could be the result of hypoperfusion to gastrointestinal mucosa and is often relieved by timely use of vasopressors and fluids. Antimuscarinic drugs such as atropine and glycopyrrolate have also been successfully used to treat nausea following spinal anesthesia. Postoperative ileus is a common side effect after abdominal surgery and account for a lot of associated morbidity. It has been shown that the duration of postoperative ileus can be shortened by neuraxial anesthesia because of the blockage of nociceptive afferent nerves and thoracolumbar sympathetic efferent fibers with functional maintenance of craniosacral parasympathetic efferent fibers.[12]

Renal and Genitourinary System

Spinal and epidural blockade are often associated with an increased risk urinary retention causing a delay in discharge of surgical patients from the Post Anesthesia Care Unit (PACU). It also increases the likelihood of prolonged bladder catheterization postoperatively.[14] Micturition is a complex neuromuscular process, and the precise mechanisms of urinary retention following neuraxial blockade is not fully understood. It is believed that reducing the concentration of local anesthetics could help reduce the risk of urinary retention; however, this has not been proven in clinical studies.[15]

Spinal Anesthesia

Technique

A good understanding of the three-dimensional anatomy of the vertebrae and surrounding structures is useful when it comes to the placement of spinal anesthesia. Neuraxial anesthesia can be challenging depending on the patient's physical characteristics, patient cooperation, and structural anatomical limitations of the spine itself. Patient education and setting up expectations is essential and helpful, and is often overlooked.

Positioning

Perhaps the most important aspect of the technique of spinal anesthesia is patient positioning, and it is often the most underestimated. Administration of the spinal anesthetic requires at least two personnel, one operator and an assistant. Spinal anesthesia is commonly placed in a sitting, lateral, or prone position. Sitting up position has the advantage of opening interspinous spaces and is also convenient in patients who do not require heavy sedation. Sitting position also has the advantage of easier identification of the bony landmarks in obese patients and those with structural abnormalities of spine. Patient's shoulders are depressed with flexion of the cervical and lumbar spine toward the operator. Clear instruction improves patient cooperation in maintaining the position during the procedure. Care must be taken to avoid malpositioning such as excessively leaning forward or with rotation of the spine.

Lateral decubitus position is useful in patients who are unable to maintain a sitting up position and in patients who require moderate amounts of sedation. The patient is positioned to the left or right lateral decubitus with the back of the patient brought closer to the edge of the bed. The assistant would maintain the position of the neck flexion with the flexion at the hip joints. The main advantage of lateral decubitus positioning is patient comfort and the ease of positioning the patient in the operating table after the placement of the neuraxial blockade.

Needle Selection

Spinal needles could be broadly classified into cutting and pencil point based on the bevel design. Examples for pencil-point needles are Whitacre and Sprotte. The risk of PDPH needs to be weighed when choosing the type of spinal needle. Pencil-point or conical shape needles are associated with less incidence compared to cutting needles. The other factors that increase the incidence to PDPH is the size of the needle. Larger gauge needles are associated with higher incidence and more symptomatic PDPHs.[16] It is worth noting, however, that even while using a smaller size needle, the number of dural punctures is also directly proportional to incidence of headache.

Procedure

Three-dimensional understanding of the anatomy of the spine is essential for the safe and efficient placement of neuraxial blockade, since it is essentially a blind procedure. Once the patient is appropriately positioned, vertebral bony landmarks are palpated. Typically, spinal anesthetic is placed between levels L3-L4 or L4-L5. Spinous processes are palpated to identify the midline. One of the most common mistakes that leads to difficult placement is misidentification of the midline. Hence, using either two-finger technique or one-finger technique to clearly identify spinous processes and the midline is of paramount importance. Once midline is identified and asepsis is ensured with topical antiseptic solution, the operator will proceed to LA infiltration typically with lidocaine 2%. The spinal needle of choice is introduced hereafter. A needle introducer is often inserted prior to the insertion of smaller gauge spinal needles, and this is because smaller gauge needles tend to bend upon advancement and is often difficult to redirect. Author recommends needle entry point on the skin toward the lower spinous process in the intervertebral space of choice. The needle is then advanced in a slightly cephalad direction.

In the midline approach, the operator may have tactile feedbacks from supraspinous and interspinous ligaments. When the needle tip goes through the dense dura typically a give is felt. If in doubt, it is important to withdraw the stylet looking for free CSF flow at any point. Once a clear CSF flow is ensured, the local anesthetic of choice is injected at a slow pace. It is highly recommended to aspirate CSF to ensure that the free flow is confirmed before injecting the LA. Aspiration of CSF is often performed in the middle of injection and at the end in order to ensure intrathecal injection of the local anesthetic agent. If the needle feels to be hitting a bony surface, the needle is withdrawn and redirected in a cephalad direction. It is also useful to recheck if the needle was placed in midline. Close communication with the patient is essential throughout the procedure. If the patient is complaining of paresthesia, locate if the paresthesia is in the back area or if it is radiating down the lower extremity. Radicular pattern of paresthesia could denote that the needle is too close to one of the spinal nerve roots. Depending on which side the paresthesia is, it is important to withdraw the needle and redirect it toward the midline. Smooth purposeful movements during spinal anesthetic is recommended. It is also useful to know the degree of angulation of the needle that is required depending on the patient's body habitus. In general, morbidly obese patients have deeper interspinous spaces, hence, smaller angle of redirection is necessary. The redirection of the spinal needle should be smooth, purposeful, and controlled.

The paramedian approach for spinal anesthesia is a useful technique especially when the patients have narrow interspinous spaces. This approach is essentially an interlaminar approach, which enables a larger window and access to the thecal sac. Spinous processes are palpated, and the needle is inserted 1-1.5 cm lateral. The needle is directed in a slightly cranial and medial trajectory, and advanced anteriorly. Note that this approach is bypassing the supraspinous and interspinous ligaments. It is very common to encounter the lamina first with this approach in which case the needle is withdrawn a few millimeters and redirected more cranially and medially until the ligament flavum is encountered. As mentioned above, the angle of redirection is essentially determined by the size of the patient and the depth of intrathecal space. The paramedian approach is a useful technique when the midline approach has failed or when it is difficult due to patient anatomy or patient cooperation. The paramedian approach does not require a full reversal of the lumbar lordosis for accessing the intrathecal space.

Ultrasound-guided (USG) neuraxial blockade has gained popularity in the recent years. USG is useful to identify the spinous processes and hence the midline. It also helps to gauge depth to the epidural space. Another useful aspect of using ultrasound is in reducing the number of needle passages though this is not proven in wider clinical studies.[17] Authors highly recommend the use of ultrasound if spinous processes are not palpable in a patient. Familiarity with sonographic anatomy of the vertebra and surrounding structures is essential. This can be challenging in special scenarios such as in patients who had spinal surgery or those with severe scoliosis. The largest interspinous and intralaminar space in the vertical column is in fact the space between L5 and S1 vertebrae. This is a useful technique to obtain CSF flow when other methods fail. This technique was described by Taylor.[18]

Continue spinal anesthesia is a useful technique with a more definite motor-sensory end point compared to epidural blockade. Concerns for postdural puncture headache and accidental overdose of local anesthetic preclude the use of this in routine practice. An epidural needle is used to achieve dural puncture through which the spinal catheter is inserted. An epidural catheter is placed 2-3 cm in the subarachnoid space. Care must be taken to avoid over insertion of the catheter, or any paresthesia during injection. Many clinicians would take extreme precautionary steps to label and intrathecal catheter to avoid accidental overdose with epidural dose of LA.

Pharmacology

Choice of local anesthetic is based on the site and type of surgery. LAs commonly used for spinal anesthesia could be classified as amides or esters. LAs are weak bases, hence the principles of drug action follow general rules in pharmacology. The nonionic portion is the active form of local anesthetic that could penetrate phospholipid bilayer. Hence, local anesthetics with lower pKa tends to have a higher amount of nonionized fraction of the drug and hence have a faster onset. As with any other form of drugs, local anesthetics with higher lipid solubility tend to be more potent. Highly protein-bound LAs have a longer duration of action.

Inside the subarachnoid space, the local anesthetics diffuse across the pia mater into the spinal cord. Additionally, LAs are believed to follow the perivascular *Virchow-Robin* spaces to diffuse into the spinal cord. LAs also diffuse across the Dura Mater into the subdural and epidural spaces, albeit at a slower rate. The drug action is terminated by systemic reabsorption of local anesthetic into the bloodstream.

The commonly used local anesthetic agents for spinal anesthesia are bupivacaine, chloroprocaine, ropivacaine, tetracaine, and less commonly lidocaine. Local anesthetics have neurotoxic properties and not all local anesthetics are routinely used for intrathecal use. Neurotoxicity is primarily related to the molecular size, concentration, and volume of the drug used. For example, the use of 5% lidocaine has been associated with transient neurologic symptoms (TNS) and is no longer used in neuraxial anesthesia.

Factors Affecting Block Height

Achieving appropriate surgical block height is a vital part in spinal neuraxial anesthesia. There are many factors that affect the block height. Perhaps the most important ones are the volume and concentration of the local anesthetic agent. The higher the volume and the dose of the drug injected, the higher the block height will be. The dose is also directly proportional to the density of the block. Baricity, which is the density of local anesthetic in relation to the CSF at body temperature, is the next important factor affecting the block distribution. A hyperbaric local anesthetic agent is essentially denser than the CSF, and when injected intrathecally, it will distribute and settle under gravity. This property could be utilized to titrate the height of the block by adjusting the patient position after the placement of the block. The hyperbaricity provides a convenient and relatively predictable block distribution. The most commonly used hyperbaric solutions are hyperbaric bupivacaine and tetracaine. Hyperbaric solutions are typically made by adding dextrose. Once a hyperbaric solution is injected intrathecally, the patient position can be adjusted at varying angles of Trendelenburg to achieve the desired level. Hyperbaric solutions are commonly used for various orthopedic surgical procedures such as total joint replacement. Bupivacaine and tetracaine are commonly used local anesthetics to make hyperbaric solutions. The hypobaric agents on the other hand have less density compared to CSF and tend to ascend against gravity whereas isobaric local anesthetics tend not to be affected by change of position of the patient, that is, gravity.

On the contrary to the popular belief that patient height affects block height, studies have shown poor correlation between patient height and the blockage. This is perhaps due to the fact that the height differences between patients are primarily due to differences in lower extremities rather than trunk length. The volume of the CSF that the local anesthetic gets mixed in may also affect the block height. This has clinical significance when dosing spinal anesthetic in patients with morbid obesity and term pregnancy. Obese and pregnant patients have decreased CSF volume and increased CSF volume displacement. This group of patients typically require less mass and volume of local anesthetic to achieve the desired block level. The level of injection of the spinal anesthetic and the needle direction may also affect the height of the block.

Local Anesthetic Uses

Bupivacaine is the most commonly used LA for spinal anesthetic. The onset of action is variable and usually ranges between 3 and 8 minutes. Bupivacaine spinal anesthetic typically last around 2-3 hours. It is important to note that there are other factors as mentioned above, which affects the duration of a spinal anesthetic. For example, a 15-mg intrathecal dose of isobaric bupivacaine may last well more than 3 hours for a total knee replacement. The same dose of drug may not last 2 hours for a total hip replacement surgery.

Chloroprocaine is commonly used for outpatient ambulatory surgery procedures. This is due to the agent's short duration of action that typically wears off within 30-40 minutes following intrathecal injection. Chloroprocaine is an ester local anesthetic with an onset time of 2-5 minutes and hence ideally suited for outpatient procedures such as rectal and perennial surgery. In the past, there has been concerns about neurotoxicity with the use of chloroprocaine, but these solutions contained sodium metabisulfite as preservative, which is believed to be responsible for the neurotoxicity. All chloroprocaine preparations currently available for clinical use are devoid of any preservatives.

The use of intrathecal lidocaine has slowly grown out a favor owing to the TNS associated with in the spinal injection of lidocaine in the past. Lidocaine has a duration of action of 1-1.5 hours and is ideal for short to intermediate procedures. Tetracaine is similar to bupivacaine in its onset and duration of action, lasting for more than 2-3 hours. It is currently prepared as a hyperbaric solution with 10% glucose that is ideal for perennial and abdominal surgery. Ropivacaine is less commonly used for spinal anesthesia. It is less potent compared to bupivacaine, and there have been case reports of TNS associated with the use of ropivacaine intrathecally, although this association has not been confirmed with more formal studies.

Adjuvant Drugs in Spinal Anesthesia

One of the most common additive drugs used intrathecally are opioids. Both morphine and fentanyl are widely used intrathecally. Hydrophilic drugs such as morphine (Duramorph) tend to ascend cranially in the CSF owing to poor systemic absorption. Lipophilic drugs such as fentanyl on the other hand are readily absorbed into systemic circulation, resulting in shorter duration of action. Intrathecal opioids act on mu receptors in the dorsal horn of the spinal cord, enhancing the quality and duration of spinal anesthesia. Intrathecal Duramorph can cause delayed respiratory depression owing to the hydrophilic nature, necessitating overnight hospital stay in most patients.

Other commonly used class of drugs that are used in conjunction with local anesthetics for intrathecal use are vasoconstrictors such as epinephrine and less commonly phenylephrine. The addition of vasoconstrictors affects the reabsorption of local anesthetic into the systemic circulation and thereby prolonging the duration of action. One concern while using vasoconstrictors in intrathecal space is the reduction of spinal cord blood flow causing cord ischemia. Cauda equina syndrome (CES) has been reported with the use of intrathecal epinephrine; however, further studies have failed to demonstrate any strong association between the use of epinephrine and CES.[19]

Alpha-2 agonists like clonidine are also used in spinal neuraxial blocks. Clonidine has been shown to increase the duration of both sensory and motor blockade. The central mechanism involved is believed to be a hyperpolarization of the central horn of the spinal cord. The side effects following intrathecal injection of clonidine parallel its systemic effects such as hypotension bradycardia and over sedation. Less commonly used class of drugs that are used intrathecally are acetyl cholinesterase inhibitors such as neostigmine. Reduction in the breakdown of acetylcholine results in analgesia when low-dose neostigmine is administered intrathecally. Systemic side effects such as nausea, vomiting, and bradycardia often limits the routine use of neostigmine for neuraxial blockade.

Epidural and Caudal Anesthesia

Technique

As with the spinal anesthesia, three-dimensional acquaintance of the anatomy of the spine and surrounding structures is crucial in performing epidural anesthesia. Patient education and cooperation are essential, since the procedure of epidural placement takes longer than spinal anesthetic. The most commonly used technique to identify epidural space is loss of resistance to either air or saline. This technique has the advantage of a definite end point in identifying the epidural space. The other technique that is less commonly used is a hanging drop technique. This technique utilizes the fact that the pressure in the epidural space is sub atmospheric. A drop of saline is placed at the end of the Tuohy needle, which would be sucked in as soon as the needle tip enters epidural space. This technique is less commonly used for thoracic and lumbar epidural these days but more commonly for cervical epidural placement.

While using the saline or air for loss of resistance, the operator needs to be aware of the differences in the tactile feedback between the two. A continuous loss of resistance technique or an intermittent loss of resistance can be used. When intermittent loss of resistance technique is used, it is important to maintain the same force applied to the syringe during each tapping. Change of resistance or loss of resistance can be very subtle. The subtleness of the loss of resistance especially when using air could make the operator advance the needle too far causing an accidental dural puncture, which is not desirable.

Positioning

Patient positioning is an important factor for successful epidural placement. Epidural can be placed in sitting position, lateral decubitus, or in prone position. The sitting position has the advantage of opening up the interspinous spaces while performing thoracic or lumbar epidural blockade. Lateral decubitus is more comfortable for patients, but the operator needs to be aware that malalignment of the hips in the lateral decubitus position can result in lateral flexion as well as axial rotation of the lumbar vertebrae. As a result of this, modification of the projection and direction of the epidural needle is often required in lateral decubitus position. Prone position is rarely used in blind epidural placement and is commonly used in conjunction with fluoroscopy or ultrasound. Caudal anesthesia in adults is typically performed in lateral position since it is easier to palpate the sacral horns in this position. Caudal anesthesia is most commonly performed in children under anesthesia and hence lateral decubitus position is preferred.

Needle and Catheter Selection

The most commonly used needle type for epidural placement is the Tuohy needle. Typically for lumbar and thoracic epidural placement, a 16-gauge or 17-gauge needle is used. Smaller size needles are used for epidural steroid injections. Note that the tip of the Tuohy needle is designed to be less traumatic. Another less commonly used needle is a Crawford needle. There are different types of epidural catheters available, most commonly used sizes are either a 19 or 20 gauge. These catheters could be single orifice or multiorifice catheters. Some catheters are wire reinforced and hence tend to be softer compared to the nonwire reinforced stiffer catheters. The stiffer epidural catheter has the advantage of easier advancement upon obtaining the loss of resistance. However, the stiffer the catheter, the higher the chance of intravascular insertion and potential for accidental dural puncture. The softer wire-reinforced catheters are associated with less incidence of vascular and dural puncture. However owing to the softer nature, these catheters could present more resistance upon advancement of the catheter. Wire-reinforced catheters are not compatible with MRI.

Procedure

Once the patient is appropriately positioned, the bony landmarks are carefully palpated. Appropriate interspinous levels are chosen either at the lumbar or thoracic level depending on which dermatomal distribution is needed for intraoperative or postoperative analgesia. In a midline epidural approach, the operator often feels the various ligaments prior to reaching the ligamentum flavum, such as supraspinous and interspinous ligaments. Often as the needle traverses the ligamentum flavum, distinct rubbery foam texture is felt through the Tuohy needle, although this tactile feedback may not be present in all patients. As the needle is advanced through the ligamentum flavum, care needs to be taken not to advance the needle too quickly to avoid an accidental dural puncture. When the needle tip passes the ligamentum flavum and reaches the epidural space, a distinct loss of resistance is felt; however, in many cases, this could be very subtle. Author recommends that if in doubt about the loss of resistance, withdraw the needle back to the interspinous ligament and advance forward again till a definite loss of resistance is encountered. The subtleness of the loss of resistance often leads to misplacement of the epidural catheter either superficial to the epidural space or too deep into the intrathecal space. Advancing the catheter is another way to ensure that the loss of resistance occurred at the true epidural space. If the epidural catheter advances with minimal resistance, it often indicates the correct target. If there is resistance in advancing an epidural catheter, it might indicate that the needle tip was outside the epidural space. Careful advancement of the epidural needle for a millimeter forward is often used to ease the insertion of the catheter; however, care needs to be taken to avoid a dural puncture with this maneuver. Another way to confirm the epidural placement is the use of a spinal needle to perform a dry tap through the Tuohy needle. If CSF flow is observed via spinal needle, it indicates that the Tuohy needle tip is in the epidural space. Note that this technique can only be used for epidural placement below the level of L2. The angle of advancement of the epidural needle varies with the level of placement. The upper thoracic vertebrae tend to have spinous processes, which are long and angled caudally, which necessitate advancement of the epidural needle at a steeper angle compared to lower thoracic vertebrae and lumbar vertebrae.

Paramedian approach to placement of epidural has the advantage of a wider interlaminar window. Paramedian technique requires practice and a three-dimensional understanding of the anatomy of thoracic and lumbar vertebrae. Note that in this approach, the operator may not feel distinct textures of interspinous and supraspinous ligament and might be aiming straight for the ligamentum flavum. Paramedian technique is especially useful for high thoracic epidural placement where the interspinous window is narrow. In this approach, the epidural needle is inserted perpendicular to the skin 1 cm lateral to the midline and advanced cranially and medially toward the ligamentum flavum. If bony resistance is met, the needle is withdrawn and redirected cranially and medially, to walk on the ipsilateral lamina, toward the ligamentum flavum.

When loss of resistance is achieved, the epidural catheter is advanced to 3-4 cm in the epidural space. This is followed by careful aspiration of the epidural catheter to confirm the absence of blood or CSF. This is followed by administration of an epidural test dose. Epidural test doses typically comprise 45 mg of lidocaine and 15 μg of epinephrine to a total volume of 3 mL. Intravascular placement is confirmed if the heart rate increases more than 20% from the baseline and the patients typically feel perioral tingling and is flushed. An intrathecal administration is confirmed when the patient develops sudden sensory and motor blockade.

Caudal epidural anesthesia is commonly performed in children under general anesthesia. In the lateral decubitus position, an equilateral triangle joining the posterior superior iliac spine is drawn and the apex of the triangle is roughly where the sacral horns can be palpated with two fingers. The needle is inserted through the sacral hiatus at an angle of 45° and advanced until a distinct pop is felt as the needle traverses the sacrococcygeal ligament.

The needle is not advanced from this point because of the risk of accidental double puncture. A small volume of saline is injected while feeling for any subcutaneous infiltration. Ultrasound can also be used to improve the accuracy of placement of caudal epidural. Typically, a 22-gauge needle intravenous catheter is used in the pediatric population. Once the caudal epidural space is accessed, the catheter is aspirated to ensure absence of CSF or blood. This is followed by injection of local anesthetic typically mixed with epinephrine. Small volume of our local anesthetic with epinephrine is injected initially as a test dose. Once intravascular and intrathecal placement are ruled out, the full volume of epidural anesthetic is injected.

Image-Guided Neuraxial Anesthesia

While ultrasound have a limited role, fluoroscopy remains the gold standard imaging technique for neuraxial interventions. Fluoroscopic guidance help visualize the bony anatomy of the spine to adjust the needle trajectory and gauge the depth. During epidural interventions, fluoroscopy is also the gold standard for confirming that the needle tip or catheter is within the epidural space through injecting small amount of radiopaque contrast. Fluoroscopic guidance, however, requires special safety settings and precautions and hence is not practical in the acute and perioperative settings and is mostly reserved for elective outpatient pain procedures. Clinical studies are testing novel techniques for confirming epidural placement. Electrical stimulation through a removal stylet and monitoring for myotomal response has been tried.[20] More recently, epidural waveform analysis has shown some encouraging results as a convenient readily available means of verifying correct placement of epidural catheters.[21,22]

Pharmacology of Epidural Anesthesia

The main site of action of local anesthetic during epidural blockage is spinal nerve root. This is different from spinal anesthesia where local anesthetics have direct access to the spinal cord and the bare nerve roots. Hence, the dose and volume of local anesthetics tend to be larger in epidural compared to spinal blocks. Studies have shown that the epidural local anesthetics do penetrate the dural sheath and diffuse into subarachnoid space albeit this diffusion may not be clinically significant. Termination of action of a local anesthetic in epidural space is primarily through reabsorption into the systemic circulation. Local anesthetic agent, being lipid soluble, are also retained in the fatty connective tissue of the epidural space. Continuous epidural blockade has the advantage of being able to titrate surgical anesthesia and postoperative analgesia by adjusting the dose and volume of local anesthetics in the epidural space. This is drastically different to the technique of a single injection spinal aesthetic.

The most commonly used local anesthetic currently for epidural blockade is ropivacaine. Although less potent than bupivacaine, it has better safety profile with less impact on myocardial function. Concentrations of 0.75% or 0.5% up to a volume of 20-30 mL could be required to achieve surgical anesthesia. Lower concentrations of ropivacaine such as 0.25% or 0.2% are used for achieving postoperative analgesia and labor analgesia. Bupivacaine is less frequently used in large doses for epidural blockade due to severe cardiotoxicity risk. Levobupivacaine is an isomer of bupivacaine that has a better safety profile in terms of cardiotoxicity.

Two percent lidocaine is an intermediate-acting local anesthetic, which is commonly used to achieve surgical anesthesia in obstetrics and nonobstetric patients. The most commonly used short-acting local anesthetic for epidural blockade is preservative-free 3% chloroprocaine. In the past, there are two distinct issues with the use of chloroprocaine for neuraxial anesthesia. The sulfites contained in previous generations of chloroprocaine were linked to severe arachnoiditis, and this practice has been discontinued. Later, it was noted that the perseverative EDTA used with chloroprocaine may have caused refractory back pain and chronic back pain following larger doses. The current generation of commercially available 3% chloroprocaine is safe in this regard. Some studies have shown that chloroprocaine could inhibit the action of a subsequent doses of opioids or other local anesthetics in the epidural space; however, this has not been proven to be clinically significant.

As local anesthetics are weak bases, adding bicarbonate can increase the unionized fraction. Small dose of bicarbonate is commonly added to chloroprocaine or lidocaine resulting in faster-onset surgical anesthesia. Bicarbonate is typically not mixed with bupivacaine since it could cause precipitation. As explained earlier, adding a vasoconstrictor such as epinephrine has been shown to prolong the duration of action of local anesthetics.

Additives to Epidural Local Anesthetics

As with spinal anesthesia, the most common additive drugs used epidurally are opioids. Morphine and fentanyl are commonly used epidurally to improve the quality of analgesia. Epidural duramorph can cause delayed respiratory depression owing to the hydrophilic nature. Fentanyl on the other hand is readily absorbed into systemic circulation, resulting in shorter duration of action.

Centrally acting alpha-2 agonists such as clonidine are often used in conjunction with a local anesthetic agent in the epidural space. The mechanism is not fully understood, but clinically significant prolongation of action of LAs have been demonstrated with drugs such as clonidine.[23] Adding clonidine may also have system side effects such as hypotension, bradycardia, and sedation. As with the spinal anesthesia, neostigmine has also been used as an additive for epidural analgesia.

Factors Affecting the Spread of Local Anesthetic

Similar to spinal anesthesia, the main factors affecting the spread of local anesthetic in epidural are the volume and concentration of local anesthetic. The epidural space is a potential space, and the volume of the epidural space varies between patients. The baricity of the local anesthetic has minimal impact on the spread of local and setting in epidural space. Patient positioning does seem to affect the spread of local anesthetic. The epidurally infused solution tends to settle by gravity to the dependent side, commonly observed in obstetric analgesia when the parturient lay on one side for a prolonged period of time, which results in wearing off of the analgesic effect and recrudesce of pain on the nondependent side. Similar to spinal anesthesia, obesity and pregnancy could augment the spread of epidural blockade. This could be attributed to the increased amount of fat tissue in the epidural space, increase of intra-abdominal pressure, which enhances the spread of local anesthetic.

Complications of Neuraxial Anesthesia

Neurological Complications

Permanent nerve injury is the most dreaded complication of neuraxial anesthesia. This complication was first reported in the mid-1940s when case reports emerged of patients suffering permanent paraplegia following spinal anesthetic. Further research revealed that the incidence of permanent nerve damage from direct trauma to the spinal cord during neuraxial anesthesia was in fact extremely rare.[24,25]

Direct trauma to the spinal cord could result from accidental insertion of needle into the spinal cord or nerve roots, or chemical inflammatory reaction resulting from local anesthetics/adjunct drugs. Many of the case reports of direct trauma to the spinal cord and cauda equina syndrome were associated with the use of epidural and intrathecal micro catheters. This was thought to be secondary to exposure of nerve roots to localized high concentration of local anesthetics that are neurotoxic. These patients presented with sensory and motor deficits of acute onset along with bowel and bladder dysfunction. Some of these patients also complained of sudden onset back pain. TNS or transient neurological syndrome was associated with the use of hyperbaric lidocaine 5% for spinal anesthesia. These patients presented with varying degrees of sensory and motor deficits. Most of these deficits were self-limiting, but some of them progressed to long term.

Reports of arachnoiditis associated with intrathecal chloroprocaine were attributed to sulfite admixed with the local anesthetics. It has also been reported after single shot spinals and epidural blood patch with accidental intrathecal injection. The pathophysiology appears to be an acute inflammation of the nerve roots at the cauda equina and meninges, resulting in matting of nerve roots and subsequent fibrosis and scarring of the neuronal tissue. Patients usually present with a sudden onset of back pain with mixed sensory and motor symptoms progressing into permanent nerve damage. Urgent MRI scan is recommended, which typically identifies matting of the nerve roots at the cauda equina region. The mainstay of treatment consists of corticosteroids, anti-inflammatory drugs, and aggressive physical therapy. However, prognosis could be poor depending on the extent of inflammatory process.

Neuraxial hematoma is the important indirect cause of spinal cord injury, which often results in partial or permanent nerve damage. The epidural space is highly vascular; hence, the risk of puncturing a blood vessel during spinal or epidural is high. The true incidence of epidural and spinal hematoma is unknown. Nevertheless, there are several retrospective studies that show similar incidences of neuraxial hematoma in the range of 1/200 000 in the obstetric population. However, the incident seems to be much higher in elderly population undergoing hip or knee surgery, in the range of 1 in 4500. This observation was replicated in other trials. Perhaps the most important cause for neuraxial hematoma is the association with coagulopathy. Any abnormalities in the coagulation cascade either hereditary or acquired could result in an epidural hematoma formation. Epidural space being a more compliant space could accumulate a larger volume of blood, and this hematoma could exert a local mass effect resulting in neural tissue injury either directly thru direct pressure or by impairing cord perfusion.

When low molecular weight heparin was introduced to clinical practice, multiple case reports started emerging, suggesting association with epidural hematoma. This prompted international regional anesthesia societies to publish guidelines pertinent to the use of neuraxial anesthesia in the setting of anticoagulants. ASRA guideline is one such example of where there are specific recommendations on insertion of epidural catheter, placement of spinal anesthesia, and removal of epidural catheter. It appears that the highest risk time points are the insertion and removal of an epidural catheter. Please refer to the latest ASRA guidelines for further details.[26] Multiple traumatic attempts at epidural or spinal have been observed to be associated with increased likelihood of neuraxial hematoma. Patients with abnormal spinal anatomy such as scoliosis and prior back surgery are also at increased risk of hematoma formation. Risk of neuraxial hematoma in the setting of anticoagulants has drawn even more attention in the last decade since the introduction of newer oral anticoagulants. Some of these new generation oral anticoagulants have direct and indirect effects on coagulation and are often hard to reverse in clinical practice. Adhering to the accepted guidelines in clinical practice may be far more important in these patients for the above reason. It is important to note that the duration of action of newer anticoagulants may be prolonged in patients with kidney and liver dysfunction. Standard coagulation tests such as APTT/PT/INR are commonly performed in patients on traditional oral anticoagulants such as warfarin. Note that these tests may not be useful in the case of newer oral anticoagulants. Although advanced coagulation tests such as TEG and factor Xa assay may be useful in selected patients, these tests are not routinely recommended for routine use.

Thrombocytopenia is often considered a relative contraindication for neuraxial blockade. However, there is no universally accepted value of platelets prior to neuraxial placement. It is a common clinical practice in the obstetric population to not perform neuraxial blockade in patients with platelet count less than 70 000. Although this is common practice, there is little to no evidence suggesting that the incidence of a clinically significant epidural hematoma is higher in patients with platelet count less than 70 000.[7] It is important to note that not only the absolute number of platelets but the quality of platelets is also important when it comes to coagulation. The timing of these coagulation tests including platelet count is also important since the level of coagulation factors could change significantly over time. The most common clinical practice is to obtain coagulation tests and platelet count closer to the placement of neuraxial blockade, especially if a coagulopathy state is suspected.

Any patient suspected of spinal or epidural hematoma needs immediate assessment. These patients could present with acute back pain followed by sensory/motor deficits and/or bladder dysfunction. These patients should immediately undergo imaging studies such as CT or MRI for evaluation of hematoma. The treatment of choice is immediate surgical decompression usually involving a laminectomy. Reversal of coagulopathy is concurrently started while evaluating the patient. The prognosis for neurological recovery is significantly worse when the delay in intervention is over 8 hours. Unfortunately, the symptoms and signs of epidural hematoma are often caught late during the progression resulting in permanent nerve damage.

Spinal stenosis has emerged as a major risk factor for spinal cord ischemia in patients receiving neuraxial blockade. This is because smaller amounts of blood in the setting of spinal stenosis could cause a spinal cord compartment syndrome resulting in spinal cord injury. Elderly patients undergoing hip and knee surgery fall into this category, and care must be taken while placing neuraxial blockade. The risks and benefits should be carefully weighed in patients with spinal stenosis while considering epidural or spinal anesthesia.

Back pain following spinal and epidural anesthesia is a common complaint. Although more commonly associated with epidural, back pain can also result from spinal anesthesia, especially where multiple attempts were performed. The injury to local structures and the inflammatory response that follows are thought to be the cause of back pain. The back pain typically lasts for 10-14 days. If it persists for a longer period, other causes should be ruled out. In the past, the use of chloroprocaine that contained preservatives was associated with severe back pain. This complication has not been reported with the use of preservative-free chloroprocaine. Conservative management with tylenol and NSAIDs is usually effective for the back pain. It needs to be noted that any worsening of back pain should raise concern for a more serious underlying pathology such as neuraxial hematoma or infection.

Postdural puncture headache

Postdural puncture headache (PDPH) is a common complication of neuraxial anesthesia. The mechanism seems to be the leakage of CSF through the dura into the epidural space. This results in a sudden loss of volume of CSF within the neuraxis and intracranial space resulting in traction on the dura, bridging vessels, and cranial nerves. The loss of CSF volume also triggers compensatory vasodilation. This cerebral vasodilation is also taught to contribute to the severity of the headache. The headache typically is related to the size of the needle, the larger the gauge of the spinal or epidural needle, the higher the likelihood of postural puncture headache. Obstetric patients in labor seem to have the highest incidence of PDPH following an accidental dural puncture, around 70%-90%. Common symptoms are frontal pulsatile headache, which is largely positional and postural. There are less classic symptoms associated such as cranial nerve palsies, Horner syndrome, and paraspinal muscle spasms. The headache typically starts within 48 hours following the dural puncture. It most commonly lasts for 10-14 days after which the severity of the headache typically tapers off. The most effective treatment for a postdural puncture headache is epidural blood patch. This is performed by drawing a sterile sample of blood and injecting into the epidural space. Typically, the epidural space is accessed caudal to the previous epidural puncture level and sterile blood is slowly injected. If the patient reports worsening of back pressure or radiating pain down the limb, the injection should be stopped. Total volume of less than 20 mL is recommended since a larger volume seems to be less effective. Epidural blood has 80%-90% success rate in terminating the PDPH and the patients often report immediate relief of headache.

PDPH is often confused with headache from pneumocephalus following injection of air into the intrathecal space. Placement of epidural blood patch (EBP) within 48 hours following an accidental dural puncture has shown to be less effective. Limited evidence shows promise in leaving an intrathecal catheter for 24 hours following accidental dural puncture. More recently, sphenopalatine block has shown to be beneficial in providing short-term symptomatic relief in patients with PDPH. Conservative measures such as bedrest, hydration, abdominal binder, and pharmacotherapy (caffeine, theophylline, and ACTH) have shown to be beneficial in a small proportion of patients. The risks vs benefits of placing a second epidural for epidural blood patch should be weighed before performing the epidural blood patch.

Cardiovascular Complications

Total spinal anesthesia usually results from accidental injection of a large volume of local anesthetic meant for epidural injection. This results in cranial spread of local anesthetics sometimes extending close to the brainstem. The patient typically presents with sudden onset of sensory motor blockade followed by severe hemodynamic compromise and apnea. The mechanism of total spinal anesthesia is thought to be mostly related to the hypo perfusion of the respiratory center and vasomotor centers in the brainstem. This could also result from the direct effect of local anesthetics on the brainstem. Immediate ventilatory and circulatory support is recommended. Support with fluids, vasopressors, and occasionally inotropes typically returns the patient's consciousness.

Local anesthetic systemic toxicity (LAST) could result from accidental intravascular injection of a large dose of local anesthetic. This typically occurs with a misplaced epidural catheter intravascularly. An epidural test dose containing epinephrine and a small dose of lidocaine is a reliable way to rule out LAST. LAST presents with acute-onset CNS symptoms initially followed by cardiovascular collapse. Bupivacaine is the most cardiotoxic among the local anesthetics. Ropivacaine and levobupivacaine are found to be less cardiotoxic compared to bupivacaine. If LAST is suspected, patients should be immediately resuscitated according to ACLS guidelines. Note that early use of Intralipid is useful in reducing the severity of cardiac involvement. The dose of epinephrine during CPR is reduced to 1 mcg/kg in these patients.

Infectious Complications

Infectious complications from neuraxial anesthesia are rare. Epidural abscess is the most important infectious complication following epidural catheter placement. This is commonly observed in immunocompromised patients and associated with prolonged use of epidural catheters. Worsening back pain with systemic symptoms such as fever should raise the suspicion of epidural abscess. In severe cases, there may be sensory motor deficits with bladder and bowel dysfunction. Note that the epidural abscess could also produce localized signs and symptoms such as purulent discharge from the catheter insertion site and local erythema. Patients with previous spinal surgery and instrumentation are at high risk. If suspected, urgent imaging is recommended followed by surgical decompression and drainage of abscess. Less symptomatic patients with small volumes of abscess may be managed by conservative measures such as systemic antibiotics and by removal of the indwelling catheter. The microbial flora associated with epidural and spinal abscess tends to be mostly on the gram-positive spectrum and rarely gram negative. The placement of epidural catheter in the setting of active systemic infection is controversial. Most clinicians would not perform in epidural if the patient has active bacteremia for concerns of introducing infection into the epidural space.

Bacterial meningitis has been reported following spinal anesthesia though the incidence is rare. The microorganisms mostly appear to be streptococci and enterococci indicating potential contamination from the nasal flora of the operator, indicating lack of a sterile barrier. Meningitis following neuraxial anesthesia has similar signs and symptoms of bacterial and viral meningitis, such as fever, neck stiffness, and headache. Early diagnosis by imaging and CSF examination is important for early systemic antibiotic therapy.

It is not uncommon for patients to report allergy to ester and/or amide local anesthetics. Most of these reactions are not true allergy that is IgE-mediated type 1 hypersensitivity. Historically, most case reports on allergy to LA were related to esters. This may be due to the structural similarity of ester metabolites to PABA. Methylparaben and metabisulfite could also contribute to the allergic reaction. Often patients report side effects to the LA adjuncts such as epinephrine, as an allergic reaction. If a true allergy is suspected, it would be prudent to avoid the use of local anesthetics. Referral to an allergy specialist may be useful in identifying and differentiating the allergen.

REFERENCES

1. Bier A. Versuche über Cocainisirung des Rückenmarkes. *Deutsche Zeitschrift für Chirurgie*. 1899;51(3):361-369. doi:10.1007/BF02792160
2. Schwarz GA, Bevilacqua JE. Paraplegia following spinal anesthesia: clinicopathologic report and review of literature. *Arch Neurol*. 1964;10(3):308-321. doi:10.1001/archneur.1964.00460150078008
3. Hebert CL, Tetirick CE, Ziemba JF. Complications of spinal anesthesia: an evaluation of the complications encountered in 5,763 consecutive spinal anesthesias. *JAMA*. 1950;142(8):551-557. doi:10.1001/jama.1950.02910260025006
4. Martinez Curbelo M. Continuous peridural segmental anesthesia by means of a ureteral catheter [in English]. *Curr Res Anesth Analg*. 1949;28(1):13-23.
5. Helander EM, Webb MP, Bias M, Whang EE, Kaye AD, Urman RD. Use of regional anesthesia techniques: analysis of institutional enhanced recovery after surgery protocols for colorectal surgery (in English). *J Laparoendosc Adv Surg Tech A*. 2017;27(9):898-902. doi:10.1089/lap.2017.0339
6. Rodgers A, et al. Reduction of postoperative mortality and morbidity with epidural or spinal anaesthesia: results from overview of randomised trials (in English). *BMJ*. 2000;321(7275):1493. doi:10.1136/bmj.321.7275.1493
7. Lee LO, et al. Risk of epidural hematoma after neuraxial techniques in thrombocytopenic parturients: a report from the multicenter perioperative outcomes group (in English). *Anesthesiology*. 2017;126(6):1053-1063. doi:10.1097/ALN.0000000000001630
8. Johansson S, Lind MN. Central regional anaesthesia in patients with aortic stenosis—a systematic review (in English). *Dan Med J*. 2017;64(9):A5407.
9. Vercauteren M, Heytens L. Anaesthetic considerations for patients with a pre-existing neurological deficit: are neuraxial techniques safe? (in English). *Acta Anaesthesiol Scand*. 2007;51(7):831-838. doi:10.1111/j.1399-6576.2007.01325.x
10. Singh B, Sharma P. Subdural block complicating spinal anesthesia? *Anesth Analg*. 2002;94(4):1007-1009. doi:10.1097/00000539-200204000-00043
11. Wink J, Veering BT, Aarts LPHJ, Wouters PF. Effects of thoracic epidural anesthesia on neuronal cardiac regulation and cardiac function. *Anesthesiology*. 2019;130(3):472-491. doi:10.1097/aln.0000000000002558
12. Clemente A, Carli F. The physiological effects of thoracic epidural anesthesia and analgesia on the cardiovascular, respiratory and gastrointestinal systems (in English). *Minerva Anestesiol*. 2008;4(10):549-563.
13. Bajwa SJ, Kulshrestha A, Jindal R. Co-loading or pre-loading for prevention of hypotension after spinal anaesthesia! A therapeutic dilemma (in English). *Anesth Essays Res*. 2013;7(2):155-159. doi:10.4103/0259-1162.118943
14. Choi S, Mahon P, Awad IT. Neuraxial anesthesia and bladder dysfunction in the perioperative period: a systematic review. *Can J Anesth*. 2012;59(7):681-703. doi:10.1007/s12630-012-9717-5

15. Baldini G, Bagry H, Aprikian A, Carli F, Warner DS, Warner MA. Postoperative urinary retention: anesthetic and perioperative considerations. *Anesthesiology*. 2009;110(5):1139-1157. doi:10.1097/ALN.0b013e31819f7aea
16. Arevalo-Rodriguez I, et al. Needle gauge and tip designs for preventing post-dural puncture headache (PDPH) (in English). *Cochrane Database Syst Rev*. 2017;4:CD010807. doi:10.1002/14651858.CD010807.pub2
17. Perna P, Gioia A, Ragazzi R, Volta CA, Innamorato M. Can pre-procedure neuroaxial ultrasound improve the identification of the potential epidural space when compared with anatomical landmarks? A prospective randomized study (in English). *Minerva Anestesiol*. 2017;83(1):41-49. doi:10.23736/S0375-9393.16.11399-9
18. Gupta K, Rastogi B, Gupta PK, Rastogi A, Jain M, Singh VP. Subarachnoid block with Taylor's approach for surgery of lower half of the body and lower limbs: a clinical teaching study (in English). *Anesth Essays Res*. 2012;6(1):38-41. doi:10.4103/0259-1162.103370
19. Hashimoto K, Hampl KF, Nakamura Y, Bollen AW, Feiner J, Drasner K. Epinephrine increases the neurotoxic potential of intrathecally administered lidocaine in the rat (in English). *Anesthesiology*. 2001;94(5):876-881. doi:10.1097/00000542-200105000-00028
20. Charghi R, Chan SY, Kardash KJ, Tran DQ. Electrical stimulation of the epidural space using a catheter with a removable stylet (in English). *Reg Anesth Pain Med*. 2007;32(2):152-156. doi:10.1016/j.rapm.2006.10.006.
21. Tangjitbampenbun A, et al. Randomized comparison between epidural waveform analysis through the needle versus the catheter for thoracic epidural blocks (in English). *Reg Anesth Pain Med*. 2019. doi:10.1136/rapm-2019-100478
22. Leurcharusmee P, et al. Reliability of waveform analysis as an adjunct to loss of resistance for thoracic epidural blocks (in English). *Reg Anesth Pain Med*. 2015;40(6):694-697. doi:10.1097/AAP.0000000000000313
23. Crespo S, Dangelser G, Haller G. Intrathecal clonidine as an adjuvant for neuraxial anaesthesia during caesarean delivery: a systematic review and meta-analysis of randomised trials (in English). *Int J Obstet Anesth* 2017;32:64-76. doi:10.1016/j.ijoa.2017.06.009
24. Hewson DW, Bedforth NM, Hardman JG. Spinal cord injury arising in anaesthesia practice (in English). *Anaesthesia*. 2018;73(Suppl 1):43-50. doi:10.1111/anae.14139
25. Ortiz de la Tabla González R, Martínez Navas A, Echevarría Moreno M. [Neurologic complications of central neuraxial blocks] (in Spain). *Rev Esp Anestesiol Reanim*. 2011;58(7):434-443. doi:10.1016/s0034-9356(11)70108-6
26. Horlocker TT, Vandermeulen E, Kopp SL, Gogarten W, Leffert LR, Benzon HT. Regional anesthesia in the patient receiving antithrombotic or thrombolytic therapy: American Society of Regional Anesthesia and Pain Medicine evidence-based guidelines (Fourth Edition) (in English). *Reg Anesth Pain Med*. 2018;43(3):263-309. doi:10.1097/AAP.0000000000000763

40

Cognitive and Behavioral Aspects of Pain

Anna M. Formanek, Vijay Kata, and Alan D. Kaye

Introduction

Pain began to be explored through a cognitive and behavioral lens in the latter part of the 1960s. Around this time, scientists came to realize that pain relates to both uncomfortable sensations within the body and unpleasant emotional experiences relating to these physical sensations.[1] The pain that individuals feel modifies the thoughts they experience, and the thoughts in turn influence the pain experience.

In this chapter, cognitive and behavioral aspects relating to pain will be explored. First, common pain perpetuating cognitive distortions and biases will be described. Second, common pain perpetuating behaviors will be described. Third, the tools available to combat these cognitive and behavioral changes will be explored, beginning with cognitive tools, and culminating with behavioral tools.

Common Pain Perpetuating Cognitive Distortions and Biases Seen in Chronic Pain Patients

Cognitive distortions and biases were first described in the 1970s and were originally used to characterize thought patterns seen in patients with depression.[2] Cognitive distortions are errors in thinking that can be seen in patients with depression and lead to worsening of their depressive state. Similar cognitive distortions are also seen in patients with chronic pain and are equivalently apt to worsen the chronic pain severity. Cognitive biases are like cognitive distortions but apply to a larger frame of relating to the world than each specific distortion. Biases are akin to "lenses" the world is seen through, while distortions are the specific thought abnormalities contributing to the overall world view. These distortions and biases are described below:

- *Black and White Thinking*: The tendency to interpret a situation as ALL bad or ALL good, that is "the pain will never go away, there is no chance of it" or "everything in my life is awful because of my pain" or "I can't live a full life if I can't participate in this activity due to my pain."
- *Mental Filtering and Discounting the Positive*: This occurs when individuals pay attention to features of their reality that are only congruent with their world view. For example, if they have pain when walking up a flight of stairs, they may think "I will never get better, this pain will continue forever." Yet, when the same individual walks the next day for 10 minutes with no pain, they may say to themselves "even though I didn't have pain this time that was just 10 minutes, I can't go up the stairs, I will never get better."

- *Catastrophizing*: A very common distortion seen in patients with chronic pain, when the stimulus of pain leads to a negative prediction for how the pain will play out, typically thinking thoughts along the lines of "the pain will never go away, this will take away all the things I love to do, I will never be happy again."
- *Personalization*: A distortion occurring when an individual comes to the conclusion that they are the cause of their fate/pain and that this pain is not something that could happen to anyone else. For example, the individual may think "I have pain because I am a bad person, and this is all my fault, this doesn't happen to anyone else."
- *Over generalization*: When an individual predicts that since something bad has happened before in a similar situation, the bad thing will happen again. For example, if a patient with chronic pain has had pain exacerbated by doing a certain activity in the past, he or she predicts that it will happen again and apply it to all similar situation. This exacerbates avoidance behavior, which will be described in the next section.
- *Emotional Reasoning*: Occurring when the emotional response to an event is valued more than the objective event itself. For example, the patient may say "I felt awful when I walked for 10 minutes, I did so badly, this was a bad event overall," rather than saying "I walked for 10 minutes, and I also had a negative emotional state during that moment."
- *Should Statements*: The habit of thinking that something "should" go a certain way, or that the result "should" be this or that. It can be seen in patients with chronic pain as "I should be feeling better by now, I shouldn't be having pain still, there must be something horribly wrong with me."
- *Recall Biases*: In this bias, patients with chronic pain will interpret health-related and illness-related stimuli more acutely and recall painful situations as more painful or more distressing than paired cohorts who do not experience chronic pain. This narrative harms patients with chronic pain and stilts their future experiences with pain to be more painful.
- *Attentional Biases*: In this bias, patients pay more attention to pain-related stimuli than non–pain-related stimuli. This has been demonstrated comparing patients with chronic pain and patients without chronic pain, and seeing the difference in attention given to pain-related words or pictures vs non–pain-related words or pictures.[3] By doing this, patients end up experiencing their pain as more pervasive and more intense, simply due to their increased attention to the pain.
- *Interpretation Biases*: In this bias, patients with chronic pain interpret situations more negatively than patients without chronic pain. For example, they will interpret a period of increased pain as a sign that they will always be in pain. They interpret the pain to align with their cognitive distortion that they will always be in pain and that they are doomed to have pain for life.

Common Pain Perpetuating Behaviors in Patients with Chronic Pain

One in five individuals across Europe and the United States report a history of chronic pain.[4] Frequent chronic pain episodes lead to a variety of behavioral manifestations that express pain-related feelings or enact protective measures to prevent bodily harm. These behaviors are indicative of the severity of pain that each person experiences and the effects that pain has on a personal and professional level. Chronic pain-related behaviors present differently in each person with varying symptoms and clinical presentations. Behavioral patterns are the results of the cognitive, emotional, psychological, and physical aspects of pain. Chronic pain patients and their providers need to distinguish between behaviors that are habitual vs ones that are associated with pain.[4] Described below are common behaviors observed in chronic pain patients:

- *Avoidance*: Avoidance behaviors are actions that prevent interaction with an unpleasant stimulus.[4] Perceptions of pain create fear and a need to escape, inducing protective behaviors. This is a natural evolutionary response to pain and is critical for the survival of the species. Exposure-based treatments, as will be described in subsequent sections, have shown promising results toward remedying these avoidance behaviors for individuals with chronic pain. Avoidance may provide short-term relief from negative emotions but will give rise to unhealthy long-term habits.
- *Fear of Movement*: Fear of movement stems from a reluctance to engage in movement that could bring about additional pain or feelings of anxiety. If this fear continues, it can lead to maladaptive responses that cause increased fear, limited exercise or physical activity, and mental duress.[5] Furthermore, the increased pain-related fear within patients can elevate ambiguous physical sensations, possibly leading to a new pain occurrence.[5] Patients who continue to experience pain may stop activities that they previously enjoyed. This begins a vicious cycle of physical deconditioning that will ultimately exacerbate pain.[5]
- *Withdrawing from Activities*: Withdrawal from activities is common in patients with chronic pain. This is often a result of both avoidance and fear of movement, as described above. When individuals remove themselves from meaningful activities, they are prone to episodes of sadness, emptiness, anger, panic, and resentment.[6]
- *Inactivity*: Many studies establish physical activity as a low-cost, helpful, and constructive way to manage chronic pain.[7] An inactive lifestyle causes health problems such as diabetes, obesity, hypertension, heart disease, and other ailments.[7] A physician should prepare patients for the dangers of prolonged inactivity with an emphasis on how pain can be managed through active lifestyle changes. Increased activity levels nurture the physiological modulation of pain experienced by a person, decreasing levels of worry, anxiety, and avoidant behaviors.
- *Immobility*: Immobility involves an inability to carry out normal bodily movements without the aid of assistive devices or people. Chronic pain contributes to limited mobility of patients, creating an environment that compromises accessibility to specialists, follow-up care, and preventative health care services.[8] Immobility poses threats to exploration of new interests and increases pain-related feelings of discomfort.

Cognitive Tools to Address Chronic Pain

Identifying cognitive distortions and biases seen in chronic pain patients is the first step toward helping alleviate maladaptive cognitive patterns. The next step is to develop tools to address these distortions and biases. Below are described three common cognitive tools directed toward patients with chronic pain. These include pain education, cognitive behavioral therapy (CBT), and acceptance commitment therapy (ACT).

Pain Education

Education regarding the nature of chronic pain and how it compares to acute pain is a commonly employed strategy for treatment of chronic pain. Describing how the body is evolutionarily programmed to respond to pain aids in understanding this difference in response to chronic vs acute pain. In the acute pain setting, humans are designed to always respond to pain with avoidance, fear, and hyperarousal, while in the setting of chronic pain, this response is not helpful. When patients with chronic pain understand how acute pain can be helpful, and how it can then devolve into a nonhelpful process, they can feel more in control of their pain. In other words, as written by Harrison et al. "pain science education teaches people about the underlying biopsychosocial mechanisms of pain, including how the brain produces pain and that pain is often present without, or disproportionate to, tissue damage" and that "understanding pain decreases its threat value which, in turn, leads to more effective pain coping strategies."[9]

Cognitive Behavioral Therapy

Cognitive behavioral therapy (CBT) originated in the late 1960s from the advancement of Ellis' rational emotive behavior therapy (REBT) and Beck's cognitive therapy (CT).[10] CBT is a goal-oriented hands-on approach that helps resolve personal problems within an individual's life. In simple terms, CBT states that people's thoughts, emotions, and behaviors influence their perceptions of events.[11] This psychotherapeutic approach has recently been applied to pain, with research showing that patients' beliefs regarding pain or disability heavily predict their level of discomfort. CBT interventions equip patients with the tools to modify dysfunctional thoughts that worsen the perceptions of pain.

Pain is a subjective response to the physical and emotional experience of a person. CBT delivers strategic individualized interventions by (1) gaining insight into all the facts present within a patient's case, (2) forming a two-way thought process that plans for obtainable goals, (3) setting schedules and motivating patients to follow treatment recommendations, and (4) evaluating all the information a patient provides to find a regimen that works.[12] Beck utilized research findings and meticulous patient studies to provide a CBT approach that focuses on a variety of pain-based themes: acceptance, cognitive fusion, commitment, and emotional regulation.[10]

- *Acceptance*: When an individual agrees that their chronic pain harms their overall well-being. The individual also agrees that there is a need to decrease the natural automatic cognitive and emotional responses to pain. The goal of acceptance is that the chronic pain state will not dominate one's self-esteem and ability to cope with the pain. Acceptance allows individuals to grow from their current state of pain without harsh judgment or negative self-criticisms.[13]
- *Cognitive Fusion*: This is a maladaptive process that results in fixation to specific patterns of thinking. When patients experience cognitive fusion, they cannot distinguish themselves from their thoughts. With respect to pain, thoughts can become fixated on the distress and suffering associated with chronic pain. Thinking that is driven by rigid rules can cause inflexibility when dealing with chronic pain that can lead to distress. Reason-driven thinking can cause a fixation on the reason for experiencing pain and can prevent a person from making meaningful changes to address that pain. Cognitive fusion that occurs with judgments of oneself in response to pain can lead to disappointment. Harmful pain-related thoughts can drive perceptions of and reactions to situations, which perpetuate chronic pain. There is a significant correlation between cognitive fusion and pain catastrophizing.[13]
- *Commitment*: The effectiveness of CBT on chronic pain involves continuous dedication from the individual to alter his or her maladaptive thoughts and behaviors. The higher the level of commitment, the more likely the individual will have diminished pain. Commitment involves regular participation in activities, therapy sessions, homework assignments, physical exercise, mental training, etc.[13]
- *Emotional Regulation*: The practice of counteracting chronic pain–related behaviors with mindfulness techniques that increase awareness and acceptance. Emotional regulation is also the acceptance that emotions are temporary, and the difficulties that result from chronic pain should not determine the patient's life outcome. Emotional regulation can be strengthened through interactions with licensed professionals and others who have experienced similar episodes of chronic pain.[13]

The approaches of CBT differ depending on each patient's needs. The goals of CBT for pain management include changing the natural approach to distressing thoughts, decreasing behaviors that avoid confronting the problem, improving the patient's function within society, and increasing the patient's self-efficacy. Based on clinical findings and treatment objectives, CBT-trained therapists use strategies such as cognitive restructuring, behavioral activation, exposure therapy, and problem solving to reduce the chronic pain experienced by patients.[12] These methods are described below:

- *Cognitive Restructuring*: The ability to recognize, evaluate, and change maladaptive thought. This CBT strategy tackles situation-specific patterns of thinking. A commonly used tool for cognitive restructuring is the thought record, which is a tool where individuals record distressing situations within their lives, the automatic thoughts that occur during pain episodes, and the types of chronic pain–based emotions that they experience. For example, a man receives an invitation to go to a party but feels that his chronic pain prevents him from engaging with others. This experience causes automatic feelings of reduced self-worth, with phrases such as "my chronic pain ruins my life" and "I cannot make friends due to my chronic pain." Cognitive restructuring allows for a patient-therapist–based alteration of thoughts that reflects a more reasonable perspective such as "my chronic pain is challenging, but I will not let it dominate my life" and "I have a lot of friends who care about me, even with my chronic pain."
- *Behavioral Activation*: The reintegration of individuals with activities or behavioral changes that target personal satisfaction and pleasure. These activities create feelings of enjoyment and work to minimize avoidance-based approaches toward pain-induced situations. The overall goal of behavioral activation is to assess individual weaknesses and find meaningful ways in which individuals can contribute to their families, their professions, and their communities while living with chronic pain. Two CBT components of behavioral activation are "activity monitoring" and "activity scheduling." Activity monitoring relies on patients tracking activities that they pursue within their daily lives that invoke feelings of accomplishment or productivity. Activity scheduling involves attending social activities rather than avoiding them due to fear of pain exacerbations.[12]
- *Exposure Therapy*: Exposure therapy has shown promising results for anxiety, obsessive-compulsive disorder, stress, trauma, and other mental conditions. Exposure therapy integrates a gradual approach to introduce situations that provoke the most pain or negative emotions into patients' lives safely. These chronic pain–based resolutions are then integrated within a patient's therapy, with an emphasis on patients correcting the maladaptive thought process and behaviors. This approach will condition patients to better resolve discomfort felt in the presence of such stressors. For example, a person may feel that chronic pain will be worse in the presence of a crowd. A therapist will try to condition the individual to accept or become habituated (remain exposed to the crowd until the situation becomes normalized) to the pain-related exposure therapy.[12]
- *Problem Solving*: The problem-solving approach to CBT enhances the identification of practical solutions to problems by obtaining information and asking others for help. It is important for a patient to define the problems that cause significant chronic stress and exacerbate his or her pain and tackle obstacles that may prevent success in overcoming these stressors. For example, a patient could have a problem with riding roller coasters due to a belief that the ride will make his or her back pain worse. This cognitive mindset may stem from a personal example of a friend who became injured after riding a roller coaster years ago. However, a problem-solving approach can allow the person to address that multiple friends have been on roller coasters without any injuries. Through a pros and cons assessment, the patient decides to ride a small roller coaster to build up confidence and solve the pain-induced challenge.[12]

In summary, CBT helps patients reconstruct their negative appraisals of chronic pain and the effect chronic pain has on their lives. A prominent focus of CBT as a pain-related treatment involves psychoeducation, which includes educating patients on the impact of their automatic thoughts and behaviors toward painful stimuli.[14] With the expansion of the field of psychology over the years, researchers will find new ways to integrate and build upon Beck's CBT approach for optimal pain-relieving results.

Acceptance Commitment Therapy

Acceptance commitment therapy (ACT) began to emerge as a modus for behavioral change in the 1980s, at first being used to focus on dietary change and tolerance of physical pain.[15] It was not until more recent years that ACT began to be thought of as a potentially superior approach as compared to CBT to decrease suffering in chronic pain patients. ACT is different than CBT in that the goal of ACT is not to alter the thoughts and experiences of patients with chronic pain, but rather to change the manner in which patients with chronic pain relate to their pain.

Patients with chronic pain can "expend enormous effort in fighting against their experience of pain," which includes physical sensations, emotions, memories, images, and thoughts about pain. They may reduce their physical activity, distract, avoid thoughts of pain or engage in excessive thoughts of pain, avoid other people, constantly check for bodily changes, ruminate about the causes of pain, complain, endlessly seek information, obsess over medication or repeatedly request second opinions or additional medical care."[16] These behaviors do not decrease the experience of pain, but rather worsen the chronic pain experience. The challenge inherent in chronic pain is that humans are evolutionarily wired to avoid pain, and to practice many of the above-quoted pain avoidant behaviors to protect from future recurrence of pain. In chronic pain, the individual must strive to rewire his or her evolutionarily programmed response to pain to something more adaptive. This is where ACT comes in.

ACT is based on the goal of decreasing the central role that pain plays in the daily life of a chronic pain patient by decreasing the impact of negative emotional and behavioral responses to pain. This goal is operationalized through a model of increasing psychological flexibility. This psychological flexibility is split further into six separate arms: defusion, acceptance, self as context, contact with the present moment, values, and committed action.[15] These arms are thought of as the goals necessary to increase psychological flexibility and will be discussed further below.

- *Defusion*: This is the opposite of fusion, where the thought or emotion is interpreted as reality. In attempting to practice defusion, the patient with chronic pain must attempt to look at their emotional thoughts in reaction to pain from an outsider's standpoint. This is an attempt to "differentiate between thoughts and the experiences to which the thoughts relate."[16]
- *Acceptance*: Many patients with chronic pain have an aversion to certain emotions or thoughts, typically those relating to pain. In the model of acceptance, the patients are encouraged to observe the thoughts and emotions as they arise and accept that they exist, without reacting to them in a behaviorally unhelpful way. For example, it may provoke fear to contemplate walking around the block. This fear can be felt and acknowledged, and the walk taken anyways. This would be an example of acceptance. For the patient with chronic pain to rather walk away from that fear, and avoid the walk, would be an example of not practicing acceptance. This acceptance of undesired and unpleasant thoughts and emotions is tolerated when the emotions are connected to experiences that should not be avoided because they "are connected to part of our goals."[16] In this example, the goal of the patient is to walk around the block or, on a larger scale, to increase daily physical movement.
- *Flexible Attention to the Present Moment, or Flexible Present-Focused Attention*: This is a practice similar to Western philosophies of Buddhism and Taoism; to be in the moment,

and practice awareness of current sensations, sounds, and realities. The goal of this practice is to help "individuals respond while [being] in touch with current environmental demands" rather than being reflective of past experiences or anxious about future experiences.[15]

- *Self as Context*: Attempting to separate "thoughts" from the person who actually experiences those thoughts; alternatively, that a person is not the thoughts that they experience. They can view their thoughts as an observer. For example, patients with chronic pain may feel that they are incapable of doing anything, and that their lives have become small and meaningless due a decreased quality of life. The "self as context" tool would challenge patients to observe this thought and separate the thought that they are useless and meaningless, from themselves; the person that exists behind the thought. This creates some psychological distance from the triggering thought and resulting emotion. For example, the patient may think "I am a doomed human who will always have pain and not be able to participate in things I want to." One way to reframe this is to say "I am *experiencing* a thought that I am a doomed human who will always have pain and will not be able to participate in things I want to do."
- *Values*: These are unique for each patient with chronic pain and are carefully brainstormed to reflect core values that the patient has. For example, these could include "being a good friend," "being a loving husband," "being trustworthy and reliable," "respecting my body and building a healthier body."
- *Committed Action*: The process by which individuals who have identified their core values then extrapolate those values into actions that put their values into life. In the examples given for values above, committed action could look like "picking up my phone when a friend calls" or "telling my wife that I love her at least once a day" or "finishing my work assignments on time" or "walking for 10 minutes every day."

Oftentimes, these above six core tenants of ACT are paired and then placed into a diagram called a "Hexaflex." The tenants are paired and described as their overarching theme: "**open** (acceptance and defusion), **aware** (contact with present and self as context), and **engaged** (values and committed action)".[16]

Behavioral Tools to Address Chronic Pain

After identifying maladaptive behavioral responses seen in chronic pain patients, it is important to identify tools to combat these responses. Below are described behavioral tools to address chronic pain, including pacing, relaxation training, biofeedback, and *in vivo* exposure.

- *Pacing*: This tool is a combination of behavioral and cognitive strategies. The concept of pacing involves a commonly observed maladaptive pattern in chronic pain patients where underactivity is followed by periods of overactivity. This leads to pain exacerbation, and then further underactivity. The goal of pacing is to break this cycle and build in regular small quantity movement that builds confidence in what the patient's body can do. When a patient practices pacing, they will very gradually add time or distance to their regimen, starting off with small goals (eg, walking a quarter of a mile daily). The patient should rank their perceived level of pain between 1 and 5, where 5 is unbearable, 1 is bearable, and 3 is the zone where the patient should take a short break. If the patient reaches a level of 3 during their short walk, they will take a short break and then resume when pain is back to a level below 3. In this way, the patient can complete the short walk without going over the pain level of 3. It does not matter how long it takes the patients to complete their goal activity; it just matters that they complete it regularly and without the pain going above a level of 3. This tool allows for building physical strength, cognitive competence, and confidence.

- *Relaxation Training*: This training encompasses practices such as tai chi, mindfulness meditation, visualization exercises, and biofeedback. The goal of these practices is to increase mindfulness to "facilitate an attentional stance of detached observation."[17] A prevailing theory suggests that this type of attentional state helps the individual with chronic pain separate his or her pain experience from the current reality, thus de-emphasizing the importance of the pain sensation in the context of other sensations being observed. This is thought to "refocus the mind on the present… allowing the individual to step back and reframe experiences."[17]
- *Biofeedback*: This is a similar approach to relaxation training; however, this includes real-time feedback of several physiologic parameters such as heart rate, skin conductance, skin temperature, and respiratory rate. The goal of biofeedback is to gradually teach chronic pain patients how to first recognize what autonomic state of arousal they are in and to eventually modulate their own emotional and autonomic state with relaxation tools.[9]
- *In Vivo Exposure*: This is a treatment that is carefully performed to avoid further reinforcement of the common cycle seen in chronic pain patients of overactivity, leading to underactivity, leading to worsening pain. This *in vivo* exposure is carefully graded in intensity and is delivered under the care of a physical or occupational therapist, as well as psychological team. The goal is to decrease pain-related avoidance behavior and decrease the catastrophizing that oftentimes accompanies the feared activities.[9] This therapy is based upon the operant behavioral theories of fear avoidance that "describes how heightened fear of pain and continued avoidance of activities that might exacerbate pain leads to prolonged disability."[9]

REFERENCES

1. Gorczyca R, Filip R, Walczak E. Psychological aspects of pain. *Ann Agric Environ Med*. 2013;Spec no. 1:23-27.
2. Rnic K, Dozois DJA, Martin RA. Cognitive distortions, humor styles, and depression. *Eur J Psychol*. 2016;12(3):348-362.
3. Lau JYF, Heathcote LC, Beale S, et al. Cognitive biases in children and adolescents with chronic pain: a review of findings and a call for developmental research. *J Pain*. 2018;19(6):589-598.
4. Volders S, Boddez Y, De Peuter S, Meulders A, Vlaeyen JWS. Avoidance behavior in chronic pain research: a cold case revisited. *Behav Res Ther*. 2015;64:31-37.
5. Turk DC, Wilson HD. Fear of pain as a prognostic factor in chronic pain: conceptual models, assessment, and treatment implications. *Curr Pain Headache Rep*. 2010;14(2):88-95.
6. Harris RA. Chronic pain, social withdrawal, and depression. *J Pain Res*. 2014;7:555-556.
7. Senba E, Kami K. A new aspect of chronic pain as a lifestyle-related disease. *Neurobiol Pain*. 2017;1:6-15.
8. Musich S, Wang SS, Ruiz J, Hawkins K, Wicker E. The impact of mobility limitations on health outcomes among older adults. *Geriatr Nurs*. 2018;39(2):162-169.
9. Harrison LE, Pate JW, Richardson PA, Ickmans K, Wicksell RK, Simons LE. Best-evidence for the rehabilitation of chronic pain part 1: pediatric pain. *J Clin Med*. 2019;8(9):E1267.
10. Ruggiero GM, Spada MM, Caselli G, Sassaroli S. A historical and theoretical review of cognitive behavioral therapies: from structural self-knowledge to functional processes. *J Ration Emot Cogn Behav Ther*. 2018;36(4):378-403.
11. Fenn K, Byrne M. The key principles of cognitive behavioural therapy. 2013;6(9):579–585. [Internet]. [cited 2021 Nov 1]. https://journals.sagepub.com/doi/full/10.1177/1755738012471029
12. Wenzel A. Basic strategies of cognitive behavioral therapy. *Psychiatr Clin North Am*. 2017;40(4):597–609.
13. Davis MC, Zautra AJ, Wolf LD, Tennen H, Yeung EW. Mindfulness and cognitive-behavioral interventions for chronic pain: differential effects on daily pain reactivity and stress reactivity. *J Consult Clin Psychol*. 2015;83(1):24-35.
14. Telekes A. [Approaching new pharmacotherapy options in pain treatment]. *Magy Onkol*. 2017;61(3):238-245.
15. Zhang C-Q, Leeming E, Smith P, Chung P-K, Hagger MS, Hayes SC. Acceptance and commitment therapy for health behavior change: a contextually-driven approach. *Front Psychol*. 2018;8:2350. https://pubmed.ncbi.nlm.nih.gov/29375451/
16. Feliu-Soler A, Montesinos F, Gutiérrez-Martínez O, Scott W, McCracken LM, Luciano JV. Current status of acceptance and commitment therapy for chronic pain: a narrative review. *J Pain Res*. 2018;11:2145-2159.
17. Hilton L, Hempel S, Ewing BA, et al. Mindfulness meditation for chronic pain: systematic review and meta-analysis. *Ann Behav Med*. 2017;51(2):199-213.

41

Peripheral Stimulation Modalities

Eileen A. Wang, Priya Agrawal, Karina Gritsenko, and Fadi Farah

Advancement of Acute to Chronic Pain

With the advancements in health care management and technology, surgical volume has increased dramatically over the last few decades. An estimated, 313 million procedures were performed worldwide in 2012.[1] This was an increase from 226 million operations performed in 2004.[2] In the United States, 28 million inpatient surgical procedures and 48 million ambulatory surgeries were reported in 2006 and 2010, respectively.[3,4] Postoperative pain is normal and expected for a temporary period after surgical procedures. However, poorly controlled and persistent postoperative pain can have serious consequences. According to the U.S. Institute of Medicine, 80% of patients undergoing surgery report postoperative pain with 88% of this group reporting moderate, severe, or extreme pain levels.[5] These numbers are expected to grow with the increasing surgical volume.

Poorly managed acute postoperative pain leads to the development of chronic pain, delayed recovery from surgery, prolonged opioid use, increased morbidity, impaired function, decreased quality of life, and increase health care economic burden.[6] The incidence of chronic postsurgical pain (CPSP) varies by type of surgery. In a 2-year Spanish prospective study of 2929 patients undergoing hernia repair, vaginal hysterectomy, abdominal hysterectomy, and thoracotomy, this ranged from 37.6% for thoracotomy to 11.8% for vaginal hysterectomy at 4 months postoperatively.[7] In a French prospective study of 2397 of patients undergoing cholecystectomy, inguinal herniorrhaphy, saphenectomy, sternotomy, thoracotomy, knee arthroscopy, breast cancer surgery, or elective cesarean section, patients reported the highest mean pain scores after knee arthroscopy and thoracotomy, and the lowest after herniorrhaphy and cesarean section.[8]

Orthopedic surgeries are commonly performed procedures both in the inpatient and ambulatory settings. These procedures can range from elective knee and shoulder arthroscopies, joint replacement surgeries to urgent fracture repair and removal of primary bone and soft tissue benign or malignant tumors. Upper and lower extremity surgeries provide the unique advantage of performing peripheral nerve blocks to provide postoperative analgesia in the acute setting. Given that poor management of acute postoperative pain is associated with progression to chronic persistent pain, every effort should be made to adequately control acute pain. In addition to surgery type, other risk factors for CPSP include younger age, female gender, high body mass index (≥25), preexisting psychological conditions such as anxiety or depression. Furthermore, intraoperative surgical technique, the extent of nerve injury and tissue ischemia, and postoperative complications increases the risk of CPSP.[9]

CPSP syndromes are difficult to treat. Thus, prevention and early intervention are key to successfully keeping the rates of progression from acute pain to chronic pain to a minimum. Peripheral nerve blocks, either single-shot or continuous techniques with a catheter; central neuraxial blockade such as epidural or spinal anesthesia; neuromodulation with peripheral nerve stimulation (PNS) or spinal cord stimulation are all potential preventative and/or therapeutic modalities to optimally manage pain in the acute postoperative setting to minimize progression chronic persistent pain.

Mechanism of Action

Understanding the mechanism of action of PNS is important in the implementation and the development of new treatment modalities using PNS. This is a topic of ongoing research, with likely both centrally and peripherally mediated effects. PNS is a method of orthodromic stimulation of nonnociceptive AB fibers. One theory suggests that the effect of PNS may be carried out via the gate control theory similar to dorsal column stimulation.[10] The PNS activates the A-beta fibers at the location of the peripheral leads.[10] This leads to excitation of inhibitory dorsal horn interneurons, which in turn inhibit the transmission of nociceptive, small-diameter A-delta and C nerve fibers.[10]

Additional theories attempted to explain the pain relief provided by PNS. They include the following:

1. Excitation failure in C fiber nociceptors and suppression of dorsal horn activity
2. Stimulation-induced blockade of cell membrane depolarization preventing axon conduction propagation
3. Decreased hyperexcitability and long-term potentiation of dorsal horn neurons
4. Depletion of excitatory amino acids (glutamate, aspartate) and increased release of inhibitory transmitters (GABA)[11]

A second paradigm focuses on the local effects at the site of peripheral stimulation.[10] Chemical mediators, such as neurotransmitters and endorphins, may play a key role in transmission of pain signals by increasing local blood flow.[10] Animal models have demonstrated that nerve injury leads to localized inflammatory changes such as edema, ischemia, and increased vascular permeability.[10] Studies have suggested that PNS may reduce the levels of these biochemical mediators thus producing their analgesic effect.[10] This theory is supported by a study that demonstrated increased latency of afferent signals via A and C nerve fibers when stimulated by electrical stimulation.[10] This effect was most significant on small-diameter fibers primarily carrying nociceptive signals.[10]

A number of studies have looked at different models to understand how PNS is effective in reducing pain. Cat models have shown that repeated direct stimulation of the sciatic and tibial nerves decreases C fiber response within the spinal cord.[12] Additionally, using a rat model, investigators found that electrical field stimulation to the dorsal root ganglion plays a key role in modulating chronic pain pathways.[12] In rats, exposure of the dorsal root ganglion to electric field stimulation for 90s at 60 Hz causes a measured decrease in somatic excitability and action potential though modulation of calcium influx.[12] Calcium influx is modulated through pathways including the calcium-sensitive potassium channels, kinases, and phosphatases.[12]

Currently, it is unknown what the optimum frequency, duration, and modulation pattern is most effective to produce analgesia in PNS. The different settings of commercially available devices are titrated to patient affect in the clinical setting.

Role of Peripheral Nerve Stimulation in Chronic Pain

Peripheral nerve stimulation involves the use of electrical current via a wire like electrode to stimulate a nerve for the purpose of eliminating or reducing the perception of pain of the affected area. Julius Althaus performed the first reported use of direct electrical stimulation of the peripheral nerve in 1859.[13] He found that electrical stimulation of a peripheral nerve in an extremity alleviated surgical pain.[13] PNS has been traditionally limited by its invasiveness and complications. However, new advances in PNS devices have permitted its increased use in the last 20 years. With novel implants that are minimally invasive, its applications in the use in the treatment of peripheral nerve pain has been expanding in the treatment of chronic pain. These new devices use neuromodulation by altering nerve impulses either through electrical or chemical mechanisms and allow for implantation of permanent nerve stimulators at the affected site.

A prospective, multicenter, randomized, double-blinded, partial crossover study performed by Deer and colleagues showed the effectiveness of PNS in the treatment of axillary shoulder pain.[14] Deer and colleagues also found that in 14 randomized control trials for a variety of painful conditions including headache, shoulder, pelvic, extremity, and trunk pain, there was moderate to strong evidence to support the use of PNS to treat pain.[14] Other studies have showed enduring analgesic affects that persist despite cessation of stimulation that occur of minutes to hours.[10]

Peripheral nerve stimulation devices have shown to be effective in the treatment of phantom limb pain. Studies indicate that more than 85% of U.S. Service members with combat-related traumatic amputations suffer from moderate to severe postamputation pain. In a randomized double-blind placebo-controlled trial, in patients who had percutaneous leads placed in the femoral and sciatic nerve, 67% of patients reported greater than a 50% reduction in average weekly pain at 12 months compared to 0% in the placebo group.[15] Patients with PNS implants also reported decreased rates of depression.[15]

Although the studies listed above are focused on lower extremity of the femoral and sciatic nerve, PNS has been successfully used in a multitude of upper extremity nerves as well including the brachial plexus and its branches including radial, median, and ulnar nerves. In a series of 26 patients suffering from chronic medically refractory neuropathic pain of the upper limb including complex regional pain syndrome, ultrasound-guided percutaneous implants were placed close to the suprascapular nerve or the cervical nerve roots of the brachial plexus depending on the patients' pain topology.[16] Seventeen patients improved by >50%, including the 12 who improved by >70%, with a mean follow-up time of 27.5 months.[16]

Peripheral nerve stimulation also has clinical implications in the treatment of urinary incontinence. McGuire et al. first described posterior tibial nerve stimulation for the treatment of detrusor instability but found that patients had concomitant improvement of pelvic pain as well.[17] In a randomized control trial for chronic pelvic pain of PNS of the posterior tibial nerve vs sham treatment group, 40% of the PNS of the posterior tibial nerve showed greater than a 50% reduction in pain.[11] Furthermore, PNS has been used in the treatment of genitofemoral neuralgia. Genitofemoral neuralgia is characterized by chronic neuropathic pain that includes symptoms such as groin pain, paresthesia, and burning sensation from the lower abdomen to the medial aspect of the leg and within the genital region. It often occurs iatrogenically from inguinal hernia repair surgery or femoral hernia repair surgery. Rosendal et al. reported a case where a patient was able to reduce the pain intensity from a 9/10 to a 2/10 7 months after implantation of two percutaneous leads in the groin and low-frequency stimulation of the cutaneous branch of the inguinal and genital branch of the genitofemoral nerves.[18]

Role of Peripheral Nerve Stimulation in Acute Pain and Perioperative Pain

For many patients undergoing surgery, the postoperative pain is highest immediately postoperatively and decreases with time.[19] Thus, most of the interventional modalities implemented to date to treat postoperative pain focus on the immediate postoperative period in combination with multimodal analgesia. These modalities include single shot nerve blocks and nerve block catheters. However, the trajectories of postoperative pain are variable, and pain can persist beyond the first week after surgery. A perineural catheter is an excellent option to treat severe postoperative pain. However, its limitations include limited duration of action, up to few weeks after surgery, as well as a risk of infection and dislodgement. In addition, the nerve blocks are associated with sensory deficits, proprioception deficits, and weakness that may hinder the participation in physical therapy and resumption of daily function. In contrast, PNS offers the opportunity to provide the patient with analgesia while minimizing the risks of sensory or motor deficits and falls. Furthermore, as an opioid-sparing technique, PNS has the potential to reduce length of stay as a function of reduced opiate-related side effects. PNS also has the potential to provide analgesia even following hospital discharge while patients recover at home.[20]

The use of neuromodulation to treat postoperative acute pain is relatively novel. The invasive nature of implanted systems initially hindered the application of PNS to acute pain. Newer technologies allowing for smaller batteries made the PNS more appealing.[21] Several studies have detailed the use of PNS in the perioperative setting (Table 41.1). These studies showed that the analgesic effect of PNS was not immediate. Significant reduction in pain scores and in opioid consumption occurred at a delay from the initiation of stimulation.[22] Moreover, the studies showed an additive effect of PNS to oral analgesia and peripheral nerve blocks. Another advantage of PNS stems from the sustained analgesia after extraction of the PNS leads up to 12 months.[23] Thus, patients who are identified to be at high risk of developing persistent postoperative pain may benefit from this technology.

Ilfeld et al., in their pilot study, described the use of PNS inserted near the femoral nerve and the sciatic nerve for postoperative analgesia following total knee arthroplasty in five patients.[24] The PNS achieved complete resolution of pain in 4/5 of patients at rest and a 90% pain relief with movement. The same group published a randomized controlled study on the use of PNS for postoperative analgesia for ambulatory hallux valgus repair surgery. The stimulator was placed adjacent to the sciatic nerve at the level of the popliteal fossa. Seven patients received either 5 minutes of stimulation or sham followed by crossover and continuous stimulation for

TABLE 41.1 PERIPHERAL NERVE STIMULATOR FOR PERIOPERATIVE PAIN

Authors	Year	Journal	Surgery	Nerves Stimulated	Number of Patients	Results
Ilfeld	2017	*Pain Practice*	Total knee arthroplasty	Femoral + sciatic	5	Pain decreased an average of 63% at rest
Ilfed	2018	*Regional Anesthesia and Pain Medicine*	Hallux valgus osteotomy	Sciatic	7	50% reduction of pain and a decrease in opioid consumption
Ilfed	2019	*Neuromodulation*	Anterior cruciate ligament reconstruction	Femoral	10	84% pain decrease
Finneran	2019	*Regional Anesthesia and Pain Medicine*	Rotator cuff repair	Suprascapular nerve or brachial plexus	16	Significant pain reduction and decreased opioid consumption from postoperative days 1-14

14-28 days. During the initial 5-minute treatment period, those in the active stimulation group experienced an improvement in their pain over 5 minutes, while those in the sham group did not. Following this 10-minute period, both cohorts were subjected to 30 minutes of active stimulation, in which pain scores decreased to ~50% of baseline. The study demonstrated a 50% reduction of pain in the treatment arm and a decrease in opioid consumption.

Additionally, Ilfeld et al. published a study on the effect of PNS for Ambulatory Anterior Cruciate Ligament Reconstruction surgery.[25] The peripheral nerve stimulator was placed at the level of the femoral nerve. Similar to the study mentioned above, 10 patients received either 5 minutes of active stimulation first followed by sham stimulation or 5 minutes of sham stimulation first followed by active stimulation. Postoperatively, 80% of patients required additional continuous adductor canal nerve block for rescue analgesia during the first 2 days after surgery. After that, both pain scores and opioid use were minimal in the active treatment group.

Finneran et al. described the use of PNS to induce neuromodulation of the suprascapular nerve or the brachial plexus for postoperative analgesia following rotator cuff repair.[20] They randomized 16 patients to PNS vs sham stimulation. The leads were placed 1 week prior to surgery but were not activated. After surgery, patients were randomized to stimulus or sham, and the stimulus was activated for 30 minutes. Afterward, opioids and nerve blocks were available to the patients. The peripheral nerve stimulator did not provide reduction of pain in the PACU. However, it achieved significant pain reduction and decreased opioid consumption from postoperative days 1-14. During postoperative days 1-14, the median pain score on the numerical rating scale was 1 or less, and opioid consumption averaged less than oxycodone 5 mg/d. This suggests that the analgesia may not be immediate but requires a prolonged duration of stimulus.

There are no studies evaluating the complication risk associated with PNS in the perioperative period. In the chronic pain setting, the risk is evaluated at <1 infection per 320 000 indwelling days. The other relevant risks include lead dislodgement and lead fracture.

REFERENCES

1. Meara JG, Leather AJ, Hagander L, et al. Global Surgery 2030: evidence and solutions for achieving health, welfare, and economic development. *Lancet*. 2015;386(9993):569-624. doi:10.1016/S0140-6736(15)60160-X
2. Weiser TG, Haynes AB, Molina G, et al. Size and distribution of the global volume of surgery in 2012. *Bull World Health Organ*. 2016;94(3):201-209. doi:10.2471/BLT.15.159293
3. Buie VC, Owings MF, DeFrances CJ, Golosinskiy A. National hospital discharge survey: 2006 annual summary. *Vital Health Stat 13*. 2010;(168):1-79.
4. Hall MJ, Schwartzman A, Zhang J, Liu X. Ambulatory surgery data from hospitals and ambulatory surgery centers: United States, 2010. *Natl Health Stat Report*. 2017;(102):1-15.
5. Institute of Medicine. *Relieving Pain in America: A Blueprint for Transforming Prevention, Care, Education, and Research*. National Academies Press; 2011.
6. Gan TJ. Poorly controlled postoperative pain: prevalence, consequences, and prevention. *J Pain Res*. 2017;10:2287-2298. doi:10.2147/JPR.S144066
7. Montes A, Roca G, Sabate S, et al. Genetic and clinical factors associated with chronic postsurgical pain after hernia repair, hysterectomy, and thoracotomy: a two-year multicenter cohort study. *Anesthesiology*. 2015;122:1123-1141. doi:https://doi.org/10.1097/ALN.0000000000000611
8. Dualé C, Ouchchane L, Schoeffler P. Neuropathic aspects of persistent postsurgical pain: a French multicenter survey with a 6-month prospective follow-up. *J Pain*. 2014;15(1):24.e21-e24.e20.
9. McGreevy K, Bottros MM, Raja SN. Preventing chronic pain following acute pain: risk factors, preventive strategies, and their efficacy. *Eur J Pain Suppl*. 2011;5(2):365-372.
10. Chakravarthy K, Nava A, Christo PJ, Williams K. Review of recent advances in peripheral nerve stimulation (PNS). *Curr Pain Headache Rep*. 2016;20(11):60. doi:10.1007/s11916-016-0590-8
11. Kabay S, Kabay SC, Yucel M, Ozden H. Efficiency of posterior tibial nerve stimulation in category IIIB chronic prostatitis/chronic pelvic pain: a Sham-Controlled Comparative Study. *Urol Int*. 2009;83(1):33-38. doi:10.1159/000224865
12. Du J, Zhen G, Chen H, et al. Optimal electrical stimulation boosts stem cell therapy in nerve regeneration. *Biomaterials*. 2018;181:347-359. doi:10.1016/j.biomaterials.2018.07.015

13. Huntoon MA, Burgher AH. Ultrasound-guided permanent implantation of peripheral nerve stimulation (PNS) system for neuropathic pain of the extremities: original cases and outcomes. *Pain Med.* 2009;10(8):1369-1377. doi:10.1111/j.1526-4637.2009.00745.
14. Deer TR, Esposito MF, McRoberts WP, et al. A systematic literature review of peripheral nerve stimulation therapies for the treatment of pain. *Pain Med.* 2020;21(8):1590-1603. doi:10.1093/pm/pnaa030
15. Cohen SP, Gilmore CA, Rauck RL, et al. Percutaneous peripheral nerve stimulation for the treatment of chronic pain following amputation. *Mil Med.* 2019;184(7-8):e267-e274. doi:10.1093/milmed/usz114
16. Bouche B, Manfiotto M, Rigoard P, et al. Peripheral nerve stimulation of brachial plexus nerve roots and supra-scapular nerve for chronic refractory neuropathic pain of the upper limb. *Neuromodulation.* 2017;20(7):684-689. doi:10.1111/ner.12573
17. Roy H, Offiah I, Dua A. Neuromodulation for pelvic and urogenital pain. *Brain Sci.* 2018;8(10):180. doi:10.3390/brainsci8100180
18. Rosendal F, Moir L, de Pennington N, Green AL, Aziz TZ. Successful treatment of testicular pain with peripheral nerve stimulation of the cutaneous branch of the ilioinguinal and genital branch of the genitofemoral nerves. *Neuromodulation.* 2013;16(2):121-124. doi:10.1111/j.1525-1403.2011.00421
19. Tiippana E, Hamunen K, Heiskanen T, Nieminen T, Kalso E, Kontinen VK. New approach for treatment of prolonged postoperative pain: APS Out-Patient Clinic. *Scand J Pain.* 2016;12:19-24. doi:10.1016/j.sjpain.2016.02.008
20. Ilfeld BM, Finneran JJ IV, Gabriel RA, et al. Ultrasound-guided percutaneous peripheral nerve stimulation: neuromodulation of the suprascapular nerve and brachial plexus for postoperative analgesia following ambulatory rotator cuff repair. A proof-of-concept study. *Reg Anesth Pain Med.* 2019;44(3):310-318. doi:10.1136/rapm-2018-100121
21. Gilmore C, Ilfeld B, et al. Percutaneous peripheral nerve stimulation for the treatment of chronic neuropathic postamputation pain: a multicenter, randomized, placebo-controlled trial. *Reg Anesth Pain Med.* 2019;44(6):637-645. doi:10.1136/rapm-2018-100109
22. Ilfeld BM, Gabriel RA, Said ET, et al. Ultrasound-guided percutaneous peripheral nerve stimulation: neuromodulation of the sciatic nerve for postoperative analgesia following ambulatory foot surgery, a proof-of-concept study. *Reg Anesth Pain Med.* 2018;43(6):580-589. doi:10.1097/AAP.0000000000000819
23. Gilmore CA, Kapural L, McGee MJ, Boggs JW. Percutaneous peripheral nerve stimulation for chronic low back pain: prospective case series with 1 year of sustained relief following short-term implant. *Pain Pract.* 2020;20(3):310-320. doi:10.1111/papr.12856
24. Ilfeld BM, Gilmore CA, Grant SA, et al. Ultrasound-guided percutaneous peripheral nerve stimulation for analgesia following total knee arthroplasty: a prospective feasibility study. *J Orthop Surg Res.* 2017;12(1):4. doi:10.1186/s13018-016-0506-7.
25. Ilfeld BM, Said ET, Finneran JJ IV, et al. Ultrasound-guided percutaneous peripheral nerve stimulation: neuromodulation of the femoral nerve for postoperative analgesia following ambulatory anterior cruciate ligament reconstruction: a proof of concept study. *Neuromodulation.* 2019;22(5):621-629. doi: 10.1111/ner.12851

42

Joint Injections for Acute Pain

Chikezie N. Okeagu, Alex D. Pham, Scott A. Scharfenstein, and Alan David Kaye

Introduction

Joints, the junctions between two or more bones in the body, are frequent sources of pain. Pain can emanate from the joint itself, termed arthralgia, or from adjacent tissues, such as muscles and tendons. Joint pain can be acute or chronic and arise from a vast array of causes, including inflammation, infection, crystal deposition, cartilage degeneration, and trauma. Regardless, the initial approach to a patient with joint pain involves developing a differential diagnosis to help identify the underlying pathophysiological process. A thorough history and physical examination in conjunction with judiciously acquired laboratory tests are imperative. Details such as the number of joints affected, the type of joint (ie, axial skeleton vs peripheral joints), the chronicity of pain, and associated symptoms can help indicate a diagnosis and guide treatment. Pain that occurs as a result of a systemic disease, such as gout or rheumatoid arthritis (RA), necessitates treatment targeted at the underlying cause. Likewise, infection-induced joint pain requires eradication of the culpable pathogen. Commonly, joint pain is found to be the result of degeneration, overuse, or acute injury. In these situations, a variety of treatment options are available. In these instances, first-line interventions include activity modification, physical therapy, and analgesics, such as acetaminophen and nonsteroidal anti-inflammatory drugs. If these treatments are inadequate, more invasive measures can be considered. One such modality, intra-articular injection, involves directly introducing medication or other substances into the joint to modulate the local environment in hopes of alleviating symptoms. Intra-articular injections are used broadly across numerous joints in the body, including those in the extremities, foot/ankle, hands, and spine. While most commonly used in the management of chronic pain conditions, such as osteoarthritis (OA) that have been refractory to other treatments, intra-articular injections are also often helpful when used as adjuncts in the treatment of acute exacerbations of chronic conditions, such as OA, gout, or RA, and to help alleviate acute pain caused by injury or surgery. This chapter will present an overview of the various agents that are available for use in intra-articular injection and their utility in the treatment of a variety of acute pain conditions.

Intra-articular Injection Agents

Corticosteroids

Corticosteroid injections are a commonly utilized method of treating painful musculoskeletal conditions such as OA and RA of the knee, hand, shoulder, hip, and other joints. Corticosteroids are a group of synthetic analogs of the natural steroid hormones produced and released by the adrenal cortex, glucocorticoids and mineralocorticoids. These hormones regulate a variety of physiological processes in our bodies, playing roles in homeostasis, metabolism, and cognition. They also have significant anti-inflammatory and immunomodulatory effects. Corticosteroids are important in the treatment of allergic and inflammatory disorders to suppress undesirable actions of the immune system.[1] The mechanism of action by which corticosteroids produce their effects is complex. The classic mechanism that leads to most of the anti-inflammatory and immunosuppressive effects are mediated through the glucocorticoid receptor in the nucleus of cells where gene transcription is altered, causing inhibition of gene expression and translation of inflammatory end products. This leads to a reduction in proinflammatory mediators involved in the inflammatory response, such as phospholipase A2, cyclooxygenase-2, macrophages, eosinophils, lymphocytes, mast cells, and other inflammatory mediators.[2]

Types of corticosteroids used

There are five main types of corticosteroids FDA approved for intra-articular injections: methylprednisolone acetate, triamcinolone acetonide, dexamethasone, betamethasone sodium phosphate, and betamethasone acetate.[3] Corticosteroids are classified as soluble or insoluble in water. The acetate/acetonide formulations are insoluble because of their hydrophobic steroid ester groups. Insoluble steroids require hydrolysis by cellular esterases to convert to their active forms, so these theoretically have a longer duration of action at the site of injection. Sodium phosphate formulations are soluble in water and do not require conversion to an active form; thus, onset of action is rapid. Soluble preparations also have a potency five times greater than ester formulations, requiring a much smaller dose to achieve similar effects. Ester compounds also contain larger size particles and tend to coalesce and form larger aggregate "crystals." Nonester compounds are freely soluble in water and do not aggregate.[4] Water-soluble formulations can also diffuse rapidly from the injected joints and tend to exert more systemic effects than their counterparts. Therefore, the duration of effect is inversely related to the solubility of the preparation.[5] According to multiple trials, there is no difference in efficacy of using any of the above corticosteroids for intra-articular injections, as long as each are being used for the correct indication, dosing, and timing.[1]

Side effects and contraindications

Side effects to corticosteroids are numerous and are usually related to dosage, duration of administration, added contaminants, and particulate size. Chronic administration of corticosteroids, even at low doses, has been shown to cause adverse physiologic effects, the most significant being suppression of the HPA axis (hypothalamic-pituitary-adrenal). Other long-term sequelae include osteoporosis, immunosuppression, growth suppression, acne, skin atrophy, cataracts, decreased wound healing, and weight gain. Short-term therapy with corticosteroids is associated with adverse effects but is usually not associated with long-term complications. Some short-term effects include hyperglycemia, hypertension, poor wound healing, edema, psychiatric sequelae, and electrolyte disturbances. Intra-articular joint injections are a great way to provide prolonged concentrations of the steroid in the synovial fluid and synovium while limiting high plasma concentrations thereby avoiding systemic effects.[2]

In general, corticosteroid joint injections are relatively safe, but contraindications do exist. The main concern with injecting into a joint is the introduction of bacteria into that joint, potentially leading to septic arthritis. *Staphylococcus aureus* is the most common organism involved, with other organisms like coagulase-negative staphylococci and anaerobes present occasionally.[6] Local cellulitis, active septic arthritis, acute fracture, bacteremia, and joint prosthesis are absolute contraindications. Some relative contraindications include minimal relief after two previous injections, bleeding risk due to a coagulopathy or a patient on blood thinners, osteoporosis of surrounding joint, and uncontrolled diabetes. If a patient is on blood thinners, clearance from cardiology should be obtained prior to stopping or bridging anticoagulants.[5]

Indications

The anti-inflammatory effects of intra-articular corticosteroids have been well established in the treatment of inflammatory disorders. OA is the most common indications for intra-articular steroid injections, especially in large weight-bearing joints with bone on bone pain, such as the knees and hips. RA, especially with persistent activity in large or medium-sized joints can slow joint erosion. Other inflammatory conditions indicated include reactive arthritis, gout, psoriatic arthritis, and other spondyloarthropathies.[5]

Effectiveness

The clinical effectiveness of intra-articular corticosteroid injections is highly debatable, and many studies showed limited if any long-term improvements in pain and functionality. A review by Cato looked at multiple studies conducted on the effectiveness of osteoarthritic knee steroid injections and concluded that intra-articular steroid injections of the knee do show statistically significant results. However, pain relief was only statistically significant within the first 2 weeks. There was only small benefit at 8 weeks and little or no benefit at 12-26 weeks.[7] Other studies have shown better results for other disease processes such as synovitis in patients with RA.[8] Overall, intra-articular steroids likely do have a significant clinical effect despite the various results by a multitude of studies. However, many factors likely contribute to clinical effectiveness, such as type of steroid used, dosage, psychosocial components, and technique. Also, patients with greater pain, presence of effusion, and less structural damage are more likely to benefit from intra-articular steroids.[7]

Frequent use of intra-articular steroid injections is usually not recommended against. One randomized trial studying patients with symptomatic knee OA injected their subjects every 12 weeks for 2 years and found that there was a minimal statistically significant difference in decreasing their pain. Long-term therapy has also been linked to intra-articular structural damage. This study also found significantly greater cartilage volume loss in patient knee joints.[9]

Hyaluronic Acid

Hyaluronic acid is a compound that can be considered for injection in the management of joint pain. Though hyaluronic acid has been used for chronic pain in the past, it may have some utility as an acute joint pain or acute exacerbations of chronic joint pain.[10] Hyaluronic acid can be bound in a variety of tissues with a high concentration in synovial fluid and articular cartilage. Hyaluronic acid is a glycosaminoglycan that is nonprotein and nonsulfated. It is naturally occurring and is created by a variety of cell types, including fibroblasts, chondrocytes, and synoviocytes. The role of hyaluronic acid is diverse and includes properties such as lubrication, viscoelasticity, shock absorption, and stabilization of joints.[11] With particular disease, such as OA, hyaluronic acid declines notably by number and molecular weight.[11] The development of OA has been associated with apoptosis of chondrocytes leading to degradation of the articular cartilage matrix.[11]

Osteoarthritis has been observed to affect various joints in the body. Most frequently affected are the feet, hands, elbow, knees, hips, and shoulders.[11] Prior reports have noted that giving hyaluronic acid intra-articular is more efficacious vs intravenous or oral route.[11] It is reported that normal human physiologic hyaluronic acid is about 0.35 g/100 mL with an MW of 4 000 000-10 000 000 Da in particular fluid. In OA, hyaluronic acid in synovial fluid is degraded and eliminated at faster rates vs nonosteoarthritic joints.[11]

The efficacy of injecting lower vs higher molecular weight hyaluronic acid was studied previously. Studies conducted by Gigis et al.[12] had shown that both high and low molecular weight hyaluronic acid produced similar beneficial effects. Other studies had shown that both were equally effective. Migliore et al.[13] had reported that injecting joints with higher molecular weight (6 000 000-7 000 000 Da) hyaluronic acid had led to improved retention of joint fluid and reportedly improved anti-inflammatory process.[11] Concoff et al. conducted a systemic review and meta-analysis and found that patients with knee OA who had received multiple hyaluronic acid (2-4 and >5 weekly increments) injections had improved pain scores vs the single shot and saline injection group.[14]

There have been some studies on intra-articular hyaluronic acid injections in patients with OA of the hip. Wu et al. conducted a meta-analysis of randomized controlled trials of intra-articular hyaluronic acid injections of the hip.[15] They found that hyaluronic acid injections lead to a reduction in pain and improved recovery; however, these effects were not noted to be significantly different from the saline group or from the other treatments studied.

Mechanism of action

Through several studies, it is known that hyaluronic acid exerts its effects through several mechanisms of action, including (1) reducing nitric oxide, superoxide, and hydroxyl radicals leading to decrease cell damage; (2) protective effect on mitochondria preventing apoptosis of chondrocytes; (3) reducing lipid peroxidation and reducing TNF-α with combination of chondroitin sulfate; (4) reduction of pain through PGE2 inhibition; (5) mechanical elastoviscous properties; (6) chondroprotective properties through attenuating IL-1β expression of lytic enzymes as well as reducing MMP-14 and ADAMTS4; and (7) promoting cartilage repair through proteoglycan synthesis.[11] Overall, hyaluronic acid has antioxidative, anti-chondropoptosis, analgesic, chondroprotective, and cartilage promoting properties[11] (Fig. 42.1).

Indications

Walker et al. reported that the only indications sanctioned by the FDA for hyaluronic acid join injections includes pain relief in patients suffering from mild to moderate OA in the knees who have failed conservative therapy[16] (Table 42.1). No other joints were approved for injection by the FDA.[16] Although the FDA has not approved hyaluronic acid injections for the hip, it has been used off-label for hip injections.[16]

Contraindications

Contraindications for intra-articular hyaluronic acid injections include hypersensitivity, anaphylaxis/detrimental allergic reaction, gram-positive bacterial protein hypersensitivity, lidocaine hypersensitivity, and disorders of bleeding.[16]

Adverse effects

Based on Walker et al., adverse effects of hyaluronic acid intra-articular injections have been reported as “mild and self-limiting.”[16] The most common event is irritation and site reactions at the injected area. It has been noted that up to 2% of patients can experience swelling and pain after injection.[16] Reactions such as these can be mitigated with ice, rest, and medications. Intra-articular fluid obtained from these patients was found to be aseptic. Angioedema and anaphylactic reactions were reported in the past with some patients experiencing nausea, muscle cramps, and joint pains.[16]

Platelet-Rich Plasma

Platelet-rich plasma (PRP) is a biologic agent that is derived from a patient’s own blood. Autologous blood is taken and centrifuged to produce a sample that contains platelet concentrations 4-5 times above baseline. Platelets contain a milieu of factors such as transforming growth factor (TGF)-β1, platelet-derived growth factor, basic fibroblast growth factor, vascular endothelial growth factor, epidermal growth factor, and insulinlike growth factor (IGF)-1, which are involved in the growth and repair of tissues. The proposed mechanism behind PRP is that delivering supraphysiologic amounts of these factors directly to sites of injury can augment the body’s natural response and enhance healing.[17,18] The principles behind PRP date all the way back to the first century BC when Aulus Cornelius Celsus described the process of inflammation and postulated its importance in the healing process.[19] In the ensuing years, continued attempts to harness the power of the body’s natural injury response led to the development of PRP, and by the early 2000s, PRP use had become commonplace to aide in healing in maxillofacial

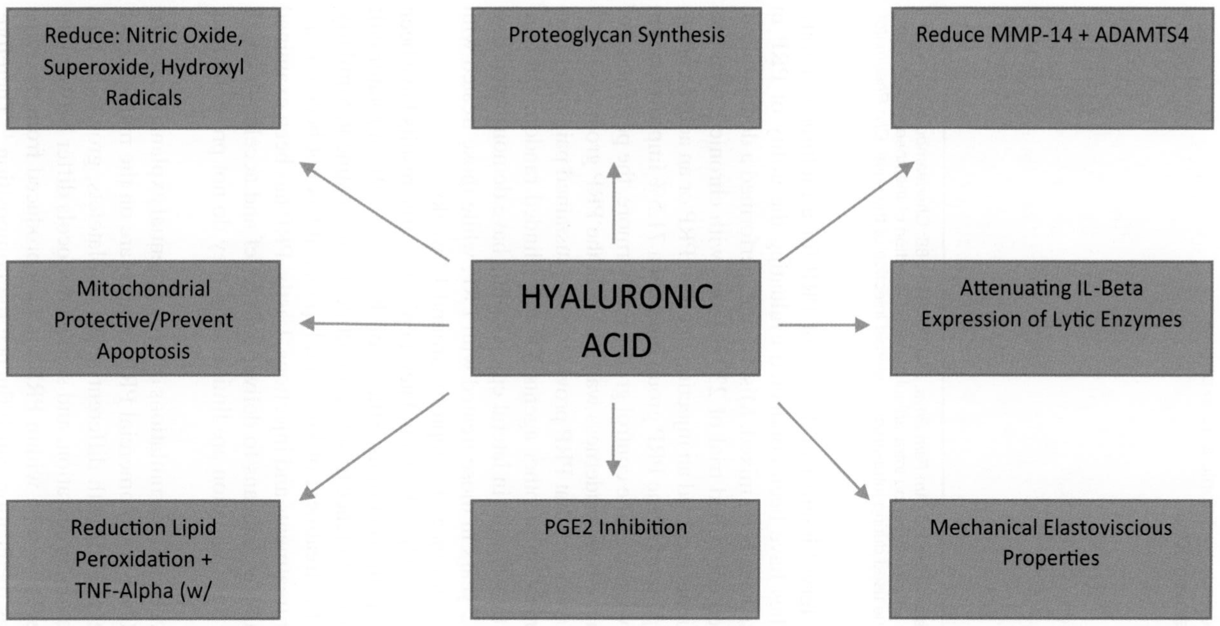

*TNF-Alpha: Tumor Necrosis Factor – Alpha

*PGE2: Prostaglandin E2

*MMP-14: Matrix Metalloproteinase-14

*ADAMTS4: ADAM Metallopeptidase with Thrombospondin Type 1 Motif 4

*IL-Beta: Interleukin Beta

FIGURE 42.1 MOA of hyaluronic acid. (From Williams DM. Clinical pharmacology of corticosteroids. *Respir Care*. 2018;63:655-670.)

TABLE 42.1 HYALURONIC ACID INJECTION

Indications: • Pain relief for mild to moderate knee osteoarthritis in patients failing conservative therapy
Contraindications: • Anaphylactic allergic reactions to previous hyaluronic acid exposure • Gram-positive bacterial protein hypersensitivity • Lidocaine hypersensitivity • Bleeding pathology
Side effects: • Site and irritation reactions at injection location • Swelling and pain • Nausea • Muscle cramps • Reported angioedema

From Cardone DA, Tallia AF. Joint and soft tissue injection. *Am Fam Phys*. 2002;66:283-288; Charalambous CP, Tryfonidis M, Sadiq S, Hirst P, Paul A. Septic arthritis following intra-articular steroid injection of the knee—a survey of current practice regarding antiseptic technique used during intra-articular steroid injection of the knee. *Clin Rheumatol*. 2003;22:386-390.

surgery.[19] Recently, there has been fervid interest in the use of PRP for a multitude of musculoskeletal maladies. Several studies have been conducted evaluating the utility of PRP in relieving joint pain; however, results have been mixed. Mishra et al. performed a double-blind, prospective, multicenter, randomized controlled trial of 230 patients with chronic lateral epicondylar tendinopathy in which patients received an injection of either PRP or an active control with local anesthetic. At 24 weeks, patients in the PRP group reported a 71.5% improvement in pain as compared to a 56.1% improvement in the control group. Furthermore, the percentage of patients reporting significant residual elbow tenderness was 29.1% in the PRP group and 54% in the control group.[20] There is also evidence that PRP provides more sustained pain relief than that achieved with intra-articular injection of other agents. Double-blinded randomized controlled trials examining PRP vs corticosteroids in lateral epicondylitis have demonstrated lasting improvement in pain for up to 2 years in those treated with PRP, while those treated with corticosteroid began to experience recurrence of symptoms around 12 weeks.[21,22]

In contrast to the relative success PRP has shown in lateral epicondylitis, results have been equivocal when used for other joint pain conditions. Studies of the use of PRP in rotator cuff tendinopathy have not produced strong evidence to suggest routine use in treatment. Similarly, though PRP has shown efficacy in the treatment of knee and hip OA, it has not been consistently shown to be superior to other treatments and injections. Lastly, PRP has been examined as a treatment for acute ankle sprains as a means to deliver pain relief and accelerate return to activity. The studies of PRP for this indication are limited, and they do not present strong evidence in favor of its use.[18]

The lack of standardization between PRP formulations offers a potential explanation for the varied results seen across studies. Over 16 commercial PRP systems are on the market. Each system is unique and therefore yields PRP with different levels of platelets, growth factors, and other cells. Additionally, collection, preparation, and storage protocols differ between the systems. Moreover, variation can even be seen within PRP samples produced from the same individual as patient factors such as medication can influence the composition.[18] Therefore, while intra-articular PRP injection has shown some promise as a treatment for joint pain, continued investigation into both its preparation and application is warranted.

Novel and Experimental Injections

Corticosteroid and hyaluronate joint injections are by far the most common injections used for joint pain. However, there are other investigational agents that are uncommonly used. Several disease-modifying antirheumatic drugs, such as methotrexate and tumor necrosis factor inhibitors, have been investigated in the use of inflammatory RA. In one study comparing the effectiveness of intra-articular methotrexate to intra-articular glucocorticoids over a 5-year period, both treatments halted radiographic progression and induced remission in the majority of patients with early RA.[23] Microspheres of gelatin, chondroitin, and liposomes have also been tested in animal models attempting to control the release of protein drugs within the injected joint. In one study, the researchers looked at creating a novel membrane-targeting complement regulatory protein that would inhibit complement activation within a joint, which is a known factor in the pathogenesis of chronic synovitis. Although done in rats, the study showed a dose-dependent therapeutic effect, with significantly milder clinical and histologic disease when compared to placebo.[24]

Stem cells have also been gaining popularity in joint arthropathies. Intra-articular injections for OA have been investigated thus far using bone marrow and adipose-derived stem cells. This normally involves harvesting fat or bone marrow from the patient, isolating the stem and regenerative cells, and administering the cells back to the patient. It is thought that stem cells can be involved in regrowth of new cartilage, subchondral bone, and synovium. The procedure itself is done with the same technique as other intra-articular injections and can be performed in the outpatient setting. Although studies are limited, some studies have shown promise with this treatment method. According to one study, injection of isolated bone marrow stem cells improved pain scores and increased range of motion up to 12 months. Increases in cartilage growth and thickness with decreases in the size of poor cartilage and edematous subchondral bone were also seen with magnetic resonance imaging.[25] Although there's great potential, studies are still very limited, and more randomized controlled trials are needed to determine their true efficacy.

Interventional Technique

Intervention technique for knee joint injections involves first preparation.[26] This includes using sterile gloves, sterile probe cover with gel for the ultrasound if being used, skin decontamination with alcohol or chlorhexidine, 1.5-in. needle that is 22-25 gauge, 1% lidocaine or ethyl chloride spray to numb the injection site, hyaluronic acid, and dressing.[26] Fluoroscopy or ultrasound can be used. If under fluoroscopy, the patient is placed in the supine position for a retropatellar and superolateral approach.[26] Mark the skin when palpating the upper third and lateral patella. Applying numbing solution. Apply medial pressure to move the patella in the lateral direction leading to opening the patellar space laterally.[26] Through fluoroscopy, one can then aim the needle medially in a transverse plan between the lateral femoral condyle and patella. Advance needle while aspirating for blood as to prevent intravenous injection.[26] Once confirmed position, inject the medication.[26]

If done under ultrasound, have the patient in the supine position. Again, palpate the upper third of the patella on the lateral side. Apply disinfectant solution and numb with topic spray or lidocaine.[26] Ultrasound can then be placed above the patella in a transverse plane. Note, while doing so, confirm depth of needle with ultrasound.[26] While maintaining a parallel view of the long axis, the operator should use an in-plane approach to insert the needle in a medial direction. This approach requires that the insertion point of the needle is superior and lateral to the patella.[26] Once confirmed in the joint, check with aspiration that administration is no intravascular and then inject the solution.[26]

Conclusion

Acute pain especially at the joints can be detrimental and excruciating. This pain can be acute or chronic in nature and can arise from a variety of mechanism including inflammation, infection, crystal deposition, cartilage degeneration, and trauma. Given the etiology, there are a variety approaches to treatment of joint pain. Currently, intra-articular injections are available including corticosteroids, PRP, hyaluronic acid, and novel components such as placental tissue matrix injections among others. It is our hope that we can shed more light on current research for available and novel intra-articular injections for acute joint pain.

REFERENCES

1. Ayhan E, Kesmezacar H, Akgun I. Intraarticular injections (corticosteroid, hyaluronic acid, platelet rich plasma) for the knee osteoarthritis. *World J Orthop*. 2014;5:351-361.
2. Williams DM. Clinical pharmacology of corticosteroids. *Respir Care*. 2018;63:655-670.
3. Pekarek B, Osher L, Buck S, Bowen M. Intra-articular corticosteroid injections: a critical literature review with up-to-date findings. *Foot*. 2011;21:66-70.
4. Freire V, Bureau NJ. Injectable corticosteroids: take precautions and use caution. *Semin Musculoskelet Radiol*. 2016;20:401-408.
5. Cardone DA, Tallia AF. Joint and soft tissue injection. *Am Fam Physician*. 2002;66:283-288.
6. Charalambous CP, Tryfonidis M, Sadiq S, Hirst P, Paul A. Septic arthritis following intra-articular steroid injection of the knee—a survey of current practice regarding antiseptic technique used during intra-articular steroid injection of the knee. *Clin Rheumatol*. 2003;22:386-390.
7. Arroll B, Goodyear-Smith F. Corticosteroid injections for osteoarthritis of the knee: meta-analysis. *Br Med J*. 2004;328:869.
8. Blyth T, Hunter JA, Stirling A. Pain relief in the rheumatoid knee after steroid injection a single-blind comparison of hydrocortisone succinate, and triamcinolone acetonide or hexacetonide. *Rheumatology*. 1994;33:461-463.
9. Maricar N, Callaghan MJ, Felson DT, O'Neill TW. Predictors of response to intra-articular steroid injections in knee osteoarthritis-a systematic review. *Rheumatol (United Kingdom)*. 2013;52:1022-1032.
10. Migliore A, Procopio S. Effectiveness and utility of hyaluronic acid in osteoarthritis. *Clin Cases Miner Bone Metab*. 2015;12(1):31-33.
11. Gupta RC, Lall R, Srivastava A, Sinha A. Hyaluronic acid: molecular mechanisms and therapeutic trajectory. *Front Vet Sci*. 2019;6:1-24.
12. Gigis I, Fotiadis E, Nenopoulos A, Tsitas K, Hatzokos I. Comparison of two different molecular weight intra-articular injections of hyaluronic acid for the treatment of knee osteoarthritis. *Hippokratia*. 2016;29:26-31. http://www.artosyal.it
13. Migliore A, Giovannangeli F, Granata M, Laganá B. Hylan g-f 20: review of its safety and efficacy in the management of joint pain in osteoarthritis. *Clin Med Insights Arthr Musculoskelet Disord*. 2010;20:55-68. doi:10.1177/117954411000300001
14. Concoff A, Sancheti P, Niazi F, Shaw P, Rosen J. The efficacy of multiple versus single hyaluronic acid injections: a systematic review and meta-analysis. *BMC Musculoskelet Disord*. 2017;18(1):1-15.
15. Wu B, Li YM, Liu YC. Efficacy of intra-articular hyaluronic acid injections in hip osteoarthritis: a meta-analysis of randomized controlled trials. *Oncotarget*. 2017;8(49):86865-86876.
16. Walker K, Basehore BM, Goyal A, Bansal P, Zito PM. Hyaluronic acid. In: *StatPearls* [Internet]. StatPearls Publishing; 2021.
17. Werner BC, Cancienne JM, Browning R, Verma NN, Cole BJ. An analysis of current treatment trends in platelet-rich plasma therapy in the Medicare database. *Orthop J Sports Med* 2020;8.
18. Le ADK, Enweze L, Debaun MR, Dragoo JL. Platelet-rich plasma. *Clin Sports Med*. 2020;38(1):17-44. doi:10.1016/j.csm.2018.08.001
19. Bashir J, Panero AJ, Sherman AL. The emerging use of platelet-rich plasma in musculoskeletal medicine. *J Am Osteopath Assoc*. 2015;115:24-31.
20. Mishra AK, Skrepnik NV, Edwards SG, et al. Efficacy of platelet-rich plasma for chronic tennis elbow: a double-blind, prospective, multicenter, randomized controlled trial of 230 patients. *Am J Sports Med*. 2014;42(2):463-471.
21. Gosens T, Peerbooms JC, Van Laar W, Den Oudsten BL. Ongoing positive effect of platelet-rich plasma versus corticosteroid injection in lateral epicondylitis: a double-blind randomized controlled trial with 2-year follow-up. *Am J Sports Med*. 2011;39(6):1200-1208.
22. Peerbooms JC, Sluimer J, Bruijn DJ, Gosens T. Positive effect of an autologous platelet concentrate in lateral epicondylitis in a double-blind randomized controlled trial: platelet-rich plasma versus corticosteroid injection with a 1-year follow-up. *Am J Sports Med*. 2010;38(2):255-262.
23. Hetland ML, Hørslev-Petersen K. The CIMESTRA study: intra-articular glucocorticosteroids and synthetic DMARDs in a treat-to-target strategy in early rheumatoid arthritis. *Clin Exp Rheumatol*. 2012;30:S44-S49.
24. Linton SM, Williams AS, Dodd I, Smith R, Williams BD, Paul Morgan B. Therapeutic efficacy of a novel membrane-targeted complement regulator in antigen-induced arthritis in the rat. *Arthritis Rheum*. 2000;43:2590-2597.
25. Orth P, Rey-Rico A, Venkatesan JK, Madry H, Cucchiarini M. Current perspectives in stem cell research for knee cartilage repair. *Stem Cells Cloning*. 2014;7:1-17.
26. Manchikanti L, Kaye AD, Falco FJE, et al. *Essentials of Interventional Techniques in Managing Chronic Pain*. Springer International Publishing AG; 2018:645-655.

43

Acupuncture

Olabisi Lane, Jamie Kitzman, and Anna Woodbury

Introduction

Acupuncture has been practiced for more than 2000 years. Its origin continues to be debated, but is generally considered an important component of traditional Chinese medicine (TCM). The word a*cupuncture* has Latin roots meaning "needle penetration" and involves the act of inserting metallic, solid thin needles through the skin to stimulate specific points on the body. The needle can be manipulated either manually or via electrical stimulation to improve pain. It is typically used for pain relief but has also been employed in treating a wide array of conditions.[1] It is believed to cause stimulation of small nerve endings and other structures around the acupoints, which results in both local and distant changes within the body.

Traditional acupuncture is based on ancient Chinese beliefs that "qi" (life force or energy) circulates throughout the body via energy carrying pathways called meridians. Twelve major meridians are thought to remain in continuous flow and in balance with two polarities yin and yang, reflecting good health and well-being. Illness occurs as a result of an imbalance between yin and yang due to a disruption of qi. Acupuncture is thought to reestablish the flow and balance by stimulating anatomical target points along the meridians in the body. The needles are typically stainless steel but may be made of gold and silver. Most needles are 1.3-12.7 cm long with a diameter of 26-36 gauge. The needles are inserted 3-15 mm under the skin.[2] A sensation, de-qi, is said to be felt when the acupuncture needle is inserted. This sensation can be described as numbness, pressure tingling, heaviness, soreness, or aching in nature. The sensation is also sensed by the proceduralist as a grasping of the needle with a sense of fullness, tightness, or even tension.[3] Most acupuncturist believe that this sensation is needed to provide the full effect of acupuncture.

Manual Acupuncture vs Electroacupuncture

Acupuncture can be administered via manual acupuncture (MA) or electrical acupuncture (EA). MA is the insertion of needles into acupoints and then manually twisting the needle up and down, whereas in EA, a stimulating current via small clips is administered to the acupoints. Stimulation may be high (100-200 Hz), medium (15-30 Hz), or low (2-4 Hz).

The frequency and intensity can be modified depending on the aim of the treatment. Needles can be stimulated in pairs for <30 minutes. EA may also be administered without the use of needles in the form of transcutaneous electrical nerve stimulation (TENS), whereby electrodes are applied to the skin to stimulate identified points. EA is also advantageous in that the needles do not have to be inserted into precise points as the stimulation of the needle affects a larger area.

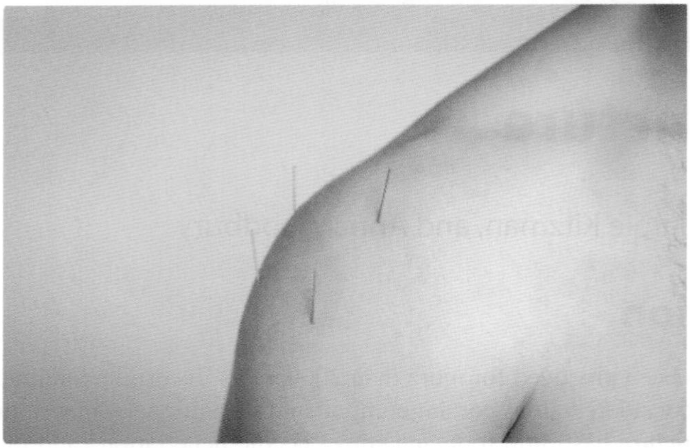

A

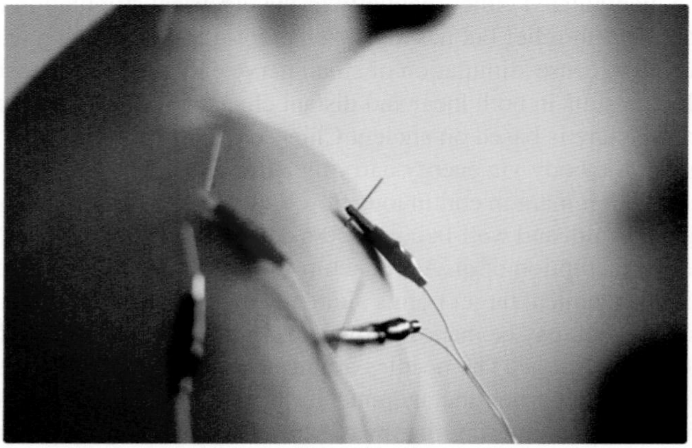

B

Electroacupuncture vs. manual acupuncture of the shoulder. Electroacupuncture has been shown to have greater efficacy than manual acupuncture in the treatment of various musculoskeletal conditions. The figure depicts **(A)** manual acupuncture at SI 12, SI 10, LI 16, and LI 15 and **(B)** electroacupuncture, where electrodes are applied to the same acupuncture points used in manual acupuncture, but current is delivered to the needles via a machine that creates an alternating current (AC) waveform from a direct current (DC) battery. Because it is AC, the placement of the *black* and *red* clips should not matter, though some acupuncturists prefer to place the *red* clips closer to the torso and the *black* clips more in the periphery. The frequency and amplitude of the current can be adjusted to stimulate release of various endogenous endorphins and produce a tingling, buzzing, or pulsing sensation. A usual treatment lasts approximately 20 minutes. (Credit: medical photo created by wavebreakmedia_micro.)

There are various techniques and methodologies to the practice of acupuncture owing to different traditions from countries including China, Japan, Korea, and Vietnam. The overall thought is that the ears, hands, and feet are “micromodels” of the body and denote acupuncture points, meridians, organs, and body parts. The unifying principal of this practice remains in the application of acupuncture to specific anatomical target points to obtain a reduction in pain and induce other beneficial effects.[2]

Auricular Acupuncture

First described in France by Paul Nogier, auricular acupuncture (AA) is similar to reflexology as it also uses a microacupuncture technique. It is believed that organs are represented on the human auricle and stimulation of identified points will have effects on the respective distant organs. Research has shown that it can be used to treat pain and anxiety, but more exploration is needed to confirm its use in the treatment of tobacco and substance abuse. Various materials such as stainless steel, sterile acupuncture needles, press-tack needles, Semen Vaccariae (SV, radish seeds), small metal pellets, or magnetized pellets have been used. Perhaps one of the best-studied auricular acupuncture protocols for acute pain is the battlefield acupuncture (BFA) protocol originally designed by Dr. Richard Niemtzow, which will be discussed in more depth later in the chapter.[4,5] Medical practitioners can now be trained specifically in battlefield acupuncture as an adjunct outside of traditional Chinese medicine training or full acupuncture accreditation.[6] A concern among modern researchers is the ability to standardize identified points in the ear and the lack of correlation with these identified areas and knowledge of anatomy and physiology. Wirx-Ridolfi discusses the likelihood of an increase in credibility of this practice if better comparable charts were available, which could be advantageous to spreading the acceptance of the practice in the scientific world as well as achieving improved patient results improved results for patients.[7-9]

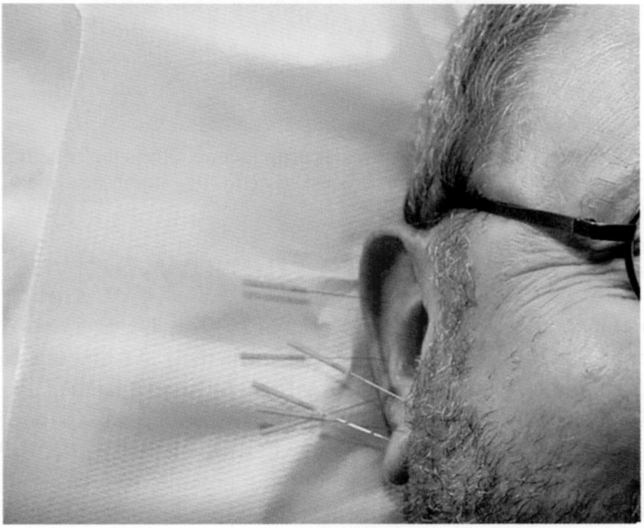

Auricular acupuncture. Auricular acupuncture involves the insertion of acupuncture needles at predefined points along the external ear. Practitioners can use a nanometer or "point finder" to measure the resistance in the ear. The point called "shen men" is typically used as a zeroing point. Auricular acupuncture is typically well-tolerated and is amenable to quicker placement due to the accessibility of the ear without the need for clothing removal. Though traditional acupuncture needles are used in the photo, semipermanent needles, press tacks, vaccaria seeds, or pellets with adhesive can also be placed, allowing the patient to receive a quick treatment and needles/seeds/pellets that they can go home with, without the typical 20-30 minute wait for needle removal. (Credit: medical photo created by Walti Goehner. Licensed via Pixabay.)

Scalp Acupuncture

Chinese scalp acupuncture is a technique that integrates traditional Chinese methods with Western medical knowledge of representative areas of the cerebral cortex. This technique has been shown to be an effective treatment of acute and chronic central nervous system disorders.

It produces excellent and almost immediate results with just a few needles. The areas identified on the scalp are based on Western medicine reflex somatotopic system, where needles are inserted subcutaneously into specific zones rather than into acupuncture points. These zones are areas within the cerebrum and cerebellum that perform motor and sensory functions, assist in vision, hearing, speech, and balance. Scalp acupuncture has been used for a variety of neurologic conditions, including Parkinson disease, stroke, and multiple sclerosis. An experienced practitioners is needed to perform this technique.[10]

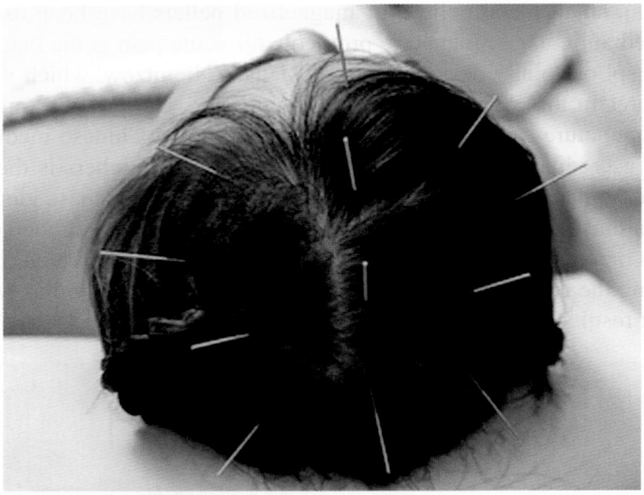

Scalp acupuncture. Scalp acupuncture, like auricular acupuncture, offers the benefit of allowing the patient to remain clothed during the treatment process. (Credit: PK Studio licensed via Adobe Stock Photo.)

Korean Hand Acupuncture Therapy

This form of acupuncture was developed in Korea in 1971 by Dr. Tae-woo Yoo. Korean hand acupuncture therapy (KHT) is grounded in the same principals of Chinese acupuncture including yin and yang, meridians systems, and energy flow. In Korean hand acupuncture, the hand is viewed as a microcosm of the body, with all body parts and organs assigned a specific point on the hand. KHT uses short, narrow diameter needles, which are inserted 1-3 mm into points on the hand. KHT can also be performed by applying pressure to precise points on the hand or using metal pellets of opposite polarities. KHT is advantageous in that less invasive techniques can be used.[11,12]

Acupuncture was introduced in the United States in the 1970s, after President Nixon's visit to China. During that visit, a member of the press corp, James Reston, a New York Times reporter, required an appendectomy. Reston's postoperative pain was treated with acupuncture and his experience was highly publicized.[13,14] Interest in this treatment modality grew in the 1970s with California being the first state to establish the need for a license to practice, with several states following suite. Research into this therapy further amplified interest, with studies delving into its mechanism of action, such as endorphin hypothesis, and the use of imaging modalities, including fMRI and positron emission tomography. The National Institutes of Health (NIH) continues to support experimental and clinical acupuncture studies and released a consensus statement in 1997, showing promise with the use of acupuncture in adult postoperative pain, chemotherapy-induced nausea and vomiting, as well as for postoperative dental pain. It also discussed the likelihood of acupuncture being used as part of a multimodal treatment regimen in patients with headaches, myofascial pain, fibromyalgia to name a few. The NIH developed an Office of Alternative Medicine now known as the National Center for Complementary and Integrative Health (NCCIH) that continues to fund clinical trials to evaluate the efficacy of acupuncture. The World Health Organization also describes a variety of medical conditions that may benefit from acupuncture, including the prevention and treatment of nausea and vomiting; treatment of addiction to tobacco, alcohol, and other drugs; and treatment of pulmonary conditions. It can be used to assist with rehabilitation after neurological damage such as those caused by a stroke. Concerns regarding study designs, sample size, the ability to properly control studies (placebo vs sham acupuncture, insertion of needle into nonacupuncture points) were highlighted.[15] For many years, acupuncture needles were classified as class III medical devices, which are considered devices with a high risk to the patient or user. In the 1990s, a group of lawyers and acupuncturist petitioned the U.S. Food and Drug Administration (FDA) to designate the needles as class II medical devices.

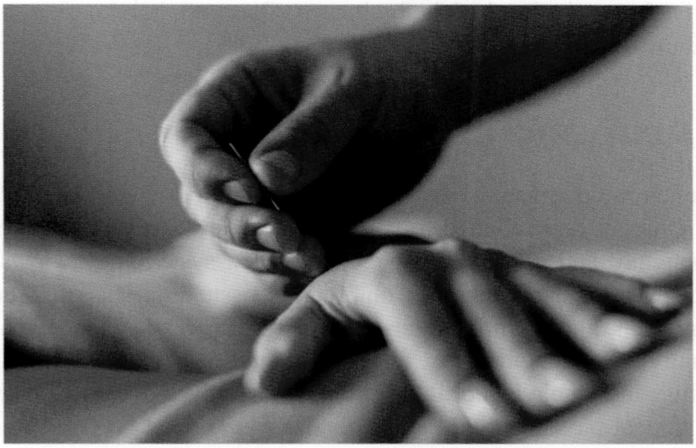

Hand acupuncture. Like auricular acupuncture and scalp acupuncture, hand acupuncture utilizes a body part that is easy to access and also has its own somatotopic mapping for body regions that can be treated via the hand. The photo depicts needle insertion at LI4 one of the most utilized acupuncture points. LI4 is traditionally used for the treatment of headaches, toothaches, and upper body pain as well as other symptomatology. (Photo Credit: https://www.freepik.com/photos/health">Health photo created by freepik—www.freepik.com)

Mechanism of Action

As previously stated, acupuncture can be delivered via MA or EA. James Kennedy describes MA as the insertion of needles into acupoints and then manually twisting the needle up and down. MA results in the stimulation of A-β, A-δ, and C fibers. EA involves the application of a stimulating current to the acupoints and is thought to excite A-β and a portion of A-δ fibers. EA has been widely studied in fMRI, compared to the gate control theory, as well as studied for its role with NMDA receptors and central sensitization.[16] Despite ongoing research, the exact mechanism of acupunctures effects continues to be debated with the endorphin theory appearing to be the most accepted. Chernyak et al. described a mechanism of action proposed by Pomeranz and Stux that involves three components contributing to the analgesic properties, with effects at the spinal cord level, the midbrain, and in the pituitary-hypothalamic complex. At the level of the spinal cord, it is thought to cause the release of enkephalin and dynorphin, inhibiting pain signals from ascending into the spinothalamic tract. In the midbrain, it stimulates the cells in the periaqueductal gray matter and the raphe nucleus, resulting in descending signals that cause the release of serotonin and norepinephrine, which lessens pain by reducing signal transmission through the spinothalamic tract. Finally, in the pituitary-hypothalamic complex, it causes release of endorphins and adrenocorticotropic hormone.[2,17] Kawakita and Okada, described a pharmacological study conducted by a group at Peking University that described endogenous opioid peptides as having a major role in electroacupuncture analgesia (EAA). This theory is further strengthened because EAA is said to be antagonized by naloxone, an opioid receptor antagonist. Han's group showed that low-frequency (2 Hz) EAA caused the release of enkephalin, β-endorphin, and endomorphin, which in turn activated μ- and δ-opioid receptors; while high-frequency (100 Hz) EAA resulted in the release of dynorphins, which affected κ-opioid receptors in the spinal cord.[18,19] Lin and Chen touched on the response of animals with hyperalgesia to acupuncture, noting that these animals may respond differently to EA. This study also highlighted the role of the inflammatory reflex and the autonomic nervous system as it pertains to antihyperalgesic properties seen with acupuncture treatment. This reflex also modulates the immune system and may explain the role of acupuncture in inflammatory states.[20] More research is needed to determine the exact mechanism for acupuncture exerting its analgesic effect, though current evidence supports the endogenous opioid response, modulation of long-term potentiation and neural plasticity through activation at the level of the brain as well as peripheral nerves, and the release of various anti-inflammatory and neuro-hormones.

Safety of Acupuncture

The use of acupuncture continues to grow, as such it is important to keep track of its safety profile. In 2016, Chan et al. evaluated all systematic reviews (SRs) for adverse events associated with acupuncture and related therapies. Seventeen systematic reviews were identified and adverse effects were categorized based on organ or tissue injuries, infections, local adverse events or reactions, and other complications such as dizziness or syncope. The most common organ or tissue injury was pneumothorax. Infections included hepatitis, tetanus, auricular infection, septic arthritis, and staphylococcal infection. Local adverse events or reactions, such as contact dermatitis, local bleeding, and pain, as well as burns and bruising were also reported, as were more systemic effects such as nausea and vomiting, dizziness or syncope, and vasovagal reactions. Chan et al. concluded that serious and minor adverse effects do occur albeit rare. However, uncommon, it is important to be able to promptly identify them as some can lead to increased mortality. The importance of referring patients to credible acupuncturist was also stressed.[21] Similarly, Park et al. investigated adverse events associated with acupuncture. Of the 2226 patients enrolled in the study, 99 reported adverse events including hemorrhage (32%), hematoma (28%), and needle pain site (13%). Sixty-four patients ended treatment with 62 of those patients with adverse events reporting diminished or a disappearance of the symptoms. Of the 35 remaining cases of adverse events in which treatment was continued, 28 patients reported a reduction or disappearance of the symptoms. Park et al. also acknowledged that acupuncture is associated with adverse events, but patients in this study did not experience serious adverse events. Again, the authors stressed the importance of referral to practitioners with experience who can perform this technique in accordance with set guidelines.[22]

Use as Part of Perioperative Multimodal Treatment Plan

Uncontrolled postoperative pain remains a challenging problem and has been shown to lead to chronic pain. The standard of care for treating postoperative pain is slowly shifting away from using opioids as the sole agent to a multimodal treatment approach. Wang et al. performed a follow-up study reviewing the use of complementary and alternative medicines (CAM) by surgery patients and discovered that most surgical patients were willing to use CAM, with 7% of these patients agreeable to the use of acupuncture for postoperative pain reduction. The authors determined that acupuncture is an effective part of regular care, is safe, and rarely causes significant adverse effects.[23] Wu et al. performed a systematic review and meta-analysis to determine the effectiveness of acupuncture and acupuncture-related techniques in treating postoperative pain. As compared to the control group, patients who received traditional acupuncture and transcutaneous electric acupoint stimulation (TEAS) reported less pain on day 1 after surgery. The TEAS group were reported to use significantly less opioids. Based on these finding, the authors support the use of acupuncture for the treatment of postsurgical pain.[24] Similarly, Sun et al. performed a systematic review to quantitatively evaluate the available evidence for the efficacy of acupuncture and related techniques in postoperative pain management. The results showed a reduction in postoperative opioid use, most evident at the 72-hour mark, as well as a reduction in postoperative pain scores at the 8- and 72-hour mark. Both the reduction in pain intensity and the reduction in absolute opioid consumption was thought to only be modest. Overall, the authors determined that acupuncture may be a good addition to postoperative analgesia.[25] Hendawy and Abuelnaga sought to determine the efficacy of ear acupuncture in patients undergoing abdominal hysterectomy with patients sorted based on who received spinal analgesia alone (control group) and spinal analgesia and electric ear acupuncture (EAA). Their findings revealed an increased threshold in somatic pain when acupuncture and TENS are employed. The study also revealed a reduction in PCA use in the first 24 hours after surgery in the treatment group and a delay in the time to request first supplemental analgesia. Again, the authors concluded that acupuncture is a useful part of a multimodal treatment regimen and improves patient satisfaction with minimal risk associated with its use.[26]

Acupuncture for Labor and Delivery

The safety of acupuncture in pregnancy is relatively well accepted. Studies have shown that acupuncture may be beneficial during pregnancy and delivery. Favorable effects during pregnancy include ameliorating nausea and vomiting, improving sleep, back pain, and depression. During childbirth and delivery, it has been reported to prevent postterm dates, promote cervical ripening, shorten time of labor, and reduce postpartum bleeding. In a recent meta-analysis of acupressure including 13 randomized controlled trials and 1586 patients, Chen et al. concluded that there is moderate quality data to support the effects of acupressure for relieving labor pain.[27] Its use to promote induction may not be supported.[28] Allais et al. highlighted acupuncture as a potential therapy for nausea, vomiting, and migraine attacks during the first trimester of pregnancy and should be considered a treatment.[29] Park et al. performed a systemic review evaluating the safety of acupuncture in pregnancy, as some of acupuncture's peripartum effects are thought to be related to oxytocin release from stimulation at specific acupoints, including those around the ankle and sacrum. The review concluded that acupuncture is associated with mild and transient adverse events, such as unspecified pain, pain at needling site, and bleeding. Of the serious adverse events identified, they were deemed to likely be unrelated to the acupuncture therapy.[22] Carr revisited the debate surrounding the possibly harm of performing acupuncture at forbidden points including in the sacral region and lower abdomen. This concern runs high among traditional acupuncturist and less so in Western medicine acupuncture since it is not based on evidence. These points have been considered to be contraindicated before 37 weeks of pregnancy, given concerns surrounding cervical ripening, uterine contraction, and risk of uterine penetration. Carr summarized that acupuncture at these identified locations is not associated and did not increase the risk of adverse events in controlled and observational trials nor did it induce miscarriage or labor. He was reassured that additional factors may contribute to adverse pregnancy outcomes.[30] Furthermore, Asher et al. performed a study where they determined that acupuncture when compared to normal medical care or sham acupuncture was not effective in inducing labor nor did it affect the rate of cesarean delivery.[31] Mansu et al. concluded that acupuncture seems to be safe and well tolerated by women in all trimesters. The authors urge practitioners to use judgment when selecting appropriate patients, selecting acupuncture points, combination, and order as well as the strength of the stimulation.[32]

Acupuncture for Acute Pediatric Pain

Acupuncture is widely accepted by pediatric patients and parents, even in the perioperative and emergency room setting.[33-36] In a study investigating the acceptability and feasibility of acupuncture for acute postoperative pain, Wu et al. found 86% of patients accepted treatment with a 14% refusal rate, and the acupuncture session was well tolerated.[36] Moreover, 70% of both parents and patients felt acupuncture helped the child's pain, and 85% of parents suggested that they would be willing to pay out-of-pocket for acupuncture in the future. Similarly, in a small study in the emergency room, 96% of patients who received acupuncture for pain were satisfied with pain relief and reported that they would have acupuncture again.[35]

The safety and efficacy of acupuncture in the pediatric population has been studied.[36-38] In a literature review from 2007, Jindal et al. concluded that it is a low-risk procedure that is most effective in the prevention of PONV, followed by the treatment of pain. In a more recent literature review, Lin et al. concluded that acupuncture is well supported as an effective treatment in pediatric procedural pain, with literature supporting its use in infant heel lancing, venipuncture, dental, tonsillectomy and adenoidectomy, myringotomy tube placement, and kidney biopsy.[38] In a small study, Wu et al. reported that postoperative pain scores decreased at 4 and 24 hours postacupuncture treatment in children having surgical procedures with planned inpatient admission, most of which were posterior spinal fusions.[36]

Considering the challenges of pain management and PONV in pediatric ENT surgery, there is growing interest in acupuncture for these patients due to the low-risk profile of acupuncture compared to existing pharmacological treatments. Much of this literature focuses on acupuncture for tonsillectomy, specifically investigating pain control, PONV prevention, and emergence agitation prevention. A literature review of the use of CAM post tonsillectomy found the greatest evidence for the use of acupuncture for pain and nausea compared to other CAM but noted methodological limitations in the studies.[39] In a meta-analysis of RCTs, Cho et al.[40] found that patients who received acupuncture treatments had decreased post-op pain up to 48 hours after tonsillectomy, decrease in analgesic requirements, and decreased incidence of PONV compared to control (conventional drug therapy or sham treatment). They concluded that perioperative acupuncture may provide pain relief, but the efficacy could not be determined due to heterogeneity of studies. Another meta-analysis that included RCTS and non-RCTs found a decrease in PONV by 23% with the use of PC-6 compared to control (conventional drug therapy or no drug therapy).[41] These findings were confirmed in a recent, randomized double-blinded trial.[42] Moeen reported that acupuncture provides a similar antiemetic effect as dexamethasone in pediatric patients undergoing tonsillectomy.[43] However, the power of the study was questioned.[44] Calcium plasters applied to acupoints were found to decrease the incidence of emergence agitation but not pain post tonsillectomy.[45] Electroacupuncture has been found to decrease analgesic requirements, pain scores, and agitation score in patients undergoing myringotomy and tympanostomy tube placement.[46]

Other potential uses of acupuncture in pediatric acute pain are beginning to be explored. Acupuncture has been used for the treatment of acute pain in pediatric emergency departments. There is also a substantial body of literature supporting the use of acupuncture for acute dental pain, demonstrating decreased VAS score and edema, albeit most are in adult populations.[47-50] Nonetheless, the use of acupuncture may be beneficial to those children who present commonly in a surgical setting for dental restorations. Tsai et al. reported improvement of acute lower back pain, carpal tunnel pain, joint pain, sprains, acute abdominal pain from appendicitis, otitis externa, dysmenorrhea, and paraphimosis with the use of BFA and traditional acupuncture.[35,51] Given the clear relationship between physical and emotional distress particularly in children, the use of acupuncture for anxiolysis could facilitate pain management. Wang et al. found single point acupressure at Yin Tang decreased preoperative anxiety reported by STAIC questionnaire (State Trait Anxiety Inventory for Children) in pediatric patients undergoing endoscopy.[52]

The actual practice of pediatric acupuncture requires special considerations, including addressing a child's fear of needles or inability to remain still once needles are in place. Needle phobia can be mitigated by developing a rapport with the patient through age-appropriate dialogue or performing a single test point (on patient or parent, if amenable). Distraction whether by conversation or an electric device can facilitate the process of needle placement and child stillness during a treatment session. If the child's acceptance to needle placement is not possible, acupressure and nonneedle adjuncts including acupuncture beads, adhesive microneedles, and lasers can be used. It may be necessary to decrease the length of the treatment in children who have a tendency to fidget. As with any procedure in a pediatric patient, it is important to obtain assent from a child to minimize emotional stress or PTSD.

Current literature shows promise for acupuncture in pain management. However, in general, study strength is limited by small sample size, and literature reviews are limited by heterogeneity of study design and acupuncture technique. There is a need for larger, more rigorously designed RCTs. Given the interdependence of pain control and anxiety, it is reasonable to use acupuncture as a safe and cost-effective adjunct to traditional management. With an adaptable qualified acupuncturist, acupuncture can be a tension-free and effective addition to the care of a pediatric patient.

Acupuncture for Acute Injury (Pain Clinic)

In 2001, battlefield acupuncture was developed by Dr. Richard Niemtzow, the name was inspired by the events surrounding 9/11 and the hopes of its application in military battlefield. It is a 5-point AA procedure using Aiguille Semi-Permanent (ASP) acupuncture needles. ASP needles are very short, penetrate only about 2 mm, and have small barbs and blunted outer ends. They are designed to remain in the skin for 3-4 days for prolonged therapeutic response but may be removed earlier.[53] Placement involves the sequential positioning of acupuncture needles into certain areas within the ears including cingulate gyrus, thalamic nuclei (anterior), omega2, Point Zero, and Shenmen with periods of allowed ambulation, during which pain is assessed. It has been shown to promote beneficial effects by affecting pain processing in the central nervous system with improvement in pain symptoms within a few minutes of application with variable duration depending on modality used. Dr. Niemtzow demonstrated effectiveness of this therapy in an outpatient clinic and emergency care setting.[54]

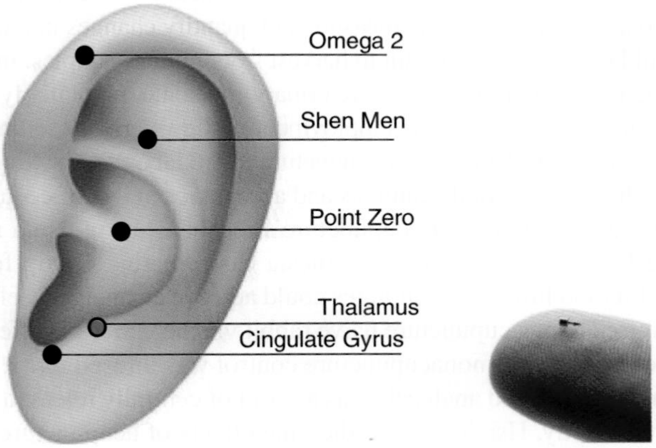

Battlefield acupuncture. Medical practitioners who seek to deliver this therapy can receive certification to perform battlefield acupuncture without the comprehensive additional training and licensure required to perform other types of acupuncture. A semipermanent gold ASP needle is depicted on an index finger in the bottom right corner. This type of needle is often used in the delivery of battlefield acupuncture because it can be rapidly delivered and will remain indwelling in the ear for up to 2 weeks. The battlefield acupuncture points are shown on the ear. The battlefield acupuncture protocol involves the rapid placement of needles at 5 points (cingulate gyrus, thalamic nuclei, omega 2, point zero, and shen men), depicted in *black*, on the external ear to quickly alleviate pain. The *red point* is on the posterior aspect of the area visualized. (Original illustration of ear by tigatelu, licensed by Adobe Stock photos. Modified by authors.)

ASP Ear needle

There is increasing interest in the use of acupuncture for acute pain injury states, such as in the emergency department, and for common sports injuries, "sideline acupuncture." Fox et al. performed a pilot feasibility study that revealed the possibility of using battlefield acupuncture for the treatment of acute lower back pain in the emergency department.[55] Liu et al. concluded that acupuncture alone or in combination with rest, ice, compression, and elevation (RICE) may be beneficial for acute ankle sprain by significantly decreasing pain and increasing cure rate when compared with RICE only. The study also showed that acupuncture plus massage could also significantly relieve pain than massage alone.[56] deWeber et al. described the outcomes of AA (battlefield acupuncture) in eight veteran athletes afflicted with various injuries including limb amputations, spinal cord injuries, traumatic brain injury, and posttraumatic stress disorder, participating in the 2010 warrior games (Paralympic sports). Acute injuries addressed with this treatment modality included ruptured anterior cruciate ligament (ACL), chronic knee pain with exacerbation due to a patellar cartilage injury with effusion, exacerbation of chronic lower back pain with and without radiculopathy, and three patients with varying degrees of hamstring sprain. All patients were initially treated by a multidisciplinary medicine team. Those athletes not improving with traditional treatments such as physical therapy, chiropractor, and standard therapies, were offered acupuncture. They demonstrated an overwhelming positive response to acupuncture and were able to continue in the competition.[53] Goertz et al. performed a pilot study in the emergency department consisting of a randomized controlled clinical trial to compare the effects of standard emergency medical care compared to standard care and AA. These authors revealed that both group had similar reductions in pain 24 hours after treatment and recommends more research to evaluate this treatment option.[57]

In regards to chronic pain, Zeliadt et al. determined battlefield acupuncture was effective, safe, and found to reduce pain intensity in a large population of veterans with chronic pain. The authors notes that the more research needs to be done to determine the duration of its effects.[58]

Animal and Basic Science Studies for Acute Pain

Animals provide a unique opportunity for the study of acupuncture due to (1) decreased susceptibility to placebo and (2) the ability to measure and quantify changes in biomarkers and biological tissues that would be otherwise difficult to harvest from human samples. In recent years, acupuncture has become increasingly utilized in veterinary medicine, particularly for pain and musculoskeletal conditions.[59] Despite its wide employment in the veterinary setting for dogs, horses, and some small animals, the utilization of acupuncture in the laboratory setting presents some unique challenges including the size of the animals and acceptance of the procedure by the animals.

Some of the earliest studies of acupuncture's mechanisms utilize a rabbit model. In 1973, Dr. Han of the Peking Acupuncture Anesthesia Coordinating Group found that acupuncture applied to a rabbit hind limb for 30 minutes could achieve an analgesic effect and that this effect could be transferred to an acupuncture naive rabbit via the CSF (this effect was not found when normal saline or CSF from a nonacupuncture control was infused into a naive rabbit), suggesting that acupuncture-induced analgesia was a result of centrally released neuromodulatory substances.[60] More recently, Hsieh et al. studied the effects of acupuncture on myofascial trigger points in rabbits and found that acupuncture applied to a gastrocnemius trigger point significantly enhanced spinal enkephalin expression and serum β-endorphin levels, with increased dosing elevating β-endorphin levels in a distal biceps femoris trigger point as well as in the spinal dorsal root ganglia; they suggested that this mechanism as a potential pathway for the distal analgesic effects of acupuncture for myofascial trigger point pain management.[61]

The morphological characteristics of acupoints has also been studied in rodents, revealing significantly higher number of subepidermal nerve fibers with a high expression of TRPV1.

Interestingly, Abraham et al. showed that TRPV1 expression increased after EA stimulation in nerve fibers projecting to the spinal cord, which may modulate central neuronal responses.[62] These points have been mapped using noxious antidromic stimulation of the tibial nerve of rats, resulting in the extravasation of Evans blue dye in receptive fields of C fibers of the foot that largely matched the distribution of human acupoints, again highlighting the high density of nerve fibers at acupoints.[63]

Acupuncture has been studied in clinically relevant animal models of osteoarthritis, as well, using stimulation of acupoints held in place with dental floss or other devices. One group successfully trained chimpanzees to accept acupuncture and measured a benefit in osteoarthritis using ST34, ST35, and ST36 points purported to alleviate inflammation in humans.[64] In a rodent model of arthritic pain, electroacupuncture (EA) applied to Zusanli (ST36), Yinlingquan (SP9), and Taichong (LR3 or LV3) significantly improved weight bearing in rats, compared to controls.[65] The commonality in these two studies is the ST36 acupoint, which is generally known to produce an immune modulatory effect. A mechanistic study in rodents applying EA at ST36 found that stimulation of this point regulated production of cytokines IFN-γ, IL-2, and IL-17 and the activation of splenic T cells. The researchers noted that regulation of extracellular and intracellular Ca^{2+} concentrations mediated this effect and suggested that EA at ST36 induces Ca^{2+} influx in spleen cells via TRPV channels.[66] EA at ST36 and LV3 has also been found to increase mesenchymal stem cell release in mice, which may exert anti-inflammatory effects and promote healing.[67]

Due to the ability to apply indwelling, semipermanent needles in a concentrated area, auriculotherapy, also known as ear acupuncture or AA, may offer a unique method to study acupuncture's effects in animals. In a study of 30 dogs with thoracolumbar disc disease, 73% recovered or improved following auriculotherapy.[68] AA has also been studied in rodent models of gastric hypersensitivity (dyspepsia) and epilepsy.[69,70]

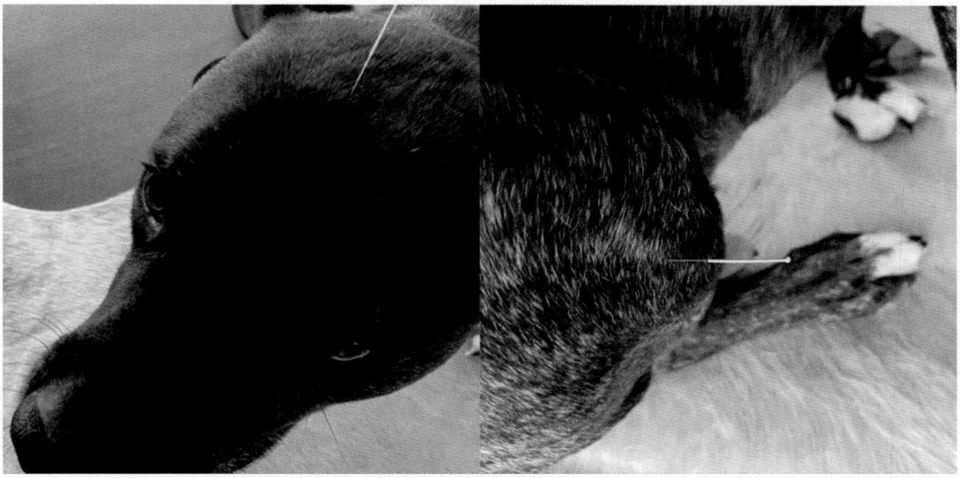

Veterinary acupuncture. Veterinary acupuncture requires additional training through veterinary medicine. It is typically well-tolerated and used for the treatment of osteoarthritis and other pain conditions in animals. Dr. Woodbury's dog is depicted in the photo receiving acupuncture at GV 20, a point commonly used for headaches and anxiety, and at ST31 for hip/thigh pain. Acupuncture administered to laboratory animals has also served to advance research in the field, as animals are less likely to be placebo responders.

Conclusions and Additional Resources

A significant amount of research has been performed regarding acupuncture for acute pain, from laboratory and mechanistic studies to clinical trials of traumatic and postoperative pain in animals, children, and adults. Though there exist challenges involved in designing acupuncture trials, researchers have overcome many of these hurdles to provide evidence of acupuncture's analgesic effects. Different modalities of acupuncture exist, and these individual modalities (AA, electroacupuncture, MA, scalp acupuncture) and the permutations of point combinations offer immense potential for further study. Electroacupuncture has shown the most potential for a positive effect, and AA is likely to be the most accessible mode of acupuncture application. Overall, acupuncture offers a minimally invasive, nonpharmacologic, low-risk, opioid-sparing option for patients and should be considered as part of an integrative approach to pain management.

Ongoing clinical trials regarding acupuncture for acute pain include research in battlefield acupuncture for acute musculoskeletal pain,[71] acupuncture for acute low back pain,[72] acupuncture analgesia for rib fractures,[73] AA for pain relief following knee arthroscopy,[74] and acupuncture vs morphine for acute pain in the emergency department.[75] For more details regarding ongoing acupuncture trials that are actively recruiting, interested participants and referring physicians can perform an advanced search on clinicaltrials.gov.

Other resources for physicians and patients to retrieve updated and evidence-based information regarding acupuncture include the National Center for Complementary and Integrative Health (https://www.nccih.nih.gov/health/acupuncture-in-depth), the American Academy of Medical Acupuncture (https://www.medicalacupuncture.org/), the World Federation of Acupuncture-Moxibustion Societies (http://en.wfas.org.cn/), and the International Association for the Study of Pain (https://www.iasp-pain.org/). Local and regional acupuncture and pain societies, as well as medical boards, can also offer resources and information regarding practice and training standards for different areas.

REFERENCES

1. Acupuncture—UpToDate. n.d. Accessed April 12, 2020. https://www.uptodate.com/contents/acupuncture?search=acupuncture&source=search_result&selectedTitle=1~150&usage_type=default&display_rank=1
2. Chernyak GV, Sessler DI, Warltier DC. Perioperative acupuncture and related techniques. *Anesthesiology*. 2005;102:1031–1049. https://doi.org/10.1097/00000542-200505000-00024
3. Yang X-Y, Shi G-X, Li Q-Q, Zhang Z-H, Xu Q, Liu C-Z. Characterization of deqi sensation and acupuncture effect. *Evid Based Complement Alternat Med*. 2013;2013:319734. https://doi.org/10.1155/2013/319734
4. Salamone FJ, Federman DG. Battlefield acupuncture as a treatment for pain. *South Med J*. 2021;114(4): 239-245. doi:10.14423/SMJ.0000000000001232
5. Yang J, Ganesh R, Wu Q, et al. Battlefield acupuncture for adult pain: a systematic review and meta-analysis of randomized controlled trials. *Am J Chin Med*. 2021;49(1):25-40. doi:10.1142/S0192415X21500026
6. Niemtzow RC. Implementing battlefield acupuncture through a large medical system: overcoming barriers. *Med Acupunct*. 2020;32(6):377-380. doi:10.1089/acu.2020.1470
7. Gori L, Firenzuoli F. Ear acupuncture in European traditional medicine. *Evid Based Complement Alternat Med*. 2007;4:13-16. https://doi.org/10.1093/ecam/nem106
8. Lee MS, Shin B-C, Suen LKP, Park T-Y, Ernst E. Auricular acupuncture for insomnia: a systematic review. *Int J Clin Pract*. 2008;62:1744-1752. https://doi.org/10.1111/j.1742-1241.2008.01876.x
9. Wirz-Ridolfi A. The history of ear acupuncture and ear cartography: why precise mapping of auricular points is important. *Med Acupunct*. 2019;31:145-156. https://doi.org/10.1089/acu.2019.1349
10. Hao JJ, Hao LL. Review of clinical applications of scalp acupuncture for paralysis: an excerpt from Chinese scalp acupuncture. *Glob Adv Health Med*. 2012;1:102-121. https://doi.org/10.7453/gahmj.2012.1.1.017
11. KHT: Korean Hand Therapy—Simple, Fast & Effective. n.d. Accessed November 1, 2020. https://www.easterncurrents.ca/for-practitioners/practitioners'-news/eastern-currents-news/2015/02/27/kht-korean-hand-therapy
12. Dan Lobash. Korean Hand Therapy: Micro-meridians. n.d. Accessed November 1, 2020. https://www.easterncurrents.ca/for-practitioners/practitioners'-news/eastern-currents-news/2016/08/03/korean-hand-therapy-micro-meridians
13. Now, About My Operation in Peking. The New York Times. n.d. Accessed November 1, 2020. https://www.nytimes.com/1971/07/26/archives/now-about-my-operation-in-peking-now-let-me-tell-you-about-my.html
14. Patil S, Sen S, Bral M, et al. The role of acupuncture in pain management. *Curr Pain Headache Rep*. 2016;20:22. https://doi.org/10.1007/s11916-016-0552-1

15. The National Institutes of Health (NIH) Consensus Development Program: Acupuncture. n.d. Accessed November 1, 2020. https://consensus.nih.gov/1997/1997acupuncture107html.htm
16. Kenney JD. Acupuncture and pain management. *Integrative Medicine*.AAEP proceedings. 2011;57:121-137.
17. Pomeranz B, Stux G, eds. *Scientific Bases of Acupuncture*. Springer-Verlag; 1989. https://doi.org/10.1007/978-3-642-73757-2
18. Han J-S. Acupuncture: neuropeptide release produced by electrical stimulation of different frequencies. *Trends Neurosci*. 2003;26:17–22. https://doi.org/10.1016/s0166-2236(02)00006-1
19. Kawakita K, Okada K. Acupuncture therapy: mechanism of action, efficacy, and safety: a potential intervention for psychogenic disorders? *Biopsychosoc Med*. 2014;8:4. https://doi.org/10.1186/1751-0759-8-4
20. Lin J-G, Chen W-L. Acupuncture analgesia: a review of its mechanisms of actions. *Am J Chin Med*. 2008;36:635-645. https://doi.org/10.1142/S0192415X08006107
21. Chan MWC, Wu XY, Wu JCY, Wong SYS, Chung VCH. Safety of acupuncture: overview of systematic reviews. *Sci Rep*. 2017;7. https://doi.org/10.1038/s41598-017-03272-0
22. Park J-E, Lee MS, Choi J-Y, Kim B-Y, Choi S-M. Adverse events associated with acupuncture: a prospective survey. *J Altern Complement Med*. 2010;16:959-963. https://doi.org/10.1089/acm.2009.0415
23. Wang S-M, Caldwell-Andrews A, Kain Z. The use of complementary and alternative medicines by surgical patients: a follow-up survey study. *Anesth Analg*. 2003;97:1010-1015. https://doi.org/10.1213/01.ANE.0000078578.75597.F3
24. Wu M-S, Chen K-H, Chen I-F, et al. The efficacy of acupuncture in post-operative pain management: a systematic review and meta-analysis. *PLoS One*. 2016;11(3):e0150367. https://doi.org/10.1371/journal.pone.0150367
25. Sun Y, Gan TJ, Dubose JW, Habib AS. Acupuncture and related techniques for postoperative pain: a systematic review of randomized controlled trials. *Br J Anaesth*. 2008;101:151-160. https://doi.org/10.1093/bja/aen146
26. Hendawy HA, Abuelnaga ME. Postoperative analgesic efficacy of ear acupuncture in patients undergoing abdominal hysterectomy: a randomized controlled trial. *BMC Anesthesiol*. 2020;20:279. https://doi.org/10.1186/s12871-020-01187-4
27. Chen Y, Xiang XY, Chin KHR, et al. Acupressure for labor pain management: a systematic review and meta-analysis of randomized controlled trials. *Acupunct Med*. 2021;39(4):243-252. doi:10.1177/0964528420946044
28. Handayani S, Balgis. Pre-labor acupuncture for delivery preparation in multiparous women past age 40. *Med Acupunct*. 2019;31:310-314. https://doi.org/10.1089/acu.2019.1357
29. Allais G, Chiarle G, Sinigaglia S, et al. Acupuncture treatment of migraine, nausea, and vomiting in pregnancy. *Neurol Sci*. 2019;40:213-215. https://doi.org/10.1007/s10072-019-03799-2
30. Carr DJ. The safety of obstetric acupuncture: forbidden points revisited. *Acupunct Med*. 2015;33:413-419. https://doi.org/10.1136/acupmed-2015-010936
31. Asher GN, Coeytaux RR, Chen W, Reilly AC, Loh YL, Harper TC. Acupuncture to initiate labor (Acumoms 2): a randomized, sham-controlled clinical trial. *J Matern Fetal Neonatal Med*. 2009;22:843-848. https://doi.org/10.1080/14767050902906386
32. Mansu S, Layton J, Shergis J. Forbidden acupuncture points and implications for inducing labor. *Integr Med Res*. 2016;5:336-337. https://doi.org/10.1016/j.imr.2016.10.003
33. Kemper KJ, Sarah R, Silver-Highfield E, Xiarhos E, Barnes L, Berde C. On pins and needles? Pediatric pain patients' experience with acupuncture. *Pediatrics*. 2000;105:941-947.
34. Ochi JW, Richardson AC. Intraoperative pediatric acupuncture is widely accepted by parents. *Int J Pediatr Otorhinolaryngol*. 2018;110:12-15. https://doi.org/10.1016/j.ijporl.2018.04.014
35. Tsai S-L, Reynoso E, Shin DW, Tsung JW. Acupuncture as a nonpharmacologic treatment for pain in a pediatric emergency department. *Pediatr Emerg Care*. 2021;37(7):e360-e366. https://doi.org/10.1097/PEC.0000000000001619
36. Wu S, Sapru A, Stewart MA, et al. Using acupuncture for acute pain in hospitalized children. *Pediatr Crit Care Med*. 2009;10:291-296. https://doi.org/10.1097/PCC.0b013e318198afd6
37. Jindal V, Ge A, Mansky PJ. Safety and efficacy of acupuncture in children: a review of the evidence. *J Pediatr Hematol Oncol*. 2008;30(6):431-442.
38. Lin Y-C, Perez S, Tung C. Acupuncture for pediatric pain: the trend of evidence-based research. *J Tradit Complement Med*. 2019;10:315-319. https://doi.org/10.1016/j.jtcme.2019.08.004
39. Keefe KR, Byrne KJ, Levi JR. Treating pediatric post-tonsillectomy pain and nausea with complementary and alternative medicine. *Laryngoscope*. 2018;128(11):2625-2634. doi:10.1002/lary.27231
40. Cho HK, Park IJ, Jeong YM, Lee YJ, Hwang SH. Can perioperative acupuncture reduce the pain and vomiting experienced after tonsillectomy? A meta-analysis. *Laryngoscope*. 2016;126(3):608-615. doi:10.1002/lary.25721
41. Shin HC, Kim JS, Lee SK, et al. The effect of acupuncture on postoperative nausea and vomiting after pediatric tonsillectomy: a meta-analysis and systematic review. *Laryngoscope*. 2016;126:1761-1767. https://doi.org/10.1002/lary.25883
42. Martin CS, Deverman SE, Norvell DC, Cusick JC, Kendrick A, Koh J. Randomized trial of acupuncture with antiemetics for reducing postoperative nausea in children. *Acta Anaesthesiol Scand*. 2019;63:292-297. https://doi.org/10.1111/aas.13288

43. Moeen SM. Could acupuncture be an adequate alternative to dexamethasone in pediatric tonsillectomy? *Paediatr Anaesth*. 2016;26:807-814. https://doi.org/10.1111/pan.12933
44. Xin J, Zhang Y, Zhou X, Liu B. Acupuncture may be an effective supplement treatment for dexamethasone in pediatric tonsillectomy. *Paediatr Anesth*. 2016;26:1213-1214. https://doi.org/10.1111/pan.13017
45. Acar HV, Yilmaz A, Demir G, Eruyar SG, Dikmen B. Capsicum plasters on acupoints decrease the incidence of emergence agitation in pediatric patients. *Paediatr Anesth*. 2012;22:1105-1109. https://doi.org/10.1111/j.1460-9592.2012.03876.x
46. Lin Y-C, Tassone RF, Jahng S. Acupuncture management of pain and emergence agitation in children after bilateral myringotomy and tympanostomy tube insertion. *Paediatr Anesth*. 2009;19:1096-1101. https://doi.org/10.1111/j.1460-9592.2009.03129.x
47. Armond ACV, Glória JCR, dos Santos CRR, Galo R, Falci SGM. Acupuncture on anxiety and inflammatory events following surgery of mandibular third molars: a split-mouth, randomized, triple-blind clinical trial. *Int J Oral Maxillofac Surg*. 2019;48:274-281. https://doi.org/10.1016/j.ijom.2018.07.016
48. Ernst E, Pittler MH. The effectiveness of acupuncture in treating acute dental pain: a systematic review. *Br Dent J*. 1998;184:443-447. https://doi.org/10.1038/sj.bdj.4809654
49. Grillo CM, Wada RS, de Sousa M, da LR. Acupuncture in the management of acute dental pain. *J Acupunct Meridian Stud*. 2014;7:65-70. https://doi.org/10.1016/j.jams.2013.03.005
50. Kitade T, Ohyabu H. Analgesic effects of acupuncture on pain after mandibular wisdom tooth extraction. *Acupunct Electrother Res*. 2000;25:109. https://doi.org/10.3727/036012900816356172
51. Tsai S-L, Fox LM, Murakami M, Tsung JW. Auricular acupuncture in emergency department treatment of acute pain. *Ann Emerg Med*. 2016;68:583-585. https://doi.org/10.1016/j.annemergmed.2016.05.006
52. Wang S-M, Escalera S, Lin EC, Maranets I, Kain ZN. Extra-1 acupressure for children undergoing anesthesia. *Anesth Analg*. 2008;107:811-816. https://doi.org/10.1213/ane.0b013e3181804441
53. deWeber K, Lynch JH. Sideline acupuncture for acute pain control: a case series. *Curr Sports Med Rep*. 2011;10:320-323. https://doi.org/10.1249/JSR.0b013e318237be0f
54. Jan AL, Aldridge ES, Rogers IR, Visser EJ, Bulsara MK, Niemtzow RC. Does ear acupuncture have a role for pain relief in the emergency setting? A systematic review and meta-analysis. *Med Acupunct*. 2017;29(5): 276-289. doi:10.1089/acu.2017.1237
55. Fox LM, Murakami M, Danesh H, Manini AF. Battlefield acupuncture to treat low back pain in the emergency department. *Am J Emerg Med*. 2018;36:1045-1048. https://doi.org/10.1016/j.ajem.2018.02.038
56. Liu A-F, Gong S-W, Chen J-X, Zhai J-B. Efficacy and safety of acupuncture therapy for patients with acute ankle sprain: a systematic review and meta-analysis of randomized controlled trials. *Evid Based Complement Alternat Med*. 2020;2020:9109531. https://doi.org/10.1155/2020/9109531
57. Goertz CMH, Niemtzow R, Burns SM, Fritts MJ, Crawford CC, Jonas WB. Auricular acupuncture in the treatment of acute pain syndromes: a pilot study. *Mil Med*. 2006;171:1010-1014. https://doi.org/10.7205/MILMED.171.10.1010
58. Zeliadt SB, Thomas ER, Olson J, et al. Patient feedback on the effectiveness of auricular acupuncture on pain in routine clinical care. *Med Care*. 2020;58:S101-S107. https://doi.org/10.1097/MLR.0000000000001368
59. Magden ER. Spotlight on acupuncture in laboratory animal medicine. *Vet Med (Auckl)*. 2017;8:53-58. https://doi.org/10.2147/VMRR.S125609
60. McGregor M, Becklake MR. Basic research in acupuncture analgesia. *Can Med Assoc J*. 1974;110:328-329.
61. Hsieh Y-L, Hong C-Z, Liu S-Y, Chou L-W, Yang C-C. Acupuncture at distant myofascial trigger spots enhances endogenous opioids in rabbits: a possible mechanism for managing myofascial pain. *Acupunct Med*. 2016;34:302-309. https://doi.org/10.1136/acupmed-2015-011026
62. Abraham TS, Chen M-L, Ma S-X. TRPV1 expression in acupuncture points: response to electroacupuncture stimulation. *J Chem Neuroanat*. 2011;41:129-136. https://doi.org/10.1016/j.jchemneu.2011.01.001
63. Li A-H, Zhang J-M, Xie Y-K. Human acupuncture points mapped in rats are associated with excitable muscle/skin-nerve complexes with enriched nerve endings. *Brain Res*. 2004;1012:154-159. https://doi.org/10.1016/j.brainres.2004.04.009
64. Magden ER, Haller RL, Thiele EJ, Buchl SJ, Lambeth SP, Schapiro SJ. Acupuncture as an adjunct therapy for osteoarthritis in chimpanzees (Pan troglodytes). *J Am Assoc Lab Anim Sci*. 2013;52:475-480.
65. Oh JH, Bai SJ, Cho Z-H, et al. Pain-relieving effects of acupuncture and electroacupuncture in an animal model of arthritic pain. *Int J Neurosci*. 2006;116:1139-1156. https://doi.org/10.1080/00207450500513948
66. Chen L, Xu A, Yin N, et al. Enhancement of immune cytokines and splenic CD4+ T cells by electroacupuncture at ST36 acupoint of SD rats. *PLoS One*. 2017;12:e0175568. https://doi.org/10.1371/journal.pone.0175568
67. Salazar TE, Richardson MR, Beli E, et al. Electroacupuncture promotes CNS-dependent release of mesenchymal stem cells. *Stem Cells*. 2017;35:1303-1315. https://doi.org/10.1002/stem.2613
68. Stephen J, Hernandez-Divers Bv. *World Small Animal Veterinary Association World Congress Proceedings, 2005*. 2015. VIN.com
69. Liao E-T, Tang N-Y, Lin Y-W, Liang Hsieh C. Long-term electrical stimulation at ear and electro-acupuncture at ST36-ST37 attenuated COX-2 in the CA1 of hippocampus in kainic acid-induced epileptic seizure rats. *Sci Rep*. 2017;7:472. https://doi.org/10.1038/s41598-017-00601-1

70. Zhou J, Li S, Wang Y, et al. Effects and mechanisms of auricular electroacupuncture on gastric hypersensitivity in a rodent model of functional dyspepsia. *PLoS One*. 2017;12:e0174568. https://doi.org/10.1371/journal.pone.0174568
71. Crawford P. Pilot Study: Effect of Battlefield Acupuncture Needle Selection on Symptom Relief and Patient Tolerance in the Treatment of Acute Musculoskeletal Pain (Clinical trial registration No. NCT04464954). 2020. clinicaltrials.gov
72. wallace L. Accessible Acupuncture for the Warrior with Acute Low Back Pain (Clinical trial registration No. NCT04236908). 2020. clinicaltrials.gov
73. Liu C-T. Analgesic Effect of Acupuncture for Patients with Rib Fractures: an Open-label, Randomized-controlled Trial (Clinical trial registration No. NCT03822273). 2020. clinicaltrials.gov
74. University Medicine Greifswald. Auricular Acupuncture Versus Placebo (Sham Acupuncture) for Postoperative Pain Relief After Ambulatory Knee Arthroscopy - a Randomized Controlled Trial (Clinical trial registration No. NCT00233857). 2011. clinicaltrials.gov
75. Nouira PS. Acupuncture Versus Intravenous Morphine in the Management of Acute Pain in the Emergency Department. An Efficacy and Safety Study (Clinical trial registration No. NCT02460913). 2020. clinicaltrials.gov

SECTION V

Subspecialty Considerations and Other Topics

44

Dental and Facial Pain

Ahmad Elsharydah

Background

Orofacial pain is a pain generated from the different structures of the face and the head. It is the most common reason for patients to seek medical care. The main source of orofacial pain is the dental and the periodontal regions.[1] The oral pain in general can be divided into odontogenic pain (tooth pain) and nonodontogenic pain. The odontogenic pain originates from the different dental structures such as tooth pulp and periodontal structures. On the other hand, the nonodontogenic pain may come from various intraoral structures such as gums and mucosa. The innervation of these components are complex, therefore may generate pain with different types of mechanisms. Detailed history, physical examination, and review of the available laboratory and imaging studies would help to differentiate the different types of orofacial pain and make a diagnosis. The first step to manage acute orofacial pain is management of the source disease or condition. Symptomatic therapies include the use of pharmacological agents, nonpharmacological treatment such as heat or cold, and nerve blocks. Table 44.1 lists the differential diagnosis of the orofacial pain (American Academy of Orofacial Pain classification).

This chapter is a concise summary for the assessment and management of patients with acute orofacial pain based on the available scientific evidence.

Epidemiology of Orofacial Pain

Orofacial pain is a very common pain problem. Some demographic studies have shown that >39 million people, 22% of the U.S. population, report pain in the orofacial region.[2] One study reported that more than 81% of the population has some type of significant jaw pain in their life time.[3] Orofacial pain is rarely an isolated complaint; it is commonly part of other conditions. The overall reported prevalence of orofacial pain is 1.9%-26%.[4,5] Orofacial pain is more prevalent in women and young adults (18-25)[4] than in men and older adults.

Neurophysiology and Neuroanatomy for Orofacial Pain

It is important for the clinician managing patients with acute or chronic orofacial pain to understand the basic neuroanatomy and neurophysiology of this type of pain. Most of the orofacial pain pathways communicate through the trigeminal nerve,[6] the largest and most complex cranial nerve. They are mostly transmitted by sensory, motor, and autonomic nerve networks. To better understand orofacial pain, it is an essential to understand the peripheral and the central connection of the trigeminal nerve system. It is out of the scope

TABLE 44.1 DIFFERENTIAL DIAGNOSIS OF OROFACIAL PAIN (AMERICAN ACADEMY OF OROFACIAL PAIN CLASSIFICATION)

Intracranial pain disorders	Neoplasm, aneurysm, abscess, hemorrhage, hematoma, edema
Primary headache disorders (neurovascular disorders)	Migraine, migraine variants, cluster headache, paroxysmal hemicrania, cranial arteritis Carotidynia, tension-type headache
Neurogenic pain disorders	Paroxysmal neuralgias (trigeminal, glossopharyngeal, nervus intermedius, superior laryngeal) Continuous pain disorders (deafferentation, neuritis, postherpetic neuralgia, posttraumatic and postsurgical neuralgia) Sympathetically maintained pain
Intraoral pain disorders	Dental pulp, periodontium, mucogingival tissues, tongue
Temporomandibular disorders	Masticatory muscle, temporomandibular joint, associated structures
Associate structures	Ears, eyes, nose, paranasal sinuses, throat, lymph nodes, salivary glands, neck

of this chapter to describe the details of these connections. In general, nociceptors in the facial and oral regions are responsible for the recognition of proprioception, mechanical stimuli, thermal stimuli, and pain perception.[7] Trigeminal nerve (via afferent fibers A, B, and C) is the dominant nerve that relays sensory impulses from the orofacial area to the central nervous system. The facial nerve, the glossopharyngeal nerve, the vagus nerve, and the upper cervical nerves (C2 and C3) also transmit sensory information from the face and surrounding area. The upper cervical nerves provide innervation to the back of the head, lower face, and neck. More importantly, they converge in the brainstem at the trigeminal nucleus. Most nociceptive orofacial pain impulses are transmitted by the somatic nerves, a significant portion is transmitted by autonomic nerves and a small portion may be transmitted by motor nerves.

Heterotopic and referred pain are common in the acute and chronic orofacial pain conditions. Orofacial heterotopic pain occurs when the source of pain is not located in the region of pain perception; and referred pain describes pain felt at a location served by one nerve, but the source of nociception arrives at the subnucleus caudalis of the trigeminal nerve by a different nerve. The heterotopic and referred phenomena explained by the complexity of the trigeminal network and the convergence of multiple sensory nerves carrying input to the trigeminal spinal nuclei from cutaneous and deep tissues located throughout the head and neck set the stage for referred pain.[8]

Acute Orofacial Pain

Acute orofacial pain is a very common complaint. In most of the cases, acute orofacial pain is a symptom of other conditions involving the face and/or the oral cavity including trauma, surgery, infections. Most of chronic orofacial pain conditions stem from untreated and poorly controlled acute orofacial pain. Postoperative orofacial pain management is similar to other acute postoperative management including the use of pharmacological agents, nonpharmacological therapies such as heat or cold, and nerve blocks. In this section, I will briefly mention the different conditions causing acute orofacial pain and the specific management for these conditions. Table 44.2 summarizes the common topical medications used for orofacial pain management.

TABLE 44.2 TOPICAL MEDICATIONS USED TO TREAT OROFACIAL PAIN

Type	Generic Name	Dosage	Form
Topical local anesthetics	Lidocaine	2%	Gel Viscous solution Ointment Spray Lozenge
		4% or 5%	Adhesive patch
	Benzocaine	20%	Aerosol Gel Lozenge Liquid Ointment Mouth strip Mouth swap
	Lidocaine/prilocaine	2.5% lidocaine/ 2.5% prilocaine	Cream Periodontal gel
Nonsteroidal anti-inflammatory drugs	Ketoprofen	10%-20%	Cream Patch
	Diclofenac	10%-20%	Gel Patch Solution
Neuropeptide	Capsaicin	0.025% or 0.075%	Cream Liquid Gel Patch Lotion
Sympathomimetic agent	Clonidine	0.01%	Gel Cream Patch
NMDA antagonist	Ketamine	0.5%	Cream
Anticonvulsant	Carbamazepine	2%	Cream
Antidepressant	Amitriptyline	2%	Gel Cream

NMDA, *N*-methyl-D-aspartate.
Modified from Halpern L, Willis P. Orofacial pain: pharmacologic paradigms for therapeutic intervention. *Dent Clin North Am*. 2016;60:381-405.

Acute Oral Pain (Odontogenic and Nonodontogenic Pain)

Odontogenic pain is divided into pulpal pain and periodontal pain. Pulpal pain is caused by condition or a disease affects the pulp of the tooth such as dental caries, pulpitis, and cracked tooth syndrome.[9] Differently, the periodontal pain is usually originated from a condition involving the teeth surroundings like periodontitis (abscess, granuloma, cyst, or trauma). Management of odontogenic pain includes treatment of the source of pain (eg, antibiotics for infection and drainage for periodontal abscess). Symptomatic therapy of the pain is also usually needed including nonsteroidal anti-inflammatory drugs, acetaminophen, and in some cases local anesthetic infiltration and nerve blocks. Table 44.3 summarized the different nerve blocks used for anesthesia and analgesia for oral/dental procedures.[10,11]

TABLE 44.3 NERVE BLOCKS USED FOR ANESTHESIA AND/OR ANALGESIA FOR ORAL AND DENTAL PROCEDURES AND PAIN

Nerve Block	Coverage Area
Supraperiosteal infiltrations	Individual teeth
Anterior, middle, or posterior superior alveolar nerve block	
Infraorbital nerve block	Lower eyelid, upper cheek, part of the nose, and upper lip
Greater palatine nerve block	Posterior two-thirds of the hard palate
Nasopalatine nerve block	Anterior hard palate and associated soft tissues
Inferior alveolar nerve block	All teeth on the ipsilateral side of the mandible, as well as the ipsilateral lip and chin via the mental nerve
Mental nerve block	Ipsilateral lower lip and skin of the chin (not the teeth)
Lingual nerve block	Anterior two-thirds of the tongue
Buccal nerve block	Mucous membrane of the cheek and vestibule and, to a lesser extent, a small patch of skin on the face

Nonodontogenic oral pain usually stems from a wide variety of conditions including oral ulcers (bacterial, viral, fungal, neoplasia, immunological diseases, drug adverse reactions, etc.).[9] Management of the oral ulcer pain includes initial treatment of the disease causing the ulcer. Symptomatic therapy of the pain includes the use of over-the-counter anesthesia agents (such as 20% benzocaine) or local steroids. Some oral ulcers respond to tetracycline-containing rinse. Other causes of the oral nonodontogenic pain are the acute pericoronitis (inflammation of the flap tissues around the erupting tooth) and acute alveolar osteitis (usually called dry socket, a complication after dental extraction). Dry socket is caused by the exposure of the bone and the nerve after inadequate formation of blood clot in the extracted tooth socket or dislodgement the formed blood clot. Minimizing the trauma related to the procedure is an important factor to prevent dry socket. Oral mucositis secondary to anticancer treatment such as chemotherapy and/or radiation therapy may generate oral pain. Different types of gingivitis also can cause this type of pain like acute necrotizing ulcerative gingivitis (severe acute infection of the gingiva associated with gingival necrosis, fever, and sometime bleeding).

Burning Mouth Syndrome

Burning mouth syndrome (BMS) presents as burning sensations within the oral cavity involving mucosa, tongue, gingiva, and lips. This sensation is continuous, and it increases throughout the day. This disorder is more common in females (6:1) during their premenopausal and postmenopausal years. Its incidence is 1%-3% of the general population. It is worse and more frequent in the anterior part of the oral cavity including the first one-third of the tongue, palate, and gingiva. Its diagnosis is a diagnosis of exclusion. Associated symptoms include dry mouth and dysgeusia. It is critical to exclude other systemic disorders such as gastroesophageal reflux disease, diabetes, and vitamin deficiencies (such as vitamin B12 and folic acid) before starting the symptomatic treatment for BMS.[12]

Musculoskeletal Orofacial Pain

Temporomandibular joints (TMJs) and associated ligaments, masticatory muscles, and tendons are a source of the one most common causes of facial pain. It is estimated that 40%-75% of individuals have at least one sign of joint dysfunction.[13] Facial pain secondary to TMJs dysfunction is usually felt in the muscles of mastication, in the front of the ear, or in the joint itself. This type of pain is usually mild and resolve over time without intervention. It is more common in women of childbearing age. In severe cases, this pain may significantly limit the range of motion of TMJ. Temporomandibular disorders in general generate three main types of acute or chronic orofacial pain including myofascial pain, arthritic pain, and more common pain caused by the TMJ dysfunction (such as clicks, crepitus, and locking).[14] A wide range of etiologies have been reported for this disorder from pure mechanistic theory to more recent biopsychosocial and multifactorial etiologies. Specific diagnostic tools have been developed for diagnosis.

Orofacial Neuropathic Pain

Orofacial neuropathic pain is defined as a pain caused by a lesion or injury of the somatosensory nerves innervate the orofacial region. For clinical purposes, it may manifest as continuous or episodic based upon its temporal presentation. Continuous neuropathic pain is constant, ongoing, and unremitting pain. Patients usually experience varying and fluctuating intensities of pain, often without total remission. Examples of continuous orofacial neuropathic pain include peripheral neuritis, peripheral trigeminal neuritis, herpes zoster/postherpetic neuralgia, atypical odontalgia/nonodontogenic toothache, and BMS. On the other hand, episodic neuropathic pain (neuralgia) is a sudden severe, shooting electric-like pain lasting only a few seconds to several minutes. Often, there exists a perioral or intraoral trigger zone whereby nontraumatic stimuli such as light touch elicit a severe paroxysmal pain.[15] Common examples of orofacial episodic neuropathic pain include trigeminal neuralgia (TN), glossopharyngeal neuralgia, and occipital neuralgia. For the purpose of this chapter, I will discuss TN in more details.

Trigeminal Neuralgia

Trigeminal neuralgia, called also *tic douloureux*, is defined as a sudden, severe, brief, stabbing, shocklike, usually unilateral and recurrent orofacial pain within one or more branches of the trigeminal nerve. TN is a chronic pain condition; however, clinicians in the acute care settings such as emergency departments may encounter these patients with uncontrolled pain. Most common triggers are mastication, touch, eating, talking, cold air on the face, and tooth brushing. Pain is most commonly distributed along the V2 and V3 branches of the trigeminal nerve.[16] This disorder is more common in females and generally rare condition (12/100 000).[17] More common in females than in males. It occurs mostly after the age of 50. The International Classification of Headache Disorders (ICHD-3) diagnostic criteria for TN include pain lasting from a fraction of a second to 2 minutes, which severe in intensity and with a quality of shock-like, shooting stabbing, or sharp. This pain must be precipitated by innocuous stimuli within the affected trigeminal distribution. The last criterion is that this pain is not better accounted by another ICHD-3 diagnosis.

TN etiology and pathophysiology is not very clear; however, the vascular compression theory of the trigeminal nerve appears the leading theory at this time.[18] TN pain is consistent of two types of pain: type 1 as intermittent and type 2 as constant pain represent distinct clinical, pathological, and prognostic entities.[19] Although multiple mechanisms involving peripheral pathologies at root (compression or traction), and dysfunctions of brainstem, basal ganglion, and cortical pain modulatory mechanisms could have role, neurovascular conflict is the most accepted theory.

Imaging studies such as MRI (magnetic resonance imaging) and MRA (magnetic resonance angiography) may help to confirm the diagnosis, detect pathological changes in affected root and neurovascular compression (NVC), and rule out secondary causes and other similar orofacial pain disorders. Pain medical therapies are needed in most patients. The goals of the treatment are to decrease the intensity of pain and decrease the frequency and the duration of the pain episodes. Furthermore, the medical treatment may help to relieve associated symptoms such as headache and depression. The drug of choice to treat TN is carbamazepine (CBZ). It is the only Food and Drug Administration–approved drug to treat TN. It is an anticonvulsant, and it inhibits the sodium channel activity and also modulates calcium channels. The starting dose is usually 100 mg bid, which may increase gradually to 200 mg twice a day or higher dose as tolerated by the patient to reach pain relief, not to exceed 1200 mg/day. Some of its common side effects are dizziness, drowsiness, and nausea. Severe adverse reactions are uncommon including aplastic anemia, hyponatremia, and abnormal liver function tests; therefore, it is recommended to routinely monitor liver function tests, sodium level, and blood counts in these patients. Other drugs used to treat TN include oxcarbazepine (analog of CBZ); however, it has better risk profile and similar efficacy for CBZ. Pregabalin, gabapentin, topiramate, valproic acid, baclofen, lamotrigine, and phenytoin are also useful. Multidrug regimens and multidisciplinary approaches are useful in selected patients. Local anesthesia, steroids, phenol, glycerol, alcohol, and botulinum toxin type A have been used to treat and diagnose TN. Patients who do not respond or tolerate medical therapy and injections may consider other interventional therapies including percutaneous trigeminal ganglion balloon compression rhizotomy, percutaneous radiofrequency gangliolysis, microvascular decompression, or Gamma Knife.

Neurovascular Orofacial Pain

Referred pain to the orofacial area from other neurovascular craniofacial pain–producing disorders is common. Clinicians may encounter this pain in its acute phase; however, most patients seek care when pain turned into recurrent and chronic pain. This pain is usually located around the eyes and the frontal regions of the face. The most common pain disorders in this group are migraine and trigeminal autonomic cephalgias. Distinct neurovascular orofacial pain does also exist; however, it is significantly less common that the above described referred pain. Clinician has to be aware of these different types of pain and be able to differentiate them from pain produced by dental pathology or referred pain from migraine or trigeminal autonomic cephalgias. Facial migraine was reported in the medical literature as lower facial pain associated with nausea, vomiting, phonophobia, photophobia, or other autonomic symptoms usually associated with migraine.[20] Treatment is similar to common migraine including preventative mediations, abortive medical therapies, and behavioral changes including good sleep hygiene.

REFERENCES

1. Renton T. Chronic orofacial pain. *Oral Dis*. 2017;23:566-571.
2. Hargreaves KM. Orofacial pain. *Pain*. 2011;152(3 Suppl):S25-S32.
3. James FR, Large RG, Bushnell JA, et al. Epidemiology of pain in New Zealand. *Pain*. 1991;44:279-283.
4. Macfarlane TV, Blinkhorn AS, Davies RM, et al. Oro-facial pain in the community: prevalence and associated impact. *Community Dent Oral Epidemiol*. 2002;30:52-60.
5. Macfarlane TV, Beasley M, Macfarlane GJ. Self-reported facial pain in UK Biobank study: prevalence and associated factors. *J Oral Maxillofac Res*. 2014;5:e2.
6. Halpern L, Willis P. Orofacial pain: pharmacologic paradigms for therapeutic intervention. *Dent Clin North Am*. 2016;60:381-405.
7. Sacerdote P, Levrini L. Peripheral mechanisms of dental pain: the role of substance P. *Mediators Inflamm*. 2012;2012:951920.
8. De Rossi SS. Orofacial pain: a primer. *Dent Clin North Am*. 2013;57:383-392.
9. Patel B. Pain of odontogenic and non-odontogenic origin. In: Patel B, ed. *Endodontic Diagnosis, Pathology and Treatment Planning*. Springer International Publishing; 2015:1-18.
10. Reichman E, Kern K. Dental anesthesia and analgesia. In: Reichman E, Simon R, eds. *Emergency Medicine Procedures*. McGraw-Hill; 2004:1353-1367.

11. Larrabee W, Makielski K, Henderson J. Facial sensory innervation. In: *Surgical Anatomy of the Face*. 2nd ed. Lippincott Williams & Wilkins; 2003:85-95.
12. Balasubramaniam R, Klasser GD. Orofacial pain syndromes: evaluation and management. *Med Clin North Am.* 2014;98:1385-1405.
13. De Leeuw R, Klasser GD, eds. *Orofacial Pain: Guidelines for Assessment, Diagnosis, and Management*. 5th ed. Quintessence Publishing Co.; 2013:312.
14. Schiffman E, Ohrbach R. Executive summary of the diagnostic criteria for temporomandibular disorders for clinical and research applications. *J Am Dent Assoc*. 2016;147:438-445.
15. Christoforou J, Balasubramaniam R, Klasser GD. Neuropathic orofacial Pain. *Curr Oral Health Rep*. 2015;2:148-157.
16. Cruccu G, Finnerup NB, Jensen TS, et al. Trigeminal neuralgia: new classification and diagnostic grading for practice and research. *Neurology*. 2016;87:220-228.
17. Majeed MH, Arooj S, Khokhar MA, et al. Trigeminal neuralgia: a clinical review for the general physician. *Cureus*. 2018;10:e3750.
18. Love S, Coakham HB. Trigeminal neuralgia pathology and pathogenesis. *Brain*. 2001;124:2347-2360.
19. Yadav YR, Nishtha Y, Sonjjay P, et al. Trigeminal neuralgia. *Asian J Neurosurg*. 2017;12:585-597.
20. Penarrocha M, Bandres A, Penarrocha M, et al. Lower-half facial migraine: a report of 11 cases. *J Oral Maxillofac Surg*. 2004;62:1453-1456.

45

Acute Pain in the Emergency Department

Stephanie Guzman, Aimee Homra, Franciscka Macieiski, and Alan David Kaye

Introduction

The most common chief complaint resulting in an emergency department (ED) visit is pain. Pain can be subdivided into acute pain, which will be the focus of this chapter, or chronic pain. Acute pain is often shorter in duration (typically <30 days) and often occurs as a part of a single and treatable event. When assessing patients for acute pain conditions, one must consider not only patient comfort and self-determined pain scores, but also patient functionality. In addition, acute pain can often be recognized with a physiologic response such as tachycardia, hypertension, and/or diaphoresis that may help guide treatment.[1] Proper treatment of pain improves patient satisfaction and mood, decreases hospital length of stay, and decreases mortality.[2]

Acute pain conditions in the ED can be traumatic or nontraumatic including bone fractures, burns, procedural pain, visceral pain (ie, appendicitis, nephrolithiasis), or acute exacerbations of recurring pain conditions such as with sickle cell crisis and migraines. Analgesia in the ED should be patient-centered and pain syndrome targeted.[1] Treatment goals include not only providing relief for the acute pain but also decreasing complications including opioid dependence; physicians are encouraged to use a multimodal approach including both pharmacologic and nonpharmacologic treatments whenever possible.[3]

Opioid Analgesics and the Opioid Epidemic

As discussed in Chapter 31, opioid analgesics, while seemingly effective in acute pain control, have many negative side effects. They are highly addictive and are associated with respiratory and CNS depression as well as risk of tolerance and development of hyperalgesia. Other side effects include euphoria, constipation, and pruritus and hypotension from degranulation of mast cells. Nonetheless, opioids may be appropriate for the treatment of traumatic injuries, vaso-occlusive crisis, and acute on chronic cancer-related pain.[4]

One of the most commonly used opioids is morphine, which is used as a baseline for which other opioids are measured.[4] Parenteral morphine dosing ranges from 0.1 to 0.15 mg/kg with reassessment of pain every 5-15 minutes, onset within 5-10 minutes, and duration of action of 3-6 hours.[2] Oral morphine has 20%-25% bioavailability and is metabolized by the liver through glucuronidation to active metabolites, morphine-6-glucuronide and morphine-3-glucuronide, with M6G being more potent than morphine and M3G having the risk of neuroexcitatory effects. Morphine metabolites are renally excreted and may accumulate in elderly and renal failure patients.[4]

Fentanyl is metabolized by the liver, which utilizes CYP3A4 to produce inactive metabolites that are renally excreted; for this reason, fentanyl is safer to use in patients with renal failure.[4] Initial IV dose is 1-1.5 μg/kg with time of onset in 1-2 minutes and typical duration of action about 30 minutes. It causes minimal histamine release, giving it a favorable hemodynamic profile, but caution should be taken at higher doses due to the risk of chest wall rigidity.[2]

Hydromorphone is a semisynthetic derivative of morphine that is seven times more potent than morphine.[2] It undergoes hepatic glucuronidation to its primary metabolite, hydromorphone-3-glucuronide, which has risks of neuro-excitatory effects, similar to M3G, and is renally excreted; hydromorphone should be used with caution in patients with renal failure.[4] Initial IV dose is 0.25-0.5 mg with onset in 5-10 minutes, and duration of action of 3-6 hours.[2]

Until recently, treating acute pain in the ED with opioid analgesics had been considered a standard of care; however, from 1999 to 2018, almost 450 000 people died from an overdose involving opioids, including both prescription and illicit opioids.[5,6] Because of the adverse effects of opioids and the worsening opioid epidemic, emergency physicians are now encouraged to avoid prescribing these medications for acute pain treatment when possible. It is important for the physician to recognize for whom opioids may be helpful as well as avoid prescribing opioids to patients at high risk of tolerance or abuse.

Some patients are considered higher risk for adverse events with opioid administration. These include older patients (65 years or older), those concomitantly taking other CNS depressant medications (ie, benzodiazepines, muscle relaxants, sleep aids), patients with a history of drug abuse or overdose, as well as patients with mental health conditions or sleep apnea.[6]

Current guidelines from the center for disease control (CDC) for pain treatment with opioid analgesics include the following:

- Prescribers should establish treatment goals with all patients receiving opioid analgesics, including realistic goals for pain control and function.
- Physicians should discuss the risks of opioid therapy and often assess if the benefit of treatment outweighs the risk throughout treatment.
- When starting opioid therapy, physicians should prescribe immediate-release opioids (avoiding extended-release/long-acting opioids), while using the lowest effective dose for the shortest duration deemed reasonable (recommended 3 days or less for acute pain).[6]

In addition, ED physicians are encouraged to order urine drugs screen tests prior to prescribing opioids as well as review the prescription-monitoring program. The prescription-monitoring program allows emergency providers to identify patients with patterns of frequent opioid use/likely opioid abuse, ultimately helping the physician limit abuse potential as well as recognize patients with drug-seeking behavior who may benefit from treatment centers for addiction.[6]

Due to the risks with opioid analgesia and the rapidly growing epidemic, all physicians, especially those working in the ED, are encouraged to utilize nonopioid analgesics when appropriate prior to resorting to opioids to treat acute pain. For this reason, the rest of this chapter will focus on nonopioid analgesics.

Nonopioid Analgesics

COX Inhibitors

Acetaminophen has antipyretic and analgesic effects through selective inhibition of COX-3, present in the brain in spinal cord.[4] It is appropriate as a sole agent for mild to moderate pain and is available in oral, IV, and rectal formulations, with doses ranging from 325 to 1000 mg (maximum dose should not exceed 4000 mg in 24-hour period), and duration of action of 4-6 hours.[4]

Traditional nonsteroidal anti-inflammatory drugs provide analgesia for mild to moderate inflammatory pain through nonselective inhibition of COX-1 and COX-2 receptors, preventing the conversion of arachidonic acid to inflammatory prostaglandins.[4] Reduced levels of prostaglandins in central and peripheral nervous system relieves pain and swelling and prevents prostaglandin-mediated stimulation of the hypothalamus resulting in lowering of body temperature.[4] Examples of these include aspirin, ibuprofen, naproxen, and ketorolac. Another group of agents remains nonselective but has higher affinity for COX-2 receptors and includes indomethacin, meloxicam, and diclofenac.

Second-generation nonsteroidal anti-inflammatory drugs (NSAIDs) are selective COX-2 inhibitors, which improves the gastric safety profile, but increases risk for myocardial infarction, stroke, and heart failure resulting from induction of a pro-thrombotic state (decreased prostaglandin I2 and increased thromboxane A2).[4] Celecoxib is the only COX-2 selective NSAID currently available. All NSAIDs exhibit an analgesic ceiling dose, which is lower than the anti-inflammatory maximal dose.[4] Depending on receptor affinity, side effects include GI irritation, platelet and renal dysfunction, bronchospasm, and delayed wound healing.[2]

Ibuprofen has an initial dose of 400 mg oral with duration of action of 8 hours and maximum dose of 1200 mg/day. Naproxen has an initial dose of 250 mg oral or 500 mg oral with duration of action of 8-12 hours, respectively, and maximum dose of 1000 mg/day. Ketorolac has an initial dose of 10-15 mg IV with duration of action of 6 hours and maximum dose of 60 mg/day. Diclofenac has an initial dose of 50 mg oral with duration of action of 8 hours and maximum dose of 150 mg/day.[4] Topical NSAIDs, which limit systemic distribution and side effects, may also be considered for localized transdermal analgesia for acute pain associated with sprain, strain, tendinopathies, bursitis, and exacerbations of osteoarthritis.[4] They can preferably accumulate in targeted areas such as cartilage and meniscus with concentrations 4-7 times greater than plasma concentrations and in tendons with concentrations one hundred times greater than plasma concentrations. Examples include diclofenac, ketoprofen, and ibuprofen with patch duration of action similar to parenteral and oral administration.[4]

NMDA Receptor Antagonists

Ketamine in sub-dissociative doses is an analgesic adjunct useful for intractable pain, neuropathic pain, and opioid-tolerant or induced hyperalgesic states.[4] Once in the bloodstream, it has a very rapid onset of action, within 30-45 seconds. A single dose of 0.1-0.3 mg/kg IV given over 10-15 minutes or a continuous infusion of 0.15 mg/kg/h should be employed.[4] At sub-dissociative doses, it acts as a noncompetitive NMDA receptor antagonist in the brain and spinal cord with additional mu receptor agonist properties.[4] Patients should be counseled on the likelihood of psychoperceptual side effects, sedation, and dizziness, which have shown to be decreased when given as an infusion vs single bolus.[3]

Sodium Channel Blockers

Sodium channel blockers function as analgesics through noncompetitive inhibition of sodium channels, which in turn, inhibits nerve signal propagation by slowing the flow of sodium across cell membranes, lessening the influx of calcium ions into nerve terminals, and inhibiting the release of glutamate.[4] They consist of two classes, esters and amides. Intravenous lidocaine has analgesic, antihyperalgesic, and anti-inflammatory properties when given as a single bolus dose of 1-2 mg/kg or as a continuous infusion of 0.5-3 mg/kg/h.[4]

Dopamine Receptor Antagonists

These medications include metoclopramide, haloperidol, chlorpromazine, and droperidol and act as analgesics by modulation of dopamine-centered pain signaling pathways.[4] They are commonly used to treat acute migraines at their respective doses: metoclopramide 10 mg IV, prochlorperazine 10 mg IV, and chlorpromazine 10 mg IV. Side effects include QT prolongation, extrapyramidal side effects (which can be decreased with diphenhydramine 25 mg IV), antimuscarinic effects, and neuroleptic malignant syndrome.[4]

Alpha-2 Receptor Agonists

Dexmedetomidine, commonly used in the ICU setting for sedation, produces analgesia by blunting the central-activated sympathetic adrenergic pathway. It is commonly given IV or intranasal with dosing of 0.5-1.0 μg/kg IV or 1-2 μg/kg IN.[4]

Anticonvulsants

Gabapentin and pregabalin both bind to the same site on the presynaptic, voltage-dependent calcium channels located throughout the peripheral and central nervous systems. They are effective for the treatment of posthepatic neuralgia, phantom limb pain, peripheral neuropathy, and nerve compression pain.[4] Although they both bind to the same receptor, the binding affinity and potency of pregabalin is six times more potent than gabapentin.[4] Although they may be initiated in the ED, the onset of pain relief is not usually seen immediately, so a slow titration to effect over several weeks is commonly used.[4]

Antidepressants

Tricyclic antidepressants and serotonin-norepinephrine reuptake inhibitors at lower doses than given for antidepressant effects can be used for chronic neuropathic pain. Some commonly used include amitriptyline, nortriptyline, and duloxetine, which work in theory, by potentiating the descending inhibitory pathways by inhibiting reuptake of serotonin and norepinephrine and increasing the release of endogenous opioids.[4] Caution should be taken with tricyclic antidepressants and the elderly due to their anticholinergic effects (dizziness, dry mouth, constipation, and cardiotoxicity).[4]

Regional Anesthesia

Regional anesthesia provides the opportunity for pain management as well as anesthesia for simple procedures in the ED. Regional anesthesia is useful particularly for patients who cannot tolerate sedation for procedures such as those with obstructive sleep apnea, advanced age, and multiple medical comorbidities. It is also useful for minimizing the use of opioids. Contraindications to regional anesthesia include infection at the site of the injection, coagulopathies, and known neural deficit in the distribution of the block.[7]

In this chapter, we will discuss digital blocks, and all other blocks will be discussed in the chapter on Regional Anesthesia. Digital nerve blocks are used for fingers and toes and are useful for repair of lacerations, nail bed injuries, and foreign bodies of the nail or digit. Contraindications to digital blocks include infection of the soft tissue where the block will be administered, compromised digital circulation, and patient refusal.[8]

Anatomy

Each digit is innervated by four digital nerves, and all four nerves must be blocked. The digital nerves of the fingers arise from the median and ulnar nerves, and the digital nerves of the toes arise from the tibial and peroneal nerves.[8]

Medication

Typically lidocaine is used for digital blocks, but multiple types of local anesthetics will be discussed separately in this book. The use of epinephrine causes local vasoconstriction, which

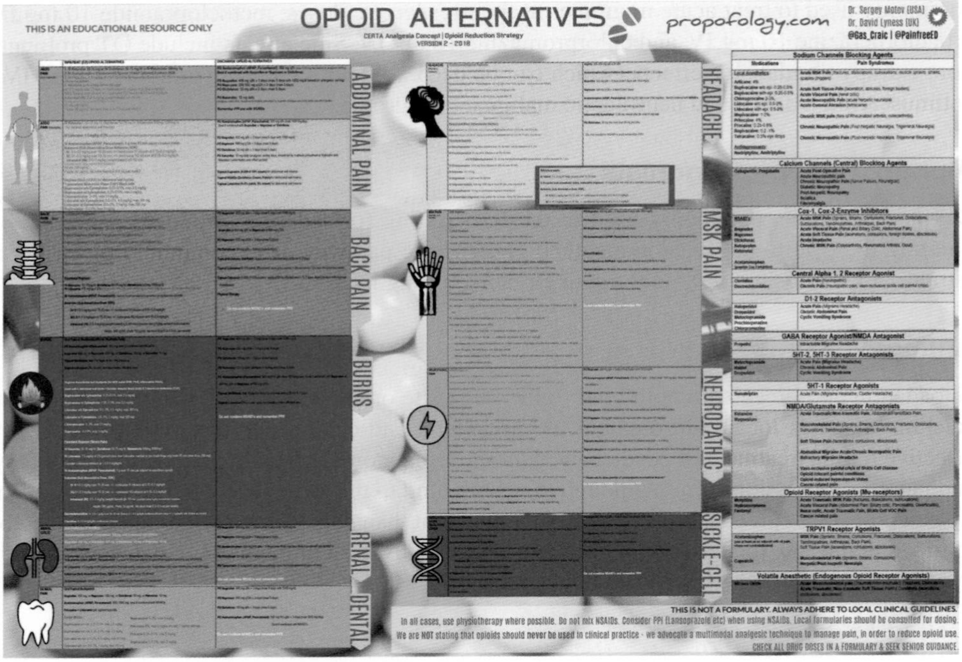

FIGURE 45.1 Opioid alternatives—CERTA analgesia concept | opioid reduction strategy—Version 2—2018.

keeps the local anesthetic in the soft tissue for a longer period of time and decreases bleeding. Epinephrine is generally used in digital blocks except in situations in which the patient has peripheral vascular disease or are at otherwise increased risk of vascular compromise. Use 3-4 mL of local anesthetic.[7]

Performing the finger web space block (traditional digital block)

Patient should be monitored with pulse oximetry, blood pressure monitoring, and electrocardiography for the placement of the block. Place the patient's hand or foot palm or plantar side down on a sterile drape. Prepare the skin with chlorhexidine or povidone iodine to decrease the risk of infection. Using a small-gauge needle (typically 25 or greater), inject local anesthetic into the subcutaneous tissue at the dorsal web space of the finger or toes, just distal to the metacarpophalangeal joint or metatarsophalangeal joint, respectively. Insert the needle deeper into the tissue toward the palmer surface and infiltrate the tissue around the palmar nerve. Remove the needle and repeat on the opposite side of the finger or toe.[8]

Channels-Enzymes-Receptors Targeted Analgesia

Emergency department physicians are encouraged to incorporate multimodal analgesia whenever treating patients with acute pain. Multimodal analgesia known as Channels-Enzymes-Receptors Targeted Analgesia (CERTA) is a method of treating pain that focuses on treating pain based on the several different physiologic pathways of pain transmission.[9] Targeting individual pain pathways allows providers to use multiple nonopioid analgesics, which leads to decreased amount of opioids overall. By targeting pain via multiple pathways, providers can also use lower doses of each medication allowing for a decreased side effect profile for the patient. Figure 45.1 is an example of the use of CERTA to treat a variety of pain syndromes seen in the ED.* Mechanism of action of these drugs is explained elsewhere in this chapter.

---

*Based on a work by Dr. David Lyness and Dr. Sergey Motov.

Emergency department physicians are challenged with the presentation of many different acute pain syndromes daily. Current treatment focuses on the cause of pain and deciphering the appropriate treatment for the specific pain syndrome to optimize pain control and function while avoiding opioid analgesia when possible. To maximize nonopioid therapeutic effects, the CERTA concept should be applied. By incorporating nonopioid analgesics with multiple mechanisms of action, emergency physicians may be able to reduce the amount of opioids prescribed, positioning them not only to be at the forefront of controlling acute pain presentations but also making them leaders in fighting the opioid epidemic.

REFERENCES

1. American College of Physicians, American Academy of Emergency Nurse Practitioners, Emergency Nurses Association, Society of Emergency Medicine Physicians Assistants. *Optimizing the Treatment of Acute Pain Win the Emergency Department.* Policy Statement 2017.
2. Samcam I, Papa L. Acute pain management in the emergency department. In: Prostran M, ed. *Pain Management.* 1st ed. InTech Open; 2016.
3. Motov S, Strayer R, Hayes B, et al. The treatment of acute pain in the emergency department: a white paper position statement prepared for the American Academy of Emergency Medicine. *J Emerg Med.* 2018;54(5):731-736. doi:10.1016/j.jemermed.2018.01.020
4. Koehl J. Pharmacology of Pain. July 2020. Retrieved September 19, 2020, from https://www.emra.org/books/pain-management/pharmacology-of-pain/
5. Sin B, et al. Comparing nonopioids versus opioids for acute pain in the emergency department: a literature review. *Am J Ther.* 2019;28:e52-e86.
6. Cdc.gov. *Opioid Overdose Drug Overdose CDC Injury Center.* 2020. Accessed September 19, 2020. https://www.cdc.gov/drugoverdose/index.html
7. Pardo M, Miller RD. *Basics of Anesthesia.* Elsevier; 2018.
8. Kaye A, Urman R, Vadivelu N, eds. *Essentials of Regional Anesthesia.* 2nd ed. Springer; 2018.
9. Cisewski D, Motov S. Essential pharmacologic options for acute pain management in the emergency setting. *Turk J Emerg Med.* 2018;19(1):1-11.

46

Anesthesia and Pain Assessment for Foot, Ankle, Knee, and Hip Surgery

Melinda Aquino, Kevin A. Elaahi, Benjamin Cole Miller, Sumitra Miriyala, Matthew R. Eng, Elyse M. Cornett, and Alan David Kaye

Introduction

Pain is often viewed as a subjective variable that can be difficult to quantify. However, it is a variable that is being viewed as increasingly more important as it pertains to postoperative care. It has been shown that patients who admit to a higher level of pain postoperative equate their surgery with a lower level of satisfaction. In one study that evaluated total knee replacements, it was found that pain was the highest reason for patient dissatisfaction postoperatively.[1] Postoperative pain not only affects the patients' operative outcome, well-being, and satisfaction from medical care but also directly affects the development of tachycardia, hyperventilation, decrease in alveolar ventilation, transition to chronic pain, poor wound healing, and insomnia. Patients typically undergo lower extremity orthopedic surgery due to pain and lack of function. Preoperatively, it is important for surgeons to discuss the expectations of the surgical outcome with the patient and be prepared to mitigate any unrealistic expectations that the patient has, related to pain relief and gain of function. Especially since pain may worsen shortly after surgery before it gets better. Severe postoperative pain has an adverse impact on early physical recovery especially in the acute setting (the first 2 days postoperative). Patients who report lower pain have a faster recovery process and return to activity. Postoperative pain is also costly as it lengthens hospital stays and requires more intensive care. After drowsiness and digestive discomfort, pain is the most common cause of delay in being discharged. The failure to provide good postoperative analgesia is multifactorial. Insufficient education, fear of complications associated with analgesic drugs, poor pain assessment, and inadequate staffing are among the most common causes.[2] To achieve maximum pain management, preoperative evaluation and planning must be just as important as postoperative care.[3] This includes directed pain history, physical exam as well as a plan control plan. To achieve an adequate postoperative pain assessment, a 10-point pain assessment scale has been implemented with 1 being no pain and 10 being the worst pain imaginable. The key to sufficient control is to reassess the patient and determine if he or she is satisfied with the outcome. Together, the pain and satisfaction ratings minimize that inadequately treated pain goes unnoticed. A multimodal approach combining localized analgesic treatments with systemic injection of analgesic drugs results in improved pain management. It is showing that in orthopedic surgery, regional analgesia is significantly shortening the period of recovery after knee and foot surgeries. In effectively treating postoperative pain, physicians will be able to prevent their patients from developing things such as chronic pain syndrome.[4] In providing patients with the access to a pain assessment by their medical team and in turn having that determine how they are cared for allows the patient to not only feel as though they are a greater part of their care team but also provide the staff with a better understanding of the patient's pain level. A true pain assessment requires not only the viewpoint of the medical team but also the patient's input as well. In doing so, the choice of appropriate pain management can be provided while simultaneously allowing patients the opportunity to be a part of their health care. In giving patients the chance to make decisions on their own behalf, they are able to feel more in control of their pain, which shows to act as a sort of psychological therapy as well.[3]

Barriers and Solutions for Improving Pain Management Practices in Foot, Ankle, Knee, and Hip Surgery Patients

Most patients who undergo surgical procedures experience acute postoperative pain, but evidence suggests that less than half report adequate postoperative pain relief.[5] Inadequate pain management affects 80% of the global population and that up to 50% of the general population could be affected by chronic pain. Barriers to pain management are multifactorial and can have significant implications for functional outcomes.[6] Health care practitioners report that one of the key barriers is a feeling of apprehension toward the appropriate use of diverse pain medications. Due to the constantly evolving field of pain management, many health care professionals do not administer state of the art treatments.[7] It is for this reason staying up to date becomes all the more vital, and it can have a tremendous outcome in the management of patients. Another barrier can be caused by a lack of communication between the patient and medical team as well as among the medical team itself. Patient participation in decision-making regarding pain management is associated with less time in severe pain, better pain relief, lower pain severity, and improved quality of care. With increasing consumer access to health care information, patients are more knowledgeable and demand greater involvement in clinical decisions. It is then through patient education that the medical team may provide the patient with the understanding of what is going on to be able to assist in their care. Through patient education prior to surgery as well as identifying and planning a pain goal, this barrier can be mitigated.[8] However, with the need for greater communication and patient education, medical care team members can find themselves struggling to find the time to undertake these crucial discussions. One critical way to aid with this issue is to adopt a policing attitude toward patients to confirm that routine medications are given at specified times. Furthermore, it is important that every member of the team be educated as well as on just how important it is to control the pain in these patients in order to provide them with the best care. With regard to lack of communication between the medical team, it is important for every member of the team, from physician to pharmacist to patient, to discuss the goals for pain management and be on the same page with how to treat it. Cultural factors are a barrier that can greatly affect treatment. In the elderly, pain can be challenging for multiple reasons, including medical problems contributing to pain and an inability to self-report due to cognitive impairment. Due to cultural beliefs, some patients may prefer nonpharmacological treatments, which may make managing pain more difficult. These instances further emphasize the need for physicians and medical team members to stay up to date on alternative approaches to pain management and to have an open dialogue in handling it. As pain management continues to evolve, so do the medications. Many of these newfound medications can play great roles in helping alleviate pain. However, they often come with their own adverse risks and can make administering them to certain patients at higher risk of side effects challenging. With more and more medications being created to help deal with pain, it makes choosing the right ones for the right patient even more of a delicate process. This can lead to physician hesitancy in prescribing new medications and can lead to specific vulnerable groups such as the elderly, pregnant or breastfeeding women, children, people with substance abuse, and the mentally ill having a greater risk for inadequate pain management. Education is the cornerstone of any effective strategy to remove the barriers toward optimal pain management. Pain management should be introduced as a core and major topic of the curriculum in any medical school and residency programs, so as to embed the importance of addressing pain early on in the career of a physician.[9]

Decreasing Severe Pain and Serious Adverse Events While Transporting Lower Extremity Orthopedic Surgical Patients

During the preoperative and postoperative period, severe pain and serious adverse events are common and strongly associated while moving ICU patients for procedures.[10] It is the responsibility of the operating room anesthesia and surgical team to move the patient from the operating room to recovery. This is usually done while simultaneously monitoring and performing additional therapeutic tasks such as manual ventilation.[11] During this time, it is important to prevent the patient from harming himself postanesthesia and to reduce movement to the surgically fixed area. Anesthesia is usually one of the first members of the medical team to talk to the patients after a surgery and can quickly and effectively administer pain medication or nerve blocks in accordance with the patients' pain. Having an anesthesia team member travel with the patient allows the patients' pain be managed immediately and therefore decrease the pain before it becomes too severe.[12] This is a vital part of the process as early pain mitigation has been shown to be correlated to better outcomes postoperatively. Studies have shown that improved pain management is associated with improved patient outcomes; however, pain remains underevaluated and undertreated. One essential factor in mitigating the pain caused in moving has been found to be when preliminary reports are provided to the receiving team members, allowing them to better prepare for the patient arrival. Not only does this allow for safer care upon arrival but also maximizes patient safety during travel. One of the most common causes of pain in the hospital setting with knee, ankle, and foot injury patients is moving patients and turning of patients for various nursing care procedures.[13] Other serious adverse effects associated with the moving of patients include cardiac arrest, arrhythmias, tachycardia, bradycardia, hypertension, hypotension, desaturation, bradypnea, or ventilatory distress. It has been shown that serious adverse events occur in up to one out of three experiences of moving patients. The moving of patients can often cause pain to the patient, which can lead to these adverse events noted to be associated with patient moving. In improving pain management prior to moving patients, there has been noted to be a decrease in the amount of serious adverse effects. This can likely be attributed to the fact that pain induces reflex responses that may alter respiratory mechanics and increase cardiac demand through tachycardia and increased myocardial oxygen consumption. To ensure safe and effective care transfers, strategies are needed to improve shared situational awareness, teamwork, patient flow, and resource efficiency. Safe transfers involve coordination, optimal timing, early mobilization, participation, and multidiscipline approach. It has been shown that differences in pain appreciation exist between different members of the medical team. Physicians have been shown to underevaluate patients' pain compared to nurses, while nurses under-evaluate patients' pain compared to assistant nurses.[14] It is with this knowledge that incorporating medical education early on in the educational process of the various disciplines so as to make medical team members more aware of pain management and the impact that it can cause in the recovery of a patient.[15]

Anesthesia for Lower Extremity Orthopedic Surgery

Hip, foot, knee, and ankle surgeries are common orthopedic procedures. Fractures of the ankle are common surgeries, while ankle arthrodesis, tendon repair, and ankle replacement are less common. Foot surgeries typically seen in ambulatory settings include bunionectomies, hammer toe repair, and metatarsal fractures. The most common knee operations include knee arthroscopies, anterior cruciate ligament (ACL) repairs, and total knee replacements. Orthopedic surgery for the hip includes hip arthroscopy as well as both elective and traumatic hip replacements. Anesthesia for these orthopedic operations can be accomplished by general anesthesia, neuraxial anesthesia, regional anesthesia, or local anesthesia.[16] If a general anesthetic is preferred, regional anesthesia can be performed for the purpose of postoperative pain relief. Ultrasound-guided regional anesthesia provides excellent analgesia postoperatively, reducing the requirements for systemic analgesics. To decide which nerve block is appropriate for the type of surgery being performed, it is critical to understand the anatomy of the lower extremity. The sensory nerve supply to the lower extremity is distributed between the branches of the femoral nerve and the sciatic nerve.[17]

The femoral nerve arises from the L2, L3, and L4 branches. The saphenous nerve, which arises from L3 to L4, gives rise to terminal branches that supply the skin over the medial malleolus and the medial aspect of the foot, and the head of the first metatarsal. The sciatic nerve divides into the common peroneal and tibial nerves at a variable location between the buttock and the popliteal fossa. Commonly, the split can be located 6-10 cm above the popliteal fossa. In up to 30% of patients, this split may occur more proximally. The common peroneal nerve winds around the head of the fibula and divides into two branches, the superficial peroneal nerve, which supplies the dorsum of the foot and ankle, and the deep peroneal nerve, which supplies the webspace of the first toe. The tibial nerve supplies motor function to the flexor muscles of the calf and foot and divides into two branches, the sural nerve and the posterior tibial nerve. The sural nerve supplies sensation to the lateral portion of the foot and heel. The calcaneal branch of the tibial nerve innervates the remaining parts of the heel. The posterior tibial nerve travels posterior to the medial malleolus, immediately posterior to the tibial artery. It then divides into the medial and lateral plantar nerves to the foot, which provide motor innervation to the foot and sensory innervation to the internal structures of the foot and the skin over the sole of the foot. See Figure 46.1.

Anesthesia for Foot and Ankle Operations

There are several combinations of anesthetic techniques that can be utilized for foot operations. General anesthesia can be used in combination with ankle blocks for postoperative pain relief. Spinal anesthesia is appropriate for those who are not candidates for general anesthesia.

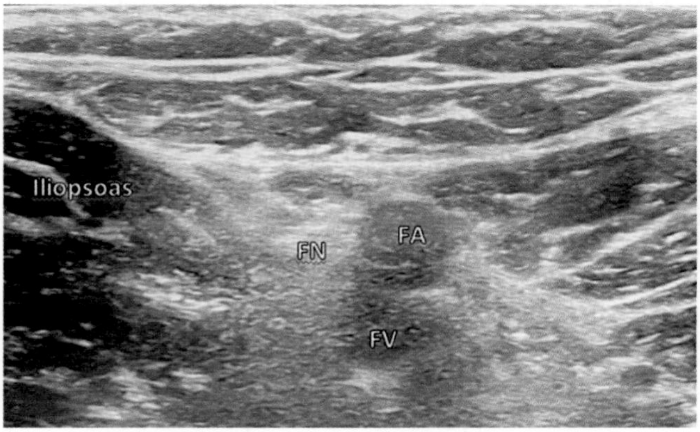

FIGURE 46.1 Femoral nerve block—the iliopsoas muscle is bordered by fascia iliaca, which can be appreciated during needle insertion. The femoral nerve (FN) can be seen located between the femoral artery (FA) and iliopsoas muscle.

Peripheral nerve blocks (popliteal and saphenous) or ankle blocks can be used as the sole anesthetic with sedation in ambulatory settings. There are several factors that should be taken into consideration when performing peripheral nerve blocks or ankle blocks. The onset time if using ropivacaine or bupivacaine is usually 10-30 minutes, so you must place a block in a timely fashion. The block placement can be uncomfortable, so sedation during the block may be required. Ropivacaine and bupivacaine can last up to 12 hours or longer, so either local anesthetic is an excellent choice when post-op analgesia is preferred. Owing to the potential for intravascular toxicity, ropivacaine would be a safer choice in all situations. The maximum dose of bupivacaine to avoid toxicity is 3 mg/kg but uptake is different depending on the nerve block employed, while ropivacaine is generally safer due to less cardiac toxicity with inadvertent intravascular injection. Furthermore, it is not advisable to add epinephrine in ankle blocks related to the risk of causing ischemia in the foot. All resuscitative equipment and airway supplies must be available in case of toxic reaction and in the setting of bupivacaine, which would include lipid emulsion. Full monitors should be in place, with IV access for both sedation and resuscitation.

There are five nerves to be injected in an ankle block. These include the posterior tibial, sural, superficial peroneal, deep peroneal, and saphenous nerves. The patient is placed in the supine position with the calf placed on a padded support. Sedation and oxygen should be administered. There must be sterile prep and draping to prevent infection. Chlorhexidine is preferred and more effective compared to previous antiseptics such as betadine. Some practitioners prefer to start with the posterior tibial nerve first. The leg must be externally rotated with the knee slightly flexed to allow the foot to be externally rotated. The technique involves locating the pulse of the tibial artery just posterior and inferior to the medial malleolus. The needle should be inserted at 30° angle to the malleolus to pass 2-3 mm posterior to the artery. Contact of the tibia should be made and then withdraw the needle 0.5 cm. Five milliliter of local anesthetic should be injected after negative aspiration for blood. A nerve stimulator can also be used as the tibial nerve is the only nerve in the ankle bock that has a major motor nerve supply. Using a 50 mm stimulator needle, you are looking for flexion of the great toe, or less commonly, flexion of the other toes.

The sural nerve block is performed by locating the lateral border of the Achilles tendon at the level of the lower border of the lateral malleolus. The needle is advanced anteriorly toward the fibula. If a paresthesia is felt, inject 3-5 mL of local anesthetic. If not, then inject 5-7 mL as the needle is withdrawn to ensure adequate infiltration of the nerve. An ankle block covers procedures of the toes, and foot distal to the ankle. It is not sufficient for procedures including surgeries on and proximal to the ankle. In many cases, the injection sites for the ankle block are likely to be at the site of the surgical incision. A more appropriate approach for ankle procedures would be to perform femoral and sciatic nerve blocks, or lower branch blocks depending on the specific surgical procedure such as utilizing a popliteal nerve block, etc. A combination of these blocks will anesthetize the leg below the knee. A proximal sciatic nerve block (eg, above the knee) will cause profound motor weakness and can be avoided by performing a tibial and common peroneal nerve block in the popliteal fossa. This block is an excellent choice for ankle surgery and midfoot surgery when combined with an adductor canal block.

The sciatic nerve block (also known as a popliteal nerve block) in the popliteal fossa is indicated for ankle and foot surgery and provides anesthesia in combination with a saphenous nerve block for all foot/ankle operations. Anatomically, the sciatic nerve lies lateral to the popliteal artery and vein and divides into the common peroneal and tibial nerves between 6 and 10 cm above the popliteal crease. In 30% of the population, the split occurs above 10 cm above the crease. The sciatic nerve in the popliteal fossa lies in a triangle—it is bordered superomedially by the semimembranosus and semitendinosus muscles, and superolaterally by the long head of the biceps femoris muscle. The base of the triangle is the popliteal crease. Most commonly, ultrasound is used for the lateral approach.[18] With the patient's knee flexed, the probe is placed in the popliteal fossa. The femur is identified and then the probe is used to locate the popliteal artery by pulsation. The sciatic nerve is hyperechoic and located superficial to the femur and lateral to the popliteal artery. In order to ensure you do not pierce the common peroneal nerve accidently, one should scan distally to observe the splitting of the sciatic nerve into both branches and then scan up to localize the point at which the sciatic nerve is formed. Nerve visualization is improved when hydrodissection with the local anesthetic is injected due to enhanced contrast between the hyperechoic nerve and the hypoechoic fluid collection. Both in-plane and out of plane techniques can be utilized, and electrical stimulation of the nerve can be utilized to confirm needle placement as well. Twenty milliliter of local anesthetic is administered under direct visualization, aiming to see circumferential spread around the nerve, known as the "Donut Sign." If there is inadequate spread, the needle may be repositioned to ensure complete nerve block. The patient should be minimally sedated, so that if an intraneural injection occurs and a paresthesia is elicited, the patient can report abnormal sensation and the needle can be repositioned. When block is completed, it is advisable to scan proximally and distally to ensure vertical spread of the local anesthetic. Complications of the block include bleeding, infection, nerve damage, failure of injection, and partial injection. Local anesthetic toxicity is a complication as well. See Figure 46.2.

The sciatic nerve block spares the medial side of the calf and the foot. For a complete regional anesthetic, we must perform a saphenous nerve block. The saphenous nerve is a terminal branch of the femoral nerve and is a pure sensory nerve. It supplies innervation on the medial aspect of the leg to the ankle and foot. There are also terminal branches—infrapatellar nerves that are sent to the knee joint. An adductor canal block, which blocks the saphenous nerve, is performed in the mid-thigh with a large volume (20 mL) of local anesthetic utilizing ultrasound technique.[19] Anatomically, the sartorius muscle crosses the anterior thigh in a lateral to medial direction and forms a roof over the adductor canal in the lower half of the thigh. The three sides of the canal are formed by the sartorius muscle, the vastus medius laterally, and the adductor longus medially. The femoral artery and vein are located in the canal and help us to locate the nerve. The nerve is a small hyperechoic structure anterior to the artery. After appropriate prep and drape, a linear ultrasound probe is placed on the anterior thigh in the transverse position to the longitudinal axis halfway between the patella and the anterior

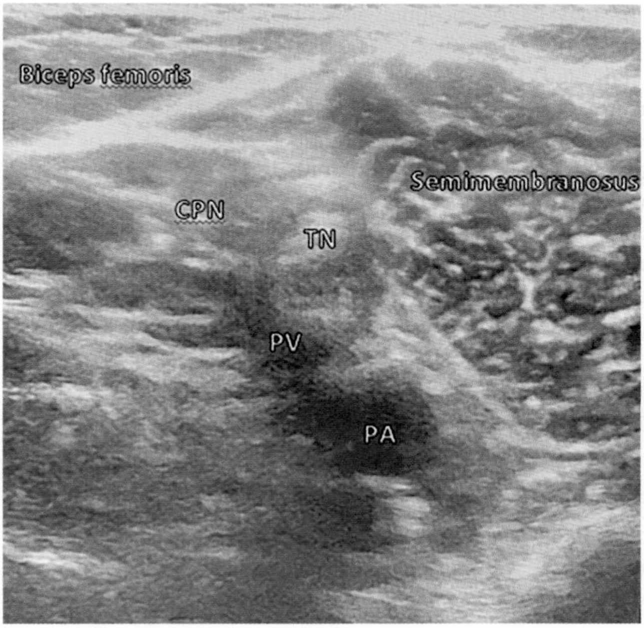

FIGURE 46.2 Popliteal sciatic block—here the common peroneal (CPN) and tibial nerves (TN) can be seen in this image captured from above the popliteal crease. It is key to identify the popliteal artery (PA), which is found deep to the nerves.

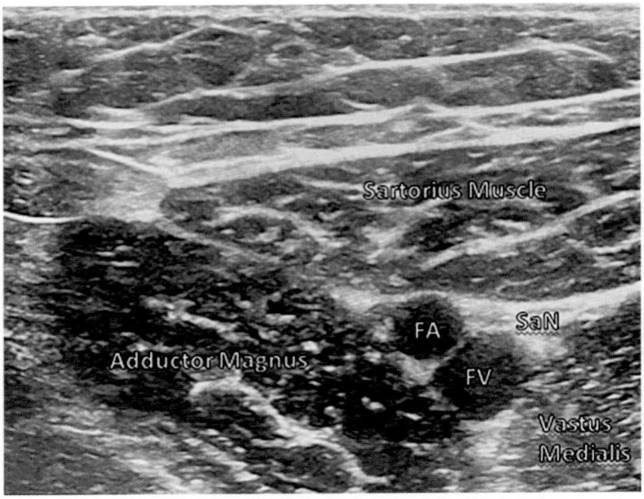

FIGURE 46.3 Adductor canal block—in this ultrasound image, the neurovascular bundle comprising of the saphenous nerve (SaN), femoral artery (FA), and femoral vein (FV) can be seen surrounded by muscle. The sartorius muscle is superficial, while the vastus medialis is anatomically medial and the adductor magnus anatomically lateral.

superior iliac spine. The femoral artery pulsation is identified, and the femoral vein is inferior. The saphenous nerve is just lateral to the artery.[6] In-plane technique is used to inject local anesthetic around the nerve. The recommended volume to inject is 10-20 mL. The risks of this nerve block are the same as the risks of other nerve blocks. See Figure 46.3.

Anesthesia for Knee Operations

The most common orthopedic operations to the knee include knee arthroscopy, ACL repair, and knee arthroplasty. Each of these operations has its unique challenges. In patients undergoing knee arthroscopy, early ambulation and resumption of normal activity is paramount. The surgical manipulation is minimally invasive to accomplish these goals, and a general anesthetic is utilized to provide optimal operating conditions. These patients benefit from a multimodal approach, utilizing nonsteroidal anti-inflammatory drugs for postoperative pain relief, as well as a regional nerve block to the saphenous distribution if postoperative pain is anticipated.

Patients undergoing ACL repairs may likely encounter more pain than knee arthroscopy. Patients are fixated in a knee immobilizer for several weeks, and therefore, a femoral nerve block or saphenous nerve block may be indicated. There is debate whether adductor canal or femoral nerve blocks may contribute to quadricep function several weeks following the operation.[20,21]

Patients undergoing total knee arthroplasty operations have become the focus of orthopedic-enhanced recovery pathways. Models have been well studied to reduce length of stay, reduce surgical complications, improve pain control, and improve patient satisfaction.[22] Unless contraindicated, patients undergoing knee arthroplasty should receive a neuraxial anesthetic, regional nerve blocks, as well as a cocktail of multimodal analgesics. A saphenous nerve block will reduce pain to the medial knee postoperatively and result in a pain reduction of ~30%-70%. Additionally, an iPACK block (innerspace to the popliteal artery and capsule of the knee) has been demonstrated to reduce postoperative pain. A combination of oral opioids, anticonvulsants (pregabalin or gabapentin), ibuprofen, and celecoxib are also utilized in a multimodal approach to postoperative pain.

Anesthesia for Hip Operations

Patients presenting for hip operations include hip arthroscopy and either elective or traumatic hip arthroplasty. For the patient undergoing a hip arthroscope, the postoperative pain can be very challenging. Often, a labral repair may cause a great amount of pain to the L1-L4 nerve distribution. Therefore, a lumbar plexus nerve block is often employed in combination with general anesthesia to manage these patients perioperatively. Patients undergoing either elective or traumatic hip arthroplasty have been well studied in enhanced recovery pathways similar to knee arthroplasty patients.[22] Both elective and traumatic hip replacement operations should be managed with neuraxial anesthetics if not contraindicated. Careful attention must be paid to patients who have recently taken anticoagulants, as this is the most common contraindication to a neuraxial anesthetic. In coordination with emergency medicine physicians, internists, and orthopedic surgeons, a fascia iliaca block should also be administered to patients who present to the hospital with hip fractures. The fascia iliaca block should be performed as soon as possible and is often completed preoperatively to reduce total opioids administered to an often geriatric age patient. The reduction of opioids greatly reduces the incidence of delirium and other sinister opioid-related complications.

Conclusion

Postoperative discomfort is extremely expensive, extending hospital stays, and necessitating more careful care. Following drowsiness and stomach problems, pain is the most often cited reason for discharge delays. The inability to give adequate postoperative analgesia has several causes. Inadequate education, fear of analgesic medication problems, poor pain assessment, and insufficient personnel are among the most prominent causes. A multimodal approach combining localized analgesic treatments with systemic injection of analgesic drugs results in improved pain management. It demonstrates that localized analgesia considerably reduces the time required to recover from knee and foot procedures in orthopedic surgery. By appropriately managing postoperative pain, physicians can help their patients avoid developing chronic pain syndrome. Finally, there are several options for pain control and anesthesia for foot, ankle, and knee surgeries. Regional anesthesia is an excellent choice, as it provides a solid anesthetic for the procedure, and will give superior postoperative pain relief. Multimodal analgesia including nonsteroidal anti-inflammatory drugs, gabapentin, and pre-emptive analgesics can also improve outcomes. Patient satisfaction, early ambulation, and early discharge are advantages of regional anesthesia. General anesthesia should be reserved for those not amenable to regional anesthesia or in whom regional anesthesia is contraindicated.

By providing patients with access to a pain assessment conducted by their medical team and using that evaluation to decide how they are cared for, the patient not only feels more connected to their care team but the staff also has a better grasp of the patient's pain level. True pain evaluation involves not just the medical team's perspective but also input from the patient. This way, patients may receive excellent pain treatment while also having a say in their health care. By allowing patients to make their own choices, they get a sense of control over their suffering, which acts as a form of psychological treatment as well.

REFERENCES

1. Baker PN, van der Meulen JH, Lewsey J, Gregg PJ. The role of pain and function in determining patient satisfaction after total knee replacement. *J Bone Joint Surg Br*. 2007;89-B(7):893-900.
2. Eriksson K, Broström A, Fridlund B, et al. *Postoperative Pain Assessment and Impact of Pain on Early Physical Recovery, From the Patients' Perspective*. Jönköping University, School of Health and Welfare; 2017.
3. Gan TJ. Poorly controlled postoperative pain: prevalence, consequences, and prevention. *J Pain Res*. 2017;10:2287-2298.
4. Shoar S, Esmaeili S, Safari S. Pain management after surgery: a brief review. *Anesthesiol Pain Med*. 2012;1(3):184-186.
5. Akbar N, Teo SP, Hj-Abdul-Rahman HNA, Hj-Husaini HA, Venkatasalu MR. Barriers and solutions for improving pain management practices in acute hospital settings: perspectives of healthcare practitioners for a pain-free hospital initiative. *Ann Geriatr Med Res*. 2019;23(4):190-196.
6. Al-Mahrezi A. Towards effective pain management: breaking the barriers. *Oman Med J*. 2017;32(5):357-358.

7. Thakur AC. Barriers to optimal pain management in the general surgery population. In: Narayan D, Kaye AD, Vadivelu N, eds. *Perioperative Pain Management for General and Plastic Surgery*. Oxford University Press; 2018. https://oxfordmedicine.com/view/10.1093/med/9780190457006.001.0001/med-9780190457006-chapter-3
8. Chou R, Gordon DB, de Leon-Casasola OA, et al. Management of postoperative pain: a clinical practice guideline from the American Pain Society, the American Society of Regional Anesthesia and Pain Medicine, and the American Society of Anesthesiologists' Committee on Regional Anesthesia, Executive Committee. *J Pain*. 2016;17(2):131-157.
9. Clarke H, Woodhouse LJ, Kennedy D, Stratford P, Katz J. Strategies aimed at preventing chronic post-surgical pain: comprehensive perioperative pain management after total joint replacement surgery. *Physiother Can*. 2011;63(3):289-304.
10. de Jong A, Molinari N, de Lattre S, et al. Decreasing severe pain and serious adverse events while moving intensive care unit patients: a prospective interventional study (the NURSE-DO project). *Crit Care*. 2013;17(2):R74.
11. Nearman HS, Popple CG. How to transfer a postoperative patient to the intensive care unit. Strategies for documentation, evaluation, and management. *J Crit Illn*. 1995;10(4):275-280.
12. Segall N, Bonifacio AS, Schroeder RA, et al. Can we make postoperative patient handovers safer? A systematic review of the literature. *Anesth Analg*. 2012;115(1):102-115.
13. Segall N, Bonifacio AS, Barbeito A, et al. Operating Room–to-ICU patient handovers: a multidisciplinary human-centered design approach. *Jt Comm J Qual Patient Saf*. 2016;42(9):400-414.
14. Manias E, Bucknall T, Botti M. Nurses' strategies for managing pain in the postoperative setting. *Pain Manag Nurs*. 2005;6(1):18-29.
15. Medrzycka-Dabrowka W, Dąbrowski S, Gutysz-Wojnicka A, Gawroska-Krzemińska A, Ozga D. Barriers perceived by nurses in the optimal treatment of postoperative pain. *Open Med*. 2017;12:239-246.
16. Lee TH, Wapner KL, Hecht PJ, Hunt PJ. Regional anesthesia in foot and ankle surgery. *Orthopedics*. 1996;19(7):577-580.
17. Shah S, Tsai T, Iwata T, Hadzic A. Outpatient regional anesthesia for foot and ankle surgery. *Int Anesthesiol Clin*. 2005;43(3):143-151.
18. Saranteas T, Chantzi C, Zogogiannis J, et al. Lateral sciatic nerve examination and localization at the mid-femoral level: an imaging study with ultrasound. *Acta Anaesthesiol Scand*. 2007;51(3):387-388.
19. Tsui BCH, Finucane BT. The importance of ultrasound landmarks: a "traceback" approach using the popliteal blood vessels for identification of the sciatic nerve. *Reg Anesth Pain Med*. 2006;31(5):481-482.
20. Christensen JE, Taylor NE, Hetzel SJ, Shepler JA, Scerpella TA. Isokinetic strength deficit 6 months after adductor canal blockade for anterior cruciate ligament reconstruction. *Orthop J Sports Med*. 2017;5(11):2325967117736249.
21. Xerogeanes JW, Premkumar A, Godfrey W, et al. Adductor canal vs. femoral nerve block in anterior cruciate ligament reconstruction: a randomized controlled trial. *Orthop J Sports Med*. 2017;5(7 suppl 6).
22. Kaye A, Urman R, Cornett E, Hart B, et al. Enhanced recovery pathways in orthopedic surgery. *J Anaesthesiol Clin Pharmacol*. 2019;35(5):35-39.

47

Acute Pain in Primary Care

Madelyn K. Craig, Devin S. Reed, and Justin Y. Yan

Introduction

Pain is one of the most common complaints seen in primary care practices; however, it is still one of the most poorly managed complaints. Back and neck pain, headaches and migraines, joint pain, musculoskeletal pain, facial pain, chest pain, and abdominal pain are several types of acute pain commonly encountered by general practitioners. Typically, the pathophysiology of acute pain is not complex. It is the perception of pain, which can be influenced by a number of psychological, cognitive, hormonal, or biological factors, that makes treating pain less straightforward. Numerous institutions cite pain management as a fundamental human right and providing effective pain management a health professional's moral obligation.[1] The initiative to make pain the "fifth vital sign" brought well deserved attention to the need for improved pain assessment and treatment; however, it also led to an overemphasis on one-dimensional pain intensity scales that lead to an overuse of opioids for treatment and adverse events such as opioid over sedation and death.[2] We must shift our attention from pain as a 5th vital sign to expanding our education and training in the assessment of pain to improve our treatment strategies.[3] Pain left untreated not only can lead to chronic pain but also has effects on mental and physical health as well. The first step in every pain management plan should be a thorough multidimensional pain assessment.[4] This chapter includes a discussion on pain assessment and education as well as pharmacologic and nonpharmacologic treatments of acute pain in the primary care setting.

Pain Assessment

The assessment of pain can be challenging as it relies on patient communication of a subjective perception of an unpleasant sensory and emotional experience. The perception of pain varies widely between patients, and it cannot be objectively quantified. The goals of pain assessment are to gather information from the patient in a standardized way in order to help determine the type of pain, the effect this pain is having on the patient and their daily activities, and a cause of the pain so the provider may develop a suitable treatment plan. Standardizing pain assessments is important to obtain reliable, reproducible data that may be used to guide treatment and determine when changes are needed. Pain intensity and pain relief are the two characteristics typically assessed in acute pain. There are several one-dimensional pain scales physicians may use to assess pain intensity.[1] The Numerical Rating Scales (NRS), Verbal Rating Scales (VRS), Visual Analog Scales (VAS), and Faces Pain Scale (FACES) are the more commonly used intensity assessment tools for acute pain. Examples of these pain scales are shown in Figure 47.1. The NRS, VRS, and FACES scales are relatively self-explanatory. The VAS requires the patient to point to an area on the line, which is then recorded in millimeters as their pain rating. When determining which scale to use, the physician should take into account the patient's age, cognitive status, and communication barriers. Pain assessment

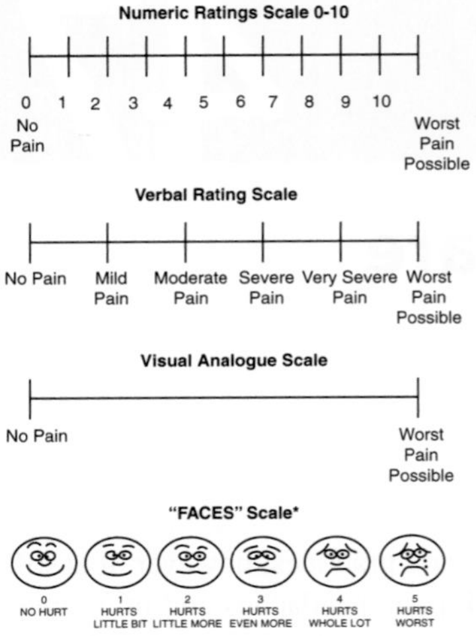

FIGURE 47.1 One-dimensional Intensity Pain Scales.

in patients with cognitive impairment or those unable to report such as unconscious or sedated patients present unique challenges. The tools recommended for these patients use behavioral and physiologic indicators to assess pain. The Critical-Care Pain Observation Tool shown in Table 47.1 incorporates facial expression, body movements, ventilator compliance for intubated patients and vocalization in extubated patients, and muscle tension to determine a pain

TABLE 47.1 CRITICAL CARE PAIN OBSERVATION TOOL

Facial expression	Relaxed/neutral	No muscle tension observed	0
	Tense	Presence of frowning, brow lowering, orbit tightening, and levator contraction	1
	Grimacing	All of the above plus eyelids tightly closed	2
Body movements	Absence of movements or normal position	Does not move at all or normal position	0
	Protection	Slow, cautious movements, touching or rubbing the pain site, seeking attention through movements	1
	Restlessness/agitation	Pulling tube, attempting to sit up, moving limbs/thrashing, not following commands, striking at staff, trying to climb out of bed	2
Muscle tension	Relaxed	No resistance to passive movements	0
	Tense, rigid	Resistance to passive movements	1
	Very tense or rigid	Strong resistance to passive movements or incapacity to complete them	2
Ventilator compliance (intubated)	Tolerating ventilator/movement	Alarms not activated, easy ventilation	0
	Coughing but tolerating	Coughing, alarms may be activated but stop spontaneously	1
	Fighting ventilator	Asynchrony: blocking ventilation, alarms frequently activated	2
Vocalization (extubated)	Talking in normal tone or no sound		0
	Sighing, moaning		1
	Crying out, sobbing		2

TABLE 47.2 BEHAVIORAL PAIN SCALE[5–8]

Facial expression	Relaxed	1
	Partially tightened	2
	Fully tightened	3
	Grimacing	4
Upper extremity movements	No movement	1
	Partially bent	2
	Fully bent with finger flexion	3
	Permanently retracted	4
Compliance with mechanical ventilation	Tolerating movement	1
	Coughing but tolerating ventilation for most of the time	2
	Fighting ventilator	4
	Unable to control ventilation	

score between 0 and 8. The Behavioral Pain Scale uses facial expression, upper extremity movements, and compliance with mechanical ventilation to compile a pain rating between 0 and 12 (Table 47.2). Infants and children present another group requiring behavioral and physiologic indicators to assess pain. The Face, Legs, Activity, Cry, Consolability (FLACC) or the Children's Hospital of Eastern Ontario Pain Scale are recommended for assessing pain in children older than 3 years. Using indicators such as facial expressions, body movements, heart rate, and oxygen saturation is recommended when assessing acute pain in infants.

It is also important to assess pain intensity at rest and during activity. Assessment while at rest indicates a patient's comfort level, while assessment during activity indicates functional ability. It is important to gather information beyond just the intensity of the pain. Multidimensional pain scales assess the impact this pain is having on the patient's emotional state and functionality such as sleep and daily activities.[1,2] The Clinically Aligned Pain Assessment (CAPA) tool shown in Table 47.3 was designed to assess pain more thoroughly and identify the impact pain is having on quality of life. It goes further than solely identifying pain intensity. It is also important to take a detailed history and identify other features relating to the onset, location, quality, and modifying characteristics of the pain. There are several mnemonics listed in Table 47.4 used to obtain a more comprehensive assessment of the patient's pain.[2]

Nonpharmacologic Treatments

Treatment of acute pain in primary care has increased focus toward nonpharmacologic options in conjunction with pharmaceuticals rather than solely opiate and other oral medications. These nonpharmacologic options include lifestyle changes, cognitive behavioral therapy (CBT), electrical stimulation, physical therapy (PT), acupuncture therapy, and massage therapy.

Lifestyle changes include recommendations such as improving nutritional habits, exercise regimens, sleep hygiene, and stress management. Anti-inflammatory foods—including nonstarchy vegetables, legumes, fruits, vegetables, healthy oils, whole grains, and a diet low in mammalian protein—is recommended. Supplementation of micronutrients such as vitamin D, magnesium, fish oils high in omega 3 fatty acids, and B12 have been shown to decrease overall pain. Lowering consumption of highly processed foods is recommended. While nutritional improvements may have limited utility in mitigating acute pain, nutrition can help improve

TABLE 47.3 CAPA TOOL

Comfort	Intolerable Tolerable with discomfort Comfortably manageable Negligible pain
Change in pain	Getting worse About the same Getting better
Pain control	Inadequate pain control Partially effective Fully effective
Functioning	Cannot do anything because of pain Pain keeps me from doing most of what I need to do Can do most things, but pain gets in the way of some Can do everything I need to
Sleep	Awake with pain most of the night Awake with occasional pain Normal sleep

chronic pain or act as a preventative measure.[1] Physical exercise has been shown to improve mood in patients and has been shown to decrease pain. Exercise regimens should be increased slowly, with goals of daily aerobic stimuli. Poor sleep and increased stress have been related to certain pain disorders and shown to aggravate pain.[2]

TABLE 47.4 MNEMONIC TOOLS FOR COMPREHENSIVE PAIN ASSESSMENTS

SOCRATES	Site: Where is the pain? Onset: When did the pain start? Sudden or gradual? Character: Describe the pain. Radiation: Does the pain spread anywhere? Associations: Any other signs or symptoms associated with the pain? Time course: Does the pain follow any pattern or vary throughout the day? Exacerbating/relieving factors: Does anything make the pain better or worse? Severity: Intensity of pain on grading scale.
OPQRSTUV	Onset: When did it begin? How long does it last? How often does it occur? Provoking/palliating: What brings it on? What makes it better? What makes it worse? Quality: What does it feel like? Can you describe it? Region/radiation: Where is it? Does it spread anywhere? Severity: What is the intensity (grading scale)? At best? At worst? Treatment: What medications and treatments have you tried or are currently taking? How effective? Understand how it impacts on you: What do you believe is causing this symptom? How is it affecting you and your family? Values: What is your comfort goal or acceptable pain level?
QISS-TAPED	Quality Impact Site Severity Temporal characteristics Aggravating/alleviating factors Past treatment, response, and patient preferences Expectations and meaning Diagnostics and physical examination

CBT involves the process of learning how to change the way the patient thinks about the pain in a more constructive way. The patient will eventually change the way they feel about the pain in order to minimize its effects.[3] CBT combined with its counterpart of mindfulness and meditation-based therapies designed to focus nonjudgmental attention on pain has been shown to be a cost-effective and cost-saving methods of pain reduction.[2] Transcutaneous Electrical Nerve Stimulation (TENS) uses low-voltage electrical currents to stimulate the skin and underlying nerve fibers. The stimulation reduces pain by activating inhibitory pain receptors. TENS has been shown to reduce acute pain when adequate stimulation frequency is applied.[4]

Physical therapy aims to target sources of pain through exercises and strengthening with hopes to alleviate areas of weakness or stiffness.[4,9] Physical therapy is effective in treating pain by targeting multiple pain mechanisms such as nociceptive, nociplastic, and neuropathic pain. It also hopes to improve motor function and psychosocial factors.[10] Cryotherapy is a method in which an external cold source reduces tissue temperature to decrease tissue edema and vascular permeability. This has been theorized to decrease pain by reducing tissue inflammation and hypoxic injury. However, there is only preliminary support for cryotherapy at this moment.[4]

Acupuncture is the insertion and manipulation of needles at targeted points throughout the body. Acupuncture is theorized to improve pain by manipulation of the interconnectedness of the organs and certain body points in order to reduce pain. Studies have shown that pain benefit with acupuncture vs controls.[2] Massage therapy helps pain by the manipulation of soft tissue around painful areas to reduce tension, stress, or spasms. Studies and reviews have shown benefit of massage therapy in reducing pain and anxiety for pain patients.[2]

Pharmacologic Treatments

Pharmacologic treatment can be controversial in discussions about pain management but are nonetheless a crucial element in treatment regimens for pain. The best approach is to incorporate pharmacologic treatments into a multimodal analgesia strategy. Nonpharmacologic treatments combined with opioid and nonopioid oral options have shown to yield the best results in patients.[2]

Initial options for pharmacologic agents are nonopioid oral analgesics. These include NSAIDs, acetaminophen, muscle relaxants, anticonvulsants, and antidepressants. The mechanism of NSAIDs is through the inhibition of cyclooxygenase (COX). Cyclooxygenase produces downstream mediators that increase inflammatory and pain signaling, thus curtailed by regimented NSAID use.[11] Examples of NSAIDs include ketorolac and ibuprofen. Some studies have even shown NSAIDs to have equivalent pain reduction responses when compared to opioids.[4] Acetaminophen works through the inhibition of CNS nociception. NSAIDs and acetaminophen are generally considered first-line nonopioid therapy for acute pain and have strong evidence for their effectiveness.[4,11]

Gabapentin works through the binding of neuronal channels, which decreases calcium entry into neurons and inhibits neuron function. Gabapentin has been shown to decrease pain scores but not opioid consumption in multimodal regimens.[4,12] Muscle relaxers—such as cyclobenzaprine and tizanidine—have been used to treat acute pain. The data behind this are inconclusive, thus muscle relaxers remain as a second-line treatment and inferior to NSAIDs and opiates.[13] Muscle relaxers have shown to be superior to placebo in certain studies.[13]

Antidepressants have also been added to the acute pain treatment regimens. They have been shown to be superior to muscle relaxers when treating certain pain disorders.[14] Antidepressants have intrinsic antinociceptive effects. In conjunction with opiates, tricyclic antidepressants have shown to have superior results. Correlation has been shown between antidepressant and concurrent opiate treatment to have enhancement of opiate analgesia, attenuation of opiate tolerance, and attenuation of opiate dependence.[14] Antidepressants have been shown to decrease opioid consumption but not pain scores in multimodal treatment regimens.[4,14] Nonopioid IV analgesia has shown to be an adequate option when trying to avoid opiates. IV ketamine, acetaminophen, and NSAIDs can reduce pain to a similar degree as opiates.[15]

Opioids are the most prescribed treatment for severe acute pain. Caution must be applied to prescribing opiates as there is risk of abuse, addiction, and overdose. Guidelines and recommendations have been implemented to allow safer prescription practice. These include the prescription of immediate-release opioids rather than extended-release, having a single prescriber per patient ensured by state databases, and using a multimodal treatment strategy rather than opioid monotherapy.[16] Extended-release opiates have been found to have a 4.6 times higher rate of abuse and 6.1 times higher rate of diversion potential when compared to short-acting opiates.[16] Opioids work by activating G-protein coupled receptors in neurons resulting in inhibition of neuronal pain signaling. Examples of commonly prescribed opioids are oxycodone/acetaminophen, hydromorphone, and tramadol.[4,16,17] The upper limits of dosing opioids is defined by morphine equivalent dosage per day (mg MEQ/d). General practitioners should not prescribe more than 50 mg MEQ/d to patients. Specialists should not prescribe more than 90 mg MEQ/d. Prescriptions over 100 mg MEQ/d are linked to 7-9 times increase in overdose risk.[16,17] Opiate-related deaths happen when excessive dosages are prescribed—particularly in opiate-naive patients, with excessive increases in prescription dosage, and inadequate patient monitoring.[17]

There is a trend in recent years toward the use of the opiates tramadol and methadone to treat pain. Tramadol treats pain by inhibiting weak binding to the mu opioid receptor sites. It also has unique action of inhibiting reuptake of norepinephrine and serotonin.[18] This can reduce pain in the same manner antidepressants cause pain reduction. Methadone and the similar medication buprenorphine work by partial agonist of opioid receptors.[19] This prevents withdrawal and prevents further use of stronger opiates. These alternative medications allow patients with opiate addiction and abuse issues to function normally. The trend of increased tramadol and methadone prescriptions shows a trend for moving away from strong opiate treatment for pain and toward safer alternatives.[18,19]

Seeking an interventional pain specialist may be considered when conservative treatment for pain does not relieve symptoms within 2-3 weeks. Before consulting a pain specialist, a few steps must be cleared: conservative therapies have failed, complete psychological clearance, no further surgical intervention indicated, no drug-seeking behavior, and pain is consistent with observed pathology. Pain specialists can offer a variety of interventional procedures that both diagnose and treat the pain. Injections with corticosteroids, local anesthetics, or a combination of the two can act to block nerve signaling and quell inflammation at targeted structures believed to contribute to the pain source. Radiofrequency neuronal ablation can provide extended relief up to 6 months to 1 year. Epidural steroid injections can also be done to relieve back pain caused by neuroclaudication. Other procedures include spinal cord stimulation and intrathecal therapy—both forms of neuromodulation. Neuromodulation is used to reduce chronic pain—likely by inhibiting interneurons in the dorsal horn of the spinal cord—as well as improve neurologic function by altering electrical and chemical communications within the central nervous system.

REFERENCES

1. de Gregori M, Muscoli C, Schatman ME, et al. Combining pain therapy with lifestyle: the role of personalized nutrition and nutritional supplements according to the simpar feed your destiny approach. *J Pain Res*. 2016;9:1179-1189. https://doi.org/10.2147/JPR.S115068
2. Tick H, Nielsen A, Pelletier KR, et al. Evidence-based nonpharmacologic strategies for comprehensive pain care: the Consortium Pain Task Force White Paper. *Explore (NY)*. 2018;14:177-211. https://doi.org/10.1016/j.explore.2018.02.001
3. Cognitive-Behavioral Therapy for Pain Management. n.d. Accessed October 25, 2020. https://wa.kaiserpermanente.org/kbase/topic.jhtml?docId=tv3092
4. Hsu JR, Mir H, Wally MK, Seymour RB. Clinical practice guidelines for pain management in acute musculoskeletal injury. *J Orthop Trauma*. 2019;33:e158e182. https://doi.org/10.1097/BOT.0000000000001430
5. Koch K. Assessing pain in primary care. *South African Fam Pract*. 2012;54:21-24. https://doi.org/10.1080/20786204.2012.10874169

6. Gordon DB. Acute pain assessment tools: let us move beyond simple pain ratings. *Curr Opin Anaesthesiol.* 2015;28:565-569. https://doi.org/10.1097/ACO.0000000000000225
7. Morone NE, Weiner DK. Pain as the fifth vital sign: exposing the vital need for pain education. *Clin Ther.* 2013;35:1728-1732. https://doi.org/10.1016/j.clinthera.2013.10.001
8. Scher C, Meador L, Van Cleave JH, Reid MC. Moving beyond pain as the fifth vital sign and patient satisfaction scores to improve pain care in the 21st century. *Pain Manag Nurs.* 2018;19:125-129. https://doi.org/10.1016/j.pmn.2017.10.010
9. Physical Therapy in Pain Management. n.d. Accessed October 25, 2020. https://www.practicalpainmanagement.com/treatments/rehabilitation/physical-therapy/physical-therapy-pain-management
10. Chimenti RL, Frey-Law LA, Sluka KA. A mechanism-based approach to physical therapist management of pain. *Phys Ther.* 2018;98:302-314. https://doi.org/10.1093/ptj/pzy030
11. Tolba R. *Nonsteroidal anti-inflammatory drugs (NSAIDs). Treatment of Chronic Pain Conditions: A Comprehensive Handbook.* Springer New York; 2017:77-79. https://doi.org/10.1007/978-1-4939-6976-0_21
12. Chang CY, Challa CK, Shah J, Eloy JD. Gabapentin in acute postoperative pain management. *Biomed Res Int.* 2014;2014:631756. https://doi.org/10.1155/2014/631756
13. See S, Ginzburg R. Choosing a skeletal muscle relaxant. *Am Fam Physician.* 2008;78(3):365-370.
14. Barakat A, Hamdy MM, Elbadr MM. Uses of fluoxetine in nociceptive pain management: a literature overview. *Eur J Pharmacol.* 2018;829:12-25. https://doi.org/10.1016/j.ejphar.2018.03.042
15. Sobieraj DM, Martinez BK, Miao B, et al. Comparative effectiveness of analgesics to reduce acute pain in the prehospital setting. *Prehosp Emerg Care.* 2020;24:163-174. https://doi.org/10.1080/10903127.2019.1657213
16. Pathan H, Williams J. Basic opioid pharmacology: an update. *Br J Pain.* 2012;6:11-16. https://doi.org/10.1177/2049463712438493
17. Shipton EA, Shipton EE, Shipton AJ. A review of the opioid epidemic: what do we do about it? *Pain Ther.* 2018;7:23-36. https://doi.org/10.1007/s40122-018-0096-7
18. Miotto K, Cho AK, Khalil MA, Blanco K, Sasaki JD, Rawson R. Trends in tramadol. *Anesth Analg.* 2017;124:44-51. https://doi.org/10.1213/ANE.0000000000001683
19. Trends in the Use of Methadone, Buprenorphine, and Extended-release Naltrexone at Substance Abuse Treatment Facilities: 2003-2015 (Update). n.d. Accessed October 25, 2020. https://www.samhsa.gov/data/sites/default/files/report_3192/ShortReport-3192.html

48

Nursing Considerations and Authorized Agent-Controlled Analgesia

Taylor L. Powell, Erica V. Chemtob, Elyse M. Cornett, and Alan David Kaye

Introduction

Since 1971, patients have been using authorized agent-controlled analgesia (AACA) to maximize pain treatment, with the first commercially marketed AACA pump emerging in 1976. AACA's objective is to efficiently give pain relief at a patient's desired dose and schedule by enabling them to give a set bolus dosage of medicine on-demand with the push of a button. Each bolus can be provided alone or in conjunction with a continuous drug infusion. Agent-controlled analgesia is used to manage acute and chronic pain, and postoperative and labor pain. These drugs can be injected intravenously, epidurally, or transdermally using a peripheral nerve catheter. Opioids and local anesthetics are frequently used; however, dissociative agents or other analgesics may also be used. Agent-controlled analgesia more successful than nonpatient opioid injections at controlling pain and to result in improved patient satisfaction.[1]

Nurses are responsible for peripheral intravenous line installation, ACAA pump setup, medicine injection into the pumps, and monitoring of the patient's pain, sedation, and breathing. They verify that the pump is operating properly and that the drugs are being administered in the most effective manner possible while preventing difficulties and minimizing adverse effects.

While ACAA can alleviate the requirement for rounding and responding to patient demands for analgesic administration, it does not alleviate their burden; this is due to the time and effort required to educate the patient, set up the machine, and evaluate its effectiveness and adverse effects. However, it has been demonstrated that this is the preferred way since nurses and patients alike have greater control over their job and suffering.[1]

Indications and Contraindications

Authorized agent-controlled analgesia may be an option for individuals with acute, chronic, postoperative, or labor pain, particularly those who are unable to accept oral drugs. AACA can be utilized to alleviate the strain on nursing staff and patients associated with adhering to a set dose schedule of as-needed analgesics that may not effectively correspond to the patient's fluctuating pain. AACA may be beneficial in the acute pain context when the first opioid dose administered in the emergency room is insufficient to manage pain, and continuous opioid dosage has been shown to enhance patient outcomes. Vasoocclusive pain crises, trauma, pancreatitis, and burns are all common instances. AACA would be used in conjunction with other therapies to alleviate pain while the underlying cause is identified and addressed. Patients with chronic conditions who have less consistent chronic pain may potentially benefit from AACA. Metastatic malignancy, phantom limb syndrome, and complicated regional pain syndrome are the most prevalent instances. AACA is also an excellent option for postsurgical patients, particularly those with indwelling nerve or epidural catheters. The capacity of a postoperative patient to titrate and give their own pain medication enables greater pain management compared to scheduled nurse doses. Additionally, it improves patient satisfaction and reduces the need for PACU and acute pain treatment staff intervention. Patients experiencing labor discomfort are also well-suited for epidural AACA. Contracture pain, which is worsened by induction drugs such as oxytocin, can be sufficiently minimized and regulated by the patient.[1] Contraindications are listed in Table 48.1.

There are many aspects to the concept of ACAA and, by extension, AACA (Fig. 48.1). However, ethical and legal considerations have become prevalent due to cases where the patient self-administering the medication is too young to comprehend the action or the patient without the capacity to self-administer the medication.[2] In many states, family nurse practitioners have "prescriptive authority," and the intent of treatment along with who is authorized to administer the treatment must be clearly defined.[3] The authorization of who will administer the treatment to the patient must be determined to minimize any unintentional risk to the patient. Administration methods include the patient themselves (patient-controlled analgesia or ACAA), authorized agent-controlled analgesia (an authorized caregiver or health care worker who has been educated in the risks and methods), or if the drugs are administered by someone not informed on the risks and methods ("ACAA by proxy"). "ACAA by proxy" is not supported by the American Society for Pain Management Nursing (ASPMN), as it is unsafe and increases the risk of harm to the patient.[2] For drug administration to be considered AACA and not "ACAA by proxy," the responsibility of education lies on nursing staff to "authorize" and educate caregivers of the methods and risks of drug administration.[4] The ASPMN determines that AACA is an acceptable option for the relief of pain. AACA is an umbrella term that encompasses both nurse-controlled analgesia and caregiver-controlled analgesia. While the benefits of AACA/ACAA are clear (such as patient autonomy, lower health care cost, and a decreased hospital stay), the candidate must be chosen appropriately to mitigate any risks to the patient.[1,3] AACA has been proven to be safe and effective method for pain management in patients from children to adults.[2] Candidates for ACAA and those who will be involved in AACA must understand the relationship between pain, pressing (activating) the analgesic delivery, and be clear on the goal of pain relief.[2] Additionally, drugs should be carefully

TABLE 48.1 CONTRAINDICATIONS OF PATIENT-CONTROLLED ANALGESIA LEGAL AND ETHICAL CONSIDERATIONS

Absolute Contraindications of AACA	Relative Contraindications of AACA
The patient does not comprehend the notion of AACA	Chronic renal insufficiency
Illnesses throughout the body as a whole or infections at the chosen location of AACA installation	The patient is now receiving antithrombotic treatment
Allergic responses to the medicine chosen	The patient is known to have a bleeding condition
Burns or damage to the region where the AACA was placed	Sleep apnea
Neurological impairments preexisting in the location of a proposed indwelling nerve catheter	
Increased intracranial pressure (ICP) with epidural catheter insertion	

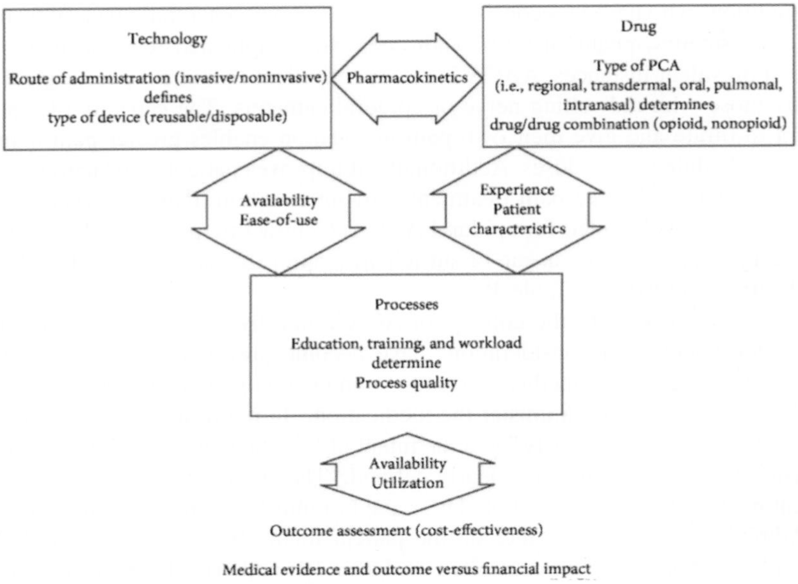

FIGURE 48.1 ACAA schematic.

considered, such as considering antiemetics or adding long-acting local anesthetics in combination with opioids.[4] The risk of including opioids is not just the physical manifestation (respiratory depression) but also must be viewed through the scope of the opioid crisis.[4] Therefore, researchers are currently evaluating nonopioid drug options to use in AACA and ACAA, but currently, opioids are still in use in decreased quantities or in combination with nonopioid analgesics.[4] As AACA and ACAA positively impact patient satisfaction, opioids are preferred due to the time of onset.[4]

Ethical Support for the Use of AACA

The Code of Ethics for Nurses states that nurses must not only provide but advocate for humane and appropriate patient care to either help restore the patient's health or provide supportive care at the end of life. AACA has the potential to have a "double effect," whereas the treatment that is being utilized to relieve suffering and provide comfort may also unintentionally cause death. Ethically and legally, the provider is not at fault for unintentional death as the intention of the treatment was to relieve the pain experienced by the patient.[2] To ensure ethical and legal administration of medications for pain management, the Joint Commission on the Accreditation of Health Care Organizations (JCAHO) issued an alert in 2004, validating the humane practice of ACAA and declaring the dangers of ACAA by prox. However, the response negatively impacted AACA via the elimination of identifying authorized agents. JCAHO states that this was not the intention of the alert and was seen as a loss of a viable method of pain management by the ASPMN.[4]

Practice Recommendations

Indications: ACAA can be used to treat acute, chronic, postoperative, and labor pain. The clinical practice guidelines from the American Pain Society and the American Society of Anesthesiologists strongly recommend the use of patient-controlled analgesia (ACAA) for postoperative pain when the parental route is required.[5] Their recommendations state that

TABLE 48.2 STANDARD ACAA PARAMETERS

Drug	Loading Dose	Bolus Dose	Lockout Interval	Continuous Infusion[a]
Morphine	3 mg	1-2 mg	10 min	<0.5 mg/h
Fentanyl	20 μg	10-50 μg	10 min	<50 μg/h
Hydromorphone	0.3 mg	0.2 mg	10 min	<0.4 mg/h

[a]Continuous (basal) infusion not recommended in opioid-naive adults or in older adults.
Adapted from: Momeni M, Crucitti M, De Kock M. Patient-controlled analgesia in the management of postoperative pain. *Drugs*. 2006;66(18):2321-2337; Craft J. Patient-controlled analgesia: is it worth the painful prescribing process? *Proc Bayl Univ Med Cent*. 2010;23(4):434-438; Hutchison RW, Anastassopoulos K, Vallow S, et al. Intravenous patient-controlled analgesia pump and reservoir logistics: results from a multicenter questionnaire. *Hosp Pharm*. 2007;42(11):1036-1044. Ref.[10-12]

ACAA is appropriate for patients 6 years of age and older who require analgesia for more than a few hours and have the cognitive function to understand and use the device. ACAA may also be used in an acute pain setting like the emergency department, in which patients require continual opioid dosing such as those with trauma or burns.[6] Patients with chronic illness, such as metastatic cancer, can also benefit from ACAA.[7]

Medications used: Opioids and local anesthetics are most used, including morphine, hydromorphone, and fentanyl.

Route: The pain medications can be given intravenously, transdermally, through a peripheral nerve catheter, or epidurally.[8] Opioids can be used alone via IV ACAA or in addition to local anesthetics given via epidural catheter ACAA.

Assessments: A preprocedure cognitive assessment should be performed to ensure that the patient has the cognitive function to understand and use the ACAA. Pain assessments, usually conducted by nursing staff, are done periodically during medication administration to assess the degree of pain management achieved. A sedation assessment is important to prevent excess sedative effects and overdose.[9]

Pump setup: An initial loading dose is typically given to achieve the minimum effective concentration of the pain medication. To maintain the MCA, a continuous (basal) infusion rate can be given in addition to the ACAA; however, it is not recommended in opioid-naive adults or older adults. A bolus (demand) dose is given when the patient presses the button. To avoid overdosing, a lockout interval ensures a specified amount of time has lapsed between each dose.[10] Time limits of 1 or 4 hours can limit the total amount of medication administered, providing additional safety to prevent overdosing. See Table 48.2.

Conclusion

ACAA is indicated for the management of acute, chronic, postoperative, and labor pain. The American Pain Society and the American Society of Anesthesiologists' clinical practice recommendations both highly urge the use of patient-controlled analgesia (ACAA) for postoperative pain when the parental route is necessary. Opioids and topical anesthetics, such as morphine, hydromorphone, and fentanyl, are the most often utilized medications. Intravenously, transdermally, through a peripheral nerve catheter, or epidurally, pain medicines may be administered. A cognitive examination should be conducted before to the surgery to verify that the patient has the cognitive ability to comprehend and utilize the ACAA. Pain evaluations, which are often undertaken by nursing professionals, are performed frequently during drug delivery to determine the degree of pain control achieved. Nurses should follow the patient closely and often for the first 24-48 hours, assessing pain and sedative levels every 1-2 hours, since the patient is most at risk of hypoventilation and nocturnal hypoxemia during this period. Agent controlled analgesia is an effective method of managing acute, chronic, postoperative, and labor pain. It does, however, need the formation of a competent interprofessional health care team composed of a physician, pharmacist, nurse, and patient. It is critical to educate health care team members on the various routes, drugs, dosage regimens, problems, pre- and postprocedure evaluations, side effects, and anticipated results associated with these procedures.

REFERENCES

1. Pastino A, Lakra A. Patient controlled analgesia. In: *StatPearls* [Internet]. StatPearls Publishing; 2021. http://www.ncbi.nlm.nih.gov/books/NBK551610/
2. Wuhrman E, Cooney MF, Dunwoody CJ, et al. Authorized and Unauthorized ("PCA by Proxy") Dosing of Analgesic Infusion Pumps: position statement with clinical practice recommendations. *Pain Manag Nurs*. 2007;8(1):4-11.
3. *APRN's Role in Ethical Prescribing Duquesne University* [Internet]. Duquesne University School of Nursing; 2018. https://onlinenursing.duq.edu/blog/aprns-role-responsibility-ethical-prescribing/
4. Nardi-Hiebl S, Eberhart LHJ, Gehling M, Koch T, Schlesinger T, Kranke P. Quo Vadis PCA? A review on current concepts, economic considerations, patient-related aspects, and future development with respect to patient-controlled analgesia. *Anesthesiol Res Pract*. 2020;2020:9201967.
5. Chou R, Gordon DB, de Leon-Casasola OA, et al. Management of postoperative pain: a clinical practice guideline from the American Pain Society, the American Society of Regional Anesthesia and Pain Medicine, and the American Society of Anesthesiologists' Committee on Regional Anesthesia, Executive Committee, and Administrative Council. *J Pain*. 2016;17(2):131-157.
6. Grass JA. Patient-controlled analgesia. *Anesth Analg*. 2005;101(5 Suppl):S44-S61.
7. Pastino A, Lakra A. Patient controlled analgesia. In: *StatPearls* [Internet]. StatPearls Publishing; 2021. http://www.ncbi.nlm.nih.gov/books/NBK551610/
8. Aguirre J, Del Moral A, Cobo I, Borgeat A, Blumenthal S. The role of continuous peripheral nerve blocks. *Anesthesiol Res Pract*. 2012;2012:560879.
9. Overdyk FJ, Carter R, Maddox RR, Callura J, Herrin AE, Henriquez C. Continuous oximetry/capnometry monitoring reveals frequent desaturation and bradypnea during patient-controlled analgesia. *Anesth Analg*. 2007;105(2):412-418.
10. Momeni M, Crucitti M, De Kock M. Patient-controlled analgesia in the management of postoperative pain. *Drugs*. 2006;66(18):2321-2337.
11. Craft J. Patient-controlled analgesia: is it worth the painful prescribing process? *Proc Bayl Univ Med Cent*. 2010;23(4):434-438.
12. Hutchison RW, Anastassopoulos K, Vallow S, et al. Intravenous patient-controlled analgesia pump and reservoir logistics: results from a multicenter questionnaire. *Hosp Pharm*. 2007;42(11):1036-1044.

49

Physical Therapy and Rehabilitative Medicine

Hannah W. Haddad, Linh T. Nguyen, Randi E. Domingue, Elyse M. Cornett, and Alan David Kaye

Introduction

Pain affects nearly everyone and is a major contributor to disability, morbidity, mortality, quality of life, and health care costs. The increase in pain prevalence has been attributed to numerous factors, including an aging population, rise in obesity, life-saving treatments in traumatic injuries, and improved surgical and medical treatments. With the prevalence of pain and the increasing incidence of chronic pain, it is essential to develop treatment plans that prevent the progression of acute to chronic pain.[1] Current treatment options for pain include oral medications, rehabilitative measures, procedural options, and finally, surgical procedures.[2] Pharmacologic interventions provide only temporary relief and lead to undesirable side effects.[3] In the case of opioid use, the risks can be subsequent substance abuse or addiction. Injections, nerve blocks, tissue ablations, spinal cord stimulators, and pain pumps are some procedural options for pain. Surgery is often the last resort for uncontrolled pain but is costly and may not provide expected results.[2]

In the acute stage of pain, rehabilitative medicine is implemented with the goals of controlling pain, restoring functionality to maintain productivity, and preventing the development of chronic pain. Common interventions include physical therapy (PT) and exercise, spinal manipulation, cognitive-behavioral therapy, meditation, acupuncture therapy, and massage therapy.[4] PT and rehabilitation have been used for the treatment of lower back pain, joint pain, neck pain, and headaches, which are some of the most common types of pain in the United States. PT and rehabilitative medicine are safe and efficacious treatment options that should be considered and incorporated into the treatment plan for managing pain.[3]

This chapter, therefore, reviews epidemiology, etiology, risk factors, and pathophysiology of pain. It also discusses efficacy of rehabilitative medicine for acute pain and reviews effects of these treatment options on the necessity of opioid use for pain control.

Etiology Epidemiology Risk Factors Pathophysiology

Epidemiology

Acute pain is one of the most common reasons why individuals seek rehabilitative care, often through PT.[5] This can be attributed to the considerable prevalence of those suffering from acute pain symptoms. Because pain is an individual, subjective experience influenced by many factors, its exact prevalence is particularly challenging to quantify. Self-reported patient surveys have been utilized to try and define pain epidemiologically. One such study in the United States documented that 126.1 million (55.7%) adults reported some pain when surveyed.[5] Additionally, pain trends among Americans have shown an increase of 10% (representing 10.5 million adults) from 2002 to 2018.[5]

Musculoskeletal pain disorders impart the largest influence on the need for rehabilitative medicine worldwide. An estimated 1.71 billion individuals across the globe suffer from musculoskeletal pain. Roughly 79% of PT in America addresses musculoskeletal pain syndromes (MPS).[6] Musculoskeletal pain encompasses a wide variety of pathologies. Frequently treated pain regions include the spine, hip, knee, and shoulder.[7] Common musculoskeletal pain disorders managed in a clinical setting are summarized in Table 49.1. Other acute pain conditions regularly managed with musculoskeletal rehabilitation include amputations, sprains, strains, joint dislocations, tears, and fractures.[5]

TABLE 49.1 LIST OF COMMON LOCALIZED MUSCULOSKELETAL PAIN DISORDERS BY ANATOMIC REGION

Head and neck			
Nonspecific neck pain		Temporomandibular disorder	
Muscle contraction headache		Cervical radiculopathy	
Torticollis		Thoracic outlet syndrome	
Thorax			
Costochondritis		Xiphodynia	
Lower rib pain syndromes		Tietze syndrome	
Upper limb			
Carpel tunnel syndrome	Rotator cuff pathology	Subacromial bursitis	Epicondylitis
Deltoid tendinopathy	Bicipital tendinopathy	Olecranon bursitis	Dupuytren contracture
Adhesive capsulitis	Cubital tunnel syndrome	Stenosing tenosynovitis	
Lower limb			
Prepatellar bursitis	Patellofemoral pain syndrome	Achilles tendinopathy	Tarsal tunnel syndrome
Iliotibial band syndrome	Shin splints	Plantar fasciitis	Morton neuroma
Baker cyst	Pes anserine bursitis	Metatarsalgia	Osgood-Schlatter disease
Hip and back			
Piriformis syndrome	Trochanteric bursitis	Iliopectineal bursitis	
Meralgia paresthetica	Ischial bursitis	Nonspecific low back pain	
Other			
Osteoarthritis		Fibromyalgia	
Rheumatoid arthritis		Myofascial pain syndrome	

From Cieza A, Causey K, Kamenov K, Hanson SW, Chatterji S, Vos T. Global estimates of the need for rehabilitation based on the Global Burden of Disease study 2019: a systematic analysis for the Global Burden of Disease Study 2019. *Lancet*. 2020;396(10267):2006-2017, Ref.[8]

Etiology

Several factors are hypothesized to contribute to the growth of acute musculoskeletal pain requiring rehabilitation. The current focus on increased involvement in physical activity has consequentially led to an increase in MPS. These exercise-related pain conditions are often a result of overuse or accidental injury.[9] The expansion of desk jobs and increased office screen time has also led to a greater incidence of musculoskeletal pain, particularly of the upper extremity. Prolonged desk and computer work have been linked to neck, wrist, and back pain as well as carpal tunnel syndrome.[10] Increased and excessive mobile phone usage has similarly been associated with higher rates of neck and upper back pain.[11] Furthermore, the increased average lifespan has led to more elderly individuals seeking rehabilitation for MPS associated with degenerative change.[12]

Risk Factors

Multidisciplinary rehabilitative medicine aims to address both the primary drivers in acute pain, anatomical or physiological pathology, as well as other contributing psychological risk factors.[13] Workplace environment and occupation present a potential biomechanical risk, as prolonged sitting, repetitive movements, awkward posturing, and excessive use of force have been indicated as workplace hazards that contribute to acute musculoskeletal pain.[14] Physical activity and participation in sports is a commonly associated risk factor for biomechanical injury resulting in acute pain.[15] Surgery frequently causes postoperative pain and stands as a risk factor for both acute and chronic pain.[16] Other common risk factors of acute pain disorders treated with rehabilitative medicine include obesity, pregnancy, childbirth, rheumatic disease, fibromyalgia, and cancer.[17]

The influence of psychological factors such as depression, stress, anxiety, fear, and catastrophizing are a factor in intensifying and prolonging pain.[18] Additionally, few studies have implicated psychosocial difficulties and adverse health behaviors in adolescents as a risk for developing musculoskeletal pain in adulthood. These risky behaviors include externalizing symptoms (poor impulse control, noncompliance, aggression), internalizing symptoms (anxiety, sadness, social withdrawal), smoking, alcohol use, and physical inactivity.[18] Emerging evidence shows that a strong therapeutic alliance between patient and practitioner may help mediate negative psychological symptoms and improve pain outcomes during rehabilitation.[19]

Pathophysiology

Musculoskeletal disorders encompass degenerative and inflammatory pathologies, which often exert adverse impacts on a variety of biological functions resulting in acute pain. Commonly, these disorders lead to reduced mobility, productivity, social interaction, and overall quality of life. Inadequately managed acute pain may induce pathophysiologic neural adaptations promoting progression to chronic pain. Here, we briefly discuss the hypothesized pathogenesis of a syndrome, highly implicated in MPS, regularly treated with musculoskeletal rehabilitation.

An estimated 30%-93% of musculoskeletal pain is reportedly of myofascial origin resulting in a collective disorder known as myofascial pain syndrome. The exact pathogenesis of myofascial pain syndrome is still unknown; however, a theory exists based on the effects of abnormal accumulation of acetylcholine at motor endplates. This accumulation is said to cause persistent muscle contraction, which disturbs the balance of available local energy resulting in local ischemia. Consequential increased expression of nociceptive mediators, such as substance P and calcitonin gene–related peptides, promote pain hypersensitivity. The resultant central excitability of neurons can be managed through a number of different rehabilitative treatments discussed later in more detail.[20]

Physical Therapy and Rehab for Acute Pain

Rehabilitation is a branch of medicine devoted to restoring health and regaining function. Rehabilitative medicine often encompasses many branches of health care through practice by an interdisciplinary team of medical professionals, including a physiatrist, neurologists, psychologists, physical therapists, occupational therapists, and speech pathologists. This branch of medicine offers targeted interventions that alleviate acute and chronic musculoskeletal pain and optimize quality of life. Rehabilitative strategies can be described by the following categories: manipulation of pain perception, stabilization of painful structures, modulation of nociceptive pathways, and reduction of soft tissue pain. The integration of rehabilitative strategies into pain management via a multidisciplinary and comprehensive approach may allow for more effective treatment of acute pain conditions.[12]

Physiatry

Physical medicine and rehabilitation (PMR), a multifaceted field, includes a subspecialized focus in pain management. Physiatrists, physicians who practice PMR, diagnose and manage acute pain disorders of the musculoskeletal and neurological system through interventional pain procedures, analgesic medications, physical therapies, and promoting integrative rehabilitation. Physiatrists are experts trained to lead the integrated, multidisciplinary rehabilitative team working to restore health and regain function in the patient.[21]

A well-organized rehabilitative program orchestrated by physiatrists delivers improved patient outcomes with speedier recoveries and decreased costs. Evidence indicates a physiatric consultation in the acute phase of low back pain significantly reduces the rate of surgical intervention and improves cost-effectiveness. Additionally, when integrated with the emergency department treating back pain, physiatrists have been linked to greater detection and diagnosis of critical conditions and significantly fewer returns to the emergency department. PMR provides an intermediary step that offers a holistic view of pain management and emphasizes the significance of shared decision-making during rehabilitation.[21]

Physical Therapy

Patients with acute or chronic pain often fear that movement and exercise will result in reinjury or exacerbation of injury and consequently worsen their pain. However, this is not always the case. PT, a division of rehabilitation that routinely incorporates physical movement, has shown to be successful in managing various types of pain and should be considered as part of a comprehensive treatment plan for acute pain management.

A pertinent goal of PT is to minimize disability, distress, and suffering through alleviating pain symptoms and increasing tolerance to movement. Some of the modalities utilized by physical therapists to modulate pain include exercise therapy, manual therapy, ultrasound, short-wave diathermy, transcutaneous electrical nerve stimulation, and neurostimulation techniques. A novel approach to identifying the most effective modality of PT to implement is based upon the identification of a patient's mechanistic category of pain. The five pain mechanisms recognized in this mechanistic-based approach include nociceptive, neuropathic, nociplastic, psychosocial, and motor. The implicated pain mechanism is determined through self-reported patient history, questionnaires, and quantitative sensory testing. The assessment of pain mechanisms by a physical therapist supports individualized patient care and offers precision medicine to those suffering from pain.[22]

Exercise and Manual Rehabilitative Therapies

Exercise and manual therapy are two of the most employed PT treatment modalities. Here, we briefly discuss the mechanism behind the clinical benefit seen from these therapies. Table 49.2 provides summaries of evidence from the literature on both modalities.

Exercise therapy has shown to be effective when treating pain derived from all five pain mechanisms.[22] Many proposed theories on how therapeutic exercise influences pain exist. Recent studies have documented that exercise diminishes nociceptor excitability through the reduction of ion channel expression and amplified release of anti-inflammatory cytokine interleukin-10 along with endogenous analgesic elements 57 (59-61). Exercise has also shown to reduce the central excitability implicated in nociplastic pain through mechanistic stimulation of descending inhibitory systems and expression of endogenous opioids.[27] Animal studies have indicated that regular exercise training can improve neuropathic pain by modulating the serotoninergic system, promoting nerve and tissue healing, and inducing analgesia through increased expression of anti-inflammatory markers such as interleukin-4 and M2 macrophages. Furthermore, improvement of many factors implicated in psychosocial pain (catastrophizing, depression, anxiety) is a well-established benefit of regular physical activity.[5]

Manual therapy encompasses techniques such as soft tissue massage, muscle manipulation, joint mobilization, and stretching. These techniques have been shown to promote the expression of anti-inflammatory mediators, reduce proinflammatory elements, stimulate the endogenous analgesic system, and promote tissue repair. The clinical benefit of manual therapies' mechanistic action has been documented as pain relief, improved function, and increased range of motion in various musculoskeletal pain disorders.[27]

Conclusion

It is estimated that 126 million Americans experience some level of pain in a year, and the prevalence continues to increase due to the aging population, obesity, and improved medical and surgical treatment. Pain has major effects on physical well-being, in addition to psychological and social impacts. In the United States alone, each year ~$560-$635 billion is lost because of chronic pain. This includes the cost of treatment as well as the loss of income due to interference with productivity and work. Aside from the economic burden, pain has been associated with inability or impairment to carry out activities of daily living, decreased quality of life, and increased suicide risk. Hence, it becomes important that acute pain is promptly controlled to prevent development of chronic pain and its additional effects on an individual.

Because of the heterogeneity of pain, development of a treatment plan for patients must be customized to meet individual needs. The current multimodal approach for pain management involves use of pharmacological, nonpharmacological, and surgical procedures. A large push for nonpharmacological options has emerged in response to the opioid crisis, ineffective procedures, and surgeries. These options include PT and rehabilitative medicine, which encompasses spinal manipulation, acupuncture, cognitive-behavioral therapy, meditation, and massage therapy. These methods have shown to be safe, efficacious, cost-effective, and reduce the need for opioid use when treating pain. Overall, PT and rehabilitation techniques should be used in conjunction with pharmacological options for pain control, and the methods implemented must tailor to the individual's needs.

TABLE 49.2 **SYSTEMATIC REVIEWS AND META-ANALYSES ON EXERCISE AND MANUAL THERAPY FOR ACUTE PAIN CONDITIONS**

First Author and Year	Objective	Database and Search Periods	No. of Included Studies and Inclusion Criteria	Key Findings	Conclusions
Haik et al. (2016)[23]	To evaluate the evidence on the efficacy of PT on pain, function, and ROM in those with subacromial pain syndrome	PubMed, Web of Science, CINAHL, Cochrane, EMBASE, LILACS, IBECS, SCIELO Inception—April 2015	64 **Study design**: RCTs and quasi-RCTs **Population**: males and females ≥ 18 years diagnosed with subacromial pain syndrome via imaging, a + painful arc, Neer, Hawkins, or Jobe test, or pain with shoulder external rotation **Intervention**: all types of active or passive PT interventions **Comparisons**: no intervention, sham, placebo, other PT modalities, or surgical intervention **Outcomes**: ≥1 of pain, function/disability, ROM	ET displayed strong evidence of effectiveness, equal to surgical intervention and superior to placebo, for improving pain, function, and ROM short- and long-term. The combination of JM and ET displayed high evidence for reducing pain and increasing function short-term. Limited evidence exists for benefits effects of isolated MT, diathermy, and TENS. Moderate to high level of evidence was concluded on lack of benefit of low-level laser, ultrasound, and taping.	ET should be the first-line therapy to improve pain, function, and ROM. Combination of JM and ET may expedite clinical benefits short-term. Low-level laser therapy, ultrasound therapy, and taping cannot be recommended based on findings.
Steuri et al. (2017)[24]	To evaluate the efficacy of conservative management for pain, function, and ROM in those with shoulder impingement	MEDLINE, CENTRAL, CINAHL, EMBASE, PEDro Inception—January 2017	200 **Study design**: RCTs **Population:** males and females ≥ 18 years with shoulder impingement diagnosed via imaging or meeting ≥1 diagnostic criteria of "complaints of shoulder pain" **Intervention**: ≥1 conservative intervention **Comparison:** any other intervention **Outcomes**: pain, function, ROM	Pain findings: ET was better than nonexercise control groups (SMD –0.94, 95% CI –1.69 to –0.19). Specific exercises were better than generic exercises (SMD –0.65, 95% CI –0.99 to –0.32). MT was better than placebo (SMD –0.35, 95% CI –0.69 to –0.01). ET + MT was better than isolated ET in the short-term (SMD –0.32, 95% CI –0.62 to –0.01).	ET should be considered for shoulder impingement. MT may be beneficial to add.

Hidalgo et al. (2017)[25]	To evaluate the evidence for different methods of MT and ET for those with nonspecific neck pain	MEDLINE, Cochrane-Register-of-Controlled-Trials, PEDro, EMBASE January 2000 to December 2015	23 **Study design:** RCTs **Population:** males and females 18-60 years with grade I or II acute (<6 weeks), subacute (6-12 weeks), or chronic (>12 weeks) neck pain localized to the posterior neck between the superior nuchal line and the spinous process of the 1st thoracic vertebra **Intervention:** ≥1 of the 4 categories of MT: MT1 = spinal manipulation with HVLA; MT2 = low-velocity mobilization, MET, soft tissue techniques; MT3 = combination of MT1 and MT2; MT4 = MWM with cervical SNAGs **Comparison:** no treatment, placebo, or other usual conservative treatment for neck pain **Outcomes**: pain, function, QoL	Acute/subacute pain findings: MT1 + ET to the cervical spine resulted in significant improvement of pain ($P < .005$, SMD > 2), disability ($P < .05$, SMD > 1), and QoL ($P < .005$; SMD of 1.14). Simple and comprehensive MT2 to the trapezius muscle showed significant improvements in pain, function, and side-bending when compared to baseline. A significant difference in pain ($P < .001$, SMD of 0.96) and disability ($P < .001$, SMD of 1.11) was seen between MT3 + ET vs MT2 + ET to the cervical and thoracic spine in favor of MT3 + ET. MT2 + ET, MT4 +ET, and isolated ET improved pain and disability over 4 weeks compared to baseline with no significant difference between groups.	The study concludes that combining various forms of MT with ET is better than MT or ET alone and that manipulation does not need to be at the symptomatic level(s) for improvement of neck pain.
Østerås et al. (2017)[26]	To evaluate the efficacy of ET compared with other interventions in those with hand OA	Cochrane Central Register of Controlled Trials, MEDLINE, EMBASE, CINAHL, PEDro, OTseeker Inception—September 2015	7 **Study design**: RCTs **Population:** males or females >18 years with physician-diagnosed OA **Intervention:** ≥ 1 ET defined as treatments targeting muscle strength, joint mobility, and joint stability **Comparison:** no exercise, different exercise programs **Outcomes**: hand pain, hand function, QoL, radiographic joint change, finger joint stiffness	ET improved hand pain (5 trials, SMD −0.27, 95% CI −0.47 to −0.07), hand function (4 trials, SMD −0.28, 95% CI −0.58 to 0.02), and finger joint stiffness (4 trials, SMD −0.36, 95% CI −0.58 to −0.15) when compared to no ET. QoL was assessed in 1 study (113 participants) which provided the effect of ET on QoL was uncertain (SMD 0.30, 95% CI −3.72 to 4.32).	This study presented low-quality evidence from five studies with low risk of bias supporting ET was moderately beneficial for hand pain, function, and finger joint stiffness.

(Continued)

TABLE 49.2 **SYSTEMATIC REVIEWS AND META-ANALYSES ON EXERCISE AND MANUAL THERAPY FOR ACUTE PAIN CONDITIONS (*Continued*)**

First Author and Year	Objective	Database and Search Periods	No. of Included Studies and Inclusion Criteria	Key Findings	Conclusions
Fredin et al. (2017)[27]	To evaluate if combined treatment with MT and ET is more effective than MT or ET alone in relieving pain and improving function in those with grade I-II neck pain	EMBASE, MEDLINE, AMED, CENTRAL, PEDro Inception—June 2017	7 **Study design**: RCTs **Population**: males and females >18 years with grade I or II neck pain without known underlying pathology **Intervention:** combination of ≥1 MT with ≥1 ET **Comparison**: isolated MT or ET **Outcomes:** pain intensity +/– neck disability	No significant differences were found between the ET only and ET + MT groups on pain intensity at rest, neck disability, and QoL at any time within 12 months posttreatment. Moderate-quality evidence was reported for pain-at-rest outcomes, and low-moderate quality evidence was reported for neck disability and QoL.	This study concludes that joint treatment of ET with MT does not appear to be more effective than ET alone in improving neck pain intensity, neck disability, or QoL in adults with neck pain.
Weerasekara et al. (2018)[28]	To evaluate the benefits of JM for ankle sprains	MEDLINE, MEDLINE In-Process, EMBASE, AMED, PsycINFO, CINAHL, Cochrane Library, PEDro, Scopus, SPORTDiscus, and Dissertations and Theses Inception—June 2017	23 **Study design:** RCTs, cross-over studies, cross-sectional studies, cohort studies, case series **Population:** males and females of any age with grade I or II acute or chronic lateral or medial ankle sprains treated with JM **Intervention**: JM to talocrural, subtalar, or inferior talofibular joint by a therapist **Comparison**: any conservative intervention (ET, elevating, icing, strapping), sham, or no intervention **Primary outcomes:** pain, ankle ROM, QoL, function	Significant immediate benefit of JM compared to other conservative treatments on improving posteromedial dynamic balance ($P = .0004$); no significant difference for short-term improvement on dorsiflexion range ($P = .16$), static balance ($P = .96$), or pain intensity ($P = .45$). JM improved weight-bearing dorsiflexion range ($P = .003$) compared with a control in the short-term.	JM may be beneficial for improving dynamic balance and dorsiflexion range in the short-term. JM does not seem to be superior to other conservative measures on pain management.

Eckenrode et al. (2018)[29]	To evaluate the efficacy of isolated or adjunctive MT, compared to standard treatment or sham for improving pain self-reported function in those with patellofemoral pain	PubMed, Ovid, Cochrane Central Register of Controlled Trials, CINAHL Inception—August 2017	9 **Study design:** RCTs with >10 participants and <20% drop-out **Population**: patients of any age or gender with a diagnosis of anterior knee pain or patellofemoral pain without other knee pathologies **Intervention:** ≥1 type of MT directed to the patellofemoral joint, LE, or lumbosacral joint used alone or adjunct to other PT treatment **Comparison:** standard treatment or sham intervention **Outcomes**: pain +/– self-reported functional questionnaire	MT in the knee region showed short-term improvement in self-reported function and pain when compared to a control or sham intervention. The effects were only clinically meaningful for pain. Based on three studies, evidence of pain improvement by lumbopelvic MT was inconclusive.	This study concludes that MT may be beneficial in reducing patellofemoral pain short-term. Improvement of self-reported function from MT was significant but not clinically meaningful.
Karlsson et al. (2020)[30]	Systematic review of systematic reviews on the effect of exercise therapy on acute low back pain	PubMed, the Cochrane library, CINAHL, PEDro, Open Grey, Web of Science, PROSPERO Inception—September 2019	24 systematic reviews with 21 RCTs on acute populations **Study design:** systematic reviews of RCTs **Population:** males and females 18-65 years with acute nonspecific low pain **Intervention:** interventions classified as ET used by physiotherapists **Comparisons**: placebo, sham, no treatment, usual care, minimal intervention, medication, other physical therapies **Outcomes**: pain, disability, recurrence, adverse effects	Pain findings: General ET: Low to moderate evidence shows general ET likely causes little to no relevant difference in pain when compared with any control treatments. Stabilization ET: Low to moderate evidence shows no relevant difference in posttreatment pain between stabilization ET and other ETs. McKenzie ET: Low to moderate evidence shows no relevant difference in pain between McKenzie ET vs usual care, spinal manipulation, educational guidance, and NSAIDs.	This study concluded that ET produces minimal difference in pain or disability in patients suffering from acute low back pain when compared with other treatments. Patient preference and practitioner capability should be considered when determining if ET should be implemented.

(Continued)

TABLE 49.2 SYSTEMATIC REVIEWS AND META-ANALYSES ON EXERCISE AND MANUAL THERAPY FOR ACUTE PAIN CONDITIONS (*Continued*)

First Author and Year	Objective	Database and Search Periods	No. of Included Studies and Inclusion Criteria	Key Findings	Conclusions
de Melo et al. (2020)[31]	To assess the efficacy of MT for the treatment of myofascial pain related to TMD	Cochrane Library, MEDLINE, Web of Science, Scopus, LILACS, SciELO	5 **Study design:** RCTs **Population:** patients of any age or gender with myofascial pain according to the Research Diagnostic Criteria for TMD **Intervention:** ≥1 MT (mobilization, soft tissue, stretching, massage, gentle isometric tension, or guided movement techniques) **Comparison:** control group with any other treatment (medication, PT, occlusal device) **Outcomes:** pain	Of the 279 patients evaluated, 156 individuals were treated with MT alone or MT + counseling, and the remaining 123 were considered a part of the control group (n = 15 botulinum toxin injection, n = 20 home PT, n = 31 no treatment, n = 57 counseling). High-quality evidence showed MT resulted in effective pain relief and improved mandibular function in all included studies. MT was not superior to educational counseling or botulinum toxin for pain relief in 2 of the 5 studies. No significant difference was seen between the counseling only and counseling + MT groups for pain relief.	Though MT was shown to be associated with improved pain relief, this study concludes that additional investigation is required before recommending MT as a treatment for TMD.

PT, physical therapy; ROM, range of motion; RCT, randomized control trial; ET, exercise therapy; MT, manual therapy; JM, joint mobilization; TENS, transcutaneous electrical nerve stimulation; SMD, standardized mean difference; CI, confidence interval; HVLA, high-velocity low-amplitude; MET, muscle energy technique; MWM, mobilization with movement; SNAG, sustained natural apophyseal glides; QoL, quality of life; OA, osteoarthritis; LE, lower extremity; NSAID, nonsteroidal anti-inflammatory drug; TMD, temporomandibular disorder.

REFERENCES

1. Institute of Medicine (US) Committee on Advancing Pain Research, Care, and Education. Pain as a public health challenge. In: *Relieving Pain in America: A Blueprint for Transforming Prevention, Care, Education, and Research* [Internet]. National Academies Press (US); 2011. https://www.ncbi.nlm.nih.gov/books/NBK92516/
2. Tick H, Nielsen A, Pelletier KR, et al. Evidence-based nonpharmacologic strategies for comprehensive pain care: the consortium pain task force white paper. *Explore (NY)*. 2018;14(3):177-211.
3. Nahin RL, Boineau R, Khalsa PS, Stussman BJ, Weber WJ. Evidence-based evaluation of complementary health approaches for pain management in the United States. *Mayo Clin Proc*. 2016;91(9):1292-1306.
4. Pergolizzi JV, LeQuang JA. Rehabilitation for low back pain: a narrative review for managing pain and improving function in acute and chronic conditions. *Pain Ther*. 2020;9(1):83-96.
5. Chimenti RL, Frey-Law LA, Sluka KA. A mechanism-based approach to physical therapist management of pain. *Phys Ther*. 2018;98(5):302-314.
6. Nahin RL. Estimates of pain prevalence and severity in adults: United States, 2012. *J Pain*. 2015;16(8):769-780.
7. Zajacova A, Grol-Prokopczyk H, Zimmer Z. Pain trends among American adults, 2002–2018: patterns, disparities, and correlates. *Demography*. 2021;58(2):711-738.
8. Cieza A, Causey K, Kamenov K, Hanson SW, Chatterji S, Vos T. Global estimates of the need for rehabilitation based on the Global Burden of Disease study 2019: a systematic analysis for the Global Burden of Disease Study 2019. *Lancet*. 2020;396(10267):2006-2017.
9. Tschopp M, Brunner F. Erkrankungen und Überlastungsschäden an der unteren Extremität bei Langstreckenläufern. *Z Für Rheumatol*. 2017;76(5):443-450.
10. Ye S, Jing Q, Wei C, Lu J. Risk factors of non-specific neck pain and low back pain in computer-using office workers in China: a cross-sectional study. *BMJ Open*. 2017;7(4):e014914.
11. Zirek E, Mustafaoglu R, Yasaci Z, Griffiths MD. A systematic review of musculoskeletal complaints, symptoms, and pathologies related to mobile phone usage. *Musculoskelet Sci Pract*. 2020;49:102196.
12. Briggs AM, Cross MJ, Hoy DG, et al. Musculoskeletal health conditions represent a global threat to healthy aging: a report for the 2015 World Health Organization World Report on Ageing and Health. *Gerontologist*. 2016;56(Suppl_2):S243-S255.
13. Marin TJ, Eerd DV, Irvin E, et al. Multidisciplinary biopsychosocial rehabilitation for subacute low back pain. *Cochrane Database Syst Rev*. 2017;6(6):CD002193. https://www.cochranelibrary.com/cdsr/doi/10.1002/14651858.CD002193.pub2/full
14. Nakatsuka K, Tsuboi Y, Okumura M, et al. Association between comprehensive workstation and neck and upper-limb pain among office worker. *J Occup Health*. 2021;63(1):e12194.
15. Igolnikov I, Gallagher RM, Hainline B. Chapter 39: Sport-related injury and pain classification. In: Hainline B, Stern RA, eds. *Handbook of Clinical Neurology*. Elsevier; 2018:423-430. https://www.sciencedirect.com/science/article/pii/B9780444639547000392
16. Rawal N. Current issues in postoperative pain management. *Eur J Anaesthesiol*. 2016;33:160-171. https://journals.lww.com/ejanaesthesiology/Fulltext/2016/03000/Current_issues_in_postoperative_pain_management.2.aspx
17. Torensma B, Oudejans L, van Velzen M, et al. Pain sensitivity and pain scoring in patients with morbid obesity. *Surg Obes Relat Dis*. 2017;13:788-795. https://www.clinicalkey.com/#!/content/playContent/1-s2.0-S1550728917300291?returnurl=https:%2F%2Flinkinghub.elsevier.com%2Fretrieve%2Fpii%2FS1550728917300291%3Fshowall%3Dtrue&referrer=
18. Michaelides A, Zis P. Depression, anxiety and acute pain: links and management challenges. *Postgrad Med*. 2019;131(7):438-444.
19. Kinney M, Seider J, Beaty AF, Coughlin K, Dyal M, Clewley D. The impact of therapeutic alliance in physical therapy for chronic musculoskeletal pain: a systematic review of the literature. *Physiother Theory Pract*. 2020;36(8):886-898.
20. Cao Q-W, Peng B-G, Wang L, et al. Expert consensus on the diagnosis and treatment of myofascial pain syndrome. *World J Clin Cases*. 2021;9(9):2077-2089.
21. Pavlinich M, Perret D, Rivers WE, et al. Physiatry, pain management, and the opioid crisis: a focus on function. *Am J Phys Med Rehabil*. 2018;97:856-860.
22. Gatchel RJ, Neblett R, Kishino N, Ray CT. Fear-avoidance beliefs and chronic pain. *J Orthop Sports Phys Ther*. 2016;46(2):38-43.
23. Haik MN, Alburquerque-Sendín F, Moreira RFC, et al. Effectiveness of physical therapy treatment of clearly defined subacromial pain: a systematic review of randomised controlled trials. *Br J Sports Med*. 2016;50:1124-1134.
24. Steuri R, Sattelmayer M, Elsig S, et al. Effectiveness of conservative interventions including exercise, manual therapy and medical management in adults with shoulder impingement: a systematic review and meta-analysis of RCTs. *Br J Sports Med*. 2017;51(18):1340-1347.

25. Hidalgo B, Hall T, Bossert J, Dugeny A, Cagnie B, Pitance L. The efficacy of manual therapy and exercise for treating non-specific neck pain: a systematic review. *J Back Musculoskelet Rehabil*. 2017;30:1149-1169.
26. Østerås N, Kjeken I, Smedslund G, et al. Exercise for hand osteoarthritis: a Cochrane systematic review. *J Rheumatol*. 2017;44:1850-1858.
27. Fredin K, Lorås H. Manual therapy, exercise therapy or combined treatment in the management of adult neck pain—A systematic review and meta-analysis. *Musculoskelet Sci Pract*. 2017;31:62-71. doi:10.1016/j.msksp.2017.07.005
28. Weerasekara I, Osmotherly P, Snodgrass S, Marquez J, de Zoete R, Rivett DA. Clinical benefits of joint mobilization on ankle sprains: a systematic review and meta-analysis. *Arch Phys Med Rehabil*. 2018;99(7):1395-1412.e5.
29. Eckenrode BJ, Kietrys DM, Parrott JS. Effectiveness of manual therapy for pain and self-reported function in individuals with patellofemoral pain: systematic review and meta-analysis. *J Orthop Sports Phys Ther*. 2018;48:358-371.
30. Karlsson M, Bergenheim A, Larsson MEH, Nordeman L, van Tulder M, Bernhardsson S. Effects of exercise therapy in patients with acute low back pain: a systematic review of systematic reviews. *Syst Rev*. 2020;9(1):182.
31. de Melo LA, Bezerra de Medeiros AK, Trindade Pinto Campos M De F, et al. Manual therapy in the treatment of myofascial pain related to temporomandibular disorders: a systematic review. *J Oral Facial Pain Headache*. 2020;34:141-148.

50

Enhanced Recovery Pathways (ERAS) and Regional Anesthesia

Simrat Kaur, Bryant W. Tran, Marissa Webber, Melissa Chao, and Anis Dizdarevic

History of Enhanced Recovery After Surgery

Enhanced recovery after surgery (ERAS) is a multimodal, multidisciplinary evidence-based perioperative care approach developed to improve recovery of patients undergoing major surgery. Dr Henrik Kehlet, a Danish colorectal surgeon, studying perioperative practices to decrease length of stay and improve outcomes after surgery, hypothesized that multimodal interventions may lead to a major reduction in the undesirable sequelae of surgical stress injury with accelerated recovery and reduction in postoperative morbidity and overall costs.[1,2] In 2001, a group of European academic surgeons, led by Ken Fearon and Olle Ljungqvist, founded an ERAS Study Group. The group aimed to develop a multimodal surgical care pathway, based on literature evidence, in order to improve quality of practice and reduce complications at their respective academic centers. The ERAS Society was officially established in 2010 in Sweden to promote and share ERAS research, improve practice protocols, expand education around perioperative care, and assist with implementation and program auditing. The Society has since hosted many symposia and facilitated the first implementation programs in Swedish medical institutions, followed by those in Switzerland, Canada, the United States, and Spain. As of 2016, implementation programs and the ERAS Interactive Audit System have further extended to France, Germany, Norway, Portugal, the Netherlands, the United Kingdom, Mexico, Brazil, Colombia, Argentina, Singapore, the Philippines, New Zealand, Israel, Uruguay, and South Africa.[3]

Components of ERAS and Goals

Enhanced recovery after surgery protocols involve comprehensive multimodal perioperative care pathways aimed at attenuating the surgical stress response and reducing end-organ dysfunction through integrated perioperative pathways. The various components of the ERAS protocol are grouped according to the timing of intervention into preoperative, intraoperative, and postoperative.[4] The key elements include counseling and nutritional strategies, including fluid and carbohydrate loading and avoidance of prolonged fasting, standardized anesthetic and analgesic regimens utilizing multimodal and regional therapies, perioperative fluid balance and normothermia maintenance, early mobilization and nutrition postoperatively and appropriate thromboprophylaxis. Details of the ERAS protocols are carefully designed based upon the specific surgical procedure that is being performed and are usually derived from high-quality published literature.

Optimizing nutrition status with correction of baseline nutritional deficiencies are critical components of ERAS protocols as poor nutrition status is detrimental to postoperative outcomes. Proper management can avoid hyperglycemia and attenuate postoperative insulin resistance, reduce protein loss, and improve muscle function as well as reduce complications such as hospital length of stay and cost.[5] The intraoperative regimens employ short-acting anesthetic agents with epidural, regional, and nonopioid pain management techniques, where appropriate. Additional components include avoidance of fluid or salt overload, prevention of nausea and vomiting, early removal of indwelling catheters, avoidance of drain placement, appropriate use of antibiotic prophylaxis and thromboprophylaxis, and maintenance of normothermia with the use of fluid warmers and body warming devices. The goals of these approaches include optimizing analgesia and recovery to mitigate ongoing nociceptive-induced stress responses while allowing early mobilization in the recovery unit and beyond, return of bowel function, and prevention of prolonged postoperative ileus.

Preoperative Patient Education, Preparation/Conditioning

Patient education plays an important role in optimizing the postsurgical outcome. Patients should be informed about the stress and deconditioning associated with surgery. ERAS protocols encourage an active role in preparation and conditioning.[6] Sleep hygiene, exercise, and preoperative carbohydrate loading have demonstrated benefits, and if patients are educated about the benefit of these modalities, they are more likely to participate in their care and outcome of surgery. In regard to these interventions, carbohydrate loading decreases preoperative nausea, perioperative insulin resistance, and hospital length of stay.[6] Smoking cessation for 4-6 weeks prior to surgery decreases airway reactivity and secretions. Smoking cessation also decreases complications such as wound infections leading to prolonged hospitalization or readmission.[6] Alcohol abuse is also associated with complications and a longer length of hospital stay.[6] Thus, alcohol cessation interventions should be utilized prior to elective surgery. Patients should also receive education in regard to postoperative rehabilitation and steps they will need to take in order to resume their presurgical activity level. If a patient's anesthetic includes regional anesthesia, they should be educated about the benefits and potential complications associated with it. Occasionally, when a patient receives continuous regional anesthesia, they might be sent home with a peripheral nerve catheter, which can potentially result in complications such as catheter dislodgement and infection if not cared for properly. Furthermore, patients should be educated about expectations in regard to pain control associated with the nerve catheters. All of these questions and concerns can be addressed at the initial preoperative visit to adequately prepare patients to actively participate in their care.

Preoperative Optimization of Patient's Medical Condition

Along with patient education, a patient's past medical history is important. Several chronic medical conditions are associated with poor perioperative outcomes if not optimized prior to surgery. Examples include poorly controlled diabetes, hypertension, unstable angina, heart failure, chronic obstructive pulmonary disease, anemia, kidney, or liver disease. Hyperglycemia is associated with poor wound healing and perioperative insulin resistance, and hypertension can significantly increase risk for stroke. Severe chronic obstructive pulmonary disease can lead to prolonged mechanical ventilation. Kidney and liver dysfunction can negatively impact the metabolism of several medications administered in the perioperative period. Thus, a surgical candidate's history can guide any further testing or interventions that are required for optimization. Examples of testing and interventions include a transthoracic echocardiogram, stress test, heart catheterization, or pulmonary function tests. While these options are available prior to elective surgery, a patient may present in emergent circumstances that do not allow for optimization.

Furthermore, a patient's past medical history can preclude them from a certain type of anesthesia. Patients with severe aortic stenosis scheduled for total knee arthroplasty tend to receive general anesthesia rather than spinal anesthesia due to risks of more profound loss of sympathetic tone and cardiac output associated with spinal anesthesia. On the contrary, patient with end-stage renal disease scheduled for arteriovenous fistula repair may benefit from regional anesthesia as it has shown to improve outcomes due to improved fistula patency and reduced failure rates.[7] It has been hypothesized that the improved fistula patency may be due to vasodilation secondary to the sympathectomy caused by regional anesthetics.[7] Thus, gathering patients' past medical history in regard to the type of surgery they are having opens conversations about what may be the most beneficial anesthetic in their situation.

Preoperative Pain Optimization and Anxiety Reduction

Mental and emotional preparation is the next step. Oftentimes, the process of undergoing surgery is anxiety-provoking. This may be more noticeable in patients with preexisting anxiety and chronic pain. Some of these patients may have had prior poor experiences with health care providers and may also have other comorbid conditions such as substance abuse. If these issues are not addressed preoperatively, it can lead to delayed discharge, poorly controlled pain, and readmissions.[8] A tailored preoperative visit provides patients with stress coping mechanisms, education about expected pain with surgery, and postoperative pain management strategies. These strategies help set real expectations of pain associated with surgery, what measures can be taken to address it, and informs the patient that they will not be completely pain free with these interventions, but the goal is to treat the pain to a tolerable level. Patients should also be educated about adverse effects of opioids and consequences of opioid dependence and addiction. If patients have substance use disorders, they can be scheduled with an addiction medicine clinic to prescribe medications such as methadone and buprenorphine, which may reduce risk of opioid withdrawal. These medications should be continued while the patient is hospitalized to treat their baseline level of pain, and additional pain medications should be scheduled for surgical pain. Preexisting anxiety or depression increases the risk for postoperative pain.[8] Thus, it is imperative that these conditions get screened and adequately treated prior to elective surgery. Hospital Anxiety and Depression Scale is a questionnaire that can be used during the preoperative visit to screen for psychological disorders that may benefit from nonpharmacologic therapy such as mindfulness and cognitive behavioral therapy.[8] Overall, a thoughtful and directed preoperative visit provides patients with additional resources prior to surgery and positively impacts both postoperative recovery as well as long-term wellness.

Preoperative Fasting Time Reduction and Optimization

Preoperative fasting guidelines were developed in order to reduce the risk of pulmonary aspiration, complications associated with aspiration, the severity and extent of hypoglycemia, and improve patient comfort and satisfaction. Guidelines focus on determining adequate time required for fasting and to utilize pharmacologic agents known to decrease gastric volume and acidity when indicated. Current guidelines require waiting 2 hours after ingestion of clear

TABLE 50.1 PHARMACOLOGIC AGENTS USED FOR ASPIRATION PROPHYLAXIS

Drug	Route	Onset	Duration	Effect
Cimetidine	PO, IV	1-2 h	4-8 h	Decrease acidity and volume
Ranitidine	PO, IV	1-2 h	10-12 h	Decrease acidity and volume
Famotidine	PO, IV	1-2 h	10-12 h	Decrease acidity and volume
Nonparticulate antacids	PO	5-10 min	30-60 min	Decrease acidity, increase volume
Metoclopramide	PO, IV	1-3 min	1-2 h	No effect on acidity, decrease volume

From Butterworth JF, Wasnick JD, Mackey DC. In: Malley J, Naglieri C, eds. *Clinical Anesthesiology*. 6th ed. McGraw-Hill Education; 2018.

liquids prior to sedation that can impair upper airway protective reflexes. Guidelines require 4 hours after breast milk ingestion, 6 hours after full liquids, nonhuman milk, infant formula and light meals, and 8 hours after heavy meals. Several studies have been performed to determine these guidelines.[9] No increased benefit was found when fasting for 2 hours after ingesting clear liquids vs 4 hours, but study participants had increased thirst and hunger with 4 hours of fasting.[9] Agents used to aid in decreasing gastric volume and/or pH include dopamine antagonists, histamine antagonists, proton pump inhibitors, and antacids. Current recommendations indicate that these agents should not be routinely administered but can be given if a patient has risk factors for aspiration.[9] It is important to understand the pharmacokinetics of these agents as summarized in Table 50.1, to ensure they are administered well in advance of the scheduled procedure to have the desired effect. Pulmonary aspiration can result in aspiration pneumonia, respiratory compromise, and significant morbidity and mortality for the patient. Thus, it is very important to preoperatively evaluate the patient and adequately prepare for a successful outcome. It is important to recognize which patients have a higher likelihood of developing aspiration based on their comorbidities such as ascites, diabetes, GERD, hiatal hernia, and ileus. These patients in particular need to be educated about their risk of aspiration and steps they can take to help minimize this risk.

Metabolic Response to Surgical Stress

Surgery results in a stress response, which leads to several hormonal and metabolic changes. These hormonal changes are summarized in Table 50.2. Important hormonal changes include high levels of cortisol, insulin resistance, high vasopressin, and low thyroid hormones.[10] Cortisol causes protein catabolism and lipolysis leading to gluconeogenesis.[10] However, glucose is unable to be utilized in these conditions, leading to hyperglycemia and poor wound healing. This stress response activates the HPA axis, which now, no longer has negative feedback mechanisms.[10] High levels of cortisol are not able to suppress release of ACTH, further exacerbating the injury. Other changes include activation of the sympathetic nervous system leading to catecholamine release resulting in tachycardia and hypertension. This can have profound consequences for patients with ischemic heart disease. Sympathetic output also results in increased renin release leading to sodium and water retention, which can be problematic for patients with volume overload.[10] Thus, the surgical stress response can have adverse effects on wound healing and lead to higher postoperative morbidity and mortality. This is where anesthesia plays a huge role. Several anesthetic modalities can help modify this surgical stress response. Regional anesthesia techniques such as paravertebral blocks have resulted in decreased stress response during mastectomy for breast cancer. Their use results in better pain control resulting in less opioid consumption.[11]

TABLE 50.2 HORMONE RESPONSES TO SURGERY

Hormone	Change in Secretion
ACTH	Increases
GH	Increases
TSH	May increase or decrease
FSH and LH	May increase or decrease
AVP	Increases
Cortisol	Increases
Aldosterone	Increases
Insulin	Decreases
Glucagon	Increases
Thyroxine, triiodothyronine	Decrease

ACTH, adrenocorticotropic hormone; GH, growth hormone; TSH, thyroid-stimulating hormone; FSH, follicle-stimulating hormone; LH, luteinizing hormone; AVP, arginine vasopressin.
From Desborough JP. The stress response to trauma and surgery. *Br J Anaesth*. 2000;85(1):109-117. doi:10.1093/bja/85.1.109

Perioperative Anesthetic Management

Anesthesia can help reduce some aspects of the surgical stress response. First, anesthesiologists determine what type of anesthesia will be the most beneficial for their patient. While regional anesthesia is useful for several surgeries including shoulder replacement, open reduction and internal fixation of several long bones, and open abdominal surgeries, its use is contraindicated in patients with local infections, severe coagulopathy, local anesthetic allergy, and patient refusal. In these instances, general anesthesia may provide a better alternative.

The next step involves determining an effective analgesic plan for the patient. Traditionally, opioids were used to help attenuate the sympathetic stimulation associated with the perception of pain. However, ongoing research demonstrated multiple adverse effects of opioids including postoperative respiratory depression, depressed consciousness, delirium, intestinal hypomotility, and ileus. This led to the development of multimodal analgesia using lidocaine, dexmedetomidine, ketamine, regional nerve blocks, and epidural analgesia in order to reduce opioid use, while still adequately treating the patient's pain. Lidocaine infusions have been studied in burn patients to reduce the inflammatory response associated with the burns and with surgery as well.[12] It acts on sodium receptors to alter cerebral perception of pain, acts peripherally on muscarinic and glycine receptors, which enhances the production of endogenous opioids, and reduces production of thromboxane limiting the inflammatory cascade.[12] Several of the commonly employed IV and PO pain medications can be found in Table 50.3. ERAS protocol utilized for pediatric laparoscopic colorectal surgery resulted in reduced perioperative opioid usage without worsening pain scores, faster return of bowel function, shorter hospital stays, and lower rates of 30 days hospital readmissions.[14]

Peripheral nerve catheters function by local anesthetic deposition either perineurally or in a muscle plane containing distal branches of nerves. Some of the most commonly employed peripheral nerve blocks include interscalene, supraclavicular, infraclavicular, femoral, popliteal, saphenous, and transversus abdominis plane blocks. These are summarized in Table 50.4. Their mechanism of action is sodium channel blockade, preventing nerve signal propagation. These nerve blocks can be utilized in surgery localized to a specific area providing analgesia both

TABLE 50.3 COMMON NONOPIOID PAIN MEDICATIONS USED IN ERAS PROTOCOLS

Analgesic Agent	Route of Administration	Mechanism of Action
Lidocaine	IV, SQ	Block sodium channels
Ketamine	IV, IM	NMDA antagonist
Dexmedetomidine	IV	Alpha-2-agonist
Acetaminophen	PO, IV, rectal	Mechanism of action unclear, some activity as a cyclo-oxygenase inhibitor
NSAIDs	PO, IV	Cyclo-oxygenase inhibitors
Gabapentinoids	PO	Calcium channel blockers
SSRIs	PO	Selective serotonin reuptake inhibitors

From Beverly A, Kaye AD, Ljungqvist O, et al. Essential elements of multimodal analgesia in enhanced recovery after surgery (ERAS) guidelines. *Anesthesiol Clin*. 2017;35(2):115-143. doi:10.1016/j.anclin.2017.01.018. Ref.[13]

intraoperatively and postoperatively. Epidural catheters function by local anesthetic or opioid deposition in the epidural space. Local anesthetic acts by blocking sodium channels at the spinal nerve. Opioids act at the mu receptor of the spinal cord. These catheters also promote both intra and postoperative analgesia allowing early mobilization, enhanced respiratory mechanics reducing atelectasis, and pneumonia. Patients undergoing liver resection surgery under the ERAS pathway with epidural analgesia had significant reductions in morphine equivalent requirements at 24 hours, 48 hours, and 72 hours postoperatively.[15] Peripheral nerve blocks allow us to target the area of concern without causing systemic side effects associated with opioids. Nerve and epidural catheters can be placed in anticipation of painful surgery such as large open abdominal surgery or joint replacement surgery. These procedures help decrease the use of opioids for several days while the catheter is in place. Often the first week after

TABLE 50.4 COMMONLY USED PERIPHERAL NERVE BLOCKS

Interscalene block	• Blocks brachial plexus nerve roots • Used for shoulder and upper arm surgery
Supraclavicular block	• Blocks brachial plexus at the level of divisions • Used for elbow or below the elbow surgery
Paravertebral block	• Blocks spinal nerves • Used for sternotomy, thoracotomy, breast surgery, and various surgeries involving the thorax or abdomen
Transversus abdominis plane block	• Blocks intercostal, subcostal, iliohypogastric, and ilioinguinal nerves • Used for open abdominal surgery
Adductor canal block	• Blocks saphenous and vastus medialis nerve • Used for knee or below the knee surgery covering the medial aspect of the lower leg
Popliteal block	• Blocks common peroneal and tibial nerves • Used for below the knee surgery

From Butterworth JF, Wasnick JD, Mackey DC. In: Malley J, Naglieri C, eds. *Clinical Anesthesiology*. 6th ed. McGraw-Hill Education; 2018.

TABLE 50.5 COMMONLY USED PONV PROPHYLACTIC AGENTS

Agent	Route of Administration	Mechanism of Action
Ondansetron	IV, PO	5-HT_3 receptor antagonists
Dexamethasone	IV, PO	Unclear
Prochlorperazine	IV, IM, PO, rectal	D_2 receptor antagonists
Scopolamine	Transdermal	Muscarinic receptor antagonist
Aprepitant	IV, PO	NK-1 receptor antagonist
Propofol	IV	Unclear

From Butterworth JF, Wasnick JD, Mackey DC. In: Malley J, Naglieri C, eds. *Clinical Anesthesiology*. 6th ed. McGraw-Hill Education; 2018.

surgery is the most painful period, and nerve blocks and epidurals help significantly during this time.

Other important factors to consider are maintenance of normothermia and prevention of postoperative nausea and vomiting (PONV). General anesthesia induces a decrease of 1-2 °C during phase one in the first hour, followed by a gradual decrease in phase two over the next 3-4 hours, reaching a steady state during phase three.[16] Hypothermia has multiple adverse effects including cardiac arrhythmias, increased peripheral vascular resistance, left shift of oxyhemoglobin curve, coagulopathy, altered mental status, impaired drug metabolism, impaired wound healing, and increased risk of infection.[16] Thus, it is imperative to employ mechanisms to maintain normothermia intraoperatively. PONV delays early nutritional intake and causes significant discomfort, and the risk should be minimized with adequate prophylaxis. Several agents can be utilized depending on patient risk factors. These agents are demonstrated in Table 50.5. Risk factors for PONV include young age, female gender, nonsmoker, history of PONV, ocular or gynecologic surgeries, and surgery lasting more than 30 minutes. If a patient has moderate risk, 1-2 interventions should be utilized for prophylaxis, and if a patient has high risk, more than 2 interventions should be utilized.[16]

Postoperative Management—Analgesia, Early Oral Intake, Mobilization

Postoperatively, several factors need to be addressed to prepare for timely discharge and avoid complications related to prolonged hospitalization such as infection and deconditioning. As discussed above, multimodal pain management strategies should be employed to reduce opioid use and opioid-related complications such as respiratory depression and opioid dependence. Use of multimodal pain medications allows targeting of multiple different receptors involved in the pain pathways, all working synergistically together to improve pain relief. Equally important is early nutritional intake. This prevents insulin resistance, reduces nitrogen loss, and decreases loss of muscle tissue. Early mobilization is also paramount to promote deep breathing exercises preventing atelectasis and associated infection, strengthen muscle tissue, and promote physical rehabilitation in order to safely discharge home in a timely manner.

Evidence has shown that peripheral nerve blocks do not impede early mobilization and thus should be incorporated into ERAS protocols whenever possible. When comparing general anesthesia vs regional anesthesia, patients had a lower rate of falls in the regional anesthesia group.[17]

TABLE 50.6 ERAS INTERVENTIONS THAT CAN IMPROVE SURGICAL OUTCOMES

Preoperative	• Patient education • Optimization of patient's medical conditions • Pain and anxiety reduction • Smoking and alcohol cessation • Carbohydrate loading and fasting
Intraoperative	• Minimally invasive surgery • Use of regional anesthesia when possible • Use of multimodal analgesics • Maintaining normothermia • PONV prophylaxis • Maintaining euvolemia
Postoperative	• Early mobilization • Early nutrition • Use of multimodal analgesics • DVT prophylaxis • Timely removal of catheters and drains

From Butterworth JF, Wasnick JD, Mackey DC. In: Malley J, Naglieri C, eds. *Clinical Anesthesiology*. 6th ed. McGraw-Hill Education; 2018.

Conclusion

In conclusion, the preoperative assessment is the most important tool to adequately prepare patients for elective surgery. Educating patients allows them the opportunity to be involved in their care and be their own advocate. It takes several steps to ensure a patient has the best outcome possible after surgery, and it all starts with a well done preoperative evaluation. Specifically in regard to regional anesthesia, oftentimes patients are awake during the regional anesthesia procedure and expectations should be set ahead of time. Table 50.6 summarizes the ERAS interventions that can improve surgical outcomes.

In conclusion, regional anesthesia has been noted to decrease intraoperative and postoperative opioid consumption, optimal pain management, and improved patient satisfaction. Thus, it should be employed whenever possible along with several ERAS interventions that have shown to improve surgical outcomes.

REFERENCES

1. Kehlet H. Multimodal approach to control postoperative pathophysiology and rehabilitation. *Br J Anaesth*. 1997;78(5):606-617. doi:10.1093/bja/78.5.606
2. Kehlet H, Mogensen T. Hospital stay of 2 days after open sigmoidectomy with a multimodal rehabilitation programme. *Br J Surg*. 1999;86(2):227-230. doi:10.1046/j.1365-2168.1999.01023.x
3. Tanious MK, Ljungqvist O, Urman RD. Enhanced recovery after surgery: history, evolution, guidelines, and future directions. *Int Anesthesiol Clin*. 2017;55(4):1-11. doi:10.1097/AIA.0000000000000167
4. Varadhan KK, Lobo DN, Ljungqvist O. Enhanced recovery after surgery: the future of improving surgical care. *Crit Care Clin*. 2010;26(3):527-547.
5. Melnyk M, Casey RG, Black P, et al. Enhanced recovery after surgery (ERAS) protocols: time to change practice? *Can Urol Assoc J*. 2011;5(5):342-348. doi:10.5489/cuaj.11002
6. Wainwright TW, Gill M, McDonald DA, et al. Consensus statement for perioperative care in total hip replacement and total knee replacement surgery: enhanced recovery after surgery (ERAS) society recommendations. *Acta Orthop*. 2019;91(1):3-19. doi:10.1080/17453674.2019.1683790
7. Jorgensen MS, Farres H, James BLW, et al. The role of regional versus general anesthesia on arteriovenous fistula and graft outcomes: a single-institution experience and literature review. *Ann Vasc Surg*. 2020;62:287-294. doi:10.1016/j.avsg.2019.05.016
8. Doan LV, Blitz J. Preoperative assessment and management of patients with pain and anxiety disorders. *Curr Anesthesiol Rep*. 2020;10(1):28-34. doi:10.1007/s40140-020-00367-9

9. Abe K, Adelhoj B, Andersson H, et al. Practice guidelines for preoperative fasting and the use of pharmacologic agents to reduce the risk of pulmonary aspiration: application to healthy patients undergoing elective procedures. *Anesthesiology*. 2017;126(3):376-393. doi:10.1097/ALN.0000000000001452
10. Desborough JP. The stress response to trauma and surgery. *Br J Anaesth*. 2000;85(1):109-117. doi:10.1093/bja/85.1.109
11. Sessler DI, Pei L, Huang Y, et al. Recurrence of breast cancer after regional or general anaesthesia: a randomised controlled trial. *Lancet*. 2019;394(10211):1807-1815. doi:10.1016/S0140-6736(19)32313-X
12. Abdelrahman I, Steinvall I, Elmasry M, et al. Lidocaine infusion has a 25% opioid-sparing effect on background pain after burns: a prospective, randomised, double-blind, controlled trial. *Burns*. 2020;46(2):465-471. doi:10.1016/j.burns.2019.08.010
13. Beverly A, Kaye AD, Ljungqvist O, et al. Essential elements of multimodal analgesia in enhanced recovery after surgery (ERAS) guidelines. *Anesthesiol Clin*. 2017;35(2):115-143. doi:10.1016/j.anclin.2017.01.018
14. Edney JC, Lam H, Raval MV, et al. Implementation of an enhanced recovery program in pediatric laparoscopic colorectal patients does not worsen analgesia despite reduced perioperative opioids: a retrospective, matched, non-inferiority study. *Reg Anesth Pain Med*. 2019;44(1):123-129. doi:10.1136/rapm-2018-000017
15. Grant MC, Sommer PM, He C, et al. Preserved analgesia with reduction in opioids through the use of an acute pain protocol in enhanced recovery after surgery for open hepatectomy. *Reg Anesth Pain Med*. 2017;42(4):451-457. doi:10.1097/AAP0000000000000615
16. Butterworth JF, Wasnick JD, Mackey DC. In: Malley J, Naglieri C, eds. *Clinical Anesthesiology*. 6th ed. McGraw-Hill Education; 2018.
17. Memtsoudis SG, Danninger T, Rasul R, et al. Inpatient falls after total knee arthroplasty: the role of anesthesia type and peripheral nerve blocks. *Anesthesiology*. 2014;120(3):551-563. doi:10.1097/ALN.0000000000000120

51

Quality and Safety Considerations in Acute Pain Management

John N. Cefalu and Brett L. Arron

Introduction

Pain is an individual experience that must be translated into quantifiable terms that clinicians can use to assess and direct medical care to safely ameliorate. Adverse consequences of acute pain increase physiologic stress, are associated with adverse cardiovascular outcomes, and limit patients' capability to cooperate in their postoperative recovery and rehabilitation. Treatment is directed at diminishing the perception of pain while, in balance, minimizing the potential adverse consequences of effective medical care. Following a review of assessment modalities to measure therapeutic success, strategic approaches to pain management are considered.

Defining Patient Safety and Quality of Care

The University of California at San Francisco-Stanford University Evidence-Based Practice Center has previously defined patient safety as "those that reduce the risk of adverse events related to exposure to medical care across a range of diagnoses or conditions."[1] This definition emphasized the importance of reducing harm in patients to provide safe care and have been demonstrated in current practices such as "Appropriate use of prophylaxis to prevent venous thromboembolism in patients at risk" and "Use of perioperative beta-blockers in appropriate patients to prevent perioperative morbidity and mortality."[1] The World Health Organization states that in order to achieve quality of care, "health care must be safe, effective, timely, efficient, equitable, and people-centered."[2]

Since 2000, safety and quality of care have been described as "indistinguishable" by the Institute of Medicine, and since this time, patient safety during delivery of health care has been gaining increasing momentum.[2] Evidence-based models of improved health care delivery and advancing information technology have significantly improved communication and delivery of safe and effective care among providers. One such model, the Donabedian model was developed to provide a framework for examining health services and evaluating quality in health care by drawing information about quality of care from three categories called structure, process, and outcomes.[3,4] While this has been useful in evaluating quality of care, the model does not account for patient, economic, or social factors.[3] Nonetheless, the Donabedian model has successfully been used for safety and quality of care assessment.

The field of acute pain management has seen exponential growth in advancement of treatment options for acute pain; however, pain continues to be poorly managed and quality and safety concerns still present health care providers with obstacles.

Management of Acute Pain

Effective pain management first begins with accurate assessment of the pain that the patient is experiencing. Only from here may a practitioner initiate strategies to alleviate the pain as well as assess the quality of the pain management. Inaccurate assessment of pain quality can lead to poor quality of pain control measures, increased risk of delirium, increased morbidity and mortality, prolonged hospital stay, and worsening patient satisfaction.

Several barriers exist to safe and effective pain management and are identified as system-related (lack of evidence-based and standardized pain management protocols, pain specialists, and pharmaceutical agents), staff-related (ineffective communication and lack of knowledge and skills), physician-related (lack of knowledge and false concerns about addiction and overdosing), patient-related barriers (reluctance to take analgesics, fear of side effects and addiction), and nursing-related barriers.[5,6] In addition, pain in itself is complex, multidimensional, and subjective in nature often requiring multidisciplinary approach to effective management.

Health care organizations are currently required to collect and review data regarding pain assessment and management while installing protocols to minimize risk associated with treatment options allowing for continual improvement in the safety and quality of acute pain management.[7]

Nurses play a pivotal role in the assessment of pain as they maintain the closest relationship with the patient within the hospital setting. In fact, nurses may play the most fundamental key role in safety and proper assessment in the acute pain setting. Some nurse-related barriers to effective pain management have been identified as inadequate knowledge, heavy workload, lack of time, and insufficient physician orders prior to procedures.[5,6,8]

Pain is multidimensional and subjective in nature. Pain assessment is challenging because the clinician must integrate relevant aspects of psychological, sensory, social, and cultural contributions to the patients' experiences. For nurses to comprehensively assess and implement the treatment plan, they must factor in patient reports of pain location, aggravating and alleviating factors, timing, duration, intensity, effectiveness of any previous pain treatment, and the effects of the patients' ability to cooperate with their rehabilitation plan. Frequency of assessment of acute pain should be standardized. This can vary greatly among institutions occurring as often as several times per hour in critical care units and to as little as once per shift within medical/surgical units.[9] It is important that timely pain reassessment be performed after each intervention to help guide treatment as some intermediate interventions may be inadequate. A uniform method of pain assessment is a foundation for quality improvement activities. An ideal program yields high sensitivity and specificity data, is automated for ease of use, and provides a useful feedback loop to the clinicians and hospital leadership. Acute pain assessment tools and programs do not translate to management of patients with chronic pain and vice versa as the source of acute pain is generally known and usually less complex to understand and manage.

A thorough, comprehensive pain history must be obtained and shared among team members who share patient care responsibilities for the patient experiencing acute pain. A thorough history of previous treatment plans, pharmacologic and nonpharmacologic modalities, and their effectiveness will help guide future treatment. The provider must understand the physical and psychosocial ramifications of the patients' acute pain experience, the patients' attitude towards opioid, anxiolytic, or other pain pharmaceutical agent used, the patients' coping response for the acute pain, and history of current psychological disorders. Finally, it is important that the clinician understand the patient and family's beliefs, knowledge of, and expectations regarding previous, current, and future treatment plans.[9]

The current gold standard for pain assessment remains direct patient feedback regardless of vital signs such as respiratory rate, blood pressure, and heart rate. Commonly used pain assessments for acute pain management include the Visual Analog Scale (VAS), Numeric Pain

TABLE 51.1 COMMON PAIN ASSESSMENT TOOLS

Common Pain Assessment Tools
Visual Analog Scale (VAS)
Numeric Pain Rating Scale (NPRS)
Verbal Rating Scale (VRS)
Faces Pain Scale Revised (FPS-R)
Wong-Baker FACES Scale
McGill Pain Questionnaire
Assessment in Advanced Dementia Scale (PAIN-AD)

Rating Scale (NPRS), Verbal Rating Scale (VRS), Faces Pain Scale Revised (FPS-R), Wong-Baker FACES scale, McGill Pain Questionnaire, and the Assessment in Advanced Dementia (PAIN-AD) scale and are discussed below (See Table 51.1).

Visual Analog Scale

The VAS is very similar to the NPRS as a measure of acute and chronic pain in which patients will select a measurement between a line drawn between 1 and 10 cm. A mark made at zero represents "no pain," while a mark made at 10 represents the "worst pain." The strength of this assessment is the ability to track pain measurements overtime similar to the NPRS. The VAS has shown to be the most common test utilized for rating endometriosis-related pain including dysmenorrhea, dyspareunia, and nonmenstrual chronic pelvic pain.[10] It has also demonstrated clinical importance in assessing skin graft site-related pain.[10] In addition, the Adamchic et al. VAS has also been used to assess loudness and annoyance of acute and chronic tinnitus.[11]

Numeric Pain Rating Scale

The NPRS is a commonly used pain scale and consists of a numeric version of the VAS. The NPRS is a subjective assessment in which the patient selects verbally or in writing a value of pain that he or she has experienced within the last 24 hours on a horizontal line showing an eleven-point scale from no pain at all (Score of 0) to the worst pain imaginable (Score of 10). The test is used for adults and children 10 years or older. Advantages include quick testing (<3 minutes to complete and score) and ability to be given verbally and in writing and that it can be used without translation between languages. Studies have shown that the NPRS has been found to be an accurate and reliable method of rating acute pain with high sensitivity in which data can be analyzed statistically.[12,13] It must be noted, however, that this method may only reliably rate pain intensity and does not take into account previous pain experiences or variations in pain intensity over time. In fact, the test may only average pain intensity experienced over the course of 24 hours.[12,13] With the use of the NPRS over the course of days to weeks, one can track a patient's progression in pain over time between health care providers allowing for better diagnoses and treatment and improving communication between providers.

Verbal Rating Scale

The VRS presents different adjectives to the patient to choose which best fits the pain intensity that the patient is currently experiencing. The adjectives are used to describe different levels of pain intensity in order from "no pain at all" to "extremely intense pain."[14] The benefit to having adjectives describe levels of pain intensity is thought to help patients and clinicians understand the nature of the acute or chronic pain in hopes of leading to a more effective treatment.

And while significantly different from VAS and NPRS, several studies have shown close correlation with these as well as other assessments of pain.[15,16] In addition, the VRS presents descriptors of pain intensity that are easy to interpret and can give researchers more information regarding the complex nature of the pain experienced by the patient. Although adjectives used can range anywhere from 4 to 15 descriptors and the list must be completely read prior to giving an answer, participants have shown to be compliant. The VRS has been found to be a reliable assessment of pain in cognitively intact and cognitively impaired geriatric population.[17]

Advantages to the VRS include quickness to administer and ease of interpretation. This assessment may be disadvantageous in that interpretation of the adjectives may be influenced by age, sex, education, and other psychological factors present within the patient prior to the assessment. In addition, patients with mental health history or poor vocabulary may lead to inaccurate pain assessment necessitating the use of demographic and clinical factors to adjust scores. Finally, the VRS has a limited number of adjectives that may not be sufficient for certain populations and, unlike the NPRS, may not be easily translatable across languages requiring adjustment.

Pictorial Pain Scales

Faces Pain Scale Revised (FPS-R) and Wong-Baker FACES Scale

Originally developed for the pediatric population, the FPS-R and Wong-Baker FACES scale are demonstrating increasing use in the adult and geriatric population.[18] The FPS-R utilizes particular facial expressions designated to particular pain scores from 0 (No pain) to 10 (Very much pain) in which the patient will choose the face they feel most likely related to their pain. It is adapted from the Faces Pain Scale (FPS) with scores added to the faces representing the sensation of pain perceived. Similarly, the Wong-Baker FACES scale uses a series of six faces ranging from a happy face (Score of 0 or no pain) to a crying face (Score of 10 or worst pain imaginable). Emotional facial expressions of pain provide the benefit of use in pediatrics and patients with cognitive dysfunction as they may not understand how to rate their pain on a linear scale. Research has demonstrated the FPS-R to be reliable assessments of pain in children and adults, but the WONG-Baker FACES scale's validity and reliability have been limited to children up to the age of 18.[19-21]

McGill Pain Questionnaire

Also known as the McGill Pain Index, the McGill Pain Questionnaire was developed in 1971 as a pain questionnaire that gives the provider a more explicit description of their pain as it consists of 78 words description of pain within 20 sections.[22] By doing this, the patients are able to give the provider a thorough description of their pain quality and intensity and attempt to answer the following questions[22]:

What does the pain feel like?
How does the pain change over time?
How strong is your pain?

The questionnaire consists of a pain rating index that is further divided into four sections of questions that represent different components of pain including sensory, affective, evaluative, and even a miscellaneous section.[22] Although this assessment may provide more descriptive and better understanding of the nature of the acute pain, the test can be lengthy and require up to 30 minutes to administer.[23] In addition, patients with limited vocabulary may have difficulty understanding the various descriptors that the questionnaire provides. However, one may resolve this issue by defining particular descriptors during the assessment.[23] Because pain had previously been assessed in terms of intensity, the McGill Pain Questionnaire brought attention to the qualitative aspect of pain. The MPQ proves to be a valid and reliable assessment of cancer pain.[24]

Almost a decade later, the short form of the MPQ (SF-MPQ) was developed in 1987 consisting of 15 descriptors related on an intensity scale of 0 = none, 1 = mild, 2 = moderate, or 3 = severe and was found to have high correlation with the original MPQ.[25,26] While the SF-MPQ had been developed for adults with chronic pain conditions, it was revised in 2009 for use in neuropathic and nonneuropathic pain conditions by adding symptoms of neuropathic pain and by changing the scale to a 0-10 numerical rating.[27] It was named the SF-MPQ-2 and has since been shown to be a valid and reliable test in acute pain conditions including acute low back pain.[28]

Assessment in Advanced Dementia (PAIN-AD) Scale

Assessing acute pain in patients with advanced dementia and delirium can present with extreme difficulty. Suboptimal acute pain management may lead to new or worsening delirium or even prolonged hospital stays.[29] For this reason, the Assessment in Advanced Dementia (PAIN-AD) scale was devised. Proper use of the PAIN-AD scale as part of a comprehensive pain management plan can help reduce the likelihood of a patient experiencing unrecognized and untreated pain.[30] The PAIN-AD can be used as this allows for scoring of the patient's behaviors on a scale of 0 to 2 that include breathing independent of vocalization, negative vocalization, facial expression, body language, and consolability. Scores of 1-3 represent mild pain, scores of 4-6 represent moderate pain, and scores of 7-10 represent severe pain.[31] Several studies demonstrate the validity and reliability of the PAIN-AD in patients unable to self-report due to cognitive impairment or advanced dementia.[32,33]

Quality Improvement in Acute Pain Management

The Joint Commission requires that health care organizations monitor acute pain management performances and implement quality improvement measures to ensure that both safety and high-quality care are met. In 1995, the American Pain Society (APS) produced the initial quality improvement guidelines that included the following[34]:

1. To recognize and treat pain promptly
2. Involve patients and families in pain management plan
3. Improve treatment patterns
4. Reassess and adjust pain management plan as needed
5. Monitor processes and outcomes of pain management

These guidelines were released to emphasize the importance of comprehensive patient assessment, preventive treatment, and prompt treatment. Further, these guidelines were based on evidence for the role that neuroplasticity has in patient recovery with an emphasis on customization of care, the participation of the patient in the treatment plan, elimination of inappropriate practices, and providing multimodal therapy. Finally, physicians should respond to pain intensity, functional status, and side effects and include new standardized quality improvement (QI) indicators and comments about forthcoming national performance indicators. These guidelines were later revised in 2005 by utilizing studies conducted on pain quality improvement.[34] Since then, the quality improvement guidelines have been further updated to include six quality indicators including the intensity of pain to be documented with a numeric or descriptive rating scale; pain intensity documented at frequent intervals; pain treated by a route other than intramuscular; pain treated with regularly administered analgesics, a multimodal approach used; pain to be prevented and controlled to a degree that facilitates function and quality of life; and that patients are adequately informed and knowledgeable about pain management.[35] The updated APS questionnaire is now known as the APS-POQ-R and could provide for valuable data needed for quality improvement in pain management in the hospital setting.

An effective health care institution might utilize a multidisciplinary approach to acute pain management with clearly defined protocols, safety measures, and data collection for quality improvement for various types of acute pain. This approach should involve clear communication between physicians, nurses, and other providers involved in the patient's care and the family. In addition, a system should be in place to monitor for poorly controlled pain management in order for future correction and continuous quality and safety improvement.

Safe Opioid Use

In 2017, 47 600 people died from opioid-related overdose. Overprescription of narcotics has continued to climb since the 1990s, yet patients still remain poorly educated on proper storage, use, and disposal at home.[36] Improper storage, use, and disposal of prescription opioids can lead to diversion and abuse as well as overdose. Health care providers involved in the care of the acute pain patient play a key role in facilitating the proper use of opioid analgesics, especially opioids in which the most safety issues have arisen such as morphine, hydromorphone, and fentanyl. Because of the safety issues with these opioids use in acute pain management, health care providers may be hesitant to administer sufficient doses out of fear of life-threatening respiratory depression and lead to ineffective pain management. Evidence-based clinical practice guidelines can help facilitate safe and effective decisions to prevent respiratory-related adverse events as well as assist in educating the practitioner in the acute pain setting.

It is known that opioid-induced respiratory depression (OIRD) varies among patients and is the result of a multitude of factors including pharmacogenetics, previous history of opioid use, and other agents that may provide additive or synergistic effects such as benzodiazepines. And because sedation precedes respiratory depression during opioid administration, monitoring sedation using sedation scales such as the Richmond Agitation and Sedation Scale (RASS) and the Pasero Opioid-Induced Sedation Scale (POSS) could provide valuable information regarding opioid-induced sedation and respiratory depression in opioid naïve and non-naïve patients experiencing moderate to severe pain. These scales provide nurses with the safe timing of opioid initiation, redosing, and whether a particular opioid should be stopped. Both the RASS and POSS have demonstrated reliability and validity for sedation monitoring during acute pain management.[37] Pasero et al. suggests using another scale, the Pasero-McCaffery scale that can be used to assess sedation and OIRD, and presents a scale from S (Sleep, easy to arouse) to 4 (Somnolent, minimal or no response to physical examination). For S, 1 (Awake and alert) and 2 (Slightly drowsy, easily aroused), supplemental opioid may be given. For 3 (Frequently drowsy, arousable, drifts off to sleep during conversation), this level of sedation is deemed unacceptable and it is recommended to decrease the opioid dose by 25%-50%, administer acetaminophen or nonsteroidal anti-inflammatory drugs (NSAIDs) if not contraindicated, and monitor sedation and respiratory status until sedation level is <3. At the level of 4, the opioid should be stopped, anesthesia provider notified, naloxone administered, acetaminophen or NSAID administered for pain control, and sedation and respiratory status monitored until less than level 3.[38] By using this scale, nurses may know when it is safe to administer more opioid, decrease the dose, or stop the opioid.

One problem that arises with opioid administration is lack of precise knowledge of individual patient onset, peak effects, and duration of action across a range of patient ages and disease states. Hydromorphone (Dilaudid), for example when given intravenous (IV), has an onset of 5 minutes with a peak analgesic effect between 10 and 20 minutes.[40] Compare these results to IV fentanyl that demonstrates an onset of ~60 seconds and a peak affect of around 2-5 minutes, and one may understand how particular orders placed by a patient's provider might overdose a patient without waiting for maximum peak effect prior to redosing.[41]

Capnography may be a great addition to sedation monitoring for OIRD as it allows for continuous observation of end tidal carbon dioxide (ETCO2) and respiratory rate. Continuous ETCO2 monitoring may allow nurses to detect respiratory depression earlier than pulse oximetry oxygen saturation (SpO_2) and intermittent respiratory rate checks and allow appropriate treatment in a more timely manner as alarms may be set to a particular respiratory rate of choice. SpO_2 desaturations can be a later sign of respiratory depression, which may be too late to treat in some circumstances. However, in most health care institutions, capnography is currently only available for 24 hours after extubation rather than for opioid monitoring, unless patients present with risk factors such as obstructive sleep apnea (OSA) or chronic obstructive pulmonary disease. In fact, one study found that the elderly, female sex, and the presence of OSA, chronic obstructive pulmonary disease, cardiac disease, diabetes mellitus (DM), hypertension, neurological disease, renal disease, obesity, opioid dependence, patient-controlled analgesia (PCA), and co-administration of other sedatives were significant risk factors for OIRD and that these patients continue to be poorly monitored regarding sedation and respiratory depression.[42] Enhanced monitoring of sedation, respiratory rate, SpO_2, and capnography is recommended in patients with these risk factors to prevent adverse events.[42]

Naloxone, an opioid antagonist for life-threatening OIRD, must be instructed on proper use. Slow titration of low doses of naloxone should be administered to avoid adverse reactions. Severe noncardiogenic pulmonary edema has been associated with rapid, large reversal doses of naloxone and have even been observed with doses as low as 0.08 mg.[43] This is thought to be due to excessive release of catecholamines upon opioid reversal. Other adverse effects of naloxone administration include hypertension, ventricular arrhythmias, cardiac arrest, and seizures. Therefore, careful administration of naloxone can reduce adverse events associated with naloxone by administering small doses of 0.04 mg at a time.

The first and perhaps most important strategic step in the management of pain is to prevent or modulate its perception. The shift to therapeutic modalities that accomplish these goals is gaining recognition for their preemptive benefits. They range from modulating the perception of pain in the central nervous system with preincisional intravenous ketamine to conductive and neuronal targeted ultrasound-guided regional anesthesia and field blocks with infiltration of long-acting local anesthetics. These opioid-sparing interventions have demonstrated pain reductions that persist long after the effects of regional anesthetics have abated.[44]

Multimodal Analgesia; Quality and Safety

The goal of multimodal analgesia is to target multiple pain pathways to reduce the perception of pain over a longer duration, effect a reduction in the opioid requirements, and maintain the desired levels of quality and safety. Successful reductions of opioid use improve the safety profile of most treatment plans. There have been variations in multimodal pain protocols designed for specific surgical procedures and general anatomic-specific surgical interventions such as intra-abdominal surgery. Creating the ideal multimodal analgesic program for a variety of surgeries is a work in progress as the protocols are subject to research studies. Many protocols also preemptively address the adverse effects of opioids including postoperative and postdischarge nausea and vomiting (PONV, PDNV), pruritus, urinary retention, and allergic reactions. Careful choice of nonopioid analgesics must be taken in order to avoid synergistic respiratory depression observed for example with co-administration of benzodiazepines and opioids. Utilization of analgesic adjuncts such as NSAIDs (Toradol), acetaminophen, alpha-2 agonists (Precedex, clonidine, tizanidine), NMDA antagonists (ketamine, magnesium), steroids (dexamethasone), and regional and neuraxial anesthetic techniques may minimize opioid use in acute pain settings.

Conductive Anesthetics

Epidurals for Thoracic and Abdominal Surgery

Thoracic and major abdominal surgeries have found success with the use of thoracic epidural anesthesia (TEA) in the perioperative and postoperative course in providing adequate analgesia. In addition to significantly reducing perioperative and postoperative opioid use, this anesthetic technique is also thought to provide the patient with an abundance of benefits including reducing the sympathetic activation of the stress response, reducing ischemia in cardiac and noncardiac surgery, increasing intestinal blood flood, and reducing tumor spread.[44] For the surgeon, these benefits include increasing intestinal motility during surgery and possibly improving anastomotic perfusion and patency.[44] However, TEA does not come without associated risks, and extreme care must be taken to prevent catastrophic complications of TEA. TEA must be performed by highly trained clinicians with the knowledge of relative and absolute contraindications to TEA. Risks of TEA include direct spinal cord injury, epidural hematoma, and epidural abscess and may be prevented by proper sterile technique, vigilant knowledge of the patient taking antiplatelet and anticoagulation therapy, platelet count, preexisting coagulopathy, and careful epidural placement with minimal attempts.

Intrathecal Opioid Anesthesia for Cesarean Sections

Intrathecal opioid anesthesia (ITOA) is a popular practice for cesarean section (C-section) and provides significant postoperative pain relief while allowing for earlier mobilization. Increased duration of action of the opioid, decreased total dose administered along with lower sedation of the mother, and earlier return of bowel function are benefits to ITOA.[45] However, ITOA has been thought to be inferior to epidural opioid anesthesia as a higher incidence of respiratory depression has been reported.[46] Opioid upward migration to the brainstem respiratory centers is thought to be the cause of respiratory depression with ITOA. Peak analgesic effects of intrathecal morphine, for example, occur between 45 and 60 minutes lasting 14-36 hours, while respiratory depression can occur in two peaks between 3.5 and 12 hours.[45] While allowing for a total reduction of overall opioid dose and lower systemic side effects, patients with preexisting diseases such as OSA and morbid obesity must be monitored in the postoperative period following ITOA particularly with morphine administration.

Human Factors Engineering, System Safety, and Commitment to Excellence

The ongoing, dramatic and myriad improvements in perioperative safety of patients is continuously fostered by identifying risks and developing risk reduction technology to improve clinical information and reduce physician and nursing team workloads. This shifts time from manual tasks to time available for cognitive assessment. Developed over the last few decades, these include monitoring end-tidal carbon dioxide, pulse oximetry, automated noninvasive blood pressure monitoring, automated safety checkout anesthesia delivery units, improved ventilator systems with flow performance monitors, and both point of care ultrasound technology and blood analysis. These allow the clinician the cognitive space to analyze the data flows and make better informed clinical assessments and decisions.

Studies of the interface between man and technology allow refinements in monitoring, alarm management practices, and clinical performance in controlled environments. Humans remain the most important monitor in the perioperative suites and the most subject to performance degradation.[47,48]

Detractors to human performance, well known from the ongoing safety analysis in aviation, aerospace, and transportation industries, are applied to examining performance in the health care setting. Production pressure, fatigue, and distraction provide substantial personal and senior management challenges to ensure the safe provision of clinical care to our patients.

Production pressure explicitly rewards efficiency at the expense of cutting safety corners including preoperative machine safety checks, thorough preoperative evaluation, and a detailed perioperative record. Turnover time between operative procedures and recovery room stays are closely tabulated, while completion of preanesthesia machine safety checks and audits for accurate perioperative records, pain assessments and adequate treatment are rare. Production pressure encourages reduced perioperative analgesia to accomplish more rapid emergence from anesthesia.

Pocket computer communicators and computers used for perioperative electronic health record data entry provide both instant access to clinically relevant information and distracting personal messages and nonclinical web surfing. They can be distractions to patient care, including pain management assessments

Pain assessment and management tools are only as effective if they are used effectively and consistently. Outcome assessment has to be reproducible and verifiable. Pain assessments when patients leave the postanesthesia care units should be compared with pain assessments on arrival to nursing units. The systems used to assess pain should be identical among nursing units. Substantial differences in reported pain assessments should be addressed within quality review systems.

Developing cultures of safety pay huge dividends to patients and organizations. Adverse outcomes, major or minor, are unavoidable in any complex system involving complex patients and health systems. Rewarding reporting of adverse outcomes to improve safety systems is far more productive than humiliating individual clinicians in continuously improving care. Adequately and safely reducing perioperative pain to achieve consistent results is an ongoing challenge across a wide spectrum of patients.[49,50]

Critical events, near miss, and adverse event reporting systems must have a reporting system that allows reports without logging into a computer system. This safeguard encourages event reporting, protecting individual or patient family member anonymity from the threat or actual retaliation. Consistent nonpunitive leadership, positive reinforcement, and a system safety approach to understanding adverse outcome lead to safer care, better outcomes, and intrinsically motivated clinicians.

Rapid access to pharmaceuticals and medical supplies is necessary to quality patient care. Diversion and unnecessary waste threaten access to high-quality care. Diversion of medications for personal use may entail substitution of saline or other fluids for analgesics needed by patients. Safety systems should reasonably balance legitimate rapid access and easy accountability for patient care with processes for medication security and accountability.[48]

Human Capital

A healthy, intrinsically motivated cadre of clinicians and staff are health systems' most valuable assets. Excessive staff turnover is expensive when costs of recruiting, training, integrating, and retaining new staff are considered. Maintaining health, safety, and a sense of value is paramount. Developing shared values regarding pain management requires time, institutional investments in staff education, and comparative performance monitoring.[50]

Conclusions

There are several methods to assess pain including the VAS, NPRS, VRS, FPS-R, Wong-Baker FACES, McGill Pain Questionnaire, and the PAIN-AD scales demonstrating the complexity of pain assessment and management by the clinician. Improving the quality of pain assessment and management will continue to present as a major obstacle; however, Joint Commission-accredited hospitals continue to improve standards of care as this is most often a requirement. Continued quality improvement in acute pain assessment and management by accredited hospitals continues to improve the current opioid crisis. High-quality acute pain management involves utilizing the most effective tools for pain assessment, treating the pain with the most effective pharmacological agent or procedure with the lowest risk of harm to the patient, and continuing to improve current treatment protocols with quality improvement. In addition, effective acute pain management involves a multidisciplinary approach with the most effective interventions and clear communication among clinicians involved in the patient's care. By utilizing effective communication among clinicians, appropriate assessment and management may be determined by analyzing previous failed interventions and treatments as well as successful ones. Patient education about safe pain management with pharmacological agents and their underlying condition may also be important to improving the quality of pain management as patients may report inadequate education on the particular pharmacological agent or intervention being used in the treatment plan. Finally, as nurses play a key role in preventing under- or overtreatment of acute pain, nurse monitoring of sedation levels when opioids or other adjunctive agents are used may improve patient safety in the hospital setting. Achieving high quality and consistent analgesic outcomes requires team building, investments in education, and continuous quality outcome assessments, reproducible across patient care units.

REFERENCES

1. Shojania KG, Duncan BW, McDonald KM, Wachter RM, Markowitz AJ. Making health care safer: a critical analysis of patient safety practices. *Evid Rep Technol Assess (Summ)*. 2001;(43):i-x, 1-668.
2. Institute of Medicine (US) Committee on Data Standards for Patient Safety; Aspden P, Corrigan JM, Wolcott J, Erickson SM, eds. *Patient Safety: Achieving a New Standard for Care*. National Academies Press (US); 2004.
3. McDonald KM, Sundaram V, Bravata DM, et al. *Closing the Quality Gap: A Critical Analysis of Quality Improvement Strategies (Vol. 7: Care Coordination)*. Agency for Healthcare Research and Quality (US); 2007. (Technical Reviews, No. 9.7.) https://www.ncbi.nlm.nih.gov/books/NBK44015/
4. Donabedian A. The quality of care. How can it be assessed? *JAMA*. 1988;260(12):1743-1748. doi:10.1001/jama.260.12.1743
5. Mędrzycka-Dąbrowska W, Dąbrowski S, Basiński A. Problems and barriers in ensuring effective acute and post-operative pain management—an International perspective. *Adv Clin Exp Med*. 2015;24(5):905-910. doi:10.17219/acem/26394
6. Al-Mahrezi A. Towards effective pain management: breaking the barriers. *Oman Med J*. 2017;32(5):357-358. doi:10.5001/omj.2017.69
7. Tighe P, Buckenmaier CC III, Boezaart AP, et al. Acute pain medicine in the United States: a status report. *Pain Med*. 2015;16(9):1806-1826. doi:10.1111/pme.12760
8. Czarnecki ML, Simon K, Thompson JJ, et al. Barriers to pediatric pain management: a nursing perspective. *Pain Manag Nurs*. 2011;12(3):154-162. doi:10.1016/j.pmn.2010.07.001
9. Wells N, Pasero C, McCaffery M. Improving the quality of care through pain assessment and management. In: Hughes RG, ed. *Patient Safety and Quality: An Evidence-Based Handbook for Nurses*. Agency for Healthcare Research and Quality (US); 2008. Chapter 17. https://www.ncbi.nlm.nih.gov/books/NBK2658/
10. Sinha S, Schreiner AJ, Biernaskie J, Nickerson D, Gabriel VA. Treating pain on skin graft donor sites: review and clinical recommendations. *J Trauma Acute Care Surg*. 2017;83(5):954-964. doi:10.1097/TA.0000000000001615
11. Adamchic I, Langguth B, Hauptmann C, Tass PA. Psychometric evaluation of visual analog scale for the assessment of chronic tinnitus. *Am J Audiol*. 2012;21(2):215-225. doi:10.1044/1059-0889(2012/12-0010)

12. Williamson A, Hoggart B. Pain: a review of three commonly used pain rating scales. *J Clin Nurs.* 2005;14(7):798-804. doi:10.1111/j.1365-2702.2005.01121.x
13. Ferreira-Valente MA, Pais-Ribeiro JL, Jensen MP. Validity of four pain intensity rating scales. *Pain.* 2011;152(10):2399-2404. doi:10.1016/j.pain.2011.07.005
14. Haefeli M, Elfering A. Pain assessment. *Eur Spine J.* 2006;15(Suppl 1):S17-S24. doi:10.1007/s00586-005-1044-x
15. Ohnhaus EE, Adler R. Methodological problems in the measurement of pain: a comparison between the verbal rating scale and the visual analogue scale. *Pain.* 1975;1(4):379-384. doi:10.1016/0304-3959(75)90075-5
16. Jensen MP, Karoly P, Braver S. The measurement of clinical pain intensity: a comparison of six methods. *Pain.* 1986;27(1):117-126. doi:10.1016/0304-3959(86)90228-9
17. Bech RD, Lauritsen J, Ovesen O, Overgaard S. The verbal rating scale is reliable for assessment of postoperative pain in hip fracture patients. *Pain Res Treat.* 2015;2015:676212. doi:10.1155/2015/676212
18. Herr KA, Garand L. Assessment and measurement of pain in older adults. *Clin Geriatr Med.* 2001;17(3):457-478. doi:10.1016/s0749-0690(05)70080-x
19. Kim EJ, Buschmann MT. Reliability and validity of the Faces Pain Scale with older adults. *Int J Nurs Stud.* 2006;43(4):447-456. doi:10.1016/j.ijnurstu.2006.01.001
20. Hicks CL, von Baeyer CL, Spafford PA, van Korlaar I, Goodenough B. The Faces Pain Scale-Revised: toward a common metric in pediatric pain measurement. *Pain.* 2001;93(2):173-183. doi:10.1016/s0304-3959(01)00314-1
21. Drendel AL, Kelly BT, Ali S. Pain assessment for children: overcoming challenges and optimizing care. *Pediatr Emerg Care.* 2011;27(8):773-781. doi:10.1097/PEC.0b013e31822877f7
22. Melzack R. The McGill pain questionnaire: from description to measurement. *Anesthesiology.* 2005;103(1):199-202. doi:10.1097/00000542-200507000-00028
23. Guttman O, Shilling M, Murali A, Mendelson AM. Quality and safety in acute pain management. In: Noe C, eds. *Pain Management for Clinicians.* Springer; 2020. https://doi.org/10.1007/978-3-030-39982-5_30
24. Ngamkham S, Vincent C, Finnegan L, Holden JE, Wang ZJ, Wilkie DJ. The McGill Pain Questionnaire as a multidimensional measure in people with cancer: an integrative review. *Pain Manag Nurs.* 2012;13(1):27-51. doi:10.1016/j.pmn.2010.12.003
25. Melzack R. The short-form McGill Pain Questionnaire. *Pain.* 1987;30(2):191-197. doi:10.1016/0304-3959(87)91074-8
26. Hawker GA, Mian S, Kendzerska T, French M. Measures of adult pain: Visual Analog Scale for Pain (VAS Pain), Numeric Rating Scale for Pain (NRS Pain), McGill Pain Questionnaire (MPQ), Short-Form McGill Pain Questionnaire (SF-MPQ), Chronic Pain Grade Scale (CPGS), Short Form-36 Bodily Pain Scale (SF-36 BPS), and Measure of Intermittent and Constant Osteoarthritis Pain (ICOAP). *Arthritis Care Res (Hoboken).* 2011;63(Suppl 11):S240-S252. doi:10.1002/acr.20543
27. Dworkin RH, Turk DC, Revicki DA, et al. Development and initial validation of an expanded and revised version of the Short-form McGill Pain Questionnaire (SF-MPQ-2). *Pain.* 2009;144(1–2):35-42. doi:10.1016/j.pain.2009.02.007
28. Dworkin RH, Turk DC, Trudeau JJ, et al. Validation of the Short-form McGill Pain Questionnaire-2 (SF-MPQ-2) in acute low back pain. *J Pain.* 2015;16(4):357-366. doi:10.1016/j.jpain.2015.01.012
29. Schreier AM. Nursing care, delirium, and pain management for the hospitalized older adult. *Pain Manag Nurs.* 2010;11(3):177-185. doi:10.1016/j.pmn.2009.07.002
30. Paulson CM, Monroe T, Mion LC. Pain assessment in hospitalized older adults with dementia and delirium. *J Gerontol Nurs.* 2014;40(6):10-15. doi:10.3928/00989134-20140428-02
31. Warden V, Hurley AC, Volicer L. Development and psychometric evaluation of the Pain Assessment in Advanced Dementia (PAINAD) scale. *J Am Med Dir Assoc.* 2003;4(1):9-15. doi:10.1097/01.JAM.0000043422.31640.F7
32. Hutchison RW, Tucker WF Jr, Kim S, Gilder R. Evaluation of a behavioral assessment tool for the individual unable to self-report pain. *Am J Hosp Palliat Care.* 2006;23(4):328-331. doi:10.1177/1049909106290244
33. DeWaters T, Faut-Callahan M, McCann JJ, et al. Comparison of self-reported pain and the PAINAD scale in hospitalized cognitively impaired and intact older adults after hip fracture surgery. *Orthop Nurs.* 2008;27(1):21-28. doi:10.1097/01.NOR.0000310607.62624.74
34. Gordon DB, Dahl JL, Miaskowski C, et al. American pain society recommendations for improving the quality of acute and cancer pain management: American Pain Society Quality of Care Task Force. *Arch Intern Med.* 2005;165(14):1574-1580. doi:10.1001/archinte.165.14.1574
35. Gordon DB, Pellino TA, Miaskowski C, et al. A 10-year review of quality improvement monitoring in pain management: recommendations for standardized outcome measures. *Pain Manag Nurs.* 2002;3(4):116-130. doi:10.1053/jpmn.2002.127570
36. Reddy A, de la Cruz M, Rodriguez EM, et al. Patterns of storage, use, and disposal of opioids among cancer outpatients. *Oncologist.* 2014;19(7):780-785. doi:10.1634/theoncologist.2014-0071
37. Nisbet AT, Mooney-Cotter F. Comparison of selected sedation scales for reporting opioid-induced sedation assessment. *Pain Manag Nurs.* 2009;10(3):154-164. doi:10.1016/j.pmn.2009.03.001

38. Pasero C. *Acute Pain Service: Policy and Procedure Guideline Manual*. Academy Medical Systems; 1994.
39. Pasero C, Portenoy RK, McCaffery M. Opioid analgesics. In: McCaffery M, Pasero C, eds. *Pain: Clinical Manual*. 2nd ed. Mosby; 1999:161-299.
40. Coda B, Tanaka A, Jacobson RC, Donaldson G, Chapman CR. Hydromorphone analgesia after intravenous bolus administration. *Pain*. 1997;71(1):41-48. doi:10.1016/s0304-3959(97)03336-8
41. Vahedi HSM, Hajebi H, Vahidi E, Nejati A, Saeedi M. Comparison between intravenous morphine versus fentanyl in acute pain relief in drug abusers with acute limb traumatic injury. *World J Emerg Med*. 2019;10(1):27-32. doi:10.5847/wjem.j.1920-8642.2019.01.004
42. Gupta K, Prasad A, Nagappa M, Wong J, Abrahamyan L, Chung FF. Risk factors for opioid-induced respiratory depression and failure to rescue: a review. *Curr Opin Anaesthesiol*. 2018;31(1):110-119. doi:10.1097/ACO.0000000000000541
43. Jiwa N, Sheth H, Silverman R. Naloxone-induced non-cardiogenic pulmonary edema: a case report. *Drug Saf Case Rep*. 2018;5(1):20. doi:10.1007/s40800-018-0088-x
44. Freise H, Van Aken HK. Risks and benefits of thoracic epidural anaesthesia. *Br J Anaesth*. 2011;107(6):859-868. doi:10.1093/bja/aer339
45. Gwirtz KH, Young JV, Byers RS, et al. The safety and efficacy of intrathecal opioid analgesia for acute postoperative pain. *Anesth Analg*. 1999;88(3):599-604 doi:10.1213/00000539-199903000-00026
46. Farsi SH. Apnea 6 h after a cesarean section. *Saudi J Anaesth*. 2018;12(1):115-117. doi:10.4103/sja.SJA_252_17
47. Petersen D. *Safety by Objectives, What Gets Measured and Rewarded Gets Done*. 2nd ed. John Wiley and Sons, Inc.; 1996.
48. Hardy TL. *The Safety System Skeptic, Lessons Learned in Safety Management and Engineering*. AuthorHouse; 2010.
49. Crutchfield N, Roughton J. *Safety Culture: An Innovative Leadership Approach*. Elsevier; 2014.
50. McSween TE. *The Values-Based Safety Process*. 2nd ed. Wiley Interscience; 2003.

Index

Note: Page numbers followed by '*f*' and '*t*' indicate figure and table page numbers respectively.

O

Q

R